NEUROLOGY

SECRETS

NEUROLOGY

SECRETS

SIXTH EDITION

JOSEPH S. KASS, MD, JD
Associate Professor
Departments of Neurology and Psychiatry & Behavioral Sciences
Center for Medical Ethics & Health Policy
Vice Chair for Education
Department of Neurology
Assistant Dean of Student Affairs
Baylor College of Medicine;
Chief of Neurology
Ben Taub General Hospital
Houston, Texas

ELI M. MIZRAHI, MD
Chair
Department of Neurology
Professor
Departments of Neurology and Pediatrics
James A. Quigley Endowed Chair in Pediatric Neurology
Baylor College of Medicine
Houston, Texas

ELSEVIER

ELSEVIER

1600 John F. Kennedy Blvd.
Ste 1800
Philadelphia, PA 19103-2899

NEUROLOGY SECRETS, 6TH EDITION ISBN: 978-0-323-35948-1

Notices

Previous editions 2010, 2005, 2001, 1998, and 1993.

Library of Congress Cataloging-in-Publication Data

Names: Kass, Joseph S., editor. | Mizrahi, Eli M., editor.
Title: Neurology secrets / [edited by] Joseph S. Kass, Eli M. Mizrahi.
Other titles: Secrets series.
Description: Sixth edition. | Philadelphia, PA : Elsevier, Inc, [2017] |
    Series: Secrets series | Includes bibliographical references and index.
Identifiers: LCCN 2016013080 | ISBN 9780323359481 (pbk.)
Subjects: | MESH: Nervous System Diseases | Examination Questions
Classification: LCC RC346 | NLM WL 18.2 | DDC 616.8--dc23 LC record
available at http://lccn.loc.gov/2016013080

Content Strategist: James Merritt
Content Development Specialist: Rae Robertson
Publishing Services Manager: Hemamalini Rajendrababu
Project Manager: Srividhya Vidhyashankar
Design Direction: Ryan Cook

Working together
to grow libraries in
developing countries

www.elsevier.com • www.bookaid.org

Printed in United States of America

Last digit is the print number: 9   8   7   6   5   4   3

CONTENTS

CONTRIBUTORS

Garima Arora, MS, MD
Assistant Professor
Department of Psychiatry and Behavioral
  Sciences
The University of Texas Health Science Center at
  Houston
Houston, Texas

Igor M. Cherches, MD
The Neurology Center
Houston, Texas

Jonathan Clark, MD, MPH
Associate Professor
Department of Neurology
Center for Space Medicine
Baylor College of Medicine
Houston, Texas

Helen S. Cohen, EdD, OTR, FAOTA
Professor
Bobby R Alford Department of Otolaryngology -
  Head and Neck Surgery
Baylor College of Medicine
Houston, Texas

Matthew D. Cykowski, MD
Adjunct Associate Professor
Department of Pathology and Immunology
Baylor College of Medicine
Staff Pathologist;
Department of Pathology and Genomic
  Medicine
Houston Methodist Hospital
Houston, Texas

Rachelle S. Doody, MD, PhD
Professor
Effie Marie Cain Chair in Alzheimer's Disease
  Research
Director, Alzheimer's Disease and Memory
  Disorders Center
Department of Neurology
Baylor College of Medicine
Houston, Texas

John D. Eatman, MD
Resident
Department of Neurology
Houston Methodist Hospital
Houston, Texas

Everton A. Edmondson, MD
Clinical Assistant Professor
Department of Neurology
Baylor College of Medicine
Houston, Texas

Randolph W. Evans, MD
Clinical Professor
Department of Neurology
Baylor College of Medicine
Houston, Texas

Daniel G. Glaze, MD, FAASM
Professor
Departments of Pediatrics and Neurology
Baylor College of Medicine;
Medical Director, The Children's Sleep Center
Medical Director, The Blue Bird Circle Rett Center
Texas Children's Hospital
Houston, Texas

Corey E. Goldsmith, MD
Assistant Professor
Department of Neurology
Director, Neurology Residency Program
Baylor College of Medicine;
Chief of Neurology Clinics
Smith Clinic, Harris Health System
Houston, Texas

Clifton L. Gooch, MD
Professor and Chair
Department of Neurology
Director
USF Neuroscience Collaborative
University of South Florida
Tampa, Florida

Pramod Gupta, MD
Fellow
Division of Vascular Neurology and
  Neurocritical Care
Department of Neurology
Baylor College of Medicine
Houston, Texas

Zulfi Haneef, MD
Assistant Professor
Department of Neurology
Baylor College of Medicine
Houston, Texas

Philip A. Hanna, MD, FAAN
Neurology
Movement Disorders
JFK Neuroscience Institute;
Associate Professor
Department of Neurology
Seton Hall University School of Health and Medical
  Sciences;
Clinical Associate Professor Department of
  Neurology
Rutgers Robert Wood Johnson Medical School;
Associate Professor
Department of Medicine
St. George's University School of Medicine
Great River, New York

Richard A. Hrachovy, MD
Distinguished Emeritus Professor
Department of Neurology
Baylor College of Medicine
Houston, Texas

Shahram Izadyar, MD
Assistant Professor
Director, Clinical Neurophysiology Fellowship
  Program
Department of Neurology
Upstate Medical University
Syracuse, New York

George R. Jackson, MD, PhD
Professor
Department of Neurology
Baylor College of Medicine;
Associate Director for Research
Parkinson's Disease Research Education and
  Clinical Center
Michael E. DeBakey VA Medical Center
Houston TX

Joseph Jankovic, MD
Professor
Distinguished Chair in Movement Disorders;
Director, Parkinson's Disease Center and Movement
  Disorders Clinic
Department of Neurology
Baylor College of Medicine
Houston, Texas

Joohi Jimenez-Shahed, MD
Assistant Professor
Associate Director, Neurology Residency Program
Director, Deep Brain Stimulation Program
Baylor College of Medicine
Houston, Texas

Joseph S. Kass, MD, JD
Associate Professor
Departments of Neurology and Psychiatry &
  Behavioral Sciences
Center for Medical Ethics & Health Policy
Vice Chair for Education
Department of Neurology
Assistant Dean of Student Affairs
Baylor College of Medicine;
Chief of Neurology
Ben Taub General Hospital
Houston, Texas

Thomas A. Kent, MD
Professor and Director
Cerebrovascular Research
Department of Neurology
Baylor College of Medicine;
Neurology Care Line Executive
Michael E. DeBakey VA Medical Center
Houston, Texas

James M. Killian, MD
Professor
Department of Neurology
Baylor College of Medicine
Houston, Texas

Doris Kung, DO
Assistant Professor
Director, Medical Student Clerkship
Department of Neurology
Baylor College of Medicine
Houston, Texas

Eugene C. Lai, MD, PhD
Professor
Departments of Neurology and Neuroscience
Robert W. Hervey Distinguished Endowed Chair in
  Parkinson's Disease
Houston Methodist Neurological Institute and
  Weill-Cornell Medical College
Houston, Texas

Atul Maheshwari, MD
Assistant Professor
Department of Neurology
Baylor College of Medicine
Houston, Texas

Jacob Mandel, MD
Assistant Professor
Department of Neurology
Baylor College of Medicine
Houston, Texas

Sharyl R. Martini, MD, PhD
Assistant Professor
Department of Neurology
Baylor College of Medicine
Staff Neurologist
Michael E. DeBakey VA Medical
  Center
Houston, Texas

Eli M. Mizrahi, MD
Chair, Department of Neurology
Chair
Department of Neurology
Professor
Departments of Neurology and Pediatrics
James A. Quigley Endowed Chair in Pediatric
  Neurology
Baylor College of Medicine
Houston, Texas

Paolo Moretti, MD
Assistant Professor
Department of Neurology and Molecular and
  Human Genetics
Baylor College of Medicine;
Staff Neurologist
Michael E. DeBakey VA Medical Center
Houston, Texas

Dennis Mosier, MD, PhD
Clinical Associate Professor
Department of Neurology
Baylor College of Medicine
Staff Neurologist
Michael E. DeBakey VA Medical
  Center
Houston, Texas

Dona K. Murphey, PhD, MD
Fellow, Clinical Neurophysiology
Department of Neurology
Baylor College of Medicine
Houston, Texas

James Owens, MD, PhD
Associate Professor
Departments of Neurology and
  Pediatrics
University of Washington
Seattle, Washington

Amee A. Patel, DO
Assistant Professor
Department of Pediatrics
Baylor College of Medicine
The Children's Sleep Center
Texas Children's Hospital
Houston, Texas

Joshua J. Rodgers, MD
Assistant Professor
Menninger Department of Psychiatry and
  Behavioral Sciences
Baylor College of Medicine
Houston, Texas

Loren A. Rolak, MD
Director, Marshfield Multiple Sclerosis Center
The Marshfield Clinic
Clinical Adjunct Professor
Department of Neurology
University of Wisconsin School of Medicine and
  Public Health;
Adjunct Professor
Department of Neurology
Baylor College of Medicine
Houston, Texas

Rohini Samudralwar, MD
Resident
Department of Neurology
Baylor College of Medicine
Houston, Texas

Paul E. Schulz, MD
Professor
Department of Neurology
Director, Memory Disorders and Dementia Clinic
Director, Neuropsychiatry and Behavioral Neurology
  Fellowship
The University of Texas Health Science Center at
  Houston
Houston, Texas

Lydia Sharp, MD
Instructor
Department of Neurology
Baylor College of Medicine
Houston, Texas

Ericka P. Simpson, MD
Associate Professor
Department of Neurology
Houston Methodist Hospital
Houston, Texas;
Associate Professor
Department of Neurology
Weill-Cornell Medical College
New York, New York

Jose I. Suarez, MD
Professor
Department of Neurology
Head, Section of Vascular Neurology and
  Neurocritical Care
Baylor College of Medicine
Houston, Texas

Colin Van Hook, MD, MPH
Fellow, Clinical Neurophysiology
Department of Neurology
Vanderbilt University
Nashville, Tennessee

Benjamin L. Weinstein, MD
Associate Professor
Menninger Department of Psychiatry and
    Behavioral Sciences
Baylor College of Medicine
Houston, Texas

Subhashie Wijemanne, MD
Assistant Professor
Department of Neurology
The University of Texas Health Science Center at
    San Antonio
San Antonio, Texas

Angus A. Wilfong, MD
Professor
Departments of Pediatrics and Neurology
Baylor College of Medicine;
Director
Comprehensive Epilepsy Program
Blue Bird Circle Clinic for Pediatric Neurology
Texas Children's Hospital
Houston, Texas

Randall Wright, MD
Mischer Neuroscience Associates;
Associate Professor of Neurology
Department of Neurosurgery
The University of Texas School of Medicine at
    Houston
Houston, Texas

PREFACE

The first edition of *Neurology Secrets* was published over 20 years ago. The subsequent editions have tracked the dramatic advances in the field of neurology. In this 6th edition, each chapter has been revised and updated to reflect the current state of the art and science of the topic. New chapters have been added that emphasize the multidisciplinary nature of the practice of neurology. The purpose of this book is to focus on the fundamental issues of the field of neurology. This edition follows the now familiar *Neurology Secrets* format with each chapter organized as a series of questions and answers. Key points are highlighted in each chapter. The chapters are developed to form a basis for further discussion with directed references and reading for more in-depth review. Each chapter is designed to provide the reader with a concise and accurate review which crystallizes the essential features of each topic.

We are indebted to the contributors of *Neurology Secrets* 6th edition. Most of these authors have some academic relationship to Baylor College of Medicine in Houston, Texas, either as current or former faculty members or trainees. This is a tradition begun with the first edition and has continued through the subsequent editions. Some are new to this edition; however, there are a number who have been contributing from the start.

The founding editor of *Neurology Secrets*, Loren A. Rolak, MD, who also edited the subsequent editions, relinquished that role for this 6th edition—although he continues as a contributor. He began this effort within the context of his role as member of the faculty and Neurology Residency Program Director, Department of Neurology, at Baylor College of Medicine in Houston, Texas. Throughout the years, Dr Rolak, who is now at Marshfield Clinic in Marshfield, Wisconsin, has been committed to medical education. The previous editions of *Neurology Secrets* are, in part, evidence of his dedication and skill as an educator, and we trust that the 6th edition does justice to the rich tradition he established.

Joseph S. Kass, MD, JD

Eli M. Mizrahi, MD

DEDICATION

To Loren A. Rolak, MD, founding editor of Neurology Secrets, expert and compassionate clinician, and skilled and dedicated medical educator.

Joseph S. Kass, MD, JD

Eli M. Mizrahi, MD

TOP 100 SECRETS

These secrets are 100 of the top board alerts. They summarize the concepts, principles, and most salient details of neurology.

1. Long-term potentiation is the synaptic mechanism of learning and memory.

2. If the facial nerve is damaged (such as from Bell's palsy), the entire side of the face is weak. If the cortical input to the facial nerve is damaged (such as from a stroke), only the lower half of the face will be weak.

3. A dilated or "blown" pupil implies compression of the III nerve.

4. Noncommunicating hydrocephalus is a medical emergency because the obstructed cerebrospinal fluid (CSF) will cause the intracranial pressure to rise.

5. To distinguish between a common peroneal neuropathy at the popliteal fossa and a L5 radiculopathy, examine for weakness in hip abduction and ankle inversion. Weakness in these muscles indicates L5 radiculopathy.

6. The first step in treating patients with neurologic disease is to localize the lesion.

7. Peripheral neuropathies often produce distal weakness, atrophy, fasciculations, sensory loss, and pain.

8. Spinal cord diseases often produce pyramidal tract deficits, sphincter problems, and a sensory level.

9. Brainstem lesions often produce cranial nerve deficits accompanied by weakness or numbness on the contralateral body.

10. Myopathies usually cause proximal symmetric weakness, with or without other symptoms.

11. Myotonic dystrophy is the most common muscular dystrophy in adults.

12. Myasthenia gravis typically presents with subacute to chronic, fatigable, proximal arm and leg weakness, ptosis, and diplopia.

13. Myasthenia gravis can cause rapid onset neuromuscular respiratory failure, which can be fatal and is therefore a neurological emergency.

14. Lambert–Eaton myasthenic syndrome is associated with cancer (typically small-cell carcinoma of the lung) in approximately 60% of cases, and may be the first manifestation of malignancy.

15. The most common causes of peripheral neuropathy are diabetes and alcoholism.

16. The most often overlooked cause of peripheral neuropathy is genetic.

17. The spinal fluid of patients with Guillain–Barré syndrome has high protein but normal cell counts (cytoalbuminologic dissociation).

18. Compression of the C6 nerve root causes radicular pain in the lateral side of the forearm and thumb, C7 compression causes pain in the index and middle fingers, and C8 compression causes symptoms in the fourth and fifth fingers.

19. Ninety-five percent of lumbar disc herniations occur at the L4/5 or L5/S1 disc spaces.

20. The dermatome for the nipple line is at T4 and the umbilicus is at T10.

21. The first seven cervical nerves exit above the vertebral body with the eight exiting below C7, and the remainder of the spinal roots exit below their corresponding vertebral body.

22. Transverse myelitis is an inflammatory process that is localized over several segments of the cord functionally transects the cord.

23. The most common metastatic tumors to the spinal cord are breast, lung, gastrointestinal tract, lymphoma, myeloma, and prostate.

24. A unilateral lesion within the brainstem often causes "crossed syndromes," in which ipsilateral dysfunction of one or more cranial nerves is accompanied by hemiparesis and/or hemisensory loss on the contralateral body.

25. Symptoms of brainstem ischemia are usually multiple, and isolated findings (such as vertigo or diplopia) are more often caused by peripheral lesions affecting individual cranial nerves.

26. Brainstem glioma is the most frequent brainstem neoplasm. Other brainstem neoplasms include ependymomas that occur in the fourth ventricle and metastatic lesions that may originate from malignant melanomas or carcinomas of the lung and breast.

27. Ménière's disease presents with the symptomatic triad of episodic vertigo, tinnitus, and hearing loss. It is caused by an increased amount of endolymph in the scala media. Pathologically, hair cells degenerate in the macula and vestibule.

28. Central pontine myelinolysis (osmotic demyelination syndrome) occurs primarily in patients suffering from malnutrition or alcoholism complicated by hyponatremia. Rapid correction of the hyponatremia has been implicated as a cause of the pathologic abnormality.

29. Cerebellar strokes and hemorrhage may result in a neurological/neurosurgical emergency by causing obstructive hydrocephalus.

30. Episodic ataxia type 2 is caused by mutations in the same gene (*CACN1A4*) as familial hemiplegic migraine and spinocerebellar ataxia type 6.

31. Differential diagnosis of cerebellar/ataxic conditions can vary by age: (1) adults are more likely to have autosomal dominant spinocerebellar ataxias, degenerative forms of ataxia, extra-axial tumors, paraneoplastic syndromes, and vascular insults to the cerebellum; (2) pediatric patients are more likely to manifest with autosomal recessive cerebellar ataxias, intra-axial cerebellar tumors, infections, or congenital/developmental abnormalities.

32. Levodopa remains the most effective therapy for Parkinson's disease, but management of levodopa-related complications continues to be a challenging probelm that often requires treatment with multiple medications and deep brain stimulation.

33. Essential tremor is a familial disorder, but the genes responsible for this alcohol-responsive action tremor have not yet been identified.

34. Cardinal symptoms of autonomic insufficiency include orthostatic hypotension, bowel and bladder dysfunction, impotence, and sweating abnormalities.

35. Autonomic failure can be seen in the setting of systemic peripheral neuropathies, the most common being diabetic neuropathy, or can be seen without involvement of the sensorimotor neurons, such as pure autonomic failure. Some dysautonomias have autoimmune etiology.

36. The diagnosis of multiple sclerosis requires lesions disseminated in time and in space: two separate symptoms at two separate times.

37. Faulty interpretation of magnetic resonance imaging is the most common error leading to the misdiagnosis of multiple sclerosis.

38. No treatment has yet been proven to alter the level of long-term disability in multiple sclerosis.

39. Dementia is a category, not a diagnosis, and Alzheimer's disease is the most common form of dementia.

40. Most causes of dementia are treatable even if not curable.

41. Frontotemporal dementia (FTD) can present with either behavioral symptoms or primary progressive aphasia.

42. Progressive supranuclear palsy and corticobasal syndrome are parkinsonian disorders associated with dementia and tau aggregation.

43. Cerebral amyloid angiopathy can cause dementia and has manifestations apart from classic lobar hemorrhage.

44. Ten to 15% of patients with amnestic mild cognitive impairment progress to development of Alzheimer's disease each year.

45. Repetitive mild traumatic brain injury can lead to a syndrome of progressive cognitive decline, behavioral and mood changes, and motor/parkinsonian symptoms known as chronic traumatic encephalopathy. The diagnosis can only be confirmed postmortem by identification of hyperphosphorylated tau protein deposits in the sulci.

46. The diagnosis of posttraumatic stress disorder requires exposure to trauma with development of symptoms (intrusive thoughts, re-experiencing, avoidance, negative alterations in cognition and mood, and marked alterations in arousal and reactivity) lasting >1 month and causing significant distress and/or impairment in functioning.

47. An acute onset of cognitive decline with fluctuations in orientation and level of alertness is the hallmark of delirium rather than indicative of dementia.

48. The main clinical feature of stroke is sudden onset of a focal neurological deficit.

49. The only Food and Drug Administration-approved treatment for acute ischemic stroke is intravenous (IV) tissue plasminogen activator, administered within 3 hours of the time the patient was last seen normal.

50. Hemorrhagic strokes often present with a diminished level of consciousness; ischemic strokes rarely do.

51. A depressed level of consciousness (Glascow Coma Scale <8) is the greatest risk factor for airway obstruction and aspiration.

52. Think of cerebral amyloid angiopathy as the most likely cause of spontaneous lobar intracerebral hemorrhage in patients age >55 years.

53. Nimodipine in aneurismal subarachnoid hemorrhage is neuroprotective as it improves outcome but has not shown to reduce vasospasm.

54. Early decompressive hemicraniectomy after large hemispheric ischemic stroke within 48 hours for patients <60 years of age improves survival and functional outcome.

55. Steroids are not recommended in Guillain–Barré syndrome.

56. Treat convulsive status epilepticus early and aggressively with benzodiazepines

57. Brain death is a clinical diagnosis.

58. Central nervous system (CNS) tumors are classified into four grades according to the World Health Organization (WHO) grading system.

59. Glioblastoma (Grade IV astrocytoma) is the most common and malignant primary brain tumor in adults.

60. Brain metastases are the most common intracranial tumors in adults, occurring nearly 10 times more often than primary brain tumors.

61. Intrathecal methotrexate use has been associated with aseptic meningitis, transverse myelopathy, encephalopathy, and leukoencephalopathy.

62. Do not prescribe opioid or butalbital-containing medications as first-line treatment for recurrent headache disorders.

63. The risk of postdural puncture headache can be greatly reduced by use of an atraumatic needle. Bedrest following the procedure is not preventive.

64. Headache or neck pain is the only symptom of cervical artery dissection in 8% of individuals.

65. A seizure is a single event, while epilepsy refers to (1) recurrent unprovoked seizures, (2) a single seizure with a high risk for recurrent seizures, or (3) recurrent reflex seizures.

66. Epilepsy surgery has the best outcomes in patients with a structural lesion (80%) or those with temporal lobe epilepsy (60% to 70%).

67. Medication-refractory (pharmacoresistant) epilepsy is diagnosed when two or three antiepileptic medications at appropriate doses fail to control seizures.

68. Sleep problems occur frequently in individuals with uncomplicated medical histories (20% to 40%) and very frequently in children and adults with complicated medical histories (40% to 80%).

69. All patients with a stroke must have screening for cardiovascular disease.

70. Patients with uremia often develop a metabolic encephalopathy with signs of neuronal depression such as lethargy as well as excitation such as myoclonus.

71. Most patients with Cushing's disease have frank weakness with myopathic findings on electromyography.

72. Decompensated hypothyroidism can cause myxedema coma with mortality rates as high as 25% to 60%.

73. Cerebrovascular ischemic events occur 13 times more frequently in pregnant women than in age-matched nonpregnant women.

74. Headache, jaw claudication, and constitutional symptoms compose the triad of clinical symptoms often found in temporal arteritis.

75. Patients suspected of having bacterial meningitis should receive adjunctive dexamethasone along with empiric antibiotics. The dosing regimen is dexamethasone 4 mg IV every 6 hours for 4 days with the first dose given either 30 minutes prior to the first dose of antibiotics or concomitantly with the first dose of antibiotics. If the CSF cultures indicate the pathogen is not *Streptococcus pneumoniae*, then dexamethasone may be discontinued.

76. Herpes simplex virus-1 (HSV-1) encephalitis should be considered in a patient presenting with fever, behavioral changes, and/or seizures and should be treated empirically with IV acyclovir. HSV polymerase chain reaction in CSF can be negative in the first few days of infection, necessitating repeating lumbar puncture 3 or more days after infection onset.

77. The differential diagnosis for a ring-enhancing lesion in a person with Acquired Immunodeficiency Syndrome includes most commonly *Toxoplasma gondii* and primary CNS lymphoma but also includes tuberculoma, cryptococcoma, histoplasmoma, and other fungal infections, bacterial brain abscess, metastatic disease, and primary brain tumor.

78. Neurocysticercosis is the most common infectious cause of epilepsy with treatment strategies varying depending on cyst life cycle stage and location within the nervous system.

79. The possibility of multiple mutation mechanisms should be considered in ordering and interpreting diagnostic test results for many neurogenetic diseases.

80. The expanding use of genome-level technologies is revealing a previously unsuspected degree of phenotypic variability in many neurogenetic diseases.

81. Causes of intrauterine infection include toxoplasmosis and other agents, such as rubella, cytomegalovirus, and herpes simplex virus.

82. Simple febrile seizures are generalized tonic or tonic–clonic seizures that typically occur between 3 months and 5 years of age. They are often accompanied by a fever greater than 38°C not associated with a CNS infection, and last less than 15 minutes with no focal features and no recurrence within 24 hours. No postictal neurologic abnormalities typically occur.

83. Headaches concerning for an intracranial mass include a recent onset of headaches or change in character of chronic headaches, headaches that awaken the patient from sleep or are present on awakening in the morning, and headaches in association with altered mental status, vomiting, constriction of visual fields, or focal neurologic deficits.

84. Psychiatric and neurologic disorders are highly comorbid and bidirectionally related, and many neurologic disorders may present first with psychiatric symptoms; neurological and medical etiologies should be considered for patients presenting with psychiatric symptoms.

85. Psychiatric disorders are debilitating but are highly treatable; all patients should be screened for common disorders and suicidality.

86. Somatic symptom disorders (including functional neurologic symptom disorder) are commonly comorbid with focal neurologic disorders and can improve with close follow-up with a single provider and psychotherapy.

87. The cardinal feature of delirium is impaired environmental awareness and ability to direct, sustain, or appropriately shift attention. No other psychiatric disorder can be diagnosed in the context of delirium.

88. Acute and chronic disorders of the vestibular system are characterized by disturbances in the behaviors mediated by the vestibular system, e.g., blurred vision, vertigo, impaired balance, nausea, and temporary changes in cardiovascular measures.

89. Most vestibular disorders can be treated. Some disorders are best treated with exercise and other aspects of rehabilitation; other disorders are best treated with medication and/or surgery.

90. The normal adult electroencephalogram (EEG), relaxed with eyes closed, is characterized by 9 to 11 cycles per second activity in the back of the brain (occipital lobes) called the alpha rhythm.

91. Periodic lateralizing epileptiform discharges on an EEG imply an acute, large lesion involving one hemisphere, such as a stroke or focal encephalitis.

92. The generalized three per second spike and wave pattern on an EEG is usually seen in patients with absence seizures.

93. The finding on an EEG that is most suggestive of focal epilepsy is a very brief (less than 70 ms) transient deflection called a spike.

94. The most common compression neuropathies are carpal tunnel syndrome (median nerve compression at the wrist) and cubital tunnel syndrome (ulnar nerve compression at the elbow).

95. The earliest conduction abnormalities in Guillain–Barré syndrome (acute inflammatory demyelinating polyneuropathy) are absent H reflexes.

96. Motor conduction abnormalities in chronic inflammatory demyelinating polyneuropathy are abnormal F waves, distal latencies delay, conduction block with dispersion of distal potential, and motor velocities >20% of normal.

97. A patient with parkinsonism, ataxia, dysautonomia, and alpha-synuclein-positive glial cytoplasmic inclusions at autopsy has multiple system atrophy.

98. *C9orf72* hexanucleotide repeat expansion is the most frequent genetic alteration underlying familial amyotrophic lateral sclerosis (ALS) including ALS with frontotemporal dementia (ALS/FTD).

99. An infiltrative (diffuse) glioma with astrocytic cytology, mitotic activity, microvascular proliferation, and necrosis is a WHO Grade IV glioblastoma.

100. Tuberculous meningitis and neurosarcoidosis both have a predilection for the basilar meninges.

CLINICAL NEUROSCIENCE

Dona K. Murphey, Dennis Mosier

CHAPTER 1

INTRODUCTION

1. Why is it important to understand the cellular, molecular, and genetic mechanisms that govern normal and abnormal nervous system function?
   - To select the most appropriate diagnostic tests and interpretation of test results
   - To optimize drug therapy by mechanisms of action, interactions, side effect profiles
   - To educate patients and their families about their diseases and prognoses
   - To aid in the critical review of rational drug design and clinical trials

2. What cellular alterations lead to neurological disease or affect management/prognosis?
   - Loss of neurons (e.g., neurodegenerative conditions)
   - Injury of axons (e.g., traumatic brain injury)
   - Reorganization of synaptic connections (e.g., deafferentation pain)
   - Disruption of the blood–brain barrier (BBB) (e.g., stroke)

3. What molecular alterations lead to neurological disease or affect management/prognosis?
   - Excitation–contraction uncoupling (e.g., channelopathies)
   - Dysfunctional volume regulation (e.g., cytotoxic edema)
   - Altered membrane excitability (e.g., epilepsy)
   - Conduction abnormalities (e.g., demyelinating conditions)
   - Oxidative stress (e.g., mitochondrial disorders)
   - Autoimmune attack of receptors (e.g., myasthenia gravis)

4. Why is the presence of genetic alterations relevant in neurologic diseases?
   - They may reveal propensity for decreased drug efficacy.
   - They may reveal susceptibility to drug toxicity.
   - They may provide presymptomatic diagnoses.
   - They may be prognostic.

CELLULAR ANATOMY

5. What are the major subcellular compartments of the canonical neuron (Fig. 1-1)?
   - Soma—body of the neuron
   - Dendrites—processes that emanate from the soma and subserve synaptic connections
   - Axon—projection from the soma that terminates on postsynaptic partners
   - Nodes of Ranvier—area between myelinated axonal segments densely populated by voltage-gated Na^+ channels that regenerate action potentials
   - Myelin—a sheath comprised primarily of lipids that electrically insulates the axon and allows for salutatory conduction at unsheathed nodes

6. How are the major subcellular compartments of the canonical neuron affected in disease?
   - Soma—site of pathological inclusions in neurodegenerative diseases
   - Dendrites—loss of dendritic spines in autism
   - Axon—susceptibility to shearing in traumatic brain injury, loss in Wallerian degeneration
   - Nodes of Ranvier—susceptibility to dysfunction in channelopathies
   - Myelin—loss in demyelinating diseases

7. What are the major cell types in the nervous system?
   - Neurons—These comprise a diverse collection of cells that marry afferent input to internal brain states to produce perception and behavior.

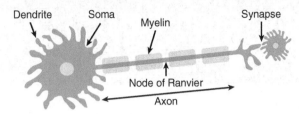

Figure 1-1. The canonical neuron consists of a soma, dendrites, and axon ensheathed in myelin and punctuated by nodes of Ranvier.

- Glia—These comprise a diverse collection of cells that support neuronal function and are believed more recently to participate actively in synaptic formation and function.

8. List the major types of neurons in the nervous system.
   - Excitatory glutamatergic pyramidal neurons—80% of neocortical neurons, long range
   - Inhibitory gamma aminobutyric acid-ergic (GABAergic) interneurons—20% of neocortical neurons, mostly local
   - Neuromodulatory neurons—neurons expressing acetylcholine, dopamine, serotonin, norepinephrine, epinephrine, histamine, and neuropeptides such as orexin/hypocretin, somatostatin that often also corelease the classical neurotransmitters glutamate or GABA.

9. List the major types of glia in the nervous system.
   - Astrocytes—establish the blood–brain barrier, flux ions, repair and form scars in injury
   - Oligodendroglia and Schwann cells—form myelin in brain/spinal cord and periphery
   - Ependymal cells—neuroepithelial cells lining the ventricles, choroid, spinal cord central canal, form cerebrospinal fluid, nonrenewing stem cell pool producing neurons in adult central nervous system (CNS) injury
   - Microglia—resident inflammatory phagocytes in infection, degeneration, demyelination

---

KEY POINTS: CELL TYPE-SPECIFIC DYSFUNCTION OR LOSS IN NEUROLOGIC DISEASE

1. Excitatory cortical neurons are preferentially lost in Alzheimer's disease (AD).
2. Inhibitory cortical neurons are preferentially affected in epilepsy.
3. Neuromodulatory neurons are preferentially lost in AD (acetylcholine), Parkinson's disease (PD) (dopamine), and narcolepsy (orexin/hypocretin).
4. Astrocytes are preferentially affected in Alexander's disease and neuromyelitis optica.
5. Oligodendroglia and Schwann cells are preferentially affected in multiple sclerosis and Charcot–Marie–Tooth disease, respectively.

---

10. What are the cellular constituents of the blood-brain barrier (BBB) (Fig. 1-2)?
    - Capillary endothelial cells—linked by tight junctions and expressing ion channels, carrier-mediated and lipid-soluble transporters, efflux pumps
    - Pericapillary astrocytes—end-feet adjacent to capillaries
    - A similar system exists for the choroidal epithelium at the blood–cerebrospinal fluid barrier (BCSFB) (Fig. 1-3).

11. Which regions of the brain lack a significant BBB?
    - Area postrema
    - Median eminence of the hypothalamus
    - Neurohypophysis

12. Under what conditions is the integrity of the BBB compromised?
    - Autoimmune inflammation or infection (e.g., multiple sclerosis)
    - Osmotic injury (e.g., rapid correction of hyponatremia)
    - Vascular overpressure (e.g., malignant hypertension, reperfusion after ischemia)

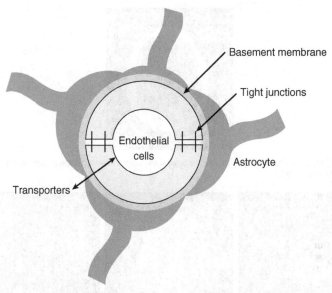

Figure 1-2. The blood–brain barrier (BBB) consists of endothelial cells bound by tight junctions and surrounded by astrocytic and pericytic (*not pictured*) processes.

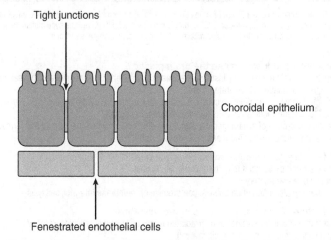

Figure 1-3. At the blood–cerebrospinal fluid barrier, choroidal cells are bound by tight junctions.

- Neovascularization (e.g., cancer)
- Neuronal hyperexcitability (e.g., seizures)

13. What are the imaging features of BBB compromise?
    - On a noncontrast computerized tomography (CT) scan, leakage of blood cells across the BBB or BCSFB is radiodense. Leakage of extracellular fluid (vasogenic edema) is radiolucent (Fig. 1-4).
    - On a T1 contrast magnetic resonance image (MRI), leakage of blood cells across the BBB or BCSFB is hyperintense. On a T2 gradient recalled echo (GRE) sequence, leakage of blood cells across the BBB or BCSFB is hypointense. On a T2 fluid-attenuated inversion recovery (FLAIR) MRI, vasogenic edema is hyperintense (Fig. 1-5).

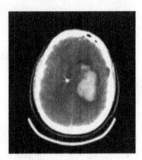

Figure 1-4. Computerized tomography (CT) scan of the brain without contrast reveals radiodense blood surrounded by radiolucent vasogenic edema.

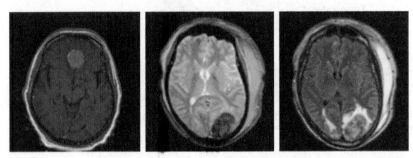

Figure 1-5. Magnetic resonance imaging (MRI) of the brain. T1 contrast reveals hyperintense enhancement of a tumor from leakage of blood across a compromised BBB. T2 gradient recalled echo (GRE) reveals hypointense hemosiderin deposition of blood. T2 fluid-attenuated inversion recovery (FLAIR) reveals hyperintense edema.

14. What cellular processes make the brain plastic?
    - Long-term potentiation—long-lasting increases in postsynaptic responsiveness to weak temporally coincident stimulation of separate inputs
    - Neuromodulation by peptidergic cells—a critical dependence of synaptogenesis on the local circuit signaling of neuromodulatory cells and their cognate receptors
    - Astrocytic secretion of synaptogenic molecules—direct selective control of synapse formation and elimination during development and in the mature adult brain

15. What features comprise necrotic neuronal death?
    - Occurs secondary to insult (e.g., trauma, stroke, toxins)
    - Typically proinflammatory
    - Cell swelling, disruption of organelles, compromise of membrane integrity, cell lysis

16. What features comprise apoptotic neuronal death?
    - Programmed "cellular suicide" (e.g., irradiated tumor cells, glucocorticoids, cytotoxic T lymphocytes, and growth factor withdrawal)
    - Not typically proinflammatory
    - Chromatin condensation, DNA fragmentation, nuclear membrane loss, cell membrane blebbing, cell fragmentation into easily phagocytosed "apoptotic bodies"

MOLECULAR NEUROBIOLOGY

17. What ionic currents support action potential generation and propagation?
    - Depolarizing phase—Na^+ currents
    - Repolarizing phase:
      - Inactivation of Na^+ currents (accounts for refractory period of action potentials)
      - Activation of K^+ currents (accounts for membrane hyperpolarization)

18. How are signals transmitted across a chemical synapse?
    - Depolarization of the presynaptic neuron by an arriving action potential
    - Activation of voltage-dependent calcium (Ca^{2+}) channels, focal entry of intracellular Ca^{2+}
    - Synchronized, quantal vesicular release of neurotransmitter from the presynaptic terminal
    - Diffusion of neurotransmitter across the synaptic cleft
    - Binding of neurotransmitter to specific receptors on the postsynaptic membrane
    - Receptor-mediated ion channel mediation of inhibitory (GABA) or excitatory (glutamate) postsynaptic potentials
    - Postsynaptic action potential initiation if the postsynaptic potentials sum to reach activation threshold

19. What are ion channels?
    Ion channels, formed from membrane-spanning proteins, allow the selective and rapid flux of ions across cell membranes. Channels respond to (are gated by) specific stimuli.

20. What are the types of ion channels?
    - Voltage-gated channels—activated by changes in the transmembrane voltage gradient
    - Ligand-gated channels—activated by binding of chemical agonists
    - Mechanical stretch or pressure

21. How do ion channelopathies present clinically?
    - Episodic clinical symptoms
    - Typically normal interictal function
    - Specific triggers for attacks (e.g., exercise, temperature changes, startle responses, drugs)

22. What are some examples of sodium channelopathies?
    - Generalized epilepsy with febrile seizures plus, a syndromic group associated with febrile seizures that may extend beyond the classic first 6 years of life, may occur without fever, and may be associated with familial epilepsies characterized by other seizure types.
    - Dravet syndrome—an early-onset epileptic encephalopathy
    - Hyperkalemic periodic paralysis—a generalized episodic flaccid weakness

23. What are some examples of potassium channelopathies?
    - Ataxia–myokymia syndrome (EA-1)—myokymia and episodic ataxia
    - Long QT syndromes—syncopal seizures and sudden cardiac death
    - Benign familial neonatal convulsions—clustered seizures at birth with spontaneous remission by 12 months and normal development, increased risk of adult epilepsy
    - Isaacs' syndrome (neuromyotonia)—an antibody-mediated autoimmune attack on K^+ channels in motor nerves

24. What are some examples of calcium channelopathies?
    - Timothy syndrome—multiorgan dysfunction, including lethal arrhythmias, immune deficiency, intermittent hypoglycemia, cognitive abnormalities, and autism
    - Familial hemiplegic migraine and episodic ataxia (EA-2)—ataxia precipitated by physical or emotional stress, gene *CACNA1A*
    - Lambert–Eaton syndrome—an antibody-mediated autoimmune attack on P/Q type voltage-gated Ca channels in the presynaptic neuron at the neuromuscular junction
    - Hypokalemic periodic muscle paralysis—mutation in gene coding for the skeletal voltage-gated Ca^{2+} channel

KEY POINTS: CERTAIN FEATURES ARE COMMON AMONG MOST ALL NEUROTRANSMITTERS

1. Presence of the substance within neuron terminals
2. Release of the substance with neuronal stimulation
3. Exogenous application of the substance at physiologic concentrations to the postsynaptic membrane reproduces the effects of stimulation of the presynaptic neuron.
4. A local mechanism exists for inactivation of the substance (e.g., enzymatic degradation, uptake into nerve terminals or glia).

25. **What is glutamate, and how is it synthesized and metabolized?**
Glutamate is the principal excitatory neurotransmitter of the CNS. It is formed by transamination of α-ketoglutarate and from glutamine by glutaminase. Metabolism involves reuptake and recycling by excitatory amino acid transporters (EAAT) expressed on neurons/glia and vesicular glutamate transporters on neurons.

26. **Through what receptors does glutamate signal?**
    - α-Amino-3-hydroxy-5-methyl-4-isoxazolepropionic acid (AMPA) receptors—open directly and pass principally Na$^+$ and K$^+$.
    - N-methyl-D-aspartate (NMDA) receptors—require depolarization from AMPA receptor activation to pass Na, K, and Ca ions. If excessively stimulated, NMDA receptors may contribute to Ca^{2+}-dependent processes that mediate neuronal injury.

27. **Name a disorder that affects glutamate transport.**
Amyotrophic lateral sclerosis (ALS)—30% to 90% loss of EAAT2, the most abundant glutamate transporter in the brain, is seen in 60% to 70% of patients with sporadic ALS.

28. **What drugs have activity at the glutamatergic synapse?**
    - Riluzole—thought to facilitate glutamate reuptake and prevent glutamate release, has shown limited efficacy in patients with ALS
    - Topiramate—antagonizes AMPA/kainate glutamate receptors
    - Memantine—NMDA-receptor blocking activity with benefit in patients with AD

29. **What comprises the excitotoxicity hypothesis?**
    - Electrochemical overstimulation of neurons (e.g., with relative excess glutamate)
    - NMDA receptor-mediated increase in intracellular calcium
    - Protease activation of catabolic processes (apoptosis)

30. **What is GABA, and how is it synthesized and metabolized?**
GABA is the principal inhibitory neurotransmitter in the CNS. It is formed from glutamate via glutamic acid decarboxylase (GAD) and is metabolized by GABA transaminase.

31. **Through what receptors does GABA signal?**
    - GABA$_A$ type (the majority of GABA receptors) acts as a fast ligand-gated chloride channel, exercising largely inhibitory effects.
    - GABA$_B$ type acts through slow G-protein coupled opening of potassium channels.

32. **Name a few disorders of GABA synthesis and signaling.**
    - Stiff-person syndrome—anti-GAD antibodies → continuous, involuntary muscle activity
    - GABA$_B$ receptor encephalitis—seizures and altered mentation

33. **What drugs have pro-GABAergic activity?**
    - Vigabatrin—an anticonvulsant that inhibits GABA transaminase
    - Barbiturates and benzodiazepines—modulate (agonize) GABA$_A$ receptors
    - Baclofen—activates GABA$_B$ receptors

34. **How is acetylcholine synthesized and metabolized?**
Acetylcholine (Ach) is formed from acetyl coenzyme A and choline by the enzyme choline acetyltransferase and degraded by acetylcholinesterase.

35. **Through what receptors does Ach signal?**
    - Nicotinic ACh receptors (nAChRs)—located at the skeletal neuromuscular junction (NMJ), in autonomic ganglia, and in the brain. Modulation of brain nAChRs is involved in reward and addiction.
    - Muscarinic ACh receptors (mAChRs)—located in parasympathetic sites and in the brain. Modulation of brain mAChRs can affect sleep–wake states, memory, and attention and modify seizure thresholds.

36. **Name a few disorders of cholinergic signaling.**
    - Myasthenia gravis—The nAChR at the NMJ is the major antigenic target of antibodies.
    - Inherited frontal lobe epilepsies—Mutations in genes encoding subunits of neuronal nicotinic receptors have been linked to these disorders.

37. What drugs are active at cholinergic synapses?
    - Donepezil, galantamine, and rivastigmine—reversible inhibitors of cholinesterase, indicated in AD
    - Pyridostigmine—reversible inhibitors of cholinesterase, useful in myasthenia gravis
    - Sarin and organophosphates—irreversible inhibitors of cholinesterase, nerve agents

38. Name the anatomy and functions of Ach in the peripheral nervous system.
    - Motoneurons innervating striated muscle
    - Preganglionic autonomic neurons innervating ganglia
    - Postganglionic parasympathetic neurons
    - Sympathetic sudomotor fibers

39. Name the anatomy and functions of Ach in the central nervous system.
    - Pedunculopontine nuclei (modulation of arousal and sleep states)
    - Projections to the neocortex from basal forebrain nuclei (particularly in the nucleus basalis of Meynert, involved in memory/attention, affected early in AD)
    - Limbic neurons expressing nAChR are involved in addiction
    - Local interneurons in the striatum (regulation of motor activity)

40. How is dopamine synthesized?
    - Tyrosine→L-hydroxyphenylalanine (L-DOPA) via tyrosine hydroxylase
    - L-DOPA→dopamine via DOPA decarboxylase
    - Dopamine→norepinephrine via dopamine β-hydroxylase
    - Norepinephrine→epinephrine via phenylethanolamine N-methyltransferase

41. How is dopamine metabolized?
    - Methylated extracellularly by catechol O-methyltransferase (COMT)
    - Inactivated intracellularly by monoamine oxidase (MAO)-mediated oxidative deamination to homovanillic acid
    - Cleared from the synapse via dopamine reuptake transporters (DAT)

42. Through what receptors does dopamine signal?
    The dopamine receptors (D1 to D5) are G-protein coupled receptors with distinct functions and neuroanatomical distributions. D1 and D2 are most important in neuropsychiatric disease.
    - D1—Gs-mediated increase in intracellular cyclic adenosine monophosphate (AMP) signaling (excitatory)
    - D2—Gi-mediated decrease in intracellular cyclic AMP signaling (inhibitory)

43. Name a few disorders of dopaminergic synthesis or signaling.
    - PD—mostly a sporadic neurodegenerative loss of dopamine neurons, characterized by bradykinesia, resting tremor, rigidity, postural instability
    - DOPA-responsive dystonia—a childhood-onset dominantly inherited deficiency in an enzyme critical for dopamine synthesis

44. What drugs are active at dopaminergic synapses?
    - COMT inhibitors such as entacapone prevent breakdown of dopamine in PD.
    - MAO-B inhibitors such as selegiline and rasagiline prevent breakdown of dopamine in PD.
    - Cocaine and other amphetamines inhibit DAT, producing euphoria.
    - Dopamine receptor (D2±D1) agonists of the ergoline (e.g., bromocriptine and pergolide) and nonergoline (e.g., ropirinole and pramipexole) classes as well as apomorphine are used in PD.
    - Dopamine receptor antagonists include antipsychotics (e.g., haloperidol, clozapine, risperidone) and antiemetics (e.g., metoclopramide).

45. What are the functions of dopamine in the CNS?
    - Motor control (via nigrostriatal projections)
    - Modulation of short-term or working memory (via projections from ventral tegmental area to prefrontal cortex)
    - Behavioral reinforcement (via mesolimbic projections)
    - Hypothalamic regulation of pituitary function (by inhibiting prolactin secretion)
    - Modulation of brain regions controlling emesis (e.g., area postrema of the medulla)

46. How is serotonin synthesized?
    Serotonin is formed from the amino acid tryptophan by the actions of two enzymes, tryptophan hydroxylase and an aromatic amino acid decarboxylase, and is produced by a small collection of neurons in the raphe nuclei of the brain stem.

47. How is serotonin metabolized?
    - Serotonin reuptake transporters (SERT) move serotonin into nerve terminals.
    - Monoamine oxidase-mediated oxidative deamination produces the major serotonin metabolite, 5-hydroxyindoleacetic acid.
    - *N*-Acetylation of serotonin by cells of the pineal gland is followed by *O*-methylation to produce the hormone melatonin.

48. Through what receptors does serotonin signal?
    - There are seven serotonin receptor subtypes.
    - With the exception of $5HT_3$, they are all G-protein coupled with diverse functions.
    - $5HT_{2-4,6,7}$ are excitatory and $5HT_{1,5}$ are inhibitory.

49. What drugs are active at serotonergic synapses?
    - Selective serotonin reuptake inhibitors act on SERT.
    - Haloperidol, quetiapine, and trazodone are selective agonists for the $5HT_{1A}$ receptor but antagonize $5HT_{2A}$. LSD agonizes the $5HT_{2A}$ receptor.
    - Ergotamine and the triptans act on the $5HT_{1B}$ and the $5HT_{1D}$ receptors.
    - 5-HT_3 receptor antagonists, such as ondansetron, and 5-HT_4 receptor agonists, such as metoclopramide, have both peripheral and central actions and suppress nausea/vomiting.

50. What is serotonin syndrome?
    Often an iatrogenic excess of serotonin results in agitation, confusion, muscle rigidity, and fever and can be life threatening.

51. What molecular features of drugs allow them to traverse the BBB?
    - Lipophilic properties
    - Small size with a molecular weight <400 kDa
    - Accessing carrier-mediated transport and receptor-mediated transport

52. What subcellular and molecular substrates make the brain plastic?
    - Dendritic spine formation and clustering
    - NMDA and AMPA receptor trafficking
    - G-protein mediated intracellular signaling

53. What molecules mediate cell injury and death?
    - Free radicals—molecules with one or more unpaired electrons, such as superoxide anion (O_2^-) and hydroxyl radical (OH), produced in ischemic stroke as well as neurodegenerative diseases such as ALS (mutations in superoxide dismutase)
    - Tumor necrosis factor-alpha—a proinflammatory cytokine → endothelial leukocyte adhesion molecule expression to support leukocyte infiltration in ischemia
    - Intercellular adhesion molecule-1—endothelial upregulation in ischemia that may potentiate injury by facilitating invasion of neutrophils

KEY POINTS: PHYSIOLOGIC FUNCTION OF CELL ADHESION MOLECULES

1. Neurite outgrowth during development
2. Cell growth
3. Cell recognition
4. Immune responses
5. Responses to mechanical stress

NEUROGENETICS

54. Distinguish among the terms *gene, allele, polymorphism,* and *mutation.*
    - Gene—the nucleic acid sequence that carries the information to build a particular protein
    - Alleles—any of the alternative forms (sequence variants) of a gene
    - Polymorphism—multiple alleles at any locus that exist across a population. A nondisease-causing genetic variant is termed a *benign polymorphism.*
    - Mutation—change in DNA sequence (with or without detectable effects)

KEY POINTS: TYPES OF GENETIC ALTERATIONS THAT CAN LEAD TO DISEASE

1. Single base-pair substitutions (may alter a single amino acid or produce a stop signal)
2. Insertion or deletion of one or more base pairs (may alter the reading frame)
3. Repetition of sequences of base pairs
4. Duplication of a gene or chromosome
5. Chromosomal deletion or translocation
6. Imprinting due to differential activity of paternal and maternal copies of a gene
7. Alterations of a regulatory protein that controls expression of downstream genes
8. Alteration in a gene with widespread effects on DNA transcription of distant genes

55. What are some specific circumstances in which single gene testing might be useful?
    - Pharmacogenetics—to determine drug efficacy (e.g., *CYP2C19* in clopidigrel oxidation), drug toxicity (e.g., *HLA-B*1502* in Stevens–Johnson syndrome susceptibility with carbamazepine, *TMPT* in bone marrow suppression with azathioprine)
    - Diagnosis and presymptomatic genetic testing (e.g., *PS1/PS2/APP* in familial and *APOE4* in sporadic AD, HD in Huntington's disease)
    - Prognosis (e.g., dystrophin in Duchenne's muscular dystrophy, *SCN1A* in Dravet's syndrome)

56. Most disease causing errors occur in the exome. What comprises the exome?
    - 180,000 exons (DNA coding regions)
    - 3% of the human genome
    - 22,000 genes

57. What information can whole exome sequencing provide?
    - Information on mutations or variants found in genes related to the clinical phenotype
    - Information on genetic aberrances found in unrelated conditions but medically actionable
    - Carrier status
    - Pharmacogenetics

58. What are some examples of neurologic trinucleotide or triplet repeat disorders?
    - Fragile X syndrome (fragile X mental retardation-1 gene)
    - Myotonic dystrophy (*DMPK* or myotonic dystrophy protein kinase gene)
    - Huntington's disease (huntingtin gene)
    - X-linked spinobulbar muscular atrophy (androgen receptor gene)
    - Dentatorubral–pallidoluysian atrophy (atrophin-1 gene)
    - Spinocerebellar atrophies (ataxin-1 gene in SCA1 and *CACNA1A* gene in SCA6)
    - Friedreich's ataxia (frataxin gene)

59. What is anticipation?
    Classically, in triplet repeat disorders longer repeat size results in earlier age of onset and/or more severe phenotype. The length of expanded repeats is characteristically unstable and often grows further with successive generations, producing the clinical phenomenon of anticipation.

FUTURE DIRECTIONS

60. Discuss the prion hypothesis and its relevance to neurological disease.
    - Altered prion proteins cause conformational changes in normal prion proteins.
    - DNA and RNA are not required for infectivity.
    - Human prion diseases classically include kuru, Creutzfeldt–Jakob disease (CJD), Gerstmann–Straüssler–Scheinker disease, fatal familial insomnia, and variant CJD.
    - Neurodegenerative diseases (e.g., AD, PD, ALS) also feature self-perpetuating protein misfolding as pathogenic.

61. Discuss the relevance of prions to normal neurologic function.
    - Memory requires persistent anatomic and functional changes at specific synapses.
    - Local protein synthesis at relevant synapses subserves these changes.

- Candidate regulators of these changes are members of the cytoplasmic polyadenylation element binding (CPEB) family.
- CPEBs maintain long-term synaptic facilitation through prion-like properties.

62. How can stem cells be useful in neurologic disease?
Induced pluripotent stem cells can be reprogrammed, allowing patient-derived cells to be used for disease modeling and potential regenerative therapies.

63. Name several potential obstacles to successful neuronal transplantation in humans.
    - Appropriate differentiation of neurons (e.g., from stem cells)
    - Maintaining stability of neuronal phenotype over time
    - Regulating neurotransmitter production and cell proliferation
    - Making connections with both upstream and downstream targets
    - Protection from ongoing disease processes

64. Describe challenges of producing successful "gene therapy" for neurologic disorders.
    - Loss of function accounts for only a small percentage of genetic disorders.
    - Most vectors for introducing DNA into cells are inefficient.
    - Expression of proteins from viral vectors on cell surfaces may trigger host immune responses.
    - Introduction of the normal protein itself may trigger host immune responses.
    - Expression of introduced DNA may be transient.
    - Vectors may introduce genes into nontarget cells.
    - Integrated DNA sequences may be regulated abnormally.

 References available online at expertconsult.com.

BIBLIOGRAPHY

1. Hille B: Ion Channels of Excitable Membranes, 3rd ed. Sunderland, MA, Sinauer, 2001.
2. Kandel ER, Schwartz JH, Jessell TM, Siegelbaum SA, Hudspeth AJ: Principles of Neural Science, 5th ed. New York, McGraw-Hill, 2013.
3. Mather JP: Stem Cell Culture (Methods in Cell Biology, vol. 86). New York, Elsevier, 2008.
4. Squire LR, Berg D, Bloom FE, du Lac S, Ghosh A, Spitzer NC: Fundamental Neuroscience, 4th ed. Waltham, MA, Elsevier, 2013.

CHAPTER 2

CLINICAL NEUROANATOMY

Igor M. Cherches

EMBRYOLOGY

1. **How is the neural tube formed?**
    Beginning around the 18th gestational day, a midline notochordal thickening anterior to the blasto-pore forms the neural plate. A midsagittal groove called the *neural groove* appears in the plate, and the sides elevate to form the neural folds. As the folds fuse, the neural tube is formed. Some cells at the edges of the fold do not fuse into the tube and become neural crest cells.

2. **What types of cells are derived from the neural crest cells?**
    Neural crest cells give rise to (1) unipolar sensory cells, (2) postganglionic cells of sympathetic and parasympathetic ganglia, (3) chromaffin cells of the adrenal medulla, (4) some microglial cells, (5) pia mater, (6) some arachnoid cells, (7) melanocytes, and (8) Schwann cells.

3. **What are the alar plate and the basal plate?**
    As the neural tube is formed, a longitudinal groove appears on each side and divides the neural tube into a dorsal half, or alar plate, and a ventral half, or basal plate. The **alar plate** gives rise to the prosencephalon; the sensory and coordinating nuclei of the thalamus; the sensory neurons of the cranial nerves; the coordinating nuclei including cerebellum, inferior olives, red nucleus, and quadri-geminal plate; and the posterior horn area (sensory) of the spinal cord. The **basal plate** stops at the level of the diencephalon and gives rise to the motor neurons of the cranial nerves and anterior horn (motor) area of the spinal cord.

4. **What is the process of formation of the ventricles, prosencephalon, mesencephalon, and rhombencephalon?**
    Around the end of the first gestational month, a series of bulges anterior to the first cervical somites appears. The first bulge is the prosencephalon, or forebrain. The cavity of this bulge forms the lateral ventricles and third ventricle. Secondary outpouchings from the forebrain are called *optic vesicles* and eventually form the retina, pigment epithelium, and optic nerve. The second bulge is the mesencephalon, or midbrain. The cavity of this bulge forms the cerebral aqueduct. The third bulge is the rhombencephalon, or hindbrain. This cavity gives rise to the fourth ventricle.

5. **Which structures arise from the prosencephalon, mesencephalon, and rhombencephalon?**
    The prosencephalon develops into the telencephalon, which includes the cerebral cortex and basal ganglia, and the diencephalon, which includes the thalamus and the hypothalamus. The mesen-cephalon gives rise to the midbrain. The **rhombencephalon** gives rise to the metencephalon (pons plus cerebellum) and myelencephalon (medulla) (Table 2-1).

MUSCLE

6. **What is the histologic organization of skeletal muscle?**
    Skeletal muscle is composed of long, thin, cylindrical, multinucleated cells called *muscle fibers* (or myofibrils). Each fiber has a motor endplate at its neuromuscular junction and is surrounded by connective tissue called *endomysium*. Groups of fibers, or a fascicle, are surrounded by a connective tissue layer called the *perimysium*. Fascicles are grouped together and surrounded by epimysium.

7. **What is found at the A band, H band, I band, and Z line?**
    The A band contains the thin filaments (actin) and the thick filaments (myosin). The **H band** is the portion of the A band that contains only myosin, and the **I band** is the portion that contains only actin. The actin is anchored at the **Z line** (Fig. 2-1).

11

Table 2-1. Embryonic Divisions of the Central Nervous System

EMBRYONIC DIVISIONS	ADULT DERIVATIVES	VENTRICULAR CAVITIES
Forebrain (prosencephalon)		
Telencephalon	Cerebral cortex	Lateral ventricles
	Basal ganglia	
Diencephalon	Thalamus	
	Hypothalamus	
	Subthalamus	Third ventricle
	Epithalamus	
Midbrain (mesencephalon)	Tectum	Aqueduct
	Cerebral peduncles	
Hindbrain (rhombencephalon)		
Metencephalon	Cerebellum	Fourth ventricle
	Pons	
Myelencephalon	Medulla	
Spinal cord	Spinal cord	No cavity

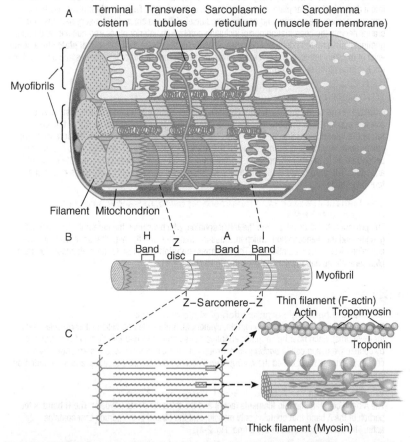

Figure 2-1. The histologic anatomy of the human skeletal muscle. (A) muscle fiber; (B) myofibril; (C) sarcomere *(Redrawn from Kandel E, Schwartz JH, Jessell TM (eds): Principles of neuroscience, 3rd ed. New York, McGraw-Hill, 1991, p. 549.)*

8. How does the muscle contract?

When the sarcoplasmic reticulum is depolarized, calcium ions enter the cell and bind to troponin. This causes a conformational change that allows exposure of the actin-binding site to myosin. The myosin attaches to the actin-binding site and flexes, causing the actin filament to slide by the myosin filament. Adenosine triphosphate is required to allow the myosin-actin crossbridge to release and the muscle to relax.

9. What is meant by the term *motor unit?*

The motor unit is one motor nerve (lower motor neuron) and all muscle fibers that it innervates.

THE MUSCLE STRETCH REFLEX

10. What is the muscle stretch reflex?

The muscle stretch reflex is a reflex arc that responds to stretching of muscle fibers to keep the muscle in an appropriate state of tension and tone, ready to contract or relax as needed. The sensory input (afferent) of the reflex is from two structures in the muscle called *spindles* and *Golgi tendon organs.* The output (efferent) is the alpha motor neuron that contracts (tightens) the muscle. (The muscle fibers are sometimes referred to as *extrafusal fibers.*)

11. What type of nerve fiber innervates the muscle?

An anterior horn motor neuron, called an *alpha motor neuron*, innervates the muscle. It is the final common pathway for muscle contraction.

12. What is the function of the Ia nerve fiber?

The Ia nerve arises from annulospiral endings within the muscle spindle. When the muscle spindle is stretched (i.e., when the muscle is relaxed), the Ia sensory nerve, through the dorsal root, mono-synaptically stimulates the alpha motor neuron, which fires and contracts (shortens) the muscle. Thus, the muscle stretch reflex maintains tone and tension in the muscle, by contracting it when it becomes too relaxed.

13. Is the Ia reflex monosynaptic or polysynaptic?

The Ia reflex is monosynaptic, but it initiates a polysynaptic inhibition of the antagonist muscle group.

14. In the spinal cord, which nerve fibers synapse on the alpha motor neuron?

Both the corticospinal tract and afferent Ia sensory nerves regulate the alpha motor neuron by snapping on it in the anterior horn of the spinal cord. Renshaw cells are interneurons that are stimulated by the alpha motor neuron and then, by a feedback mechanism, inhibit the alpha motor neuron, causing autoinhibition.

15. What is the role of the gamma efferent nerve?

The muscle spindle is kept tense and responsive by tiny muscle fibers inside it, called *intrafusal fibers.* The gamma efferent nerve fibers keep the muscle spindles "tight" by innervating and contracting the intrafusal fibers in the muscle spindle. This process ensures that the spindle remains sensitive to any stretch.

16. Where does the Ib fiber originate?

The Ib fiber originates from the Golgi tendon organ, another structure that monitors muscle stretch and acts to inhibit muscle contraction (not shown in the diagram).

17. Where does the Ib neuron synapse?

At the spinal cord level, the Ib sensory nerve polysynaptically inhibits the alpha motor neuron to prevent muscle contraction and also stimulates the gamma efferent nerve to the intrafusal fiber to reset the muscle spindle.

LUMBOSACRAL PLEXUS AND LEG INNERVATION

18. Which roots make up the lumbar plexus?

Roots of L1, L2, L3, L4, and sometimes T12 make up the lumbar plexus.

19. What are the two largest branches of the lumbar plexus?

- **Obturator nerve (L2, L3, L4).** It leaves the pelvis through the obturator foramen and supplies the adductors of the thigh.

- **Femoral nerve (L2, L3, L4)**. It exits the pelvis with the femoral artery and supplies the hip flexors and knee extensors. Distally, it continues as the saphenous nerve to supply sensation to the medial anterior knee and medial distal leg, including the medial malleolus (Fig. 2-2).

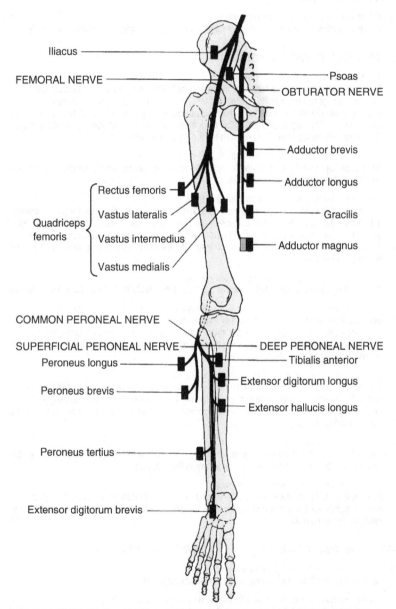

Figure 2-2. Diagram of the nerves and muscles on the anterior aspect of the lower limb. *(From Medical Research Council: Aids to the examination of the peripheral nervous system. London, 1976.)*

20. What are the other branches of the lumbar plexus?
    - **Iliohypogastric nerve (L1)**—sensation to skin over hypogastric and gluteal areas; to abdominal muscles
    - **Ilioinguinal nerve (L1)**—sensation to skin over groin and scrotum or labia
    - **Genitofemoral nerve (L1, L2)**—enters the internal inguinal ring and runs in the inguinal canal
    - **Lateral femoral cutaneous nerve (L2, L3)**—sensation to skin over anterior and lateral parts of the thigh

21. Which nerve is at risk during appendectomy (McBurney's incision)?
    The iliohypogastric nerve may be inadvertently cut as it passes between the external and internal oblique muscles. This results in weakness in the inguinal canal area, putting the patient at risk for direct inguinal hernia.

22. What is meralgia paresthetica?
    Meralgia paresthetica is numbness and tingling in the lateral thigh secondary to compression of the lateral femoral cutaneous nerve as it runs over the inguinal ligament. It commonly occurs in obese or pregnant patients. It can also be caused by placing hard objects in the pockets of pants with a low waistline such as so-called low rider jeans.

23. Which nerve supplies the gluteus maximus?
    The inferior gluteal nerve (L5, S1, S2) supplies the gluteus maximus muscle.

24. What is the largest nerve in the body?
    The sciatic nerve (L4, L5, S1, S2, S3), the largest nerve in the body, is composed of the common peroneal nerve (L4, L5, S1, S2) in its dorsal division and the tibial nerve (L4, L5, S1, S2, S3) in its ventral division (Fig. 2-3).

25. What is the only nerve in the sacral plexus that emerges through the greater sciatic foramen, superior to the piriformis muscle?
    The superior gluteal nerve (L4, L5, S1) supplies the gluteus medius and minimus and tensor fascia lata (abduction and medial rotation of the thigh).

26. Which nerve supplies the inferior buttock and posterior thigh?
    The posterior femoral cutaneous nerve (S1, S2, S3), which runs with the inferior gluteal nerve, supplies the inferior buttock and posterior thigh.

27. Which nerve supplies the structures in the perineum?
    The pudendal nerve (S2, S3, S4) supplies the perineum.

28. What is the only muscle supplied by the sciatic nerve that receives innervation exclusively from the dorsal division (i.e., peroneal component) of the sciatic nerve?
    The biceps femoris has only dorsal innervation. This is important clinically to differentiate lesions caused by damage to the common peroneal nerve versus the sciatic nerve itself.

29. Which muscles are supplied by the tibial nerve?
    The tibial nerve supplies plantar flexors and invertors of the foot.

30. What are the two divisions of the common peroneal nerve?
    - **Deep peroneal nerve**—dorsiflexion of the foot and toes and sensation to a small area of skin between the first and second toes.
    - **Superficial peroneal nerve**—evertors of the foot and sensation to the skin of the dorsal and lateral foot.

BRACHIAL PLEXUS AND ARM INNERVATION

31. The brachial plexus comprises which roots?
    The brachial plexus comprises the ventral rami of C5, C6, C7, C8, and T1 (Fig. 2-4).

32. Which nerves arise from the ventral rami of the roots before formation of the brachial plexus?
    - **Dorsal scapular nerve**, from C5 to rhomboid and levator scapula muscles; responsible for elevation and stabilization of the scapula.
    - **Long thoracic nerve**, from C5, C6, and C7 to serratus anterior; responsible for abduction of the scapula.

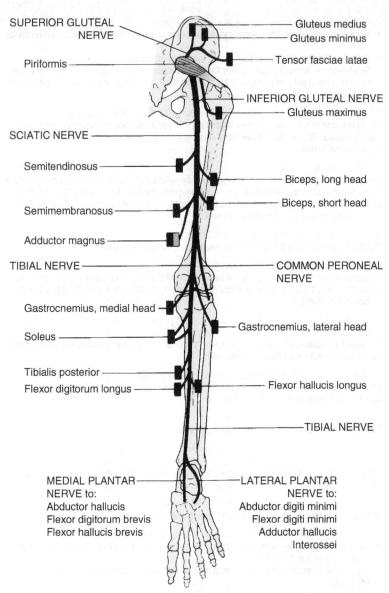

Figure 2-3. Diagram of the nerves and muscles on the posterior aspect of the lower limb. *(From Medical Research Council: Aids to the examination of the peripheral nervous system. London, 1976.)*

Testing these nerves is useful in differentiating between root and plexus lesions. If there is a deficit in one of these nerves (clinically or electrically), the lesion is proximal to the plexus.

33. Which roots form the three trunks of the brachial plexus?
   (1) Superior trunk, formed by C5 and C6; (2) middle trunk, formed by C7; and (3) lower trunk, formed by C8 and T1.

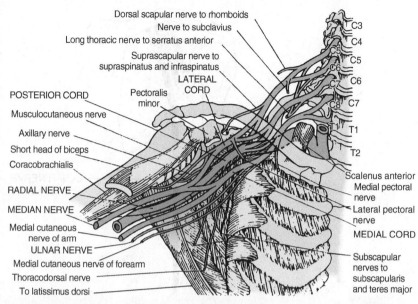

Figure 2-4. The brachial plexus. *(Redrawn from Tindall B: Aids to the examination of the peripheral nervous system. London, W.B. Saunders, 1990.)*

34. What is the only nerve from the trunks of the brachial plexus?
    The suprascapular nerve (C5) comes off the upper trunk and supplies the supraspinatus (abduction) and infraspinatus (external rotation) of the shoulder.

35. Which vascular structure is associated with the three cords of the brachial plexus?
    The lateral cord (C5, C6, C7), medial cord (C8, T1), and posterior cord (C5, C6, C7, C8) are named in relationship to the axillary artery.

36. What are the nerves off the cords of the brachial plexus?
    Lateral cord:
    - Lateral pectoral nerve (C5, C6, C7)—to pectoralis minor
    - Musculocutaneous nerve (C5, C6)—to brachialis and coracobrachialis (elbow flexion)
    - Median nerve (partial; C6, C7)—to pronator teres, flexor carpi radialis, part of flexor digitorum superficialis, part of palmaris longus

    Medial cord:
    - Medial pectoral nerve (C8, T1)—to pectoralis major (shoulder adduction)
    - Ulnar nerve (C8, T1)—ulnar wrist and long finger flexors
    - Median nerve (partial; C8, T1)—long finger flexors and small hand muscles
    - Medial brachial cutaneous nerve—skin over medial surface of arm and proximal forearm
    - Medial antebrachial cutaneous nerve—skin over medial surface of forearm

    Posterior cord:
    - Upper subscapular nerve (C5, C6)—to subscapularis (medial rotation of the humerus)
    - Thoracodorsal nerve (C6, C7, C8)—to latissimus dorsi (shoulder adduction)
    - Lower subscapular nerve (C5, C6)—to teres major (adducts the humerus)
    - Axillary nerve (C5, C6)—to deltoid (abduction of the humerus) and teres minor (lateral rotation of humerus)
    - Radial nerve (C5, C6, C7, C8, T1)—to extensor muscles of upper limb (Figs 2-5 and 2-6)

37. What is Erb's palsy?
    Erb's palsy is an injury to the upper brachial plexus (C5, C6) resulting from excessive separation or stretch of the neck and shoulder (such as from a sliding injury or from pulling on an infant's neck

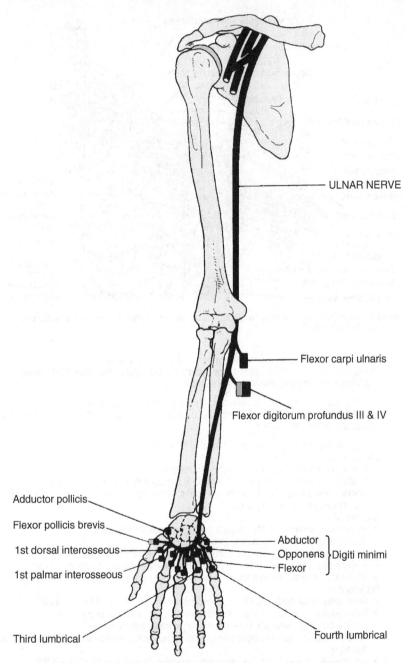

Figure 2-5. Diagram of the ulnar nerve and the muscles that it supplies. *(From Medical Research Council:* Aids to the examination of the peripheral nervous system. *London, 1976.)*

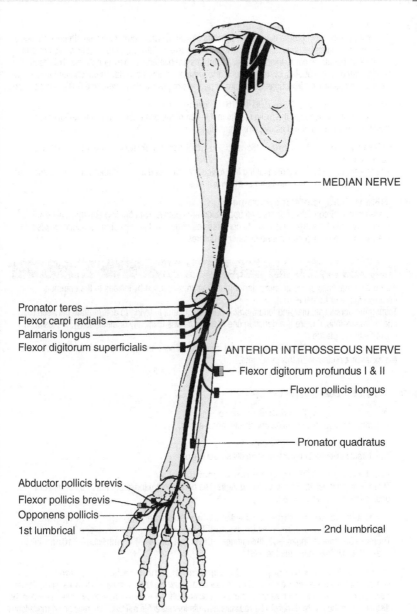

MEDIAN NERVE

Pronator teres
Flexor carpi radialis
Palmaris longus
Flexor digitorum superficialis

ANTERIOR INTEROSSEOUS NERVE

Flexor digitorum profundus I & II
Flexor pollicis longus

Pronator quadratus

Abductor pollicis brevis
Flexor pollicis brevis
Opponens pollicis
1st lumbrical

2nd lumbrical

Figure 2-6. Diagram of the median nerve and the muscles that it supplies. *(From Medical Research Council: Aids to the examination of the peripheral nervous system. London, 1976.)*

during delivery). The result is decreased sensation in the C5 and C6 dermatomes and paralysis of scapular muscles. The arm may be held in adduction, with the fingers pointing backward, so-called waiter's tip position. Distal strength in the upper extremity remains intact.

38. What is Klumpke's palsy?

Klumpke's palsy is an injury to the lower brachial plexus (C8, T1) leading to weakness and anesthesia in a primarily ulnar distribution, which may be the result of maximal abduction of the shoulder.

39. **What is Parsonage–Turner syndrome?**
    Parsonage–Turner syndrome is an acute brachial plexus neuritis, commonly also affecting the long thoracic, musculocutaneous, and axillary nerves. It causes patchy upper extremity weakness and numbness, usually accompanied by pain. Symptoms are bilateral in 20% of patients. This condition is associated with diabetes, systemic lupus erythematosus, and polyarteritis nodosa and may follow immunizations or viral infections. One-third of patients recover within 1 year and 90% within 3 years.

40. **What deficit results from poorly fitting crutches?**
    Pressure from crutches in the axilla results in a lesion of the posterior cord or the radial nerve, leading to weakness of the elbow, wrist, and digits.

41. **Which nerve is commonly affected in shoulder dislocation or fracture of the humerus?**
    The axillary nerve is affected, resulting in a lesion that causes decreased abduction of the shoulder and anesthesia over the lateral part of the proximal arm.

42. **What is thoracic outlet syndrome (TOS)?**
    Classically, TOS consists of decreased upper extremity pulses, with tingling and numbness in the medial aspect of the arm secondary to compression of the medial cord of the brachial plexus and the axillary artery by a cervical rib or other structures.

KEY POINTS: INNERVATION OF LEG AND ARM

1. Foot drop (weakness of the tibialis anterior muscle) can be caused by lesions to the common peroneal nerve or L5 nerve root.
2. Testing the dorsal scapular and long thoracic nerves is useful in trying to differentiate between root and plexus lesions. If there is a deficit in one of these nerves (clinically or electrically), the lesion is proximal to the plexus.
3. The median nerve is involved in carpal tunnel syndrome. There are typically no objective findings in the exam of a patient with this syndrome.

ROOTS AND DERMATOMES

43. **What is found in the ventral nerve root?**
    The ventral nerve root contains principally motor axons.

44. **What is found in the dorsal nerve root?**
    The dorsal nerve root contains principally sensory axons.

45. **What synapse is found in the dorsal root ganglia?**
    There is no synapse in the dorsal root ganglia. The dorsal root ganglia are made up of unipolar cell bodies for the sensory system.

46. **What are the dermatomes of the following landmarks: thumb, middle finger, little finger, breast nipple, umbilicus, medial knee, big toe, and little toe?**
    Thumb—C6, middle finger—C7, little finger—C8, breast nipple—T4, umbilicus—T10, medial knee—L4, big toe—L5, little toe—S1.

47. **What are the common signs and symptoms of lumbar radiculopathies?**
    Lumbar radiculopathies cause back pain with radiation below the knee. The pain increases with a Valsalva maneuver or leg stretch (such as the straight leg raising test). Weakness or numbness may develop in the distribution of the involved root. An S1 radiculopathy diminishes ankle reflexes, whereas an L4 radiculopathy decreases knee reflexes. Statistically, an L5 radiculopathy is more common than S1, followed by L4. This is because the intervertebral discs at these levels are under greatest pressure from the curvature of normal lumbar lordosis and thus are most vulnerable to herniation and compression of the spinal roots.

48. **What are the common signs and symptoms of cervical radiculopathies?**
    Cervical radiculopathies usually involve the lower cervical roots (C6, C7, C8). Patients typically complain of pain in the back of the neck, frequently with radiation to the arm in a dermatomal distribution. Paresthesias are often present in one or two digits. Absent biceps, brachioradialis, or triceps reflexes suggest lesions of C5, C6, and C7, respectively, and these muscles also may lose strength.

SPINAL CORD: GROSS ANATOMY

49. How is the spinal cord organized?

Sections of the spinal cord cut perpendicular to the length of the cord reveal a butterfly-shaped area of gray matter with surrounding white matter. The white matter consists mainly of longitudinal nerve fibers, carrying the ascending and descending tracts up and down the cord. Midline grooves are present on the dorsal and ventral surfaces (the dorsal median sulcus and ventral median fissure). The gray matter of the cord contains dorsal and ventral enlargements known as *dorsal horns* and *ventral horns*.

50. In a given transverse section of the spinal cord, how is the gray matter subdivided?

The gray matter can be subdivided into groups of nuclei. When the spinal cord is cut along its length, these nuclei appear to be arranged in cell columns or laminae. Rexed divides the cord into 10 laminae. Each lamina extends the length of the cord, with lamina I at the most dorsal aspect of the dorsal horn, lamina IX at the most ventral aspect of the ventral horn, and lamina X surrounding the central canal. Lamina II is also called the *substantia gelatinosa* and is the area of synapse for the spinothalamic tract. Lamina IX is the site of the cell bodies for the anterior horn motor cells.

51. What are the major ascending tracts in the spinal cord?

(1) Dorsal columns; (2) spinothalamic tract; (3) dorsal spinocerebellar tract ; and (4) ventral spinocerebellar tract.

52. What are the major descending tracts in the spinal cord?

(1) Intermediolateral columns; (2) lateral corticospinal tract; (3) lateral reticulospinal tract; (4) lateral vestibulospinal tract; (5) medial longitudinal fasciculus (MLF); and (6) ventral corticospinal tract.

53. Going from rostral to caudal, what are the five divisions of the spinal cord?

Cervical, thoracic, lumbar, sacral, and coccygeal are the five divisions of the spinal cord.

54. In the adult, at what vertebral level does the spinal cord end?

The spinal cord ends at vertebral level L1 to L2.

55. How many spinal nerves exit from each region of the spinal cord?

Spinal nerves exit the spinal cord in pairs: 8 cervical, 12 thoracic, 5 lumbar, 5 sacral, and 1 coccygeal. Each spinal nerve is composed of the union of the dorsal sensory root and the ventral motor root.

56. What is the filum terminale?

Although the spinal cord ends at the lower border of vertebral level L1, the pia mater continues caudally as a connective tissue filament, the filum terminale, which passes through the subarachnoid space to the end of the dural sac, where it receives a covering of dura and continues to its attachment to the coccyx.

57. What is the cauda equina?

The lumbar and sacral spinal nerves have very long roots, descending from their respective points in the spinal cord to their exit points in the intervertebral foramina. These roots descend in a bundle from the conus, termed the *cauda equina* for its resemblance to a horse's tail.

58. Describe the blood supply of the spinal cord.

The one anterior spinal artery and the two posterior spinal arteries travel along the length of the cord to supply blood to the cord. These arteries originate from the vertebral arteries. Other arteries replenish the anterior and posterior spinal arteries and enter the spinal canal through the intervertebral foramina in association with the spinal nerves. They are called *radicular arteries* if they supply only the nerve roots, and *radiculospinal arteries* if they supply blood to both the roots and the cord. Each radiculospinal artery supplies blood to approximately six spinal cord segments, with the exception of the great radicular artery of Adamkiewicz, which usually enters with the left second lumbar ventral root (range T10 to L4) and supplies most of the caudal third of the cord.

SENSORY: DORSAL COLUMNS AND PROPRIOCEPTION

59. What type of information is carried in the dorsal columns?

The dorsal columns convey tactile discrimination, vibration, and joint position sense.

60. What types of receptors are stimulated to sense this information?
Muscle spindles and Golgi tendon organs perceive position sense, Pacinian corpuscles perceive vibration, and Meissner corpuscles perceive superficial touch sensation needed for tactile discrimination. Pacinian and Meissner corpuscles are examples of mechanoreceptors.

61. What type of peripheral nerve fiber is involved with transmission of dorsal column information?
Large, myelinated, fast-conducting nerve fibers carry dorsal column-type information.

62. What is the pathway by which this information reaches the cerebral cortex?
Sensation on skin→afferent sensory nerve→dorsal column on ipsilateral side (fasciculus gracilis and cuneatus)→lower medulla→synapse in nucleus gracilis and cuneatus→arcuate fibers→cross to the contralateral side into the medial lemniscus→ascend to the ventral posterolateral (VPL) nucleus of the thalamus→synapse→through the posterior limb of the internal capsule→postcentral gyrus of the cortex.

63. Where do dorsal column fibers decussate? At what locations do they synapse?
The dorsal columns decussate in the lower medulla, after synapsing in the nucleus gracilis and cuneatus. They also synapse in the VPL of the thalamus before going to the cortex.

SENSORY: SPINOTHALAMIC

64. What type of information is carried in the spinothalamic tract?
The spinothalamic tract conveys pain, temperature, and crude touch.

65. What type of peripheral nerve fiber is involved with transmission of spinothalamic information?
Small, myelinated, and unmyelinated fibers carry spinothalamic-type information.

66. What is the pathway by which this information reaches the cerebral cortex?
Sensation on skin→afferent sensory nerve→substantia gelatinosa of the ipsilateral dorsal horn→synapse→cross via the anterior white commissure→contralateral spinothalamic tract→ascend to the VPL nucleus of the thalamus→synapse→through the posterior limb of the internal capsule→postcentral gyrus of the cortex.

67. Where do the spinothalamic fibers decussate? At what locations do they synapse?
These fibers decussate at the level they enter the spinal cord, after synapsing in Rexed's lamina II (substantia gelatinosa). They also synapse in the VPL of the thalamus before going to the cortex.

68. What types of receptors are stimulated to sense this information?
Pain and temperature are perceived by naked terminals of A delta and C fibers and by many specialized chemoreceptors that are excited by tissue substances released in response to noxious and inflammatory stimuli. Substance P is thought to be the neurotransmitter released by A delta and C fibers at their connections with the interneurons in the spinal cord.

69. Where in the internal capsule do the afferents travel from the VPL thalamic nucleus?
The sensory tracts from the VPL travel in the posterior aspect of the posterior limb of the internal capsule.

70. To which anatomic locations do the afferents from the VPL project?
They project to the postcentral gyrus (Brodmann's area 3, 1, 2; also called *somatosensory I*) and to somatosensory II (the posterior aspect of the superior lip of the lateral fissure).

SENSORY: SPINOCEREBELLAR

71. Which pathway carries proprioception from the lower limbs to the cerebellum?
Proprioception travels from the legs to the cerebellum in the dorsal columns.

72. Where does cerebellar proprioception for the lower limb synapse?
These fibers synapse in the midthoracic level of the spinal cord in the nucleus dorsalis of Clarke.

73. Where is the spinocerebellar tract located?
The spinocerebellar tract lies lateral to the corticospinal tract in the cord.

MOTOR: CORTICOSPINAL

74. Where do the motor fibers originate?
The motor fibers originate from the precentral gyrus (Brodmann's area 4). Initiation of movement arises from the premotor cortex (Brodmann's area 6), which lies anterior to the precentral gyrus.

75. Where do the motor fibers travel in the internal capsule?
The corticospinal fibers travel in the anterior portion of the posterior limb of the internal capsule. The motor fibers to the face (corticobulbar fibers) travel in the genu of the internal capsule.

76. Which cranial nerve exits the midbrain in close proximity to the corticospinal fibers?
Cranial nerve III exits the midbrain in close proximity to the corticospinal fibers, which explains the symptoms of a common vascular syndrome. In Weber's syndrome, a stroke in this location causes an ipsilateral third nerve palsy with contralateral hemiparesis.

77. Where do the motor fibers decussate?
The corticospinal tract decussates in the lower ventral medulla, and most fibers continue in the cord as the lateral corticospinal tract, with a small percentage descending in the ventral corticospinal tract.

78. On what types of neurons in the spinal cord do the corticospinal fibers synapse?
In the spinal cord, the corticospinal fibers synapse on the alpha and gamma motor neurons in Rexed's lamina IX.

MOTOR: OTHER TRACTS

79. What is the reticulospinal tract?
The reticulospinal tract also originates in the precentral gyrus, but instead of descending uninterrupted to the spinal cord, these fibers synapse in the reticular formation of the brain stem as they descend to the spinal cord. They mainly have an inhibitory effect on the alpha and gamma motor neurons.

80. What is the vestibulospinal tract?
The vestibulospinal tract is the efferent from the lateral vestibular nucleus. This tract descends the spinal cord, residing lateral to the spinothalamic tract, and coordinates motor and vestibular performance.

81. What is the MLF?
The MLF is primarily an efferent of the lateral vestibular nucleus. This tract ascends to the sixth, fourth, and third cranial nuclei. Other major components of the MLF are interneurons originating from the paramedian pontine reticular formation (see Question 149).

BRAIN STEM: CRANIAL NERVES

82. What are the three parts of the brain stem?
The brain stem consists of the midbrain, pons, and medulla.

83. What is the reticular formation?
The reticular formation is a loosely organized longitudinal collection of interneurons that fill the central core of the brain stem, which is concerned with modulating awareness and behavioral performance.

84. Name the 12 cranial nerves.

I. Olfactory	IV. Trochlear	VII. Facial	X. Vagus
II. Optic	V. Trigeminal	VIII. Auditory	XI. Spinal accessory
III. Oculomotor	VI. Abducens	IX. Glossopharyngeal	XII. Hypoglossal

85. What are general somatic afferent nerves? Which cranial nerves carry them?
General somatic afferent fibers carry exteroceptive (pain, temperature, touch) and proprioceptive impulses. Cranial nerves for proprioception: III, IV, V, VI, XII; for pain, temperature, and touch: V, VII, IX, X.

86. **What are general visceral afferent nerves? Which cranial nerves carry them?**
General visceral afferent fibers carry impulses from the visceral structures, and cranial nerves IX and X contain these fibers.

87. **What are special somatic afferent nerves? Which cranial nerves carry them?**
Special somatic afferent fibers carry sensory impulses from the special senses (vision, hearing, equilibrium), and cranial nerves II and VIII contain these fibers.

88. **What are special visceral afferent nerves? Which cranial nerves carry them?**
Special visceral afferent fibers carry impulses from the olfactory and gustatory senses, and cranial nerves I (olfactory), VII, IX, and X (gustatory) contain these fibers.

89. **What are general somatic efferent nerves? Which cranial nerves carry them?**
General somatic efferent fibers carry motor impulses to somatic skeletal muscles. In the head, the tongue and extraocular muscles are of this type. Cranial nerves III, IV, VI, and XII carry these fibers.

90. **What are general visceral efferent nerves? Which cranial nerves carry them?**
General visceral efferent fibers carry parasympathetic autonomic axons. The following cranial nerves carry general visceral efferent fibers:
- **Cranial nerve III** (Edinger–Westphal nucleus): the preganglionic fibers from the Edinger–Westphal nucleus terminate in the ciliary ganglion, and the postganglionic fibers innervate the pupil.
- **Cranial nerve VII** (superior salivatory nucleus): the preganglionic fibers from the superior salivatory nucleus terminate in the pterygopalatine and submandibular ganglion. The postganglionic fibers innervate the lacrimal gland (from the pterygopalatine ganglion) and the submandibular and sublingual gland (from the submandibular ganglion).
- **Cranial nerve IX** (inferior salivatory nucleus): the preganglionic fibers from the inferior salivatory nucleus terminate in the otic ganglion, and the postganglionic fibers innervate the parotid gland.
- **Cranial nerve X** (dorsal motor nucleus): the dorsal motor nucleus innervates the abdominal viscera.

91. **What are special visceral efferent nerves? Which cranial nerves carry them?**
Special visceral efferent fibers innervate skeletal muscle derived from the branchial arches. They are carried by the following cranial nerves: V (muscles of mastication, first branchial arch), VII (muscles of facial expression, second branchial arch), IX (stylopharyngeus muscle, third branchial arch), X (muscles of the soft palate and pharynx, fourth branchial arch), and XI (muscles of the larynx/sternocleidomastoid (SCM)/trapezius, sixth branchial arch).

MIDBRAIN

92. **What are the three anatomic subdivisions of the midbrain?**
The midbrain can be divided into the tectum, tegmentum, and cerebral crus (Fig. 2-7).

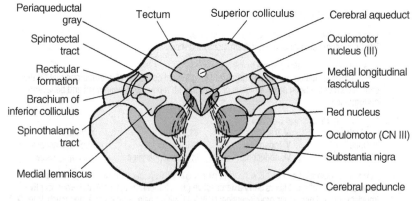

Figure 2-7. Diagram of the midbrain.

93. **What is the quadrigeminal plate?**
The quadrigeminal plate is formed by the tectum and the superior and inferior colliculi.

94. **What is the substantia nigra?**
The substantia nigra, a motor nucleus in the basal ganglia system, lies anterior to the tegmentum but posterior to the crus (pyramidal tract) in the midbrain.

95. **Which disease affects the substantia nigra? What is the pathology?**
The primary efferent neurotransmitter from the substantia nigra is dopamine. Parkinson's disease damages the substantia nigra. Pathologically, the neurons lose their melanin and the nucleus becomes depigmented. Many neurons also contain inclusion bodies called *Lewy bodies*.

96. **What is the red nucleus?**
The red nucleus is a globular mass located in the ventral portion of the tegmentum of the midbrain. It is a relay center for many of the efferent cerebellar tracts. The crossed fibers of the superior cerebellar peduncle (SCP) pass through and around its edges.

97. **What is the Edinger–Westphal nucleus?**
The Edinger–Westphal nucleus, in the posterior midbrain, supplies parasympathetic fibers that terminate in the ciliary ganglion via cranial nerve III. It is mainly involved in pupillary constriction and the light accommodation reflex.

98. **What is the function of cranial nerve III?**
Cranial nerve III innervates all the extraocular muscles except for the lateral rectus and superior oblique. It innervates the medial rectus, superior rectus, inferior rectus, and inferior oblique muscles.

99. **Where does cranial nerve III exit the brain stem?**
Cranial nerve III, the oculomotor nerve, exits the brain stem medially from the midbrain between the posterior cerebral artery and the superior cerebellar artery. This is important because the nerve can be affected by aneurysms of these arteries.

100. **What is the function of cranial nerve IV?**
Cranial nerve IV, the trochlear nerve, innervates the superior oblique muscle.

101. **What is the route of cranial nerve IV?**
Cranial nerve IV travels posteriorly and medially, crosses the midline, wraps around the midbrain, and exits the brain stem laterally between the posterior cerebral artery and superior cerebellar artery. It has the longest intracranial route (approximately 7.5 cm) of any cranial nerve. It then travels through the cavernous sinus and enters the orbit through the superior orbital fissure. Because it crosses the midline, the right trochlear nerve innervates the left superior oblique muscle.

102. **In a superior oblique palsy, which way would the patient tilt his or her head?**
If the left superior oblique muscle is weak, then tilting the head to the right would reduce the diplopia, and tilting the head to the left would worsen the diplopia. So a patient tilts his or her head away from the affected eye (Fig. 2-8).

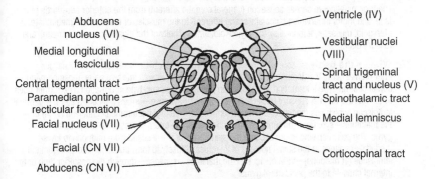

Figure 2-8. Anatomy of the medulla.

PONS

103. Which cranial nerves exit at the pontomedullary junction?
Cranial nerve VI exits medially, and cranial nerves VII and VIII exit laterally (Fig. 2-9).

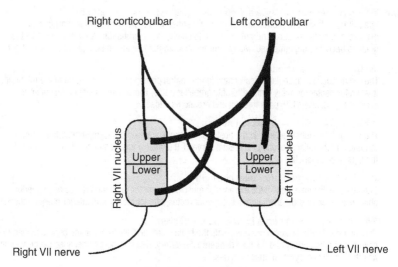

Figure 2-9. Anatomy of the pons.

104. Where does cranial nerve V exit the brain stem?
Cranial nerve V, the trigeminal nerve, exits the brain stem laterally at the midpons level. It divides into three main branches: V1 (ophthalmic), V2 (maxillary), and V3 (mandibular).

105. What are the four subdivisions of the trigeminal nucleus?
- Mesencephalic nucleus (which is a nucleus of unipolar cell bodies similar to the dorsal root ganglion, with no synapse)
- Chief sensory nucleus
- Descending spinal nucleus
- Motor nucleus

106. What type of information does cranial nerve V carry?
The trigeminal nerve carries sensation (general somatic afferent) from the anterior two-thirds of the face, and motor innervation (special visceral efferent) to the muscles of mastication (medial/lateral pterygoid, masseter, temporalis), the mylohyoid, anterior belly of the digastric, tensor tympani, and tensor palati.

107. What is the pathway by which sensation from the face reaches the cortex?
After cranial nerve V enters the brain stem, the afferent nerves split into two parts: those carrying dorsal column-type information and those carrying spinothalamic-type information. The former goes to the ipsilateral chief sensory nucleus of V (midpons)→synapse→enters the contralateral trigeminal lemniscus (which lies medial to the medial lemniscus)→ventral posteromedial nucleus (VPM) of the thalamus→synapse→through the posterior limb of the internal capsule to the postcentral gyrus. The pain-carrying fibers become the spinal tract of V→descend from midpons to lower medulla→synapse in the spinal nucleus of V→cross diffusely to form the contralateral trigeminal lemniscus (at midpons)→VPM nucleus of the thalamus→synapse→through the posterior limb of the internal capsule to the postcentral gyrus.

108. **What is the function of cranial nerve VI?**
Cranial nerve VI, the abducens nerve, abducts the eye.

109. **What is the function of cranial nerve VII?**
Cranial nerve VII, the facial nerve, innervates the muscles of facial expression (special visceral efferent); innervates the lacrimal, submandibular, sublingual, and parotid glands (general visceral efferent); supplies taste sensation to the anterior two-thirds of the tongue (special visceral afferent); and supplies sensation to the external ear (general somatic afferent).

110. **How does the nucleus for cranial nerve VII receive higher cortical input?**
The innervation to the muscles of facial expression can be separated into the muscles of the upper part of the face and the muscles of the lower part of the face. The supranuclear input responsible for the movement of the upper facial musculature is a bilateral input from the cortex to the nucleus. The supranuclear input responsible for the movement of the lower facial musculature is only a contralateral input from the cortex to the facial nucleus (Fig. 2-10).

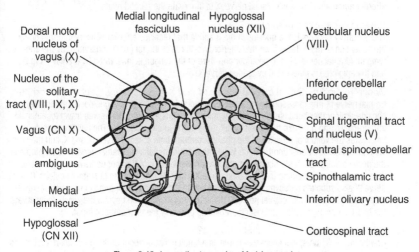

Figure 2-10. Innervation to muscles of facial expression.

111. **What is the difference between an upper motor neuron (central) and lower motor neuron (peripheral) facial weakness?**
If the patient with a facial droop can move the upper facial muscles (i.e., wrinkle the forehead), the lesion is supranuclear on the contralateral side. The lesion is somewhere in the contralateral corticobulbar tracts above the facial nerve nucleus (e.g., in the crus or in the genu of the internal capsule). If the patient cannot voluntarily move any muscle involved in facial expression (either upper or lower facial musculature), the lesion is localized to the facial nucleus or the peripheral facial nerve on the ipsilateral side.

112. **What is Möbius syndrome?**
Möbius syndrome is congenital absence of both facial nerve nuclei, resulting in a facial diplegia. Patients also may have associated absence of the abducens nuclei.

113. **What is the function of cranial nerve VIII?**
Cranial nerve VIII, the vestibulocochlear nerve, has two functionally distinct sensory divisions: the vestibular nerve and the cochlear (or auditory) nerve. The vestibular nerve responds to position and movement of the head, serving functions often identified as equilibrium. The cochlear nerve mediates auditory functions.

MEDULLA

114. What is the nucleus ambiguus?

The nucleus ambiguus is a cigar-shaped nucleus that lies in the depths of the medulla. It innervates the volitional muscles of the pharynx by way of both cranial nerves IX and X and the larynx (for phonation) via cranial nerve X. The larynx and pharynx have bilateral cortical input.

115. What is the nucleus solitarius?

The nucleus solitarius is the nucleus in the medulla that receives afferent information from the larynx (via cranial nerve X) and posterior pharynx and mediates the gag and cough reflexes (cranial nerves IX and X). Pain sensation from these areas enters the brain stem through cranial nerves IX and X but terminates in the descending spinal tract of the trigeminal nerve.

116. What is the salivatory nucleus?

The superior salivatory nucleus sends efferent autonomic fibers (general visceral efferent) through cranial nerve VII to innervate the lacrimal, submandibular, and sublingual glands as well as the mucous membranes of the nose and hard and soft palate. The inferior salivatory nucleus sends efferent autonomic fibers via cranial nerve IX to innervate the parotid gland.

117. What is the gustatory nucleus?

The gustatory nucleus is the nucleus in the medulla that receives afferent sensory information for the sensation of taste. Taste from the anterior two-thirds of the tongue is innervated by the chorda tympani (cranial nerve VII), the posterior one-third of the tongue is innervated by cranial nerve IX, and the epiglottis is innervated by cranial nerve X.

118. Describe the function of cranial nerves IX and X (glossopharyngeal–vagal complex).

Cranial nerve IX (the glossopharyngeal nerve) and cranial nerve X (the vagus nerve) are usually considered together because of their overlapping functions. Both cranial nerves travel together intracranially, and both exit the cranial vault through the jugular foramen. The nucleus ambiguus innervates the volitional muscles of the pharynx through both cranial nerves IX and X, and the larynx via cranial nerve X. Sensation from the larynx enters the medulla via cranial nerve X to terminate in the nucleus solitarius. Taste fibers from the posterior one-third of the tongue travel via cranial nerve IX, and taste from the epiglottis via cranial nerve X. They terminate in the gustatory nucleus. Cranial nerve IX also supplies parasympathetic innervation to the parotid, originating in the inferior salivatory nucleus. Branches of cranial nerve X, the vagus nerve, continue beyond the larynx to innervate the heart, lungs, and abdominal viscera, providing primarily parasympathetic input.

119. What is the function of cranial nerve XI?

Cranial nerve XI, the spinal accessory nerve, is a small nerve of about 3500 motor fibers that arises from the upper cervical and lower medullary anterior horn cells and supplies the sternocleidomastoid (SCM) and trapezius muscles. It exits the cranial vault via the jugular foramen.

120. What is jugular foramen syndrome?

Because cranial nerves IX, X, and XI exit the cranial vault through the jugular foramen, jugular foramen syndrome is a constellation of symptoms arising from a lesion (typically a tumor) at the level of the jugular foramen that compromises the function of these cranial nerves. Symptoms include loss of taste to the posterior one-third of the tongue; paralysis of the vocal cords, palate, and pharynx; and paralysis of the trapezius and SCM muscles.

121. If the left spinal accessory nerve is cut, which functions are lost?

Because cranial nerve XI supplies the SCM and the trapezius, these muscles are weakened. Because the left SCM is involved in turning the head to the right, a lesion of the left cranial nerve XI results in an inability to turn the head to the right. The left trapezius also loses function, and the patient would not be able to shrug the left shoulder.

122. If the left hypoglossal nucleus is injured, which way does the tongue deviate?

Lesioning the nucleus is similar to lesioning the peripheral nerve. The left hypoglossal nerve innervates the left tongue muscles, which, if acting alone, pushes the tongue to the right. The right hypoglossal nerve innervates the right tongue muscles, which, if acting alone, pushes the tongue to the left. Usually, these muscles work together to push the tongue forward without deviation. If the left hypoglossal nucleus is lesioned, the right hypoglossal muscles act unopposed. The tongue thus deviates to the left, or, in other words, the tongue deviates toward the affected side.

KEY POINTS: CRANIAL NERVE REFLEXES

1. Critical in establishing level of damage in coma
2. Critical to finding a cause (focal—structural lesion; nonfocal—metabolic)
3. Pupil reaction: II input, III output
4. Doll's eyes or cold water calorics: VIII input; III, IV, VI output
5. Gag: IX input, X output
6. Able to breathe: medulla function

BREATHING

123. **What is Cheyne–Stokes breathing? Where is the lesion that causes it?**
Cheyne–Stokes breathing is a crescendo-decrescendo pattern of periodic breathing in which phases of hyperpnea regularly alternate with apnea. Cheyne–Stokes respirations are seen most often with lesions affecting both cerebral hemispheres.

124. **What is central neurogenic hyperventilation? What causes it?**
Central neurogenic hyperventilation is a sustained, rapid, deep hyperpnea. It is produced by lesions in the low midbrain to upper one-third of the pons.

125. **What is apneustic breathing? What causes it?**
Apneusis is a prolonged respiratory cramp, a pause at full inspiration. Apneustic breathing may occur after damage to the mid or caudal pons.

126. **What is cluster breathing? When does it occur?**
Cluster breathing, a disorderly sequence of breaths with irregular pauses between the breaths, may result from damage to the lower pons or upper medulla.

127. **What is ataxic breathing? Where is the lesion that causes it?**
Ataxic breathing is a completely irregular pattern of breathing in which both deep and shallow breaths occur randomly. The respiratory rate tends to be slow. The lesion that causes it is in the central medulla.

POSTURING

128. **What is decorticate posturing? What causes it?**
Decorticate posturing is a stereotyped response to noxious stimuli. In the upper extremity, it consists of flexion of the arm, wrist, and fingers; in the lower extremity, it consists of extension, internal rotation, and plantar flexion. Decorticate posturing most often occurs in comatose patients with lesions below the thalamus but above the red nucleus.

129. **What is decerebrate posturing? In whom does it occur?**
Decerebrate posturing is a stereotyped response to noxious stimuli. It consists of extension, adduction, and hyperpronation in the upper extremity and extension with plantar flexion in the lower extremity. Comatose patients with lesions below the red nucleus but above the vestibular nucleus may have decerebrate posturing.

VESTIBULAR APPARATUS

130. **What are the five receptors of the vestibular apparatus, and what do they sense?**
Three semicircular canals that are oriented 90 degrees to each other sense rotational acceleration in all three planes. One horizontally oriented utricle and one vertically oriented saccule sense linear acceleration.

131. **Where does the vestibular information synapse?**
The vestibular nerve, carrying sensory data from the receptors, divides and synapses in four vestibular nuclei grouped together in the medulla: the superior, inferior, medial, and lateral vestibular nuclei.

132. **What is the output from these nuclei?**
The vestibulospinal tracts and the MLF are the two efferent tracts from the vestibular nuclei.

133. **Where do the vestibular nuclei project?**
Vestibular nuclei project to (1) the oculomotor nuclei (cranial nerves III, IV, and VI), (2) cranial nerve XI, (3) cervical nuclei for head and neck position, (4) fastigial nuclei of the cerebellum, and (5) reticular formations of the brain stem.

134. **What is the response of a normal person to cold water injected in the left ear?**
Injecting cold water into the left ear causes slow eye movements toward the left, followed by a fast phase of nystagmus back to the right.

135. **What is the expected response of a comatose patient with an intact brain stem to cold water in the left ear?**
The patient will have slow eye deviation toward the left ear. The fast-phase nystagmus is absent.

HEARING

136. **Which structures constitute the external ear, middle ear, and inner ear?**
The external ear is composed of the pinna, the external auditory canal, and the tympanic membrane. The middle ear is composed of the tympanic membrane, ossicles (malleus, incus, stapes), and oval window. The ossicles function as an impedance matching device between air and fluid during the travel of the sound wave. The inner ear is composed of part of the oval window, the cochlea, and the round window.

137. **Which compartments of the cochlea are filled with perilymph?**
- **Scala vestibuli**. It is separated from the scala tympani by Reissner's membrane.
- **Scala tympani**. It is separated from the scala media by the basilar membrane.
- **Scala media**. The third compartment is filled with endolymph and is located between Reissner's and the basilar membranes (Fig. 2-11).

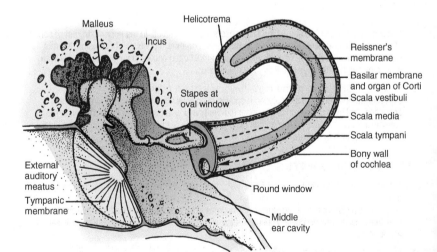

Figure 2-11. Anatomy of the hearing apparatus. (*Redrawn from Kandel E, Schwartz JH, Jessell TM (eds):* Principles of neuroscience, *3rd ed. New York, McGraw-Hill, 1991, p. 369.*)

138. **What is the pathway traveled by the cochlear fluid pressure wave initiated by a sound wave?**
The stapes transmits the pressure to the round window and from it to the perilymph of the scala vestibuli, which, in turn, sets up vibrations of Reissner's membrane, resulting in a wave in the scala media. The basilar membranes move next and transmit the pressure to the scala tympani and from there to the oval window.

139. **What is the arrangement of the neuroepithelial cells of the organ of Corti?**
    - The outer hair cells (arranged in three rows) rest on the basilar membrane, with their stereocilia inserted into the tectorial membrane; these cells are able to contract and initiate the flow of endolymph toward the inner hair cells.
    - The inner hair cells (one row) sit on the bone; they do not contract. These cells respond to the movement of endolymph and provide most of the afferent input to the spiral ganglion.

140. **How does the organ of Corti serve as an audiofrequency analyzer?**
The anatomic arrangement allows frequency analysis of sounds:
    - The basilar membrane responds to high frequencies at its base and to low frequencies at its apex.
    - The hair cells in the base of the cochlear duct have short and fat stereocilia, which are stimulated by high frequencies.
    - The hair cells in the apex of the cochlea have long and thin stereocilia, which respond best to low frequencies.

141. **What is the anatomy of the auditory pathway?**
Spiral ganglion→auditory nerve (cranial nerve VIII)→dorsal and ventral cochlear nuclei at the junction of the medulla and pons→trapezoid body (at this point 50% of the axons cross over to the other side)→superior olivary nucleus→lateral lemniscus→inferior colliculus→medial geniculate body→transverse gyrus of Heschl (area 41, partly buried in the sylvian fissure).

142. **At what level is there crossing of information between the left and right ascending tracts?**
The crossing of axons occurs on every level from the trapezoid body to the medial geniculate body.

143. **To produce unilateral deafness, where could the lesion be?**
The lesion must be at the cochlear nucleus or more peripheral because of multiple crossovers above the cochlear nucleus.

144. **What is a Weber's test?**
A vibrating tuning fork is placed in the middle of the forehead. In patients with conduction deafness, the sound is localized to the affected ear (bone is greater than air conduction). In patients with sensorineural deafness, the signal is localized to the healthy ear.

145. **What is Rinne's test?**
A vibrating tuning fork is placed on the mastoid bone; when the patient can no longer hear it, it is removed and placed next to the ear. Thus, bone conduction is compared with air conduction. In conduction deafness, bone is greater than air conduction. In sensorineural deafness, air is greater than bone conduction.

146. **What is the innervation of the external ear canal?**
The external ear canal is supplied by cranial nerves V3, VII, IX, and X.

147. **Damage to which structures results in hyperacusis?**
    - **Facial nerve (VII)**—innervates the stapedius muscle, which retracts the stapes from the round window.
    - **Trigeminal nerve (V)**—supplies the tensor tympani, which inserts into the malleus and tenses the tympanic membrane, thus preventing it from vibrating.

148. **What is the pathway for the feedback loop?**
When auditory input reaches the superior olive, it sends signals to the olivocochlear bundle through the VIII nerve; the signals then terminate on the outer hair cells or afferent fibers in the spiral ganglia.

EYE MOVEMENTS

149. **What is the paramedian pontine reticular formation (PPRF)?**
The PPRF is a collection of cells lying in the pons adjacent to the nucleus of cranial nerve VI, and is an important center for horizontal gaze. Efferent fibers from the PPRF project to the ipsilateral abducens (VI) nucleus, and to the contralateral oculomotor (III) nucleus through the MLF, stimulating both eyes to move horizontally.

150. **What is the difference between saccades and smooth pursuit movements?**
Saccades are fast conjugate eye movements that are under voluntary control. Saccades are generated in the contralateral frontal lobe (Brodmann's area 8). Smooth pursuits are slow involuntary movements of eyes fixed on a moving target. Pursuit movements to one side are generated in the ipsilateral occipital lobe (Brodmann's areas 18 and 19).

151. **What is the pathway for saccades?**
Fibers from the frontal eye field (Brodmann's area 8) pass through the genu of the internal capsule, decussate at the level of the upper pons, and synapse in the PPRF.

152. **What is the pathway for smooth pursuit?**
The pathway for smooth pursuit is not clearly defined but appears to arise in the anterior occipital lobe (Brodmann's areas 18 and 19) and travel to the ipsilateral PPRF.

153. **What is the brain stem area for vertical gaze?**
Near the superior colliculus, there are subtectal and pretectal centers that control vertical eye movements and project to cranial nuclei III, IV, and VI.

154. **What are the pathways for voluntary vertical eye movements?**
Vertical movements are driven symmetrically from both frontal lobes. When activated bilaterally, fibers from Brodmann's area 8 project via the frontopontine tract to act upon bilateral cranial nuclei III, IV, and VI, which then innervate their respective muscles.

CEREBELLUM

155. **Describe the anatomic divisions of the cerebellum.**
The cerebellum is anatomically divided into the two hemispheres, the midline vermis and the flocculonodulus.

156. **What are the functions of each cerebellar "lobe"?**
The hemispheres are involved in appendicular control, the vermis is involved in axial control, and the flocculonodular lobe is involved in vestibular balance.

157. **What are the three layers of the cerebellar cortex?**
- Outermost molecular cell layer
- Middle Purkinje cell layer
- Innermost granular cell layer

158. **What types of cells are located in each of these layers?**
The molecular layer contains (1) stellate cells, (2) basket cells, (3) dendrites of Purkinje cells, (4) dendrites of Golgi type II cells, and (5) axons of granule cells. The Purkinje layer contains the cell bodies of Purkinje cells. The granular layer contains (6) granule cells, (7) Golgi type II cells, and (8) glomeruli (synaptic complexes that contain mossy fibers, axons and dendrites of Golgi type II cells, and dendrites of granule cells).

159. **What is the afferent fiber from the inferior olives? Through which peduncle does it reach the cerebellum?**
The afferent fiber from the inferior olives is the climbing fiber. It enters the cerebellum through the inferior cerebellar peduncle.

160. **What is Mollaret's triangle?**
Mollaret's triangle is a physiologic connection between the red nucleus, inferior olives, and dentate nucleus of the cerebellum. A lesion in this pathway can cause palatal myoclonus.

161. What are the deep nuclei of the cerebellum (medial to lateral)?
Medial to lateral, the cerebellar deep nuclei are fastigial, globus, emboliform, and dentate.

162. What are the primary inputs and outputs of the cerebellum?
Cerebellar function can be conceptualized as a feedback loop, with input arriving from an origin, synapsing in a cerebellar nucleus, and then projecting back, often to the same origin (Table 2-2).

Table 2-2. Cerebellar Connections

CEREBELLAR PEDUNCLE		CONNECTED TO		TRACTS THAT RUN IN THE PEDUNCLE	
Superior (SCP)		Midbrain		DRT and VSC	
Middle (MCP)		Pons		CPC	
Inferior (ICP)		Medulla		All other tracts to/from the cerebellum	

ORIGIN	INFLOW TRACT	INFLOW PEDUNCLE	CEREBELLAR NUCLEUS	OUTFLOW PEDUNCLE	OUTFLOW TRACT	DESTINATION
Precentral gyrus	CPC	MCP	Dentate	SCP	DRT	Precentral gyrus
Spinal cord	SC	ICP	Fastigial	ICP	—	Vestibular nucleus
Vestibular nucleus	VC	ICP	Vestibular	ICP	LVS (MLF)	Spinal cord

SCP, Superior cerebellar peduncle; MCP, middle cerebellar peduncle; ICP, inferior cerebellar peduncle; DRT, dentatorubrothalamic; VSC, ventral spinocerebellar; CPC, corticopontocerebellar; SC, spinocerebellar; VC, vestibulocerebellar; LVS, lateral vestibulospinal; MLF, medial longitudinal fasciculus.

163. What type of fiber originating in the cerebellar cortex is inhibitory on the deep cerebellar nuclei?
Purkinje fibers originate in the cerebellar cortex and synapse on the deep nuclei as an inhibitory neuron.

164. Where does the dentatorubrothalamic tract synapse?
These fibers synapse in the ventrolateral (VL) nucleus of the thalamus before ascending to the cortex.

BASAL GANGLIA

165. What are the basal ganglia?
The basal ganglia are a collection of nuclei, largely concerned with motor control, composed primarily of the corpus striatum and the lenticular complex (see Fig. 11-1).

166. What are the parts of the corpus striatum?
The corpus striatum is composed of the putamen and caudate.

167. What is the lenticular complex?
The lenticular complex, or lentiform nucleus, is composed of the globus pallidus and putamen.

168. Which structure is the lateral border of the caudate?
The anterior limb of the internal capsule is the lateral border of the caudate.

169. What is the major outflow of the basal ganglia?
The major outflow of the basal ganglia projects from the medial globus pallidus as a fiber bundle known as the *lenticular fasciculus* (Forel's field H2). Another bundle from the medial globus pallidus loops around the internal capsule as the ansa lenticularis. It then merges in Forel's field H with the lenticular fasciculus and with fibers from the dentatorubrothalamic tract. These fibers then continue

as the thalamic fasciculus (Forel's field H1) and synapse in the thalamic nuclei: centromedian, ventral lateral, and ventral anterior. These thalamic nuclei then relay information up to the motor cortex.

170. **Is there any other output from the medial globus pallidus?**
Yes. Apart from the lenticular fasciculus and the ansa lenticularis, a third fiber tract leaves the medial globus pallidus as the pallidotegmental tract and descends onto the pedunculopontine nucleus in the midbrain, where neurons help to regulate posture. This is the only descending tract from the basal ganglia.

171. **Is there any output from the basal ganglia that does not originate in the medial globus pallidus?**
The only other output is a small tract (pallidosubthalamic fibers) that leaves the lateral globus pallidus to synapse in the subthalamic nucleus.

172. **What is the major input to the basal ganglia?**
The major input is from the motor cortex and the thalamic nuclei. The basal ganglia function, simplistically, as a feedback loop: cerebral cortex→basal ganglia→thalamus→cerebral cortex.

THALAMUS

173. **Which structure lies lateral to the thalamus and medial to the thalamus?**
The posterior limb of the internal capsule is the lateral border of the thalamus. The third ventricle lies medial to the thalamus.

174. **What is the anatomy of the thalamus?**
The intermedullary lamina divides the thalamus into anterior, medial, and lateral groups. The lateral group is further divided into ventral and dorsal tiers. Each group contains specific nuclei:
- **Anterior group:** anterior nucleus
- **Medial group:** dorsomedial (DM) nucleus
- **Lateral group:**
  - Dorsal tier
  - Lateral dorsal (LD) nucleus
  - Lateral posterior (LP) nucleus
  - Pulvinar
  - Ventral tier ventral anterior (VA) nucleus
  - VL nucleus
  - VPL nucleus
  - VPM nucleus
  - Lateral geniculate (LG)
  - Medial geniculate (MG)

  Other nuclei that are often considered part of the thalamus include (1) reticular nucleus—a small group of neurons that projects to other thalamic nuclei and may help regulate cortical activity; (2) midline nuclei—diffuse neurons connected to the hypothalamus; and (3) centromedian (CM)—an intralaminar nucleus that is part of the reticular formation that activates the cortex.

175. **What are the inputs to and from the main thalamic nuclei?**
See Table 2-3.

176. **What is the limbic lobe?**
The limbic lobe is not a true lobe of the brain but rather a functional collection of structures that regulate higher activities such as memory and emotion. It is commonly said to include (1) cingulate gyrus, (2) parahippocampal gyrus, (3) hippocampal gyrus, and (4) uncus.

177. **What is Papez's circuit?**
Papez's circuit is a route by which the limbic system communicates between the hippocampus, thalamus, hypothalamus, and cortex. It forms a circuit from the hippocampal formation→fornix→mammillary body→mammillothalamic tract→anterior group of thalamus→cingulate gyrus→cingulate bundle→hippocampus. (Note: the amygdala is not part of the classic Papez circuit.)

Table 2-3. Connections of the Thalamic Nuclei

THALAMIC NUCLEUS	PRINCIPAL INPUT	PRINCIPAL OUTPUT	FUNCTION
LP	Parietal lobe	Parietal lobe	Sensory integration
LD	Cingulate gyrus	Cingulate gyrus	Emotional expression
Pulvinar	Association areas of cortex	Association areas of cortex	Sensory integration
DM	Amygdala, olfactory, and hypothalamus	Prefrontal cortex	Limbic
MG	Auditory relay nuclei (from inferior colliculus)	Auditory cortex—area 41, 42	Hearing
LG	Optic tract	Visual cortex—area 17	Vision
Anterior	Mammillary body	Cingulate gyrus	Limbic
VA	Globus pallidus	Premotor cortex	Motor
VL	Cerebellum	Premotor and motor cortices	Motor
VPM	Trigeminal lemniscus	Postcentral gyrus	Somatic sensation (face)
VPL	Medial lemniscus and spinothalamic	Postcentral gyrus	Somatic integration (body)
CM	Reticular formation, globus pallidus, hypothalamus	Basal ganglia (striatum)	Sensory integration, smell, limbic

LP, Lateral posterior nucleus; *LD,* lateral dorsal nucleus; *DM,* dorsomedial nucleus; *MG,* medial geniculate; *LG,* lateral geniculate; *VA,* ventral anterior nucleus; *VL,* ventrolateral nucleus; *VPM,* ventral posteromedial nucleus; *VPL,* ventral posterolateral nucleus; *CM,* centromedian.

OLFACTION

178. **What are the olfactory receptor cells?**
     The receptor cells are bipolar neurons that pass from the olfactory mucosa through the cribriform plate to the olfactory bulb. Collectively, the central processes of the olfactory receptor cells constitute cranial nerve I.

179. **What is the anatomy of the olfactory pathway?**
     - In the olfactory bulb, the axons of receptor cells synapse on dendrites of mitral and tufted cells (forming a glomerulus).
     - The axons of mitral and tufted cells compose the olfactory tract, which soon divides into medial and lateral stria. Medial stria fibers cross to the contralateral side via the anterior commissure, while the lateral stria fibers terminate in the anterior perforated substance, amygdaloid complex, and lateral olfactory gyrus (which is the primary olfactory cortex).
     - From the lateral olfactory gyrus (prepiriform area), fibers project to the entorhinal cortex, the medial dorsal nucleus of the thalamus, and the hypothalamus.

180. **What is unique about the projection of olfactory information to the cerebral cortex?**
     Unlike other sensory modalities, olfaction reaches the cortex without relay through the thalamus.

181. **What are the most common causes of anosmia?**
     - Rhinitis/nasal congestion
     - Smoking
     - Head injury
     - Craniotomy

- Subarachnoid hemorrhage
- Meningiomas of the olfactory groove
- Zinc and vitamin A deficiency
- Hypothyroidism
- Congenital disorders (Kallmann's syndrome)
- Dementing diseases (Alzheimer's, Parkinson's)
- Multiple sclerosis

VISION

182. **What is the arrangement of cones and rods in the retina?**
The 6 million cones are concentrated toward the center, and the 120 million rods are in the periphery of the retina. In the fovea, located centrally within the macula, each cone is served by a single ganglion cell, resulting in very high resolution. In the periphery, many rods project to a single ganglion cell, giving high sensitivity but lower resolution.

183. **What are the primary functions of rods?**
Rods are concerned with night vision and are most sensitive between the blue and green wavelengths.

184. **What are the primary functions of cones?**
Cones are concerned with color vision and daytime vision. The three types of cones are tuned, via visual pigments, to different frequencies in the blue, green, and red wavelength ranges.

185. **What is the afferent pathway for the pupillary light reflex?**
Retinal ganglion cells concerned with the light reflex travel with the optic nerve and tract and then break away to project down to the midbrain pretectal nucleus. From the pretectal nucleus, fibers project bilaterally, decussating via the posterior commissure to each Edinger–Westphal nucleus.

186. **Which nucleus mediates pupil constriction?**
The Edinger–Westphal nucleus, or preganglionic parasympathetic nucleus of cranial nerve III, mediates pupillary constriction.

187. **What is the pathway for pupillary dilatation?**
This pathway has three neurons. First-order fibers descend from the ipsilateral hypothalamus through the brain stem and cervical cord to T1 to T2. They synapse on ipsilateral preganglionic sympathetic fibers, exit the cord, travel up the sympathetic chain as second-order neurons to the superior cervical ganglion, and then synapse on postganglionic sympathetic fibers. The third-order neurons travel via the internal carotid artery to the orbit and innervate the radial smooth muscle of the iris.

188. **What is Horner's syndrome?**
Horner's syndrome is an interruption of the sympathetic supply to the eye, resulting in the classic triad of ptosis, miosis, and anhidrosis.

189. **Describe the pharmacologic tests to diagnose Horner's syndrome.**
Instill 2% cocaine solution in both eyes, which dilates the pupils by preventing the reuptake of the sympathetic neurotransmitter norepinephrine. If one eye fails to dilate, a diagnosis of Horner's syndrome can be made because failure to dilate indicates an interruption of the sympathetic supply (norepinephrine) to that eye. To further localize the lesion, one can use amphetamine in the affected eye, which displaces norepinephrine from the nerve terminal and dilates the pupil. If the pupil dilates in response to this test, the lesion affects the third-order neuron, causing denervation hypersensitivity. Otherwise, the lesion is in the first- or second-order neurons.

190. **What is the anatomy of the lesion that causes an afferent pupillary defect?**
An afferent pupillary defect means the pupil will not react to light. The lesion must be prechiasmal and almost always involves the optic nerve.

191. **What is the test for an afferent pupillary defect (Marcus Gunn pupil)?**
The swinging flashlight test determines an afferent pupillary defect. Shine a light into the normal eye and the pupil constricts (the affected eye also constricts consensually). Quickly move the light onto

the opposite affected eye, and the pupil dilates. Removing the light from the normal pupil causes it and the affected pupil, responding consensually, to dilate. The affected pupil thus seems to dilate when the swinging light hits it.

192. What is the value of the pupillary reflex for diagnosing third-nerve palsies?
Because the parasympathetic fibers travel along the outside of the third nerve, they are usually damaged by nerve compression, resulting in pupillary dilatation. Third-nerve palsies that cause pupillary dilatation are usually masses (e.g., tumors, aneurysms), whereas palsies that do not involve the pupil are usually medical (e.g., ischemia, vasculitis).

193. What is the pathway for pupillary constriction that occurs with convergence?
The pathway begins in the occipital lobe (Brodmann's area 18) and projects to the Edinger–Westphal nucleus bilaterally. The details of how pupils constrict during convergence are poorly understood.

194. What is an Argyll Robertson pupil?
An Argyll Robertson pupil, one form of light-near dissociation, is an irregular pupil that does not constrict to light but does constrict to accommodation. This finding is quite specific for central nervous system (CNS) syphilis. Light-near dissociation with a regular pupil can be found in many diseases and is not specific for CNS syphilis.

195. What is the pathway of the optic nerve?
The ganglion cells from the nasal half of the retina travel in the optic nerve, where they decussate in the optic chiasm and join the contralateral optic tract to the lateral geniculate body. The ganglion cells from the temporal half of the retina travel in the optic nerve, stay in the ipsilateral optic tract, and project to the lateral geniculate body. Thus, the contralateral visual field is projected from each eye to the lateral geniculate body.

196. What thalamic nucleus is concerned with vision?
The lateral genicular body is the thalamic nucleus that handles vision.

197. What is the pathway of the optic radiation?
Second-order neurons from the lateral geniculate body project to the calcarine cortex (Brodmann's area 17). The superior visual field fibers wrap around the temporal horn on their way to the inferior lip of the calcarine fissure. The macular area is served by the most medial area of the calcarine cortex.

VISUAL FIELDS

198. Where is the lesion that causes a field defect in only one eye?
If only one eye is affected, the lesion must be prechiasmal.

199. Where are the lesions that cause each of the following: left homonymous hemianopsia, bitemporal hemianopsia, and binasal hemianopsia?
Left homonymous hemianopsia can arise from the right optic tract, right lateral geniculate body, right optic radiations, or the right occipital cortex. **Bitemporal hemianopsia** is caused by midline chiasmal lesions such as pituitary lesions (from below) or craniopharyngeal tumors (from above). **Binasal hemianopsia** can be caused only by simultaneous lesions on the lateral optic nerves or chiasm, such as bilateral internal carotid artery aneurysms.

200. What is a junctional scotoma?
A junctional scotoma results from a lesion at the junction of the optic nerve and chiasm. It causes an ipsilateral central scotoma and a superior temporal defect in the other eye. It occurs because some optic nerve fibers from the inferior temporal retina travel forward for a few millimeters in the contralateral nerve when they decussate in the chiasm; they are thus affected by a lesion in that nerve.

201. Where is the lesion that causes superior quadrantanopsia?
Superior quadrantanopsia usually results from damage to the inferior optic radiations. This may occur in Meyer's loop, which is the bundle of inferior optic radiations that swings forward into the temporal lobe.

202. What visual field results from a right occipital lobe infarction?
A right occipital lobe infarction causes a left homonymous hemianopsia with macular sparing.

CORTEX

203. **What are the layers of the cerebral cortex?**
The layers of the cerebral cortex are:

I. Molecular layer
II. Outer granular layer
III. Outer pyramidal layer

IV. Inner granular layer
V. Inner pyramidal or ganglion layer
VI. Multiform layer

    Afferent fibers activated by various sensory stimuli terminate in layers IV, III, and II. These signals are then transmitted to adjacent superficial and deep layers through multiple interconnections. All the efferent fibers originate in layer V (Figs. 2-12 and 2-13).

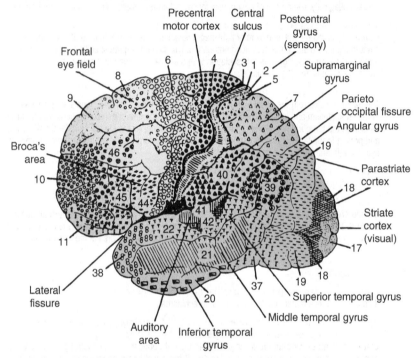

Figure 2-12. The superficial anatomy of the cerebral cortex showing Brodmann's areas. *(Redrawn from Garoutte B: Survey of functional neuroanatomy, 2nd ed. Greenbrae, CA, Jones Medical Publications, 1992, p. 144, with permission.)*

204. **What is the columnar organization of the cortex?**
Cortical neurons are arranged in cylindrical columns, each containing 100 to 300 neurons, which are heavily interconnected up and down through the cortical layers. Throughout the somatosensory system, cells responding to one modality are grouped together in the columns. All neurons in the column receive input from the same area and therefore comprise an elementary functional module of cortex.

205. **What is the line of Gennari?**
The fourth layer of the occipital cortex in area 17 is divided by a greatly thickened band of myelinated fibers, which is grossly visible and is called the *line of Gennari*. This stripe also gives the name of *striate cortex* to that area of the brain. Brodmann's areas 18 and 19 lack the line of Gennari.

206. **In what cortical cell layer are the Betz cells located?**
Betz cells give rise to efferent motor tracts (corticospinal fibers) and lie in cortical layer V.

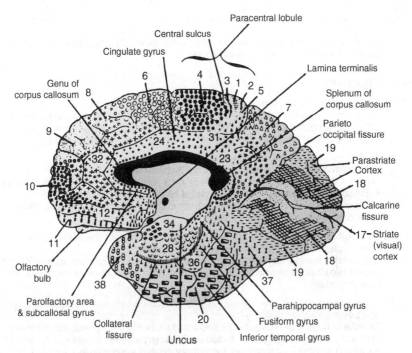

Figure 2-13. The superficial anatomy of the cerebral cortex showing Brodmann's areas. *(Redrawn from Garoutte B: Survey of functional neuroanatomy, 2nd ed. Greenbrae, CA, Jones Medical Publications, 1992, p. 144, with permission.)*

207. **What is the function of the frontal lobe?**
The frontal lobes (both right and left) are involved in voluntary eye movements, somatic motor control, planning and sequencing of movements, and emotional effect. The left frontal lobe is crucial for motor control of speech (Broca's area).

208. **What is the function of the temporal lobe?**
The temporal lobes (both right and left) handle auditory and visual perception, learning and memory, emotional effect, and olfaction. The dominant temporal lobe influences comprehension of speech (Wernicke's area). The nondominant temporal lobe mediates prosody and spatial relationships.

209. **What is the function of the parietal lobe?**
The parietal lobes (both right and left) handle cortical sensation, motor control, and visual perception. The dominant parietal lobe also handles ideomotor praxis. The nondominant parietal lobe controls spatial orientation.

210. **What is the function of the occipital lobe?**
The occipital lobes (both right and left) mainly handle visual perception and involuntary smooth pursuit eye movements.

211. **In which lobe is visual–spatial information processed?**
Visual–spatial information is mainly processed in the nondominant parietal lobe.

212. **Where is language processed?**
Language is primarily processed in Broca's area (posterior inferior frontal gyrus, Brodmann's area 44) and Wernicke's area (posterior part of the superior temporal gyrus, posterior part of Brodmann's area 22) in the dominant hemisphere.

213. **Where is the lesion that causes achromatopsia (inability to match colors and hues)?**
Achromatopsia results from a lesion of the dominant occipital lobe (Brodmann's area 18) and is a feature of the syndrome of alexia without agraphia.

CIRCULATION

214. **What is meant by the terms *anterior* and *posterior circulation*?**
Anterior circulation refers to the common carotid and its distal ramifications, including the internal carotid, middle cerebral, and anterior cerebral arteries. The posterior circulation refers to the vertebral and basilar arteries and their branches, including the posterior cerebral artery.

215. **Which vessels make up the circle of Willis?**
   - The **anterior circulation,** which is composed of the middle cerebral arteries, anterior cerebral arteries, and the anterior communicating artery, which connects the two anterior cerebral arteries.
   - The **posterior circulation,** which is composed of the posterior cerebral arteries.
   - The **posterior communicating artery,** which connects the middle cerebral with the posterior cerebral arteries, thus forming a true circle.

216. **If the right anterior cerebral artery is occluded proximally, how does the circle of Willis protect the patient from becoming symptomatic?**
If the occlusion is slow enough for the blood flow to accommodate, the right anterior cerebral artery receives blood from the contralateral internal carotid via the left anterior cerebral and anterior communicating arteries.

217. **What regions are supplied by the anterior cerebral artery, middle cerebral artery, and posterior cerebral artery?**
The **anterior cerebral artery** supplies the medial (midline) cerebral hemispheres, superior frontal lobes, and superior parietal lobes. The **middle cerebral artery** supplies the inferior frontal, inferolateral parietal, and lateral temporal lobes. The **posterior cerebral artery** supplies the occipital lobes and medial temporal lobes.

218. **What is the first intracranial branch off the internal carotid artery?**
The ophthalmic artery.

219. **What is the blood supply to the deep brain nuclei?**
The basal ganglia are supplied by small lenticulostriate arteries arising from the middle cerebral artery, whereas the thalamus is supplied by perforating thalamogeniculate arteries from the posterior cerebral artery. The blood supply of the thalamus comes from the posterior circulation.

220. **What is the name of the artery that supplies the genu of the internal capsule?**
The recurrent artery of Heubner, which is one of the named anteromedial lenticulostriate arteries, supplies the genu of the internal capsule.

221. **Which artery is the first branch off the basilar artery?**
The anterior inferior cerebellar artery (AICA).

222. **What is the blood supply to the brain stem?**
The brain stem receives its blood supply exclusively from the posterior circulation, including the vertebrals and basilar artery. The medulla receives its blood supply from the vertebrals via medial and lateral perforating arteries. The pons and midbrain receive their blood from the basilar via the medial and lateral perforating arteries.

223. **What is the blood supply to the cerebellum?**
The cerebellum receives its blood supply from the three cerebellar vessels:
   - Posterior inferior cerebellar artery, off the vertebrals.
   - AICA, the first branch off the basilar.
   - Superior cerebellar artery, the last branch off the basilar.

224. **Which nerves exit the brain stem area between the posterior cerebral artery and superior cerebellar artery?**
Cranial nerve III exits between the vessels medially, whereas cranial nerve IV exits between them laterally. Aneurysms of these blood vessels may thus damage these cranial nerves.

CEREBROSPINAL FLUID

225. What anatomic structure or structures produce cerebrospinal fluid (CSF)?
The majority of CSF is produced by the choroid plexus. A small amount of CSF is also produced by the blood vessels in the subependymal region and pia.

226. Where is the choroid plexus located?
The choroid plexus is located within the ventricular system, mainly in the lateral and fourth ventricles.

227. What is the rate of CSF production?
The rate is approximately 25 cc/hr (approximately 500 cc/day).

228. How much CSF does an average adult normally have?
The average male adult has approximately 100 to 150 cc of CSF.

229. What is communicating hydrocephalus? Noncommunicating hydrocephalus?
Communicating hydrocephalus occurs when there is dilatation of the ventricles due to obstruction of CSF flow outside the ventricular system (i.e., distal to the foramen of Magendie), so the CSF communicates with the subarachnoid space. Noncommunicating hydrocephalus occurs when there is dilatation of the ventricles due to an obstruction of CSF flow within the ventricular system at or above the foramen of Magendie.

230. What is the route of CSF from production to clearance?
Choroid plexus→lateral ventricle→interventricular foramen of Monro→third ventricle→cerebral aqueduct of Sylvius→fourth ventricle→two lateral foramina of Luschka and one medial foramen of Magendie→subarachnoid space→arachnoid granulations→dural sinus→venous drainage.

231. What space is invaded by a lumbar puncture?
During a lumbar puncture, the needle enters the subarachnoid space.

232. What is the ideal spinal level to do a lumbar puncture?
The ideal level for a lumbar puncture is below the conus medullaris at approximately vertebral level L4 to L5.

References available online at expertconsult.com.

WEBSITE

http://www.biostr.washington.edu/

BIBLIOGRAPHY

1. Garoutte B: Survey of Functional Neuroanatomy, 3rd ed. Mill Valley, CA, Mill Valley Medical Publishers, 1994.
2. Gilman S, Newman SW: Manter and Gatz's Essentials of Clinical Neuroanatomy and Neurophysiology, 10th ed. Philadelphia, FA Davis, 2002.
3. Haines D: Neuroanatomy in Clinical Context, 9th ed. Baltimore, Wolters Kluwer Health, 2015.
4. Kandel E, Schwartz JH, Jessell TM, Siegelbaum SA, Hudspeth AJ (eds): Principles of Neuroscience, 5th ed. New York, McGraw-Hill, 2013.
5. O'Brien M: Guarantors of Brain: Aids to the Examination of the Peripheral Nervous System, 5th ed. Edinburgh, Saunders, 2010.
6. Patten JP: Neurological Differential Diagnosis, 2nd ed. London, Springer-Verlag, 1996.
7. Posner JP, Saper CB, Schiff N, Plum F: Plum and Posner's Diagnosis of Stupor and Coma, 4th ed. London, Oxford University Press, 2008.

CHAPTER 3

APPROACH TO THE PATIENT WITH NEUROLOGIC DISEASE

Loren A. Rolak

1. **What is the first question to be answered in any patient with neurologic disease?**
   Where is the lesion? The neurologist, unlike most physicians, approaches patients from an anatomic perspective, leaving issues of physiology and etiology to be addressed later. The first step in evaluating patients with neurologic symptoms is to localize the lesion to a specific part of the nervous system.

2. **What is the best way to localize a lesion?**
   The history and physical examination accurately localize most lesions of the nervous system. The brain is unique among organs for its high degree of specialization. Because each part of the peripheral nerves, spinal cord, and brain has such specialized functions, damage to each region produces unique clinical effects. Identification of specific signs and symptoms, therefore, permits localization, sometimes within a millimeter, to discrete parts of the nervous system. Pioneer neurologists of the past century referred to the brain as "eloquent"—it speaks directly to the clinician.

3. **What are the most important regions for anatomic localization?**
   For clinical purposes, the great complexity of neuroanatomy can be simplified to a few major regions. Lesions should be localized to one of the following regions:
   - Muscle
   - Neuromuscular junction
   - Peripheral nerve
   - Root
   - Spinal cord
   - Brain stem
   - Cerebellum
   - Subcortical brain
   - Cortical brain

4. **How are symptoms localized to these neuroanatomic regions?**
   The history is the most important part of the neurologic evaluation of a patient. Although precise localizing information can be gleaned from the neurologic physical examination, asking the proper questions during the history accurately localizes most neurologic lesions.
   A helpful system for diagnosis is to begin distally and ask patients questions about each part of the neurologic anatomy, working proximally through the muscle, neuromuscular junction, peripheral nerve, root, spinal cord, cerebellum, brain stem, and subcortex and ending with the cortex of the brain. By sequentially asking about each of these areas, the patient can be "examined" thoroughly. If localization of the lesion is still not clear after a careful history directed at each anatomic region, do not begin the physical examination yet—go back and take a better history.

5. **Which clinical features of muscle disease can be elicited by history?**
   Muscle disease (myopathy) causes proximal symmetric weakness without sensory loss. Questions, therefore, should elicit these symptoms:
   - **Proximal leg weakness:** Can the patient get out of a car, off the toilet, or up from a chair without using the hands?
   - **Proximal arm weakness:** Can the patient lift or carry objects, such as grocery bags, garbage bags, young children, school books, or briefcases?
   - **Symmetric weakness:** Does the weakness affect both arms or both legs? (Although generalized processes such as myopathies are often slightly asymmetric, weakness confined to one limb or one side of the body is seldom caused by a myopathy.)

- **Normal sensation:** Is there numbness or other sensory loss? (Although pain and cramping may occur in some myopathies, actual sensory changes should not occur with any disease that is confined to the muscle.)

6. After a history of muscle disease is elicited, what findings can be expected on physical examination?

   The examination should show proximal symmetric weakness without sensory loss. The muscles are usually normal in size, without atrophy or fasciculations, and muscle tone is usually normal or mildly decreased. Reflexes are also normal or mildly decreased.

7. Which clinical features of neuromuscular junction disease can be elicited by history?

   Fatigability is the hallmark of diseases affecting the neuromuscular junction, such as myasthenia gravis. Because strength improves with rest, fatigability does not usually manifest as a steadily progressive decline in function; rather, it presents as waxing and waning weakness. When the muscles fatigue, the patient must rest, leading to recovery of strength, which permits further use of the muscles, causing fatigue, which necessitates rest and recovery again. This cycle of worsening with use and recovery with rest produces a variability or fluctuation in strength that is highly characteristic of neuromuscular junction diseases.

8. After a history of neuromuscular junction problems is elicited, what findings can be expected on physical examination?

   Examination should show fatigable proximal symmetric weakness without sensory loss. Repetitive testing weakens the muscles, which regain their strength after a brief period of rest. The weakness is often extremely proximal, involving muscles of the face, eyes (ptosis), and jaw. The muscles are normal in size, without atrophy or fasciculations, with normal tone and reflexes. There is no sensory loss.

9. Which clinical features of peripheral neuropathies can be elicited by history?

   Unlike myopathies and neuromuscular junction disease, weakness caused by peripheral neuropathies is often distal rather than proximal. It is also often asymmetric and accompanied by atrophy and fasciculations. Sensory changes almost always accompany neuropathies. The history should elicit the following symptoms:

   - **Distal leg weakness:** Does the patient trip, drag the feet, or wear out the toes of shoes?
   - **Distal arm weakness:** Does the patient frequently drop things or have trouble with the grip?
   - **Asymmetric weakness:** Are symptoms confined to one localized area? (Some neuropathies cause a symmetric stocking-and-glove weakness and numbness, especially those due to metabolic conditions such as diabetes. However, most neuropathies are asymmetric.)
   - **Denervation changes:** Is there a wasting or shrinkage of the muscle (atrophy) or quivering and twitching within the muscle (fasciculations)?
   - **Sensory changes:** Has the patient felt numbness, tingling, or paresthesias?

10. After a history of peripheral neuropathy is elicited, what findings can be expected on physical examination?

    Examination should reveal distal, often asymmetric weakness with atrophy, fasciculations, and sensory loss. Muscle tone may be normal but is often decreased. Reflexes are usually diminished. Because involvement of autonomic fibers is common in peripheral neuropathies, trophic changes, such as smooth, shiny skin, vasomotor changes (e.g., swelling or temperature dysregulation), and loss of hair or nails, may occur.

11. Which clinical features of root diseases (radiculopathies) can be elicited by history?

    Pain is the hallmark of root disease. Otherwise, radiculopathies often resemble peripheral neuropathies because of their asymmetric weakness with evidence of denervation (atrophy and fasciculations) and sensory loss. The weakness, while asymmetric, may be either proximal or distal, depending on which roots are involved. (The most common radiculopathies in the legs affect the L5 and S1 roots, causing distal weakness, whereas the most common radiculopathies in the arms affect the C5 and C6 roots, which innervate proximal regions.) The history, therefore, should elicit symptoms similar to a neuropathy with the added component of pain. The pain is usually described as sharp, stabbing, hot, and electric, and it typically shoots or radiates down the limb.

KEY POINTS: PERIPHERAL NERVOUS SYSTEM

1. The first step in treating patients with neurologic disease is to localize the lesion.
2. Myopathies cause proximal symmetric weakness without sensory loss.
3. Neuromuscular junction diseases cause fatigability.
4. Peripheral neuropathies cause distal asymmetric weakness with atrophy, fasciculations, sensory loss, and pain.
5. Radiculopathies cause radiating pain.

12. **After a history of a radiculopathy is elicited, what findings can be expected on physical examination?**
As is the case with a peripheral neuropathy, the physical examination shows asymmetric muscle weakness with atrophy and fasciculations. Tone is normal or decreased, and the reflexes in the involved muscles are diminished or absent. Weakness is confined to one myotomal group of muscles, such as those innervated by the C6 root in the arm or the L5 root in the leg. Similarly, sensory loss occurs in a dermatomal distribution. Maneuvers that stretch the root often aggravate the pain, such as straight leg raising or neck rotation.

13. **Which clinical features of spinal cord disease can be elicited by history?**
Spinal cord lesions usually cause a triad of symptoms:
   - **A sensory level is the hallmark of spinal cord disease.** Patients usually describe a sharp line or band around their abdomen or trunk, below which there is a decrease in sensation. The symptom of a sensory level is essentially pathognomonic for spinal cord disease.
   - **Distal, symmetric, and spastic weakness.** The muscle, neuromuscular junction, nerves, and roots make up the peripheral nervous system, but the spinal cord is in the central nervous system and so has special motor properties. Damage to the spinal cord produces upper motor neuron lesions, affecting the pyramidal (or corticospinal) tract. The weakness is distal more than proximal. In actual clinical practice, almost all processes affecting the cord are symmetric. Upper motor neuron lesions cause spasticity, but this increase in tone may cause few noticeable symptoms—it is best extracted from the history by asking about stiffness in the legs.
   - **Bowel and bladder problems.** Sphincter dysfunction commonly accompanies cord lesions because of involvement of the autonomic fibers within the cord.

14. **Which questions should be asked during the history to elicit the symptoms of spinal cord disease?**
   - **Distal leg weakness:** Does the patient drag the toes or trip?
   - **Distal arm weakness:** Does the patient drop things or have trouble with the grip?
   - **Symmetric symptoms:** Does the process involve the arms and/or legs approximately equally?
   - **Sensory level:** Is a sensory level present? Patients often describe it as a band, belt, girdle, or tightness around the trunk or abdomen.
   - **Sphincter dysfunction:** Is there retention or incontinence of bowel or bladder? (The bladder is usually involved earlier, more often and more severely than the bowel in spinal cord lesions.)

15. **After a history of spinal cord disease is elicited, what findings can be expected on physical examination?**
The physical examination in a patient with spinal cord disease usually shows a sensory level below which all sensory modalities are diminished. The sensory (and motor) tracts in the spinal cord are somatotopically organized; distinctive anatomic layering and lamination to the pathways result in greatest damage to fibers from the legs and lower part of the body in the majority of spinal cord lesions. Because most leg fibers lie laterally and are easily compressed, spinal disease usually affects the legs more than the arms. In addition, the level of the symptoms detected clinically does not always correspond to the true anatomic site of the damage. For example, a mass pressing on the spinal cord may cause a sensory level and weakness any place below the actual anatomic level of the lesion.

The patient also may have urinary retention or incontinence and may lose superficial reflexes, including the anal wink, bulbocavernosus, and cremasteric reflexes. The examination shows evidence of the following upper motor neuron damage:
   - Distal weakness greater than proximal weakness
   - Greater weakness of the extensors and antigravity muscles than of the flexors

- Increased tone (spasticity)
- Increased reflexes
- Clonus
- Extensor plantar response (positive Babinski sign)
- Absent superficial reflexes
- No significant atrophy or fasciculations

16. **Which clinical features of brain stem disease can be elicited by history?**

Cranial nerve symptoms characterize brain stem disease. The brain stem is essentially the spinal cord with embedded cranial nerves. Thus, brain stem lesions cause many of the symptoms of spinal cord disease accompanied by symptoms of cranial nerve impairment.

Like the spinal cord, the brain stem contains "long tracts" or pathways that extend from the brain down through the spinal cord. The major long tracts are the pyramidal (corticospinal) tract for motor function, the spinothalamic tract carrying pain and temperature sensations up to the thalamus, and the dorsal columns carrying position and vibration sense up to the thalamus. Because of the decussation of these tracts, lesions in the brain stem do not produce a horizontal motor or sensory level as they do in the spinal cord but rather produce a vertical motor or sensory level—that is, hemiparesis or hemianesthesia affecting one side of the body.

Lesions affecting the cranial nerves in the brain stem often produce symptoms referred to as the "Ds" (Table 3-1).

17. **Which questions elicit symptoms of combined cranial nerve and long tract dysfunction?**

- **Long tract signs:** Does the patient have hemiparesis or hemisensory loss?
- **Cranial nerve signs:** Does the patient have diplopia, dysarthria, dysphagia, dizziness, deafness, or decreased strength or sensation over the face?
- **Crossed signs:** Because the long tracts cross, but the cranial nerves generally do not, brain stem lesions often produce symptoms on one side of the face and the opposite side of the body. For example, a lesion in the pons that affects the pyramidal tracts and the facial (VII) nerve will cause weakness of that side of the face and the opposite, crossed side of the body. Brain stem disease often produces bilateral or crossed findings.

18. **After a history of brain stem disease is elicited, what findings can be expected on physical examination?**

Examination of the cranial nerves may reveal ptosis; pupillary abnormalities; extraocular muscle paralysis; diplopia; nystagmus; decreased corneal and blink reflexes; facial weakness or numbness; deafness; vertigo; dysarthria; dysphagia; weakness or deviation of the palate; decreased gag reflex; or weakness of the neck, shoulders, or tongue.

Long tract abnormalities may include hemiparesis, which shows an upper motor neuron pattern of distal extensor weakness with hyperreflexia, spasticity, and a positive Babinski sign. Hemisensory loss may occur to all modalities.

Table 3-1. Symptoms of Cranial Nerve Damage

CRANIAL NERVE	SYMPTOMS
III	Diplopia
IV	Diplopia
V	Decreased facial sensation
VI	Diplopia
VII	Decreased strength and drooping of the face
VIII	Deafness and dizziness
IX	Dysarthria and dysphagia
X	Dysarthria and dysphagia
XI	Decreased strength in neck and shoulders
XII	Dysarthria and dysphagia

19. **Which clinical features of cerebellar disease can be elicited by history?**
    Cerebellar disease causes incoordination, clumsiness, and tremor because the cerebellum is respon-
    sible for smoothing out and refining voluntary movements. Questions, therefore, should focus on the
    following symptoms:
    - **Clumsiness in the legs:** Does the patient have a staggering, drunken walk? (Most laymen
      describe cerebellar symptoms in terms of alcohol and drunkenness, probably because drinking
      alcohol impairs the cerebellum. The characteristic ataxic, wide-based, staggering gait of the person
      intoxicated by alcohol is a reflection of cerebellar dysfunction.)
    - **Clumsiness in the arms:** Does the patient have difficulty with targeted movements, such as
      lighting a cigarette or placing a key in a lock? (Cerebellar tremor is worse with voluntary, intentional
      movements that require accurate placement.)
    - **Brain stem symptoms:** Are brain stem symptoms present? (Because the cerebellar inflow and
      outflow must pass through the brain stem and the blood supply to the cerebellum arises from the
      same vessels that supply the brain stem, cerebellar disease is almost always accompanied by
      some brain stem abnormalities as well, and vice versa.)

20. **After a history of cerebellar disease is elicited, what findings can be expected on
    physical examination?**
    The patient's gait is staggering, wide based, and ataxic, causing difficulties especially with tandem
    walking. Fine coordinated movements of the legs are impossible, such as sliding a heel down
    a shin or tracing patterns on the floor with the foot. The cerebellar tremor is most visible in the
    upper extremities, which waver and wobble with attempts to touch a specific target, such as the
    examiner's finger or the patient's own nose. Rapid alternating movements are irregular in rate and
    rhythm.

21. **How can the history determine whether disease of the brain is subcortical or
    cortical?**
    The history can differentiate subcortical from cortical disease by focusing on the following four major
    areas:
    - The presence of specific cortical deficits
    - The pattern of motor and sensory deficits
    - The type of sensory deficits
    - The presence of visual field deficits

22. **What specific deficits are seen with cortical lesions?**
    The most useful symptom of cortical disease in the dominant (usually left) hemisphere is aphasia. The
    history, therefore, should focus on any difficulties with language functions, including not only speech
    but also writing, reading, and comprehension. A lesion affecting the left side of the brain that does not
    affect language function is unlikely to be cortical.
    In the nondominant (usually right) hemisphere, cortical dysfunction is more subtle, but usually
    causes visual–spatial problems. Patients with nondominant cortical lesions often have neglect and
    denial, including inattention to their own physical signs and symptoms. This finding can be difficult
    to elicit on history, however, and sometimes depends on the physical examination. Note also that
    seizures are almost always cortical in origin.

23. **How does the pattern of motor and sensory deficits differentiate cortical from
    subcortical involvement?**
    The motor homunculus in the primary and supplemental motor strips is spread upside down over
    a vast expanse of gray matter. Neurons controlling the lower extremities reside between the two
    hemispheres, in the interhemispheric fissure, whereas neurons moving the trunk, arms, and face are
    draped upside down over the superficial cortex. Cortical lesions, therefore, often involve the face, arm,
    and trunk, but spare the legs, which are protected in the interhemispheric fissure. Cortical lesions thus
    cause an incomplete hemiparesis, affecting the face and arm but not the leg.
    Of course, fibers to the leg descend and merge with those to the face and arm as the pyramidal
    tract forms deep within the brain, subcortically, to run in the internal capsule, cerebral peduncles, and
    the pyramids themselves. Therefore, even a small subcortical lesion can affect all of these conjoined
    fibers. Subcortical lesions thus cause a complete hemiparesis, affecting face, arm, and leg.
    The sensory homunculus has a similar somatotropic arrangement that results in an analogous
    pattern of localization.

24. **How does the type of sensory deficit differentiate cortical from subcortical lesions by history?**

Most of the primary sensory modalities reach "consciousness" in the thalamus and do not require the cortex for their perception. A patient with severe cortical damage can still feel pain, touch, vibration, and position. A history of significant numbness or sensory loss, therefore, suggests a subcortical lesion.

Cortical sensory loss is more refined and usually involves complicated sensory processing such as two-point discrimination, accurate localization of perceptions, stereognosis, and graphesthesia. These symptoms can be difficult to elicit by history alone.

25. **How do visual symptoms differentiate cortical from subcortical disease by history?**

Visual pathways run subcortically for most of their length. Visual impulses in the optic nerves may cross in the chiasm and run through the optic tracts, lateral geniculate bodies, and optic radiations before synapsing in the occipital cortex. Cortical lesions, such as those affecting the motor strip, sensory strip, or language areas, are too superficial to affect these visual fibers and thus do not cause visual field deficits. Subcortical lesions often affect the visual fibers, producing visual field cuts. There-fore, a history of visual field loss suggests a subcortical lesion. (Of course, a strictly cortical lesion in the occipital lobes produces visual symptoms, but it does not affect motor, sensory, or other functions and so does not cause confusion with the typical picture of a subcortical lesion.)

KEY POINTS: CENTRAL NERVOUS SYSTEM

1. Spinal cord disease causes a "triad" of distal symmetric weakness, sphincter problems, and a sensory level.
2. Brain stem disease causes abnormalities of cranial nerves plus long tracts.
3. Cerebellar disease causes ataxia and an action tremor.
4. In the brain, cortical lesions may cause aphasia, seizures, and partial hemiparesis (face and arm only), while subcortical lesions may cause visual field cuts, dense numbness of primary sensory modalities, and more complete hemiparesis (face, arm, and leg).

26. **After a history of cortical or subcortical disease is elicited, what findings can be expected on physical examination?**

Physical examination findings parallel the historical deficits:
- **Cortical dysfunction:** The patient may show aphasia, visual–spatial dysfunction, or seizures.
- **Motor involvement:** Physical examination shows upper motor neuron weakness affecting the face and arm in a cortical lesion and the face, arm, and leg in a subcortical lesion.
- **Sensory dysfunction:** In subcortical disease, the examination shows problems with primary sen-sory modalities, such as decreased pinprick and vibration, but in cortical disease, it shows relatively normal sensation with impaired higher sensory processing, such as graphesthesia and stereognosis.
- **Visual dysfunction:** Patients with subcortical disease may have visual field cuts, but patients with cortical disease do not.

27. **How accurate are the history and physical examination for diagnosing neurologic disease?**

The clinical examination is highly accurate in localizing neurologic disease. Once a lesion has been localized to one of the broad anatomic regions, an etiology usually suggests itself. For example, if a lesion can be localized to the peripheral nerve, it is usually easy to develop a differential diagnosis for peripheral neuropathies (such as diabetes, alcoholism) and a diagnostic plan (e.g., blood testing, nerve conduction studies). The anatomy usually implies an etiology.

Organized questioning and examination of the nervous system in this fashion are excellent ways to approach the neurologic patient.

 References available online at expertconsult.com.

WEBSITES

http://www.neuroguide.com
http://www.neuroland.com

BIBLIOGRAPHY

1. Alpert JN: The Neurologic Diagnosis: A Practical Bedside Approach. New York, Springer, 2012.
2. Brazis P, Masdeu JC, Biller J: Localization in Clinical Neurology, 6th ed. Philadelphia, Lippincott Williams & Wilkins, 2011.
3. Campbell W: Dejong's The Neurologic Examination, 7th ed. Philadelphia, Lippincott Williams & Wilkins, 2012.
4. Caplan L: The Effective Clinical Neurologist, 3rd ed. Boston, Butterworth-Heinemann, 2010.

CHAPTER 4

MYOPATHIES

Corey E. Goldsmith, Lydia Sharp

INTRODUCTION

1. **What is a myopathy?**
   A myopathy is a disorder in which there is a primary functional or structural impairment of skeletal muscle.

2. **What signs and symptoms are suggestive of a myopathy?**
   - Proximal symmetric weakness, which may be acute, subacute, or chronic
   - Reduced, preserved, or enlarged muscle bulk
   - Muscle pain or discomfort with palpation (myalgia)
   - Muscle stiffness or cramps
   - Fatigue
   - Myoglobinuria

3. **Define myoblast, myotube, myofiber, and myofibril.**
   A myoblast is a postmitotic, mononucleated cell capable of fusion and contractile protein synthesis. Myotubes are long, cylindrical, multinucleated (syncytial) cells formed from the fusion of myoblasts. When their central nuclei are shifted to a subsarcolemmal position in the later stages of development, they are called *myofibers*. The appearance of central nuclei within an otherwise normal adult muscle is a useful sign of muscle regeneration. Each adult myofiber is packed with numerous myofibrils, largely composed of hexagonal arrangements of thick and thin contractile filaments. Myosin is the major constituent of the thick filaments, whereas actin is the contractile protein of the thin filaments.

4. **What is a motor unit?**
   A motor unit consists of a motor neuron, its single axon, the associated neuromuscular junctions and terminal axon branches, and the many muscle fibers that they supply. All muscle fibers belonging to a single motor unit are of the same histochemical and physiologic type.

5. **What are the general categories of myopathies?**
   - Inflammatory myopathies (e.g., polymyositis [PM], dermatomyositis [DM], inclusion body myositis)
   - Toxic myopathies (e.g., alcohol, zidovudine)
   - Endocrine myopathies (e.g., hypothyroidism, hypoadrenalism)
   - Infectious myopathies (e.g., trichinosis, AIDS)
   - Muscular dystrophies (e.g., Duchenne, myotonic, limb-girdle)
   - Congenital myopathies (e.g., central core, centronuclear myopathy)
   - Metabolic myopathies (e.g., myophosphorylase deficiency, phosphofructokinase deficiency)
   - Mitochondrial myopathies (e.g., Kearns–Sayre syndrome)

6. **How do we grade functional weakness?**
   The most widely used system was developed by the Medical Research Council (MRC) of Great Britain. The MRC system grades strength from 0 to 5. The addition of a plus (+) or minus (−) further quantifies strength:
   0. No movement
   1. Trace movement
   2. Able to move, but not against gravity
   3. Able to move full range against gravity
   4. Able to move against some resistance
   5. Normal strength

   In addition, the clinician may observe the patient performing the following maneuvers to look for subtle weakness:
   - Arise from a chair with arms folded
   - Walk the length of the examining room on toes, on heels, and tandem

- Hop on either foot
- Perform deep knee bends
- Climb a step
- Horizontally abduct arms and reach the vertex of the head
- Lift up the head from a table
- Arise from supine position with hands overhead
- Lift head and shoulders, and extend the neck while in a prone position

7. **What is Gower's sign?**
This term describes the maneuver of rising from a supine position in the presence of marked proximal weakness. In order to rise to standing, the patient rolls to a prone position, pushes off the floor, locks the knees, and pushes the upper body upward by "climbing up" the legs with the hands. Although Gower's sign is usually seen in children with myopathies, it may be present in any patient with marked proximal weakness (Fig. 4-1).

DIAGNOSIS

8. **What are the most common causes of muscle pain?**
Most muscle pains are caused by a nonmuscular condition, such as vascular insufficiency, joint disease, or neuropathy. The vast majority of myopathies are painless. Myopathies that may be associated with pain include inflammatory myopathies, metabolic myopathies, mitochondrial myopathies, and some muscular dystrophies (limb-girdle, Becker muscular dystrophy [BMD]). In general, in patients with a normal exam and a normal serum creatine kinase (CK) level, muscle pain is usually not myopathic in origin.

9. **What are the most valuable tests for evaluating patients with suspected muscle disease?**
A diagnosis often can be established by supporting the clinical findings with results from three key tests: (1) serum CK levels, (2) electromyography (EMG), and (3) muscle biopsy.

10. **Which myopathies are associated with elevated serum CK levels?**
CK catalyzes the reversible reaction of adenosine triphosphate (ATP) and creatine to form adenosine diphosphate and phosphocreatine. It is elevated in many myopathies due to myofiber disruption or degeneration. Serum CK is especially high in limb-girdle muscular dystrophies (dysferlinopathies and sarcoglycanopathies), Duchenne and Becker muscular dystrophies, inflammatory myopathies, and rhabdomyolysis. However, CK levels may be normal in some patients with an ongoing myopathy. Examples include profound muscle wasting and selected conditions such as hyperthyroidism.

11. **What is rhabdomyolysis?**
Rhabdomyolysis is a condition of severe acute muscle injury causing myalgia, muscle weakness, muscle swelling, myoglobinuria, and very elevated CK levels (>5 times upper limit of normal), which develops over hours to days. Acute renal failure and its sequelae need to be treated. Then, the etiology needs to be determined. Causes include crush injuries, ischemia, alcohol/drugs/medications, metabolic disturbances, toxic exposures, infections, or myositis. If either an acquired cause is not clear or there are recurrent episodes, a muscle biopsy in search of metabolic or congenital myopathies or a muscular dystrophy may be indicated.

12. **What conditions other than myopathies are associated with an elevated CK level?**
Normal CK levels vary by race and gender with African American men having the highest values. HyperCKemia is defined as asymptomatic or paucisymptomatic elevations in CK level. Elevated CK could be a sign of a latent neuromuscular disease but there are many causes for this including:
- Exercise (especially if vigorous or unaccustomed)
- Increased muscle bulk
- Muscle trauma (needle injection, EMG, surgery, seizures, edema, or contusion)
- Viral illnesses
- Acute kidney disease
- Metabolic disturbances (hyponatremia, hypokalemia, hypophosphatemia)
- Drug use (including alcohol and cholesterol-lowering agents)
- Eating licorice
- Endocrine disorders (hypo/hyperthyroidism, hypoparathyroidism)
- Malignant hyperthermia

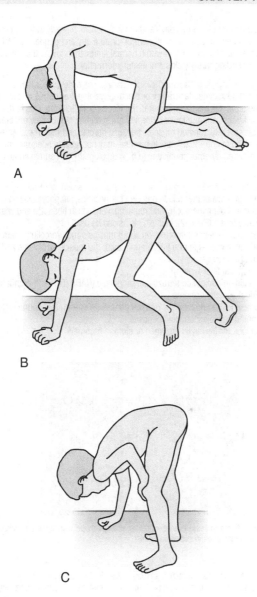

A

B

C

Figure 4-1. Gower's sign.

- Neurogenic disease (e.g., amyotrophic lateral sclerosis)
- Benign hereditary CK elevation

 Typically CK levels are increased less than threefold in these conditions, whereas CK levels greater than fivefold often suggest an underlying myopathic etiology.

13. **What is the approach to evaluating a persistent but incidental elevation of serum CK?**
 Perform an EMG if symptoms of weakness, myalgia, cramps, or tenderness are present. If the EMG findings are suggestive of a myopathy, a muscle biopsy may be considered. If the examination is

normal, have the patient rest for 3 to 4 days and recheck serum CK early in the morning. If levels are still greater than 1.5 times the upper limit of normal for ethnicity and gender, an EMG and a muscle biopsy might be beneficial. If serum CK is within normal limits, then follow the patient clinically. A muscle biopsy in this setting rarely yields any useful information.

14. **When is a muscle biopsy indicated? How is the muscle site chosen?**
   Muscle weakness with associated laboratory or electrophysiologic evidence of a myopathy is an indication to pursue a muscle biopsy. In general, the biceps or deltoid muscles in the upper extremity or the vastus lateralis muscle in the lower extremity are selected. Moderately affected muscles are better to biopsy than severely affected muscles because fibrosis and fatty replacement of the muscle, which are characteristic of end-stage muscle disease, may not provide adequate information. In addition, muscles affected by other conditions (e.g., radiculopathy or trauma) should be avoided if possible.

15. **What morphologic features of a myopathy may be seen on biopsy?**
   Morphologic features of a myopathy include muscle fiber necrosis, phagocytosis and regeneration, increased central nuclei, fiber hypertrophy and rounding, variation in fiber size and shape, and increased endomysial connective tissue (Fig. 4-2). Multiple stains can be used.
   - Hematoxylin and eosin—general information about muscle structure/cellular details
   - Modified Gomori trichrome—general information about the muscle structures and cellular details; ragged red fibers; rimmed vacuoles
   - ATPase—histochemical fiber type
   - Nicotinamide adenine dinucleotide tetrazolium reductase (NADH-TR)—differentiates type 1 and type 2 fibers, oxidative activity, cores
   - Cytochrome oxidase (COX) and succinic dehydrogenase (SDH)—mitochondrial activity
   - Congo red—rimmed vacuoles, amyloid deposits
   - Other stains can look for glycolytic enzymes or storage materials.

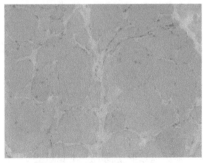

Figure 4-2. Note hypertrophic fibers, increased variation in fiber size and shape, and increased nuclei in a patient with limb-girdle muscular dystrophy (hematoxylin and eosin stain).

16. **How many fiber types are recognized by muscle histochemistry?**
   Type 1 fibers are slow-twitch, red fibers; type 2 fibers are fast-twitch, white fibers. The two major subtypes of type 2 fibers are types 2A and 2B. The histochemical and physiologic properties of each fiber type are determined by the anterior horn cell that innervates it.

17. **What are ragged red fibers?**
   Ragged red fibers are muscle fibers with an accumulation of subsarcolemmal and intermyofibrillar material that stains red with modified Gomori trichrome stain (Fig. 4-3). This red-stained material is actually mitochondria that are abnormal in number, size, and structure when viewed by electron microscopy. If there is mitochondrial dysfunction, muscle fibers with ragged red fibers also show excessive SDH staining and reduced or absent COX staining. Although ragged red fibers are typically seen in mitochondrial myopathies, they may occur in other conditions such as inclusion body myositis or could be normal.

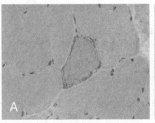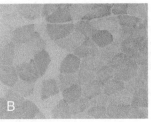

Figure 4-3. A, A ragged red fiber in a patient with progressive ophthalmoplegia (modified trichrome stain). **B,** Note cytochrome oxidase (COX)-negative fibers corresponding with ragged red fibers (cytochrome C oxidase stain).

INFLAMMATORY MYOPATHIES

18. How are inflammatory myopathies classified?
    - Dermatomyositis
    - Polymyositis
    - Immune-mediated necrotizing myopathy
    - Inclusion body myositis (IBM)

19. What are the clinical features of polymyositis (PM) and dermatomyositis (DM)?
    Although PM is an adult disease, DM occurs in both children and adults. Patients with PM or DM develop symmetric proximal muscle weakness progressive over weeks to months. Pharyngeal or diaphragmatic weakness is common. EMG shows low-amplitude, small myopathic units with evidence of fibrillation potentials and/or positive sharp waves. CK is usually markedly elevated. Magnetic resonance imaging of affected muscles can show increased T2 signal secondary to edema, inflammation, or fibrotic replacement.

    Unique to DM are cutaneous manifestations that typically present at the same time as the weakness. A purplish discoloration involving the eyelids, cheeks and nose (heliotrope rash), or an erythematous rash often seen on the knuckles (Gottron's papules), are both pathognomonic for DM. A rash on the neck and upper chest (V sign), shoulders (shawl sign), or extensor surfaces of elbows, knees, hips, and medial malleoli (Gottron's sign) can also be seen. The rash often worsens with exposure to sunlight. Skin may become scaly and atrophic, and the nail beds may appear shiny and red. Subcutaneous calcification over pressure points is more common in juvenile-onset DM.

    Patients can develop symptomatic systemic involvement, including fever, weight loss, cardiac arrhythmias and conduction abnormalities, interstitial lung disease (10% to 20%), conjunctivitis/uveitis, calcinosis, and gastrointestinal (GI) abnormalities. Myositis-specific autoantibodies (Table 4-1), found in 60% to 80% of patients with autoimmune myopathies, can help diagnose as well as predict systemic involvement. The most common is antisynthetase syndrome, most associated with the presence of anti-Jo-1 antibody. These patients have a constellation of clinical symptoms including autoimmune myopathy, interstitial lung disease (ILD), nonerosive arthritis, fever, and "mechanic's hands," hyperkeratotic lesions on the palmar fingers.

    Both PM and DM also have been associated with malignancies, in particular lung, GI, breast, and ovarian cancers. All patients with DM or PM should be screened for malignancy.

Table 4-1. Autoantibodies in Dermatomyositis

ANTIBODY	PHENOTYPE
Jo-1 (PL-7, PL-12, EJ, OJ)	Antisynthetase syndrome
Mi-2	Classic DM, more rash, less malignancy
TIF-1γ, TIF-1α	Cancer-associated DM
NXP-2	Juvenile DM, more calcinosis
SAE	Severe skin findings, mild myositis
MDA5	More severe ILD, mild myositis, Asians

DM = Dermatomyositis, ILD = Interstitial lung disease

20. What are the major pathologic changes on light microscopy in the muscle biopsies of patients with PM and DM?

Both PM and DM have the following (Figs 4-4 and 4-5):
- Variation and rounding of muscle fibers; occasional angular and atrophic fibers
- Fiber necrosis, phagocytosis
- Inflammatory infiltrate:
    - In DM, perivascular and perimysial inflammation composed of macrophages, B cells, and CD4+ dendritic cells
    - In PM, nonnecrotic endomysial inflammation composed of CD8+ T cells and macrophages

Figure 4-4. Polymyositis, endomysial inflammation showing rounding of fibers (hematoxylin and eosin stain).

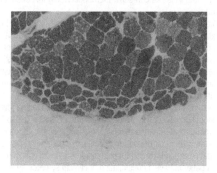

Figure 4-5. Dermatomyositis—perifascicular atrophy (ATP 9.6 stain).

21. What does the muscle biopsy in Fig. 4-5 signify?

This is the typical finding of perifascicular atrophy. The muscle fibers at the periphery of the muscle fascicles are smaller, whereas the fibers in the deepest part of the fascicle are of normal size. This type of atrophy is suggestive of DM. Even in the absence of inflammation, this biopsy is characteristic.

22. How are DM and PM treated?

Corticosteroids are considered first-line treatment usually starting with 1 mg/kg/day followed by a taper 4 weeks to several months after initiation. If there is either no improvement with steroids or the steroids cannot be tapered, treatment with a second-line agent, usually intravenous immunoglobulin (IVIG), azathioprine, or methotrexate should be started. Mycophenolate mofetil, tacrolimus, rituximab, cyclosporine, and cyclophosphamide can be used as well. The choice often depends on extramuscular involvement as well as side effects.

23. What is inclusion body myositis (IBM)?

IBM is the most common cause of acquired chronic myopathy in patients age 50 years and older. Characteristically, there is insidious onset of painless weakness and atrophy involving the quadriceps, finger flexors, and foot dorsiflexors. Dysphagia is common. There is early loss of patellar reflexes, and a mild neuropathy may be present. CK levels are either normal or only mildly elevated. Electrodiagnostic evaluation reveals mixed myopathic and neurogenic changes. Muscle biopsy shows invasion of nonnecrotic fibers by mononuclear cells, cytoplasmic "rimmed" vacuoles and eosinophilic inclusion bodies, and small angular atrophic and denervated fibers sometimes with mitochondrial dysfunction (Fig. 4-6). Despite the evident inflammation, IBM is resistant to conventional immunotherapies and is felt to be more likely a myodegenerative condition. One-third of cases appear stable or show improvement for periods of 6 months or more. Cricopharyngeal myotomy might be beneficial in cases of dysphagia and might delay the need for a percutaneous endoscopic gastrostomy.

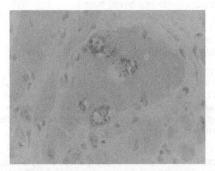

Figure 4-6. Inclusion body myositis, rimmed vacuoles (hematoxylin and eosin stain).

24. **What is immune-mediated necrotizing myopathy?**
Patients present with acute or subacute proximal weakness and myalgia with markedly elevated CK and scattered necrotic muscle fibers with only sparse inflammatory cell infiltration on muscle biopsy. The myopathy may be secondary to an underlying connective tissue disease (most commonly sclero-derma or mixed connective tissue disease) or cancer but most are likely triggered by statin use. These patients require treatment with immunosuppressive agents.

TOXIC MYOPATHIES

25. **What are the most common myotoxic agents?**
   - Statins and fibrates—myalgias, rhabdomyolysis, necrotizing myopathy
   - Steroids—type 2 fiber atrophy
   - Alcohol—rhabdomyolysis, proximal myopathy with type 2 fiber atrophy
   - Chloroquine—vascular myopathy
   - D-Penicillamine—drug-induced DM
   - Protease inhibitors (saquinavir, ritonavir, indinavir, nelfinavir, amprenavir)—rhabdomyolysis, risk is increased with concurrent use of statins
   - Nucleoside-analog reverse transcriptase inhibitors (mainly zidovudine [AZT])—mitochondrial myopathy with ragged red fibers
   - Amiodarone
   - Colchicine, vincristine
   - Snake venoms

26. **What is statin myopathy?**
Statin-associated myalgias and cramps occur in up to 20% of statin users and are dependent on dose and associated medications. Rhabdomyolysis occurs at a rate of 0.44 per 10,000 patient-years. Usually the statin myopathy is self-limited and, after discontinuation of the statin, will resolve in a few weeks to months.

However, in a minority of patients, statins stimulate a necrotizing autoimmune myopathy that progresses even after the statin is discontinued. These patients present with proximal muscle weakness, markedly elevated CK levels, an irritable myopathy on EMG, and muscle edema. Muscle biopsy shows a necrotizing myopathy with minimal inflammation. Most of these patients have developed anti-HMG-CoA reductase antibodies and often require aggressive immunosuppressive therapy.

27. **What neuromuscular conditions are associated with human immunodeficiency virus (HIV) infection?**
    A large percentage of patients with HIV report myalgias and fatigue. However, one must also evaluate for other myopathic pathologies:
    - HIV-associated polymyositis
    - IBM
    - Nemaline myopathy
    - Mitochondrial myopathy due to antiretroviral drugs
    - Diffuse infiltrative lymphocytosis syndrome
    - HIV-wasting syndrome
    - Vasculitic processes
    - Lactic acidosis, hepatic steatosis, and myopathy

28. **What is steroid myopathy?**
    Steroid myopathy is progressive painless proximal weakness in the context of steroid treatment. CK is not elevated, and EMG may either be normal or show minimal myopathic changes. Muscle biopsy shows type 2 fiber atrophy. Typically the myopathy is related to chronic use but can occur with only a few weeks of exposure. Chronic steroid myotoxicity can be prevented in part by exercise, and symptoms improve if the dose is reduced or discontinued.

29. **What is critical illness myopathy?**
    Critical illness myopathy is a primary myopathy that develops acutely over days in critically ill patients usually with sepsis or multiorgan failure. It is characterized by severe flaccid paralysis that can affect all muscles, including respiratory muscles. EMG may show reduction in compound muscle action potential amplitudes with prolonged durations and normal sensory nerve action potentials, reduced muscle excitability on direct stimulation, and myopathic motor unit action potentials. Muscle biopsy shows loss of thick myosin filaments and necrosis. Critical illness polyneuropathy can be concurrent. With supportive care, the prognosis for recovery is variable (weeks to 1 year), but there may be considerable morbidity.

30. **What is the neuroleptic malignant syndrome (NMS)?**
    The cardinal features of NMS are hyperthermia, rigidity, autonomic instability, and altered consciousness in the setting of a markedly elevated CK level and recent exposure to a triggering agent. Delirium, mutism, dysphagia, tremor, and dysautonomia can occur. NMS is most often associated with use of either typical or atypical neuroleptics. However, it can be seen with other anti-dopaminergic drugs such as metoclopramide and promethazine as well as with an abrupt withdrawal of pro-dopaminergic drugs such as levodopa and dopamine agonists. Treatment includes discontinuation of the offending agent, aggressive hydration, and initiating therapy with either bromocriptine or dantrolene.

MUSCULAR DYSTROPHIES

31. **Describe the salient features of the Duchenne muscular dystrophy (DMD) gene.**
    The gene is large (2.3 Mb), located in the short arm of the X chromosome, and codes for a structural protein called *dystrophin*. It is by far the largest gene characterized to date, consisting of 2.3 million base pairs and occupying approximately 1% of the human X chromosome. Dystrophin is a protein located in the subsarcolemmal region of the muscle fiber, which functions in linking the extracellular matrix to the sarcomere. Mutations that result in complete absence of dystrophin result in the severe DMD, whereas mutations found with the milder BMD lead to variable amounts of partially functioning dystrophin.

32. **How do Duchenne and Becker muscular dystrophy present? What organs other than skeletal muscle are involved in DMD?**
    Duchenne and Becker muscular dystrophy present in males with progressive proximal muscle weakness as well as pseudohypertrophy of the calf muscles associated with markedly elevated CK levels and myopathic features on EMG. Symptoms begin in infancy or early childhood in DMD while BMD presents later. Many patients develop heel contractures and skeletal deformities as a result of weakness.
    About 90% of patients have electrocardiogram abnormalities, but symptomatic involvement occurs in less than 1% of patients. Although the heart may be enlarged with minimal fibrosis, the myocardial

muscle fibers do not undergo necrosis or other myopathic changes. There is also an increased incidence of GI hypomotility that may lead to intestinal pseudo-obstruction and gastric dilatation. Finally, pachygyria and smaller-than-normal brains have been noted in some patients with DMD. In addition, an association between mental retardation and mutations causing central exon deletions has been observed.

33. **What pharmacologic treatment is available for DMD?**
Steroids are currently the only medication that has been proven to be beneficial for patients with DMD. Treatment can improve muscle strength, prolong the ability to walk, and may improve cardiac function. Regimens include prednisone 0.75 mg/kg/day, prednisone 5 mg/kg on Friday or Saturday (less weight gain and fewer behavioral side effects but fewer data of effectiveness) or deflazacort 0.9 mg/kg/day (not available in the United States, associated with less weight gain).

34. **What is fascioscapulohumeral muscular dystrophy (FSHD)?**
FSHD is characterized by progressive, often asymmetric, descending weakness involving the face, shoulders, arms, and distal legs. It is the third most common inherited disease of muscle. The majority of cases are autosomal dominantly inherited and result from a decrease in the number of DNA repeat sequence (D4Z4), located on chromosome 4q35. Age of onset varies from the first to the fifth decade. Patients have characteristic clinical findings including facial weakness manifesting as transverse smile and scapular winging (Fig. 4-7). With shoulder elevation, the scapula rides into the trapezius muscle (the trapezius hump sign). Deltoids are initially well preserved, while biceps muscles are atrophied (Popeye appearance). Additionally, ankle dorsiflexors are weaker than toe dorsiflexors. Beevor's sign, or the vertical movement of the umbilicus on flexion of the neck in the supine position due to abdominal muscle weakness, is present in a majority of patients. Pain can be a predominant feature. FSHD might be associated with either sensorineural hearing loss or visual loss (Coat's disease). Serum CK may be raised.

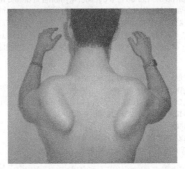

Figure 4-7. Patient with fascioscapulohumeral muscular dystrophy (FSHD) showing scapular winging.

35. **What are the limb-girdle muscular dystrophies? How are they classified?**
The limb-girdle muscular dystrophies are genetically heterogeneous disorders grouped together because they commonly present with slowly progressive, limb-girdle (or shoulder and pelvic muscle) weakness. Symptoms onset may occur from childhood to adulthood. However, one gene may cause variable phenotypes, even within the same family (e.g., mutations in dysferlin may cause proximal or distal weakness). CK levels can range from normal to severely elevated. Muscle biopsy will show dystrophic changes. Disorders are classified as type 1 (autosomal dominant) or type 2 (autosomal recessive). Letters are used to identify the specific genes involved and are assigned in the order of gene discovery.

36. **What are the most common limb-girdle muscular dystrophy subtypes in the United States?**
- **LGMD 2A:** Secondary to mutations in calpain, a calcium activated protease. Patients develop progressive proximal muscle weakness beginning in late childhood to adulthood. May have prominent scapular winging. CK may be mildly to severely elevated.
- **LGMD 2B:** Due to mutations in dysferlin, a protein involved in membrane repair. Patients develop progressive proximal muscle weakness from late childhood to adulthood, and may have normal exercise history prior to symptom onset. The same gene, and even same mutation, may also cause predominantly distal leg weakness (a.k.a. Miyoshi myopathy).

- **LGMD 2C–F:** Secondary to mutations in sarcoglycans, a complex of proteins involved in bridging the muscle cytoskeletal to the extracellular matrix. Severe, progressive, proximal muscle weakness usually begins in childhood. These patients may also develop cardiac and respiratory dysfunction.
- **LGMD 2I:** Due to mutations in Fukutin-related protein. Affected patients develop proximal weakness usually in the second decade. Patients may also develop cardiac and respiratory dysfunction. Additionally, some patients also develop scapular winging, tongue and calf hypertrophy, and cognitive dysfunction.

37. Describe oculopharyngeal muscular dystrophy (OPMD).

OPMD is a late onset muscular dystrophy, which is characterized by progressive ptosis and dysphagia and commonly presents in the fifth to sixth decades. Over time, patients may also develop tongue, laryngeal, facial weakness, and proximal muscle weakness. Diplopia is uncommon, though patients may also develop extraocular dysfunction. Due to the founder effect, the prevalence is higher in certain geographical areas including Quebec, Canada, Israel, and New Mexico. The disease results from a GCG triplet repeat expansion in the poly(A) binding protein nuclear (*PABN1*) gene and is usually inherited in an autosomal dominant fashion. CK is most often normal. Diagnosis is made by genetic testing.

38. Which dystrophies are associated with contractures?
- Dystrophinopathies
- Limb-girdle muscular dystrophy 1G and 2A
- Emery–Dreifuss muscular dystrophy

MYOTONIA

39. Define myotonia.

Myotonia is the phenomena of impaired relaxation of muscle after forceful voluntary contraction and most commonly involves the hands and eyelids. Myotonia is due to repetitive depolarization of the muscle membrane. Patients may complain of muscle stiffness or tightness resulting in difficulty releasing their handgrip after a handshake, unscrewing a bottle top, or opening their eyelids if they shut their eyes forcefully. Myotonia classically improves with repeated exercise, while in contrast, paramyotonia is typically worsened by exercise. Exposure to cold makes both myotonia and paramyotonia worse.

40. What are the inherited myotonic disorders?
- Myotonic dystrophy type 1 (DM1)
- Myotonic dystrophy type 2 (DM2) (formerly known as proximal myotonic myopathy or PROMM)
- Myotonia congenita (Thomsen disease, Becker's disease*)
- Paramyotonia congenita
- Periodic paralysis (hypokalemic, normo/hyperkalemic)
- Chondrodystrophic myotonia* (Schwartz–Jampel syndrome)

41. What is the most common muscular dystrophy in adults? How does it present?

Myotonic dystrophy type 1 (DM1) is most common muscular dystrophy in adults. DM1 is a multisystem disorder with an autosomal dominant pattern of inheritance, but severity and degree of systemic involvement vary considerably. The most common form of the disease presents in the second decade of life, but there is also a congenital form. The most common presenting symptom of adult-onset DM1 is myotonia which is most prominent in facial and distal arm muscles. Over time, patients also develop distal muscle weakness and atrophy. Facial weakness and temporalis muscle atrophy give rise to a characteristic narrow, hatchet-faced appearance. In addition, patients develop frontal baldness, ptosis, and neck muscle atrophy early in the disease.

42. What systems are involved in DM1?
- **Cardiac.** Conduction problems are a major cause of morbidity and mortality. About 90% of patients have ECG abnormalities, and complete heart block and sudden death are well recognized. Prophylactic pacemaker implantation is needed in patients with conduction block.
- **Respiratory.** Excessive daytime sleepiness is common because of a combination of weakness of the diaphragm and intercostal muscles, decreased response to hypoxia, alveolar hypoventilation, hypercapnia, and abnormalities of brain stem neuroregulatory mechanisms.

---

*Autosomal recessive inheritance; all other conditions are autosomal dominant inheritance.

- **Gastrointestinal.** Smooth muscle involvement results in many symptoms, including abdominal pain, dysphagia, emesis, diarrhea, and bowel incontinence.
- **Central nervous system.** Symptoms include impaired intelligence, apathy, and personality disorders.
- **Skeletal muscle.** Symptoms include atrophy, weakness, and myotonia.
- **Endocrine.** Testicular atrophy and insulin resistance are common; overt diabetes is uncommon.
- Other symptoms include frontal balding, cranial hyperostosis, air sinus enlargement, and minor sensory neuropathy.

43. **What are the characteristics of the *DM1* gene?**
The mutation in *DM1* is an expansion of a trinucleotide (CTG) repeat in the protein kinase gene on the long arm of chromosome 19. The size of the expanded repeat correlates with severity and age of onset of symptoms and generally increases in successive generations within a family, providing a molecular basis for the clinical observed phenomenon known as *anticipation* (progressively earlier onset of the disease in successive generations).

44. **How does DM2 differ from DM1?**
In DM2, muscle weakness is usually proximal and facial weakness is minimal. Myotonia is usually absent on examination but is present on EMG testing. There is no congenital form. Systemic involvement closely resembles DM1. The mutation is due to a CCTG expansion in a specific zinc-finger gene (*ZNF9*) localized to chromosome 3q. Anticipation is less marked when compared to DM1. DM2 should be considered in any atypical progressive disorder with proximal muscle weakness.

PERIODIC PARALYSIS

45. **What are the periodic paralysis (PP) disorders?**
PP disorders are muscle channelopathies that consist of hyperkalemic (potassium sensitive) PP, hypokalemic PP, and Andersen–Tawil syndrome (ATS). All are inherited in an autosomal dominant fashion. All present with recurrent attacks of weakness, ranging from mild and focal to severe generalized weakness. Over time, patients might develop fixed weakness. ATS patients have dysmorphic features (e.g., hypertelorism, mandibular hypoplasia, clinodactyly, syndactyly, scoliosis, short stature, high-arched palate) and cardiac arrhythmias (commonly long QT syndrome). During attacks, serum CK is usually elevated with serum potassium levels being variable (high, low, or normal). Between attacks, EMG may show myotonia in hyperkalemic PP patients, while muscles are electrically silent in all types during an episode of weakness.

46. **Compare the PP disorders.**
See Table 4-2.

Table 4-2. Differentiating Periodic Paralysis Disorders

	HYPER PP	HYPO PP	ATS
Gene	*SCN4A*	*CACNA1S* > *SCN4A*	*KCNJ2*
Triggers of weakness	Rest after exercise	Stress	Rest after exercise
	Fasting	EtOH	Carbohydrates
	High K+ food	Carb-rich food	Potassium
		Rest after exercise	
Duration of weakness	Minutes to hours	Hours to days	Hours to days
Associated features	Myotonia		Dysmorphic
			Cardiac arrhythmias
Number of episodes per month	10-20	<10	Variable

hypoPP = hypokalemic periodic paralysis, hyperPP = hyperkalemic periodic paralysis, ATS = Andersen Tawil Syndrome

47. **What is the treatment for PP?**
Acetazolamide and dichlorphenamide, both of which are carbonic anhydrase inhibitors, are effective in some patients with each form of PP. In patients with hypokalemic PP, potassium-sparing diuretics

such as spironolactone and triamterene might be used in addition to oral potassium supplements and a low-carbohydrate and low-sodium diet. Beta-adrenergic agents or ingestion of a high-carbohydrate, low-potassium diet may alleviate the attacks in hyperkalemic PP. Antiarrhythmics, beta-blockers, or cardioverter-defibrillators should be considered in ATS.

CONGENITAL MYOPATHIES

48. Describe the congenital myopathies.

The congenital myopathies are a group of inherited myopathies with early onset of weakness, manifesting as infant hypotonia or delayed motor milestones in children. These disorders are commonly either nonprogressive or only slowly progressive. Classification is based on muscle histological appearance (e.g., central clearing on NADH staining has been called *central core disease*). More than one genetic mutation may cause similar histological findings, and mutations in some genes may cause multiple histological changes, even in the same family. The most common congenital myopathies are central core disease, nemaline myopathy, centronuclear myopathy, and congenital fiber type disproportion.

49. Describe the phenotypic and histologic heterogeneity associated with mutations in the ryanodine receptor (*RYR1*) gene.

The ryanodine receptor (*RYR1*), which functions in skeletal muscle excitation–contraction coupling, is the most common cause of congenital myopathy and has been implicated in a wide spectrum of diseases ranging from mild, nonprogressive, proximal muscle weakness, to severe congenital muscular dystrophy. Additionally, mutations in *RYR1* are also known to cause malignant hyperthermia in response to anesthesia or heat, exercise-induced rhabdomyolysis, and isolated hyperCKemia. Histologically, mutations in *RYR1* may result in central core disease, multiminicore disease, centronuclear myopathy, and congenital fiber type disproportion. Inheritance may be autosomal dominant or recessive.

METABOLIC MYOPATHIES

50. What features are suggestive of a metabolic myopathy?

Clinical features suggestive of a metabolic myopathy include acute, recurrent, and usually reversible exercise-related muscular pain, stiffness, or cramps and myoglobinuria. Some disorders are associated with fixed or progressive weakness. The metabolic myopathies can be further classified by the metabolic pathway that is disrupted (glycolytic metabolism, lipid metabolism, or oxidative phosphorylation, which takes place in the mitochondrial matrix).

51. What is acid maltase deficiency disease?

Acid maltase deficiency (type II glycogenosis) is an autosomal recessive disorder caused by deficiency of the lysosomal enzyme alpha-glucosidase (acid maltase), a hydrolase that degrades glycogen to glucose. It can be subdivided into three different forms by age of onset. The infantile form (Pompe disease) presents with cardiomegaly, macroglossia, hepatomegaly, and hypotonia. The juvenile form presents with slowly progressive weakness. Some cases might have calf or tongue hypertrophy. The adult patient usually becomes symptomatic in the third or fourth decade with insidious painless limb-girdle weakness. The respiratory muscles are disproportionately affected.

52. How is acid maltase deficiency diagnosed and treated?

CK level is usually mildly elevated (2 to 10 times normal). The EMG shows abundant complex repetitive discharges, myopathic changes, and spontaneous activity, including myotonia, especially in thoracic paraspinal muscles. Characteristic findings on muscle biopsy are those of a vacuolar myopathy. For definite diagnosis, enzyme activity is first measured in dried blood spots, followed by confirmatory testing of acid maltase activity in cultures of fibroblasts, muscle tissue, or by genetic testing. Enzyme replacement therapy with recombinant alpha-glucosidase has shown significant clinical response in infantile form and modest response in juvenile and adult forms.

53. What is McArdle disease? How is it treated?

McArdle disease (glycogen storage disease type V) is an autosomal recessive disorder caused by deficiency of myophosphorylase, the enzyme responsible for liberating glucose molecules from glycogen in skeletal muscle. Patients present with a lifelong history of poor exercise tolerance, and minimal physical exertion may cause muscle pain, muscle contractures, and rhabdomyolysis. Muscle contractures are described as muscles "locking up." During a muscle contracture, the muscle is electrically silent, and, unlike common neural cramps, cannot be improved with stretching or massage. Another characteristic feature of McArdle disease is the "second wind" phenomenon, where patients experience improved exercise capacity after briefly resting after initiating exercise. This phenomenon is attributed to muscle metabolism of fatty acids or extramuscular-derived glucose. Patients should be counseled to avoid high intensity exercise. Additionally, moderate, regular endurance exercise has been shown to improve exercise tolerance.

54. **What is the most common disorder of lipid metabolism in muscle?**
Carnitine palmitoyltransferase 2 deficiency is the most common disorder of lipid metabolism in muscle and a major cause of hereditary recurrent myoglobinuria, which is precipitated by fasting, prolonged submaximal exercise, and fever. It has three phenotypes: (1) adult myopathic form; (2) infantile hepatocardiomuscular form, which is life threatening; and (3) fatal neonatal form, which presents shortly after birth with respiratory distress, seizures, cardiohepatomegaly, dysmorphic features, and neuronal migration deficits. The adult myopathic form is the most frequent type, and usually has a benign course. Between episodes of myoglobinuria, muscle strength and serum CK are normal.

55. **Describe the differential diagnosis of exercise-induced rhabdomyolysis.**
    - Disorders of muscle carbohydrate metabolism (e.g., McArdle disease, phosphofructokinase deficiency)
    - Disorders of muscle fatty acid metabolism (e.g., carnitine phosphatidyltranferase II deficiency)
    - *RYR1*-related myopathies
    - Muscular dystrophies (excluding BMD)
    - Severe form of delayed-onset muscle soreness in healthy individuals after unaccustomed exercise

56. **What features can help to distinguish exercise-associated muscle soreness and rhabdomyolysis associated with metabolic myopathies from exercise-associated muscle soreness seen in healthy individuals?**
    - **Exercise history:** Metabolic myopathies are associated with life-long exercise intolerance.
    - **Type of exercise preceding onset of symptoms:** In healthy individuals, muscle soreness typically occurs after unaccustomed, eccentric exercise, which is defined as exercise involving lengthening of contracting muscles (e.g., walking down stairs).
    - **Timing to symptom onset:** Pain occurs immediately during exercise in patients with metabolic myopathies and can be associated with myoglobinuria with the next urination after exercise. In contrast, pain usually develops after 8 to 36 hours following exercise in healthy individuals.

MITOCHONDRIAL MYOPATHIES

57. **What symptoms are classic for a mitochondrial myopathy?**
Although the degree of impairment varies, most mitochondrial myopathies are associated with non-fluctuating, insidiously progressive ptosis and ophthalmoplegia. Actual diplopia is rare. Other involved organ systems include the following:
    - Cardiac (conduction abnormalities and cardiomyopathy)
    - Gastrointestinal (pseudo-obstruction)
    - Endocrine (diabetes, goiter, short stature)
    - Central nervous system (ataxia, deafness, seizures, cerebrovascular ischemia, neuropathy)
    - Skin (lipomas)
    - Eye (retinitis pigmentosa, cataracts)
    - Ear (deafness)

58. **Describe the types of genetic mutations that lead to mitochondrial myopathies.**
    - Primary mitochondrial DNA mutations
    - Nuclear mutations that impair replication or maintenance of mitochondrial DNA
    - Nuclear mutations in genes encoding subunits of the respiratory chain
    - Nuclear mutations that impair mitochondrial protein synthesis

59. **What are the most important myopathies due to point mutations in tRNA genes of mitochondrial DNA?**
    - Myoclonic epilepsy with ragged red fibers (MERRF)
    - Mitochondrial encephalomyopathy with lactic acidosis and stroke-like episodes (MELAS)
    - Some myopathies with cardiomyopathy

60. **How are mitochondrial myopathies diagnosed?**
CK can be normal. EMG may show myopathic units. Serum lactate to pyruvate ratio may be greater than 20. Muscle biopsy may show fibers that stain positive for succinate dehydrogenase (SDH) but negative for COX. Respiratory chain enzymatic activity may also be measured on muscle tissue. Definitive diagnosis may require genetic testing.

CONTINUOUS MUSCLE ACTIVITY SYNDROMES

61. **What is myokymia?**
Myokymia is the continuous undulation of a group of muscle fibers caused by the successive sponta-neous contraction of motor units. On EMG, they appear as groups of 2 to 10 potentials, firing at 5 to 60 Hz and recurring regularly at 0.2- to 1-second intervals. Myokymia, frequently observed in facial muscles, occurs in a number of brainstem diseases, especially multiple sclerosis, radiation-induced nerve damage, Guillain–Barré syndrome, chronic peripheral nerve disorders, timber rattlesnake envenomation, gold therapy, and Isaacs' syndrome.

62. **What is neuromyotonia?**
Neuromyotonia is the continuous muscle rippling and stiffness resulting from bursts of discharges from the peripheral nerve. It is neurogenic in origin and is due to an immune-mediated neurogenic hyperexcitability. On EMG, bursts of spontaneous motor unit activity firing at 40 to 300 Hz and lasting for several seconds are observed. Antibodies against voltage-gated potassium channels are found in many cases. Myotonia differs from neuromyotonia in that myotonia is thought be of myogenic origin. This theory is supported by the failure of curare to inhibit myotonia.

63. **What is Isaacs' syndrome?**
Isaacs' syndrome (also known as myokymia with impaired muscle relaxation, neuromyotonia, pseu-domyotonia, quantal squander, armadillo disease, and continuous muscle fiber activity) is a disorder characterized by muscle cramps, twitches, myokymia, weight loss, and hyperhidrosis. If central nervous system dysfunction such as encephalitis is also present, then it is called *Morvan's fibrillary chorea*. Either myokymia or neuromyotonia can be observed on EMG. Antibodies against the voltage-gated potassium channel or neuronal ganglionic acetylcholine receptor are found in some patients. Symptomatic treatment has been achieved with phenytoin (300 to 400 mg/day) or carbamazepine (200 mg, three or four times/day). Some patients may respond favorably to plasma exchange or intra-venous immunoglobulin. Isaacs' syndrome can be associated with thymoma, small cell lung cancer, and Hodgkin's lymphoma, or other autoimmune disorders.

64. **What is stiff-person syndrome (SPS)?**
SPS is a fluctuating motor disturbance characterized by persistent muscular stiffness due to coactiva-tion of agonist and antagonist muscles with superimposed spasms. The classical form predominantly affects the axial and proximal limb muscles and is aggravated by emotional, somatosensory, or acoustic stimuli. Antiglutamic acid decarboxylase (GAD) antibodies are present in the serum and cerebrospinal fluid at high levels. SPS can be a paraneoplastic condition more commonly associated with antiamphiphysin autoantibodies. EMG demonstrates a continuous low-frequency firing of normal motor unit potentials that persists at rest. A significant symptomatic improvement is achieved by oral administration of benzodiazepines, primarily diazepam (10 to 100 mg/day). Baclofen and valproic acid also may help the symptoms. Immunomodulation by corticosteroids, plasmapheresis, or IVIG may be necessary in some patients.

65. **What are other anti-GAD-associated neurologic disorders?**
    - GAD-antibody-associated cerebellar ataxia is the other common presentation (in isolation or concurrent with SPS). Ataxia can evolve over weeks to years and be associated with dysarthria and nystagmus.
    - Progressive encephalomyelitis with rigidity and myoclonus is a rare variant that presents with axial and lower limb stiffness followed by myoclonus, long tract, and brain stem signs (i.e., ataxia, deaf-ness, oculomotor impairment, dysarthria, and dysphagia).
    - Epilepsy can be isolated or occur in conjunction with these other syndromes.

CLINICAL FEATURES

66. Which myopathies cause respiratory failure?
    - Some muscular dystrophies (Duchenne, Becker, limb-girdle, Emery–Dreifuss, myotonic,[†] congenital)
    - Acid maltase deficiency[†]
    - Carnitine deficiency
    - Nemaline myopathy[†]
    - Mitochondrial myopathy
    - Centronuclear myopathy[†]
    - PM/DM

KEY POINTS: MYOPATHIES

1. Myopathies usually cause proximal symmetric weakness, with or without other symptoms.
2. The diagnosis of myopathies often rests upon CK levels, EMG findings, and muscle biopsy.
3. Muscles contain both slow (type 1 red) and fast (type 2 white) fibers.
4. Myotonic dystrophy is the most common muscular dystrophy in adults.
5. The possibility of respiratory failure is the most serious concern in the management of most patients with myopathies.
6. Drug toxicity should always be considered in the differential diagnosis.

---

67. Which myopathies are associated with dysphagia?
    - OPMD
    - IBM
    - Myotonic muscular dystrophy
    - Mitochondrial myopathy
    - PM and DM

68. Which myopathies are associated with cardiac disease?
    - **Arrhythmias:** Kearns–Sayre disease; Anderson's syndrome; PM; muscular dystrophies: myotonic; limb-girdle type 1B, 2C–F, 2G, 2I; and Emery–Dreifuss
    - **Congestive heart failure:** muscular dystrophies: Duchenne; Becker's; Emery–Dreifuss; myotonic; limb-girdle 1B, 2C–F, 2G, 2I; nemaline myopathy; acid-maltase deficiency; carnitine deficiency; PM

69. Which myopathies are associated with ptosis or ophthalmoplegia?
    Ptosis usually without ophthalmoplegia:
    - Myotonic dystrophy
    - Congenital myopathies
    - Centronuclear myopathy
    - Nemaline myopathy
    - Central core myopathy
    - Myofibrillary (desmin subtype) myopathy
    Ptosis with ophthalmoplegia:
    - OPMD
    - Oculopharyngodistal myopathy
    - Chronic progressive external ophthalmoplegia (mitochondrial myopathy)

70. Which myopathies are characterized by predominant distal weakness?
    - Late adult-onset distal myopathy type 1 (Welander) and type 2 (Markesbery)
    - Early adult-onset distal myopathy type 1 (Nonaka), type 2 (Miyoshi), and type 3 (Laing)
    - Late adult-onset distal dystrophinopathy
    - Myofibrillary myopathy
    - Childhood-onset distal myopathy

[†] Respiratory failure may be the presenting feature.

- Myotonic dystrophy
- Fascioscapulohumeral dystrophy
- Scapuloperoneal myopathy
- Oculopharyngeal dystrophy
- Emery–Dreifuss humeroperoneal dystrophy
- Inflammatory myopathies: inclusion body myositis
- Metabolic myopathy: Debrancher deficiency, acid-maltase deficiency
- Congenital myopathy: nemaline myopathy, central core myopathy, centronuclear myopathy

Acknowledgments

The authors would like to acknowledge the contributions of Dr. Yadollah Harati who authored this chapter in the previous edition.

 References available online at expertconsult.com.

WEBSITES

http://www.mdausa.org/disease.
http://neuromuscular.wustl.edu/

BIBLIOGRAPHY

1. Carpenter S, Karpati G: Pathology of Skeletal Muscles, 2nd ed. New York, Oxford University Press, 2001.
2. Engel AG, et al.: Myology, 3rd ed. New York, McGraw-Hill, 2004.
3. Harati Y, Nawasipirong O: Cramps and myalgias. In Jankovic J, Tolosa E, (eds): Movement disorders, Baltimore, Williams & Wilkins, 2003.
4. Katirji B, Kaminski HJ, Ruff RL, et al.: Neuromuscular Disorders in Clinical Practice, 2nd ed. Boston, Butterworth-Heinemann, 2014.
5. Ciafaloni E, Chinnery P, Griggs RC, (eds): Evaluation and Treatment of Myopathies, 2nd ed. London, Oxford University Press, 2014.
6. Amato A, Russell J: Neuromuscular Disorders, New York, McGraw-Hill, 2008.

NEUROMUSCULAR JUNCTION DISEASES

Clifton L. Gooch

CHAPTER 5

ANATOMY AND PHYSIOLOGY

1. **What happens in the motor nerve terminal (presynaptically) during neuromuscular transmission?**

   When a wave of depolarization (the action potential) travels down the motor nerve and reaches its tip (the presynaptic nerve terminal), voltage-gated calcium channels in the neuronal membrane open, allowing influx of calcium ions (Ca^{2+}). This triggers the fusion of acetylcholine (ACh)-filled vesicles with the membrane and the release of ACh into the space between the nerve and muscle membranes (the synaptic cleft) (Fig. 5-1).

2. **What happens in the muscle (postsynaptically) during neuromuscular transmission?**

   The binding of two ACh molecules to each ACh receptor (AChR) in the muscle (postsynaptic) membrane opens a Na^+ channel within the receptor, allowing Na^+ influx, which generates subthreshold depolarizations known as *miniature endplate potentials (MEPPs)*. The MEPPs in each muscle fiber summate to form the endplate potential (EPP) for that fiber. When a sufficient number of receptors are activated simultaneously, the EPP becomes large enough to trigger an action potential, which then propagates along the muscle sarcoplasmic membrane to the T-tubule system, leading to the release of Ca^{2+} from the sarcoplasmic reticulum and muscle contraction.

3. **What happens in the synaptic cleft during neuromuscular transmission?**

   After ACh molecules bind to and activate AChRs, they are released back into the synaptic cleft. Acetylcholinesterase (AChE) in the cleft then decomposes ACh into choline and acetic acid within a fraction of a millisecond, and choline reuptake by the presynaptic nerve terminal provides material for the synthesis of new ACh via the enzyme choline acetyl transferase.

4. **What is the structure of the nicotinic AChR?**

   The human AChR consists of five subunits: two alpha, one beta, one epsilon (or gamma in fetal form), and one delta subunit. ACh binds to the extracellular domain of the alpha subunit. Two ACh molecules must bind with the receptor (one on each alpha subunit) to open its Na^+ channel (Fig. 5-2).

5. **What is the "safety margin" for neuromuscular transmission?**

   In the normal subject, the amount of ACh released from the presynaptic nerve terminal decreases with each repeated nerve depolarization at a slow rate. This means fewer receptors are activated at the muscle endplate, generating fewer MEPPs and a lower EPP. However, the number of receptors is still high enough that this slight decline in ACh output does not drive the EPP below the depolarization threshold for the muscle fiber, and full contraction still occurs. This functional redundancy is known as the *safety margin* for neuromuscular transmission.

MYASTHENIA GRAVIS

6. **What autoimmune diseases primarily affect the neuromuscular junction (NMJ)?**

   Myasthenia gravis (MG), in which most antibodies are directed against the AChR on the postsynaptic muscle membrane, and Lambert–Eaton myasthenic syndrome (LEMS), in which antibodies are directed against the voltage-gated calcium channel in the nerve terminal, primarily affect the NMJ.

7. **How is the safety margin for neuromuscular transmission altered in MG?**

   In MG, antibodies decrease the number of functional AChRs. Because fewer AChRs are available for activation, the safety margin for neuromuscular transmission is lowered. Fewer MEPPs are generated when ACh output falls and the EPP is lower. With repeated activation of the nerve and further declines

65

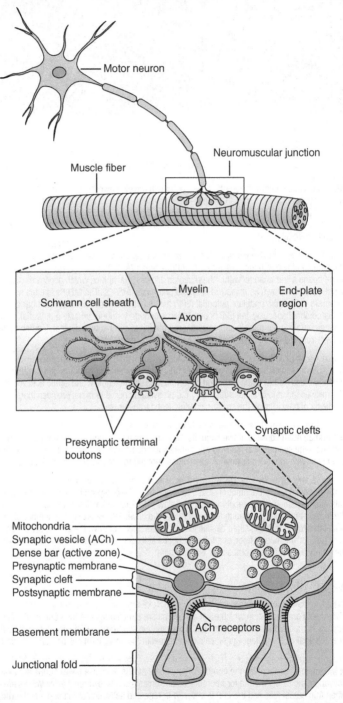

Figure 5-1. The neuromuscular junction. *ACh*, acetylcholine. *(From Kandel ER, Schwartz JH, Jessel TM (eds): Principles of neural science, 3rd ed. New York: Elsevier, 1991, p 136.)*

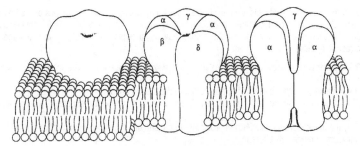

Figure 5-2. Diagram of the molecular structure of the acetylcholine receptor at the neuromuscular junction. *(From Kandel ER, Schwartz JH, Jessel TM (eds): Principles of neural science, 3rd ed. New York: Elsevier, 1991, p 146.)*

in ACh output, the EPP eventually falls below the threshold necessary to trigger depolarization and contraction of the muscle fiber (blocking of neuromuscular transmission). With continued activation of the nerve, this happens at an increasing number of NMJs and many muscle fibers fail to activate, causing weakness. With extrinsic repetitive electrical stimulation of the nerve at low frequencies, the size of the electrical response accompanying muscle contraction (the compound motor action potential or CMAP) decreases due to this same phenomenon. After a period of rest, ACh content is restored, and these abnormalities may improve.

8. What are the clinical manifestations of MG?
   Patients with MG often have variable degrees of weakness and easy fatigability of voluntary skeletal muscle. This weakness may or may not be noticeable with simple activity, but appears or worsens after sustained exercise and typically improves after a short rest. Weakness and fatigability of extraocular muscles (diplopia), bulbar muscles (dysarthria, dysphagia), and limb muscles is often easily detectable on clinical examination. The most critical manifestation is respiratory weakness, a potentially fatal complication, which can develop over hours in severe cases.

9. What is the epidemiology of MG (i.e., incidence, sex differences, age of onset, inheritance, mortality, and natural history)?
   The incidence of MG is approximately 1 in 20,000. It affects more women than men by a ratio of 3:2 and has a bimodal age distribution (affecting more women in the third decade and more men in the fifth decade), although it may appear at any age from birth to late adulthood. Five to seven percent of cases are familial, but no Mendelian inheritance pattern has been identified. Prior to the advent of effective immunomodulatory therapy and artificial ventilation, 20% to 30% of MG patients died due to respiratory failure, 20% experienced persistent symptoms, 25% experienced spontaneous improvement, and a final 25% experienced spontaneous remission. In the modern era, MG is eminently treatable, and death in the properly treated and adherent patient is rare.

10. What is the scientific evidence that AChR antibodies cause MG?
    MG is the prototypic antireceptor antibody disease and is one of the best understood of any of the autoimmune diseases at the basic science level. Animals immunized with AChRs develop serum antibodies against the receptor and exhibit both the clinical and electrophysiologic features of human MG. This model is known as *experimental autoimmune myasthenia gravis* or EAMG. Passive transfer of human MG IgG to animals also causes EAMG, and immunocytochemical studies have demonstrated IgG at the postsynaptic membrane of motor endplates in myasthenic skeletal muscle. AChR antibodies decrease the number of available AChRs in cultured muscle cells in vitro.

11. What is the clinical evidence that AChR antibodies cause MG?
    More than 90% of patients with MG have circulating antibodies against nicotinic AChR. Removal of the antibodies by plasmapheresis often improves the symptoms and signs of MG. Decreased titers after therapy also may correlate with improved symptoms. Favorable responses to immunotherapy are also consistent with autoimmune, antibody-mediated injury.

12. What is the thymus gland? What is a myoid cell?
    The thymus gland is a small gland located in the fat pad beneath the sternum. It plays a critical role in the maturation of immunologically active cells and in the development of immune self-tolerance in

the healthy patient. Myoid cells are muscle-like cells found mainly within the medulla of the thymus. Myoid cells express nicotinic AChRs, and given their location within this critical site for the development of the global immune response, these cells may play a pivotal role in autosensitization against the receptor in MG.

13. **What evidence suggests that the thymus gland has a major role in the pathogenesis of MG?**
    - Removal of the thymus seems to improve MG in the majority of patients.
    - The majority of patients with MG have an abnormal thymus, demonstrating either hyperplasia or thymoma.
    - Thymic myoid cells express AChRs proximate to the site of T-lymphocyte maturation (which includes immune self-tolerance).
    - AChRs in the thymic myoid cells in MG express the fetal gamma subunit, making them potential targets for antibody sensitization.
    - Thymic B lymphocytes from patients with MG produce more anti-AChR antibodies than other antibodies.
    - Thymic cells selectively increase the production of anti-ACh antibodies when added to myasthenic B lymphocytes in the laboratory.
    - MG thymus tissue transplanted to immunodeficient mice produces anti-AChR antibodies, which deposit at skeletal muscle endplates.

14. **What is the role of thymectomy in the treatment of MG?**
    Although prospective, randomized, controlled trials have not been performed, the beneficial effects of thymectomy in patients with MG (with or without thymic tumor) have been demonstrated in a plethora of studies. Over 75% of patients experience some benefit, which may include a reduced requirement for immunomodulatory therapy, a greater likelihood of successful taper of immunosuppressant medication with continued control, and a greater chance of permanent symptomatic remission. The extended transsternal approach (sternal split with removal of the thymus and visual exploration of the mediastinum for removal of ectopic thymic tissue) appears to confer the best balance between benefit and risk, and is extremely safe in experienced hands. Benefits in children and patients over 60 years of age are less clear, and these groups may be at greater risk for the procedure. The congenital myasthenic syndromes do not appear to be immune-mediated and do not respond to thymectomy.

15. **What is the association between thymoma and MG?**
    Approximately 15% of patients with MG have a thymoma, most of which are epithelial rather than lymphocytic in origin. Ninety percent are benign and easily treated with resection, whereas 10% are malignant, carrying an average survival of 5 to 10 years. Benign thymic hyperplasia is seen in about 50% of patients with MG.

16. **What diagnostic tests can help identify a thymoma in patients with MG?**
    Imaging studies are the gold standard for the diagnosis of thymoma in patients with MG, and all MG patients should undergo either a computed tomography (CT) or magnetic resonance imaging (MRI) scan of the chest with contrast. The sensitivity and specificity of chest CT for the identification of thymoma are 85% and 99%, respectively. Other adjunctive studies may also suggest thymoma, and antiskeletal muscle antibodies have a sensitivity of 94% in patients with MG and a thymic mass. Antiskeletal muscle antibody titers fall with successful treatment of the thymoma and rise with recurrence, making them useful screening tools for patient follow-up.

17. **What is transient neonatal MG?**
    Approximately 12% of neonates born to mothers with MG are "floppy" babies who have difficulty with breathing and sucking. This "transient neonatal myasthenia" likely results from the transfer of maternal AChR antibodies to the infant through the placenta. It typically lasts for several weeks and then spontaneously resolves but should not persist for more than 12 weeks. Neither the severity of maternal disease nor the titers of maternal antibody reliably correlate with the development of neonatal MG. Severely affected mothers may have normal infants, and mothers in clinical remission may have affected infants. Regardless, physicians caring for a myasthenic mother must be aware of this disorder and must be prepared to provide respiratory support to the newborn, if needed.

18. **What are the congenital myasthenic syndromes?**
    The congenital myasthenic syndromes are a group of extremely rare disorders typically caused by genetic mutations affecting the structure and/or function of the NMJ. They manifest as extraocular,

Table 5-1. The Congenital Myasthenic Syndromes

Presynaptic	Familial infantile congenital MG + episodic apnea
	Decreased synaptic vesicles and reduced ACh quantal release
	Congenital Lambert–Eaton-like episodic ataxia 2
	Reduced quantal release
Synaptic basal lamina defects	AChE deficiency at NMJs
Postsynaptic	
Kinetic AChR abnormalities	Reduced numbers of AChRs at NMJs
	Slow AChR channel syndromes with increased response to ACh
	Fast-channel syndromes with reduced response to ACh
	Normal numbers of AChRs at NMJs with reduced response to ACh
	Fast-channel syndrome: AChR ε subunit dysfunction
	Fast-channel syndrome: AChR α subunit dysfunction
	High conductance and fast closure of AChRs
	Increased numbers of AChRs at NMJs
	Slow-channel syndrome: AChR β subunit dysfunction
Nonkinetic AChR abnormalities	Reduced numbers of AChRs at NMJs due to AChR mutations
	Usually ε subunit abnormality
	Rarely, α, β, ε subunit abnormalities
Other postsynaptic defects	Rapsyn mutations causing reduced numbers of AChRs at NMJs
	Plectin deficiency
	Weakness + episodic apnea, and bulbar dysfunction

ACh, acetylcholine; AChR, acetylcholine receptor; AChE, acetylcholinesterase; MG, myasthenia gravis; NMJ, neuromuscular junction.
Washington University Neuromuscular Online Reference: http://www.neuro.wustl.edu/neuromuscular/synmg.html.
From Nogajski JH, Kiernan MC, Ouvrier RA, Andrews PI: Congenital myasthenic syndromes. J Clin Neurosci 16:1-11, 2009.

facial, bulbar, and/or limb weakness and fatigability beginning in early life and persisting into adulthood. These syndromes have been characterized by site of dysfunction within the NMJ and are the subject of ongoing investigation, with new syndromes described each year. Patients with these disorders do not respond to thymectomy or other immunotherapies. The presynaptic disorders involve defective release or synthesis of ACh and account for 8% of the congenital syndromes. The synaptic basal lamina disorders are due to mutations in the collagen tail of AChE, and account for 16%. The postsynaptic disorders are caused primarily by mutations in various AChR subunits, altering receptor number and/or receptor ion channel kinetics. They account for the majority of cases (76%) (Table 5-1).

19. **What are the most common diagnostic tests for MG?**
The diagnosis of MG is a clinical one but may be supported by several different tests. Electrophysiologic tests are often the first step after clinical examination, and typically include repetitive nerve stimulation (RNS) studies, which have a sensitivity of 40% to 90% depending on disease severity. A more advanced test, single-fiber electromyography (SFEMG), is the single most sensitive assay in MG with a sensitivity of 90% to 95% even in mildly symptomatic patients. The AChR binding antibody assay (using serum samples) is 90% sensitive in generalized disease and 70% in pure ocular disease, but the blocking and modulating AChR antibody assays are less sensitive, particularly in pure ocular disease. Administration of the short-acting AChE inhibitor edrophonium (the Tensilon test) may transiently improve strength and can also aid in diagnosis but must be properly performed in a patient having clearly discernible weakness on examination to serve as a gauge for response.

20. **What is RNS, and what does it show in MG?**
RNS involves the repeated transcutaneous electrical stimulation of all the motor fibers within a peripheral nerve, which generates successive impulses. These impulses travel down the nerve, across the NMJ, and into the muscle, from which consecutive electrical responses (CMAPs) are recorded. In MG, progressive failure of transmission across an increasing number of NMJs with repeated

stimulation results in activation of fewer muscle fibers, and progressively smaller CMAPs. This decrement in CMAP size with low-frequency (2 to 3 Hz) RNS confirms NMJ dysfunction. Decrement may be transiently repaired and CMAP amplitude transiently restored by brief voluntary exercise of the tested muscle between rounds of RNS (repair of decrement and postexercise facilitation). Decrement may also improve with anticholinesterase inhibitor administration.

21. What is SFEMG, and what does it show in MG?

SFEMG is a technique that enables the recording of single muscle fiber discharges, either during volitional contraction or during electrical stimulation of the axon branch to the muscle fiber. Mathematical analysis of consecutive SFEMG signals enables quantitation of the variability in transmission time across the NMJ from discharge to discharge, a value known as *jitter*. In MG, LEMS, and other NMJ disorders, jitter is increased and may be associated with intermittent failure of transmission across certain NMJs ("blocking" of neuromuscular transmission). SFEMG is the single most sensitive test for MG and is positive in 95% of generalized cases and 90% of pure ocular cases. Increased jitter also occurs in myopathic and neuropathic diseases, so careful routine electromyography and nerve conduction studies are imperative to rule out these causes before SFEMG can be interpreted.

KEY POINTS: CAUSES AND DIAGNOSIS OF MYASTHENIA GRAVIS

1. MG is caused by different sets of antibodies directed against the AChR and its associated functional proteins.
2. The thymus plays a major role in the immunopathogenesis of MG, and its removal improves chances for remission and response to medical therapy.
3. Diagnostic tests for MG include RNS, AChR antibody assays, the Tensilon test, and SFEMG.
4. Fifteen percent of MG patients have a thymoma, and 10% of thymomas in MG patients are malignant; therefore, every MG patient requires CT or MRI of the chest.
5. SFEMG has the greatest sensitivity of any test for MG (90% to 95%) and is particularly useful in mild or pure ocular cases when other assays are more likely to be negative or indeterminate.

22. How is the edrophonium (Tensilon) test performed?

The patient must have readily observable weakness (e.g., ptosis) or weakness that is easily quantified on examination. The test must be performed in a controlled setting, with emergency resuscitation equipment and trained personnel available, because there is a small risk of precipitating cardiac arrhythmia. Both a syringe containing normal saline (the placebo) and a syringe containing edrophonium (10 mg) must be prepared. The placebo is always administered first, and the same protocol should be used for both IV preparations. A test dose of 1 mg is given, and the patient is observed for side effects over 5 minutes (i.e., flushing, palpitations, tearing). In some patients, clinical effect appears at this small dose. In most of them, however, the remaining 10 mg will be required. Each minute for the next 5 minutes after administration, the patient should be observed and tested for improvement, and the results documented. Unequivocal improvement occurring only with edrophonium and not with placebo supports the diagnosis of MG.

23. What is the Mary Walker phenomenon?

Fatigue and weakness of the forearm muscles develop in myasthenic patients when the forearm muscles are exercised with a cuff around the upper arm, inflated above systolic pressure to occlude circulation (ischemic exercise). After the cuff is deflated, myasthenic symptoms in the rest of the body may worsen within minutes in some patients. This phenomenon is named after Mary Walker, the physiologist who first described it in 1938, and is also present in the myasthenic dog. Although its mechanism is not clear, it may be due to transient lactic acidosis, because lactic acid binds calcium and reduces available ionized and serum calcium. Experimentally, lactate infusions increase weakness in patients with MG much more than in controls.

24. What is pyridostigmine? Why is it the most widely used anticholinesterase medication in MG?

Pyridostigmine (Mestinon) is slightly longer acting (with a half-life of 4 hours) and has fewer cholinergic side effects than neostigmine bromide and other anticholinesterase preparations. Unlike physostigmine, pyridostigmine has no unwanted central nervous system effects because it does not cross the blood–brain barrier. However, some cases of MG may be refractory to pyridostigmine but respond to other anticholinesterases. A long-acting preparation, Mestinon Timespan 180 mg, may alleviate difficulty in swallowing medication in the morning when taken before bedtime but is not as useful for therapy while awake. A parenteral preparation is also available (2-mg parenteral dose = 60-mg oral dose).

25. What is a cholinergic crisis?

    Overdosing with anticholinesterase may result in excessive ACh in the synaptic cleft, causing a depolarizing block of AChRs. The end result is defective neuromuscular transmission causing symptoms similar to those of a myasthenic crisis. Fasciculations are also common. Establishing an airway, supporting respiration, and withholding anticholinesterase medications are the mainstays of treatment. This complication is rarely seen today because lower doses of anticholinesterase are typically utilized due to successful primary immunomodulatory therapy.

26. What are the chronic adverse effects of anticholinesterases on NMJ?

    Chronic excess ACh may also damage the muscle endplate, cause simplification of the postsynaptic folds and loss of AChRs, similar to the endplate changes seen in MG. These changes may be superimposed on the primary damage caused by MG itself. However, as with cholinergic crises, this complication is rarely seen today because successful primary immunotherapy makes the chronic use of high doses of anticholinesterases unnecessary in most patients.

27. Which drugs may worsen MG?

    Many routinely used drugs have adverse effects on the NMJ, which may not be significant in normal patients but can seriously worsen MG. The list is extensive, and the practitioner should be certain that a given drug does not have these effects before starting therapy in a myasthenic patient. The list includes many antibiotics, particularly the aminoglycosides; cardiac drugs, particularly the beta-blockers (even Timoptic eye drops); chloroquine; phenytoin; lithium; magnesium; and excess doses of the anticholinesterases (cholinergic crisis). Of course, neuromuscular blocking agents worsen symptoms and may prolong recovery and weaning from ventilation postoperatively, especially the depolarizing agents. Rarely, drugs such as D-penicillamine may precipitate MG in previously unaffected patients (Table 5-2). A more complete list can be found on the website for the Myasthenia Gravis Foundation of America (MGFA) at www.myasthenia.org.

Table 5-2. Drugs That Adversely Affect Neuromuscular Junction Function

ANTIBIOTICS	NEUROMUSCULAR BLOCKERS	OTHER DRUGS
Aminoglycosides	Cardiac drugs	Phenytoin
Neomycin	Quinine	Chloroquine
Streptomycin	Quinidine	Trimethadione
Kanamycin	Procainamide	Lithium carbonate
Gentamicin	Trimethaphan	Magnesium salts
Tobramycin	Lidocaine	Meglumine diatrizoate
Other peptide antibiotics	Beta-adrenergic blockers	Methoxyflurane
Polymyxin B	—	Oxytocin
Colistin	—	Aprotinin
Other antibiotics	—	Propanidid
Oxytetracycline	—	Diazepam
Rolitetracycline	—	Ketamine
Lincomycin	—	D-Penicillamine
Clindamycin	—	Carnitine
Erythromycin	—	—
Ampicillin	—	—

28. **What is drug-induced autoimmune MG?**

Approximately 1% of patients taking D-penicillamine for the treatment of diseases such as rheumatoid arthritis or Wilson's disease develop clinical myasthenia. The disease is six times more common in women, first striking the ocular muscles and then becoming generalized. Patients have autoantibodies against AChRs, which usually slowly disappear (along with MG symptoms) after discontinuation of the drug. Trimethadione, an anticonvulsant, also may induce myasthenia. These patients have high titers of antimuscle antibodies and antinuclear factor, and symptoms suggestive of systemic lupus erythematosus.

29. **Which temporizing therapies can rapidly improve MG?**

Both plasma exchange (PE) and intravenous immunoglobulin (IVIG) induce improvement in most MG patients within 1 to 2 weeks. Typical courses of therapy might include six exchanges every other day over 2 weeks, or 400 mg/kg/day of IVIG for 5 days. Improvement usually peaks at 2 to 4 weeks and then gradually abates at 6 to 8 weeks. These therapies seem to have equivalent efficacy in general, though some patients may respond better to one or the other. There are no data suggesting that combined therapy is any more beneficial than treatment with either agent alone. They are helpful when rapid improvement is needed (i.e., myasthenic crisis), to prepare symptomatic patients for steroid induction, and for surgical procedures such as thymectomy. In rare instances, patients refractory to chronic oral therapies may require indefinite courses of treatment with these temporizing therapies on a regular schedule.

30. **What are the side effects of PE and IVIG?**

PE induces fluid shifts and can cause electrolyte imbalance, anemia, and thrombocytopenia. In addition, PE often requires a central line, which carries some placement and infection risk. IVIG can rarely precipitate renal failure, especially in diabetics, and may cause aseptic meningitis, resulting in headache. It increases blood viscosity, and may increase cardiac and stroke risk in elderly subjects. It also causes transient myelosuppression, though this is usually mild. Unlike PE, IVIG may be protective against infection.

31. **What drugs are effective as chronic immunosuppressives in MG?**

Oral prednisone is the single most effective treatment for MG, resulting in dramatic improvement in 90% of cases within 4 weeks. Azathioprine and mycophenolate are also often effective as sole agents but take longer to begin to work (3 to 6 months). They have a primary role as adjunctive therapy for patients in whom steroids cannot be effectively tapered, and may be drugs of first choice in patients with mild, nonprogressive disease. Methotrexate, cyclosporine, rituximab, eculizumab, and cyclophosphamide may also be of benefit.

KEY POINTS: TREATMENT OF MYASTHENIA GRAVIS

1. Steroids, PE, IVIG, and other immunosuppressive drugs can dramatically improve and successfully control MG.
2. Up to 40% of MG patients experience a transient exacerbation after starting high-dose steroids, usually within 5 to 7 days.

32. **What is a steroid-induced exacerbation?**

In addition to the usual side effects of corticosteroids, patients with MG may become acutely weaker 1 to 3 weeks (average 5 to 7 days) after initiation of oral prednisone therapy (steroid-induced exacerbation) for 24 to 48 hours. Pretreatment with PE and/or IVIG or, alternatively, gradually increasing doses of oral prednisone, from 25 mg orally every other day to 100 mg orally every other day, may alleviate this phenomenon. Consequently, respiratory functions should be carefully monitored during the acute phase of steroid induction.

33. **What is the usual chronic course of patients treated with steroids?**

Patients may be successfully tapered to very low doses over approximately 12 months in most cases, especially when thymectomy has been performed. However, a significant minority of patients will experience an exacerbation (usually mild) as steroids are tapered below a certain point. This is treated by slight, recurrent increases in dosage. However, should a second attempt at steroid taper fail, the introduction of an adjunctive agent, such as azathioprine, is often necessary before taper can be successfully resumed. Excessively rapid steroid tapers are responsible for many severe exacerbations in patients with MG.

34. **What is a myasthenic crisis?**
Myasthenic crisis is an acute exacerbation of MG with severe weakness and/or bulbar and/or respiratory dysfunction. The maintenance of adequate ventilation is paramount, and patients should be hospitalized with close monitoring of pulmonary functions, especially forced vital capacity and forced expiratory volume in 1 second, which often decline before blood gases deteriorate. Early intubation with mechanical ventilatory support is lifesaving in a myasthenic crisis.

35. **After respiratory function is secured, how is a myasthenic crisis treated?**
A thorough work-up for intercurrent infection or other acute disease is needed, along with careful review of the patient's medication list and recent history (for potential agents contributing to NMJ dysfunction or recent changes in MG treatment regimen). Temporizing therapy with plasmapheresis or IVIG should be instituted as soon as possible, followed by chronic immunosuppressive therapy if not contraindicated by other intercurrent illness. If infection is present, IVIG is the temporizing therapy of choice. Anticholinesterases are problematic. If cholinergic crisis is suspected (i.e., very high daily doses used), anticholinesterases should be discontinued with careful respiratory monitoring.

36. **What is the value of the edrophonium test to differentiate myasthenic crisis from cholinergic crisis?**
The edrophonium (Tensilon) test improves myasthenic crisis but aggravates cholinergic crisis. However, interpretation of the result is often difficult and misleading because one group of muscles may deteriorate while others may improve. Securing respiratory function and discontinuing all anticholinesterase drugs in a monitored hospital environment is a safer and more practical solution.

37. **What is anti-muscle-specific kinase (anti-MuSK) antibody syndrome?**
A new population of antibodies has been identified in MG patients in recent years, directed against MuSK. MuSK is a tyrosine kinase, which has an important role in regulating and maintaining AChRs and their functional clusters at the NMJ. Anti-MuSK antibodies may be found in 40% to 60% of patients with clinical MG who are seronegative for antibodies directed against the AChR, and passive transfer of these antibodies produces physiologic effects at the NMJ similar to that caused by anti-AChR IgG (i.e., reduced MEPP amplitude). Initial clinical studies suggest that these patients have a syndrome of generalized myasthenia, often with prominent neck, shoulder, or respiratory muscle weakness with little or delayed ocular muscle involvement. Responses to cholinesterase inhibitors are variable, but PE is effective, and most patients also respond to other immunotherapies including oral steroids, azathioprine, cyclosporine, and mycophenolate. The benefits of thymectomy remain unclear at present.

LAMBERT–EATON MYASTHENIC SYNDROME

38. **What are the primary manifestations of LEMS?**
In LEMS, weakness and fatigability of proximal muscles, especially in the thighs and pelvic girdle, with depressed or absent tendon reflexes are the primary manifestations. Muscle strength and/or reflexes may increase for a short while after exercise (postexercise facilitation and facilitation of reflexes). Although ptosis may be present in LEMS, extraocular and bulbar muscles are minimally involved. Mild autonomic dysfunction may be prominent in LEMS, manifesting primarily as dryness of the mouth.

39. **Which tumor is associated with LEMS?**
About 50% to 66% of patients with LEMS have cancer, usually small-cell carcinoma of the lung, at the time of presentation or will ultimately be diagnosed with it, usually within 2 years. Although immunologic evidence suggests that this tumor may play an important role in the pathogenesis of LEMS, a substantial minority of patients with LEMS never develop malignancy.

40. **What experimental evidence suggests an autoimmune pathogenesis of LEMS?**
Passive transfer of IgG from patients with LEMS to animals produces electrophysiologic defects characteristic of LEMS. The LEMS IgG contains autoantibodies against voltage-gated calcium channels.

41. **Describe the autoimmune pathophysiology involved in LEMS.**
The primary antigen for the LEMS antibodies is found both at the presynapse and in small-cell carcinoma of the lung. LEMS antibodies cross-react with N-type and L-type voltage-gated Ca^{2+} channels and with synaptotagmin in the presynapse. This decreases the number of voltage-gated Ca^{2+} channels, which reduces activation of the cascade, thus leading to the release of fewer ACh vesicles. Decreased ACh release decreases depolarization at the muscle endplate, and threshold for activation of the muscle fiber is not reached.

42. **Explain the mechanism of incremental response after high-frequency RNS in patients with LEMS.**
Decreased Ca^{2+} influx into the presynaptic nerve terminal (due to antibody attack) results in insufficient release of ACh. When the nerve is stimulated at sufficiently high frequencies (either by extrinsic high-frequency RNS or by brief volitional exercise), recurrent depolarization of the nerve terminal causes such a high rate of calcium influx that it overwhelms the nerve cell's mechanisms for calcium clearance, temporarily increasing intracellular calcium levels and normalizing the release of ACh. This manifests as a dramatic increase in compound muscle action potential size. However, low-frequency RNS results in decrement, which may be confused with the decrement of MG.

43. **What are the morphologic changes at the NMJ in LEMS?**
In the normal subject, the freeze-fracture technique shows submicroscopic bumps arrayed in parallel rows in the portion of the presynaptic membrane where calcium channels are clustered. These "active zone protein particles" correspond with the voltage-gated calcium channels, and show reduced numbers and disruption of their normal parallel arrays in patients with LEMS.

44. **What is the treatment for LEMS?**
Release of ACh from the presynaptic nerve terminal is facilitated by guanidine hydrochloride, 4-aminopyridine (4-AP), and 3,4-diaminopyridine. The aminopyridines, particularly 4-AP, decrease the seizure threshold. Anticholinesterases may improve symptoms in some patients. In paraneoplastic cases, successful treatment of the underlying neoplasm is the best therapy and may cause full remission of symptoms. Although improvement after IVIG also has been reported and other immunomodulatory therapies have been utilized (i.e., PE, oral steroids), the results of these interventions are often disappointing.

45. **What precautions must be taken for surgical procedures that require general anesthesia in patients with MG and LEMS?**
Delayed recovery from neuromuscular blocking agents must be anticipated in both LEMS and MG. Nondepolarizing, short-acting neuromuscular blockers at minimal necessary doses are preferred. Intravenous steroids equivalent to oral maintenance doses should be given until oral steroids can be resumed. An additional bolus during surgery may also be helpful. Anticholinesterase therapy is usually unnecessary during surgery but is started postoperatively as needed when the patient regains consciousness. The differences between parenteral and oral doses of anticholinesterase should be recognized. Maintain normal serum electrolytes, calcium, phosphorus, and magnesium. Avoid unnecessary medications to minimize drug-related complications, especially those that may worsen neuromuscular transmission (see Question 27, Table 5-2).

KEY POINTS: OTHER NEUROMUSCULAR JUNCTION DISEASES

1. Antibodies against the presynaptic voltage-gated calcium channel cause LEMS, which is paraneoplastic in 60% of cases.
2. MG and LEMS both cause decrement on low-frequency RNS, but LEMS also causes dramatic increment on high-frequency RNS (often greater than 100%).
3. Botulism can often be distinguished from the aggressive onset of MG by the presence of dilated, minimally reactive pupils.

OTHER NEUROMUSCULAR JUNCTION DISEASES

46. **What are the clinical characteristics of botulism?**
Two to forty-eight hours after ingesting improperly prepared or preserved foods contaminated with *Clostridium botulinum*, ocular and bulbar muscle paralysis begins, with difficulty in convergence of the eyes, diplopia, ptosis, weakness of the jaw muscles, dysphagia, and dysarthria. Nausea, vomiting, and

diarrhea may precede these symptoms. Constipation, urinary retention, and nonreactive dilation of the pupils may occur because of autonomic dysfunction. Respiratory failure and total limb paralysis may ensue without sensory loss or mental status changes. Infantile botulism may result in poor sucking and difficulty with feeding, weak cry, loss of head control, and bilateral ptosis, with subsequent generalized flaccid paralysis. The course depends on the amount of toxin absorbed, ranging from death within 4 to 8 days without respiratory support to mild symptoms with complete recovery.

47. **What is the infectious process in botulism?**

   Botulinum toxin is an exotoxin of *C. botulinum*. The presence of common bacteria inhibits the growth of *C. botulinum*, but infection occurs when the victim ingests improperly prepared canned or bottled foods in which the common bacteria are killed, but the more resistant *Clostridium* spores are spared. In infants, the intestinal bacterial flora may not effectively inhibit the growth of *C. botulinum*. Human botulism is usually caused by exotoxin produced by types A, B, and E, which interfere with ACh release.

48. **What is the pharmacologic action of black widow spider venom?**

   Black widow spider venom promotes rapid release of ACh from the presynaptic nerve terminal, depleting its stores. The venom also inhibits choline uptake. Clinically, this causes painful muscle spasms with severe gastrointestinal symptoms, followed by weakness.

49. **What is the pharmacologic action of curare?**

   Curare is a classic antagonist of nicotinic AChRs and competes with ACh for the binding site, which is effective as a neuromuscular blocking agent (nondepolarizing blocker) for general anesthesia.

50. **Which snake venom causes a neuromuscular disorder?**

   Alpha-bungarotoxin, a potent toxin produced by the banded krait of Taiwan (*Bungarus multicinctus*), binds to the AChR at multiple sites on the alpha subunit, blocking ACh binding in a manner similar to MG.

51. **What is the importance of alpha-bungarotoxin in experimental studies of MG?**

   Because of its high affinity for the receptor, it is a useful marker for basic scientific investigation. Envenomation and clinical disease have become rare as the numbers of these snakes have steadily declined.

Acknowledgment

Previous editions of this chapter were coauthored by Tetsuo Ashizawa, MD.

 References available online at expertconsult.com.

WEBSITES

http://www.myasthenia.org.
http://www.neuro.wustl.edu/neuromuscular/synmg.html.

BIBLIOGRAPHY

1. Amato A, Russell J: Neuromuscular Disorders, 2nd ed. New York, McGraw-Hill, 2008.
2. Gooch CL, DiMauro S: Myasthenia gravis. In Greenamyre JT, DiMauro S, Rowland L, et al.: MedLink Neurology, 10th ed. San Diego, Arbor Publishing Corporation, 2014. www.medlink.com.
3. Jayawant S, Parr J, Vincent A: Autoimmune myasthenia gravis. Handb Clin Neurol 113:1465-1468, 2013.
4. Sanders DB, Guptill JT: Myasthenia gravis and Lambert–Eaton myasthenic syndrome. Continuum (Minneap Minn) 20 (5 Peripheral Nervous System Disorders):1413-1425, 2014.

CHAPTER 6

PERIPHERAL NEUROPATHIES AND MOTOR NEURON DISEASES

Corey E. Goldsmith, Doris Kung

1. **What are the most common diseases affecting the peripheral nerve?**
   - Alcohol
   - Amyloid
   - Diabetes
   - Environmental toxins and drugs
   - Guillain–Barré
   - Hereditary
   - Infections
   - Nutritional
   - Paraneoplastic
   - Rheumatic (collagen vascular)
   - Systemic disease
   - Trauma
   - Tumors

2. **What is the anatomy of a peripheral nerve?**
   The outer layer of a peripheral nerve is called the epineurium. Each nerve is made up of a bundle of nerve fibers called fascicles and each fascicle is surrounded by a perineurium. Each fascicle is made up of a number of axons and each axon is sheathed in the endoneurium.

3. **How does a nerve's size and structure contribute to its speed of conduction? How are the peripheral fibers classified?**
   The larger the fiber, the less the electrical resistance and the faster the speed of conduction. Myelin increases a nerve's diameter and also insulates the current between nodes of Ranvier, increasing the overall conduction velocity. In myelinated nerves, the conduction velocity can be estimated to be 6 m/s/μm (e.g., a nerve that is 10 μm in diameter will conduct at approximately 60 m/s). In unmyelinated nerves, the velocity is approximately 1.7 m/s/μm. Peripheral nerve fibers are classified according to diameter and conduction velocity (Table 6-1).

4. **What are the patterns of peripheral nerve damage?**
   The nerve can be damaged by injury to the myelin, axon, cell body, or vasa nervorum. Four basic pathologic mechanisms underlie nerve injury (Fig. 6-1):
   1. **Wallerian degeneration** develops after injury to the axon and myelin, as in transection of the nerve. Distal to the transection, the axon and then myelin degenerate, followed within 3 to 5 days by failure to generate and conduct a nerve action potential. The axon may regrow within the architecture provided by the basement membrane of Schwann cells, but the degree and efficiency of regrowth depend on good approximation of the nerve ends.
   2. **Segmental demyelination** develops after damage to the myelin sheath or Schwann cell. Because the muscle is not denervated, no atrophy develops. Prognosis for complete recovery is good.
   3. **Axonal degeneration** develops from damage to the axon resulting in distal dying of the axon and subsequent loss of myelin. Once the distal nerve dies, the muscle is denervated; hence, muscle atrophy develops. The denervated muscle fibers can be reinnervated by surrounding nerves, but recovery may not be complete.
   4. **Neuronopathy** develops when damage to the cell body of the neuron results in the breakdown of the entire nerve, peripherally and centrally, involving the anterior horn cell or dorsal root ganglion.

Table 6-1. Peripheral Nerve Fibers

CLASSIFICATION	ALTERNATE CLASSIFICATION	MYELINATED?	TYPE	CONDUCTION VELOCITY
A		Yes	Somatic nerves	
α	I	Yes	Subset of afferent nerves supplying the muscle spindle Sensitive to the rate of change in fiber length Also efferent motor neurons	80-120 m/s
	Ia		Afferent fibers from the muscle spindle	
	Ib		Afferent fibers serving the Golgi tendon organ at the junction between muscle and tendon	
β	II	Yes	Subset of afferent nerves supplying the muscle spindle Respond to the overall length of the muscle spindle fiber Fastest cutaneous afferent fibers, supplying the hair and skin follicles	35-75 m/s
δ	III	Yes	Convey "fast pain" sensation from skin and muscle	5-30 m/s
B		Yes	Preganglionic efferent fibers of the autonomic nervous system	3-15 m/s
C	IV, afferent	No	Postganglionic efferent nerves of the autonomic nervous system Convey afferent "slow pain" sensation in somatic nerves	1-2 m/s

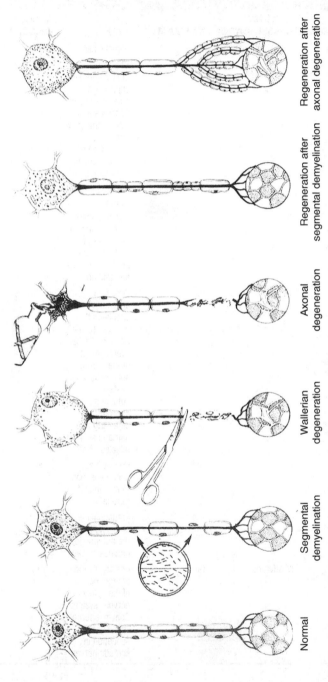

Figure 6-1. Segmental remyelination may follow segmental demyelination. The remyelinated segments are shorter and have a smaller diameter. Axonal regeneration is associated with the formation of clusters of small and thin myelinated fibers.

Normal — Segmental demyelination — Wallerian degeneration — Axonal degeneration — Regeneration after segmental demyelination — Regeneration after axonal degeneration

In acute nerve injuries, the extent and degree of damage can be graded using Sunderland's classification Grade I-V or Seddon's classification of neuropraxia, axonotmesis, and neurotmesis. Neuropraxia (Grade I) occurs when the myelin alone has been damaged with good prognosis for recovery within hours to weeks. Axonotmesis (Grades II-IV) refers to varying degrees of damage to the axons and surrounding connective tissues. Neurotmesis (Grade V) involves injury to the entire nerve including the epineurium (e.g., in a nerve transection). Usually both axonotmesis and neurotmesis result in incomplete or no recovery of function.

5. What are the electrophysiologic mechanisms that correlate with weakness in peripheral neuropathy?
Conduction block, denervation with loss of motor units, and failure of neuromuscular transmission. One or more of the above are needed. Slowing of motor conduction velocity in itself, even if severe, does not result in weakness.

6. What is conduction block?
Conduction block is a focal abnormality across a nerve segment that results in failure to conduct an action potential typically due to focal disruption of the myelin sheath. Distal to the block, conduction is preserved. In conduction block, a compound muscle action potential (CMAP) drop of 30% to 50% is recorded between the distal and proximal stimulation sites.

7. What is the significance of conduction block in peripheral neuropathy?
Conduction block occurs only in certain limited acquired settings of acute reversible ischemic injury, compression-induced demyelination, and acquired demyelinative neuropathies but not in hereditary neuropathies, with one major exception—hereditary neuropathy with liability to pressure palsy (HNPP). Clinically, conduction block is important because it implies a potentially reversible defect-causing weakness.

8. Define an "onion-bulb" formation.
An onion-bulb formation is the pathologic hallmark of the hypertrophic neuropathies, in which repeated segmental demyelination and remyelination have occurred (Fig. 6-2). When viewed in transverse sections, onion-bulb formations are multiple concentric layers of intertwined, attenuated Schwann cell processes surrounding the remaining nerve fibers. The Schwann cell processes are separated from each other by layers of collagen fibers. The onion-bulb formations may be seen in any condition with chronic segmental demyelination and remyelination but are frequently seen in Charcot–Marie–Tooth (CMT) disease, Dejerine–Sottas syndrome, Refsum's disease, and chronic relapsing idiopathic (inflammatory) demyelinating neuropathy.

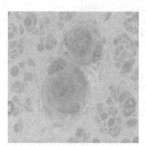

Figure 6-2. Semithin section. Note proliferation of Schwann cells with onion-bulb formation.

9. Which nerves are commonly used for biopsy?
The most common and best nerve to use is the sural nerve, a purely sensory nerve located lateral to the lateral malleolus. The nerve can be biopsied at this level or at a higher level between the heads of the gastrocnemius muscles. The superficial peroneal and radial cutaneous nerves can be sometimes used as well.

10. **What are the indications for sural nerve biopsy?**
Sural nerve biopsy is most helpful when the underlying condition is multifocal and asymmetric—mainly when a vasculitic etiology is suspected. It may be obtained in chronic demyelinating neuropathies with the aim of confirming the diagnosis when the clinical and electrophysiologic findings have been inconclusive, especially in patients who may be candidates for therapies with potentially harmful side effects. With the advent of genetic and other testing modalities, nerve biopsy is less necessary but may be of value as a final resort in patients with progressive, disabling peripheral neuropathy of undetermined etiology. The yield of nerve biopsy when vasculitis is suspected ranges from 50% to 60% while the yield in unknown neuropathy is in the 15% to 25% range.

11. **What are the common pathological findings on teased nerve fiber preparations?**
With teased nerve fiber preparation, segmental demyelination, remyelination, or axonal degeneration is identified. In segmental demyelination, the diameter of demyelinated segments is reduced. In remyelination, the internodal length varies. Axonal degeneration causes breakdown of myelin into "ovoids and balls" (Fig. 6-3).

12. **What is the outcome of the evaluation of patients with "peripheral neuropathy of undetermined etiology" when referred for a second opinion to a peripheral nerve expert at a tertiary referral center?**
Forty-two percent of patients have a hereditary neuropathy, 21% have an inflammatory neuropathy, and other conditions are discovered in 13% of patients. In 24% of the cases, even after extensive evaluation, no etiology for the neuropathy is identified.

COMMON NEUROPATHIES

13. **What is the most common cause of peripheral neuropathy in the world?**
Diabetes mellitus. Approximately 150 million people have diabetes and up to half of them have symptomatic diabetic neuropathy. The prevalence of diabetes is increasing every year. Alcoholic neuropathy is the second most common cause of peripheral neuropathy. Therefore, all patients with distal symmetric polyneuropathy should be screened for diabetes mellitus as well as unhealthy alcohol use. Leprosy was once the most common cause of neuropathy worldwide, but its incidence has dramatically decreased since 1982.

14. **What are the clinical forms of diabetic neuropathy?**
Diabetic neuropathies include distal symmetric sensory or sensorimotor polyneuropathy, small fiber neuropathy, diabetic neuropathic cachexia, hypoglycemic neuropathy, treatment-induced neuropathy (insulin neuritis), polyradiculopathy, diabetic lumbosacral radiculoplexus neuropathy (diabetic amyotrophy), mononeuropathies, and cranial neuropathies.

    Distal symmetric sensory polyneuropathy, the most common form, is a slowly progressive length-dependent axonal sensory polyneuropathy that presents with numbness and paresthesias in the feet, usually minimal motor weakness, and possibly autonomic changes.

15. **Which diabetic neuropathies are painful?**
    - Third cranial nerve neuropathy
    - Acute thoracoabdominal neuropathy
    - Acute distal sensory neuropathy
    - Acute lumbosacral radiculoplexus neuropathy
    - Chronic distal small-fiber neuropathy

16. **What are the risk factors for developing diabetic peripheral neuropathy?**
    - Duration of diabetes
    - Degree of glycemic control
    - Older age
    - Male sex
    - Excessive alcohol consumption
    - Nicotine use
    - Dyslipidemia
    - Angiotensin-converting enzyme D allele

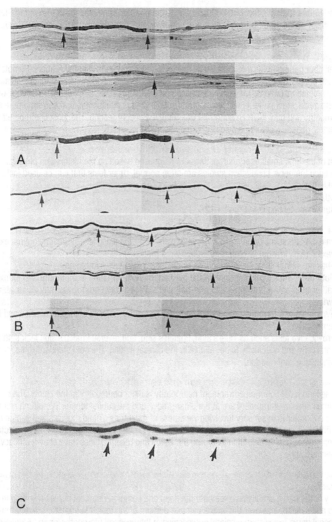

Figure 6-3. Teased nerve fiber preparation. **A,** Segmental demyelination. **B,** Remyelination. **C,** Axonal degeneration.

17. Describe alcoholic neuropathy.

Between 10% and 50% of alcoholics develop alcoholic neuropathy though in many it is asymptomatic. Usually it develops in alcoholics with prolonged and severe (>100 g/day) alcohol use. As a result, it is difficult to distinguish the direct effects of alcohol from the secondary effects of chronic malnutrition. Clinically, alcoholic neuropathy presents with dull aching or burning in the feet, hyperesthesia and/or sensory loss, distal hyporeflexia, and thin muscles with mild weakness in the feet sometimes with associated autonomic symptoms. Electromyography/nerve conduction velocity (EMG/NCV) would show a length-dependent axonal neuropathy. Symptoms can slowly improve with reduced alcohol intake and a balanced diet.

18. How does the global importance of leprous neuropathy compare to its importance in the United States?

The global registered prevalence of leprosy at the beginning of 2012 was 181,941 cases. In 2011, the number of new cases detected worldwide was 219,075. In contrast, the prevalence of leprosy in the United States is low (<10,000). In 2011, the number of new cases in the United States was 173. Most cases in the United States are in immigrants, but endemic areas include Texas, Louisiana, Florida, and Hawaii.

19. **What is small fiber neuropathy?**
Small fiber neuropathies affect the small myelinated A δ and unmyelinated C fibers. Symptoms usually consist of pain, numbness, burning, "pins and needles-like" sensations, and autonomic disturbances. On examination, patients may have decreased pinprick and temperature sensation with allodynia and hyperalgesia. Most patients will have normal sensory nerve conduction studies with a pure small fiber neuropathy and may have an abnormal Quantitative Sensory Testing. The most common etiologies are diabetes, genetic including amyloidosis, and idiopathic.

20. **What are the tests used to diagnose small fiber neuropathy?**
Most of the time small fiber neuropathies are diagnosed based on the history and physical examination since the nerve conduction studies are often normal. Other tests that can be used include:
- Skin biopsy
- Quantitative sensory testing
- Autonomic testing (see Chapter 12)

21. **Which clinical features aid in the diagnosis of carpal tunnel syndrome?**
- Pain, paresthesias, or numbness worse at night or during activities that maintain wrist extension or flexion (e.g., driving) or require repetitive wrist motion
- Shaking, wringing, or flicking motions of the hands to relieve symptoms
- Numbness often involving only partial median nerve innervation (e.g., thumb and index finger) rather than entire first three and one-half digits. Pain but not numbness may occur above the wrist.
- Symptoms of intermittent hand weakness before overt weakness of thenar muscles and lateral lumbricals
- Provocative tests such as Tinel's sign, Phalen's sign, and reverse Phalen's sign lack sufficient sensitivity and specificity to be reliable in the clinical setting. The gold standard remains electrodiagnostic confirmation.

22. **What is the second most common entrapment neuropathy?**
The second most common entrapment neuropathy is ulnar neuropathy at the elbow. The two most common sites of entrapment are at the ulnar groove and the cubital tunnel. Symptoms commonly are more motor than sensory involving weakness of the intrinsic hand muscles and sensory loss in the fifth digit, medial fourth digit, and hypothenar region, but not proximal to the wrist. Electrodiagnostic studies can be helpful in localizing the lesion and recent studies have shown efficacy using ultrasonography.

23. **What are the symptoms of peroneal (fibular) nerve compression at the fibular neck?**
Injury of the nerve usually involves both the deep and common peroneal nerves resulting in a foot drop and sensory loss over the lateral calf and dorsum of the foot. It is important to differentiate a peroneal nerve lesion from a sciatic nerve lesion, a lumbosacral plexopathy, or an L5 radiculopathy. Common causes of injury are trauma, stretch, or compression of the nerve.

24. **What are the three most common neurogenic causes of winging of the scapula?**
1. **Long thoracic nerve palsy:** The long thoracic nerve innervates the serratus anterior muscle. Serratus anterior weakness leads to the most pronounced winging, which is accentuated with forward flexion of the arms and decreased with the arms at rest. The superior (medial) angle of the scapula is displaced closer to the midline, whereas the inferior angle swings laterally and away from the thorax.
2. **Spinal accessory nerve palsy:** The spinal accessory nerve innervates the trapezius muscle. Trapezius muscle weakness leads to mild winging of the scapula at rest, which is accentuated by arm abduction to 90° and decreased by forward flexion to 90°. The superior (medial) angle of the scapula is displaced away from the midline, but the inferior angle is medially rotated. The shoulder is lower on the affected side because of atrophy of the trapezius muscle.
3. **Dorsal scapular nerve palsy:** The dorsal scapular nerve innervates the rhomboid muscle. Weakness of this muscle produces minimal winging at rest, which is accentuated by slowly lowering the arm from the forward overhead position and decreased by elevation of the arms overhead. The superior (medial) angle is displaced away from the midline, and the inferior angle is laterally displaced.

In addition, there are many nonneurogenic causes of winging of the scapula, including myopathies and muscular dystrophy (e.g., facioscapulohumeral muscle dystrophy).

25. **Which peripheral neuropathies may have cranial nerve involvement?**
See Table 6-2.

Table 6-2. Neuropathies with Cranial Nerve Involvement

NEUROPATHY	MOST COMMONLY INVOLVED CRANIAL NERVES	LESS COMMONLY INVOLVED CRANIAL NERVES
Diphtheria	IX	II, III
Sarcoid	VII	I, III, IV, VI
Diabetes	III*	IV, VI, VII
Guillain-Barré syndrome (GBS)	VI, VII	
Miller–Fisher variant of GBS	III, IV	
Sjögren's syndrome	V	
Celiac disease		V
Polyarteritis nodosa	VII, III, VIII	
Wegener's granulomatosis	VIII	
Lyme disease	VII, V	All but I
Porphyria	VII, X	III, IV, V, XI, XII
Refsum's disease	I, VIII	
Primary amyloidosis	VII, V, III	VI, XII
Syphilis	III	IV, V, VII, VIII
Arsenic	V	

*Pupil is usually not affected.

26. **Which neuropathies begin proximally rather than distally?**
Guillain–Barré syndrome (GBS), chronic inflammatory demyelinating neuropathy (CIDP), diabetic lumbosacral radiculoplexus neuropathy/diabetic amyotrophy, porphyric neuropathy, idiopathic acute brachial plexus neuropathy (Parsonage–Turner syndrome), and Tangier disease.

27. **Which neuropathies can begin in the arms rather than the legs?**
- Compression/entrapment syndromes (e.g., carpal tunnel syndrome, ulnar neuropathy at the elbow)
- Diabetes
- Vasculitic neuropathy
- GBS
- Multifocal motor neuropathy
- Lead toxicity
- Porphyria
- Sarcoidosis
- Leprosy
- CMT disease (rare)
- Tangier disease
- Inherited recurrent focal neuropathies
- Some forms of familial amyloid polyneuropathy

28. **Which neuropathies are often predominantly motor?**
GBS, diphtheric neuropathy, dapsone-induced neuropathy, porphyria, and multifocal motor neuropathy are often predominantly motor.

29. Which neuropathies are often predominantly sensory?
    - Drug toxicity: pyridoxine, doxorubicin, cisplatin, thalidomide, metronidazole
    - Autoimmune: Miller–Fisher syndrome, sensory variants of acute and chronic inflammatory demyelinating polyneuropathy, IgM paraproteinemia, paraneoplastic syndrome, Sjögren's syndrome
    - Infectious: diphtheria, human immunodeficiency virus (HIV), Lyme disease
    - Deficiency: vitamin E, pyridoxine
    - Inherited: neuropathies associated with abetalipoproteinemia and spinocerebellar degeneration

30. Which neuropathies are demyelinating?
    - Toxic/metabolic/infectious: diphtheria, buckthorn, hepatic, Creutzfeldt–Jakob disease (CJD), Hansen's disease (mixed)
    - Autoimmune: GBS, CIDP and variants, multifocal motor neuropathy (MMN), POEMS (polyneuropathy, organomegaly, endocrinopathy, monoclonal protein, skin changes)
    - Inherited: CMT syndromes, storage disorders (Krabbe, metachromatic leukodystrophy, Niemann–Pick, Farber's), Pelizaeus–Merzbacher, Refsum, Cockayne
    - Drug toxicity: chloroquine, tacrolimus, procainamide, amiodarone (mixed), gold (mixed), taxol (mixed)

31. What are the causes of multiple mononeuropathy (mononeuritis multiplex)?
    - Trauma or compression
    - Diabetes
    - Vasculitis, with or without connective tissue diseases; also virus associated (HIV, hepatitis B and C)
    - Leprosy
    - Lyme disease
    - Sarcoidosis
    - Sensory perineuritis
    - Tumor infiltration
    - Lymphoid granulomatosis
    - Demyelinating idiopathic and paraproteinemic neuropathies (MMN, multifocal acquired demyelinating sensory and motor neuropathy [MADSAM])
    - Hereditary neuropathy with liability to pressure palsies (HNPP)

32. In which conditions are the peripheral nerves palpably enlarged?
    - Hereditary motor and sensory neuropathies (HMSN) or CMT disease (demyelinative type) and Dejerine–Sottas syndrome (HMSNIII)
    - Amyloidosis
    - Refsum's disease
    - Leprosy
    - Acromegaly
    - Neurofibromatosis

GUILLAIN–BARRÉ SYNDROME

33. What is the typical presentation of GBS?
    The most common motor neuropathy is GBS. Symptoms often begin 1 to 3 weeks after a viral upper respiratory or gastrointestinal infection, immunization, or surgery. A typical patient with GBS reports a numb or tingling sensation in the arms and legs, followed by rapidly progressive ascending symmetric muscle weakness sometimes to the point of flaccid quadriplegia and inability to speak or swallow. Up to 30% of patients require artificial respiration. Paralysis is maximal by 2 weeks in more than 50% of patients and by 4 weeks in more than 90%. The patient may have mild impairment of distal sensation, but significant sensory loss is not seen. Hyporeflexia or areflexia is invariably present. Preservation of reflexes in a severely weakened patient should seriously challenge the diagnosis of GBS. Pain is present in 50% of patients. Over 50% of patients develop facial weakness, and 5% have extraocular muscular paralysis. Many patients also have autonomic dysfunction, including tachycardia, dysrhythmias, and very labile blood pressures. There are several symptomatic variants of GBS that probably form a continuous spectrum of disease including Miller–Fisher syndrome (the triad of ataxia, areflexia, and ophthalmoplegia often associated with GQ1b antibodies), Bickerstaff brainstem encephalitis, and the pharyngeal–cervical–brachial variant of GBS.

34. What are the two main pathologically distinct presentations of GBS?
    1. Acute inflammatory demyelinating polyradiculoneuropathy (AIDP) due to an immune attack on Schwann cell membrane or myelin sheath sometimes with secondary axonal damage.
    2. Acute (motor or motor-sensory) axonal neuropathy (AMAN or AMSAN) due to an immune attack against the axolemma/axoplasm. AMAN is much more common in Asia and occurs mainly in children. AMSAN may occur anywhere and affects adults preferentially. AMSAN has a much worse prognosis than AMAN, with only 20% of patients with the former ambulating at 1 year.

35. What are the typical laboratory and electrophysiologic findings in GBS?
    Classically, the CSF in patients with GBS demonstrates cytoalbuminologic dissociation, though in the first week this may not have manifested. CSF pleocytosis should bring to mind HIV, cytomegalovirus (CMV), Lyme disease, and sarcoid, lymphomatous, or carcinomatous polyradiculopathy.

    NCVs are slowed in AIDP, but may be normal within the first two weeks of onset. In early AIDP, absent or prolonged H-reflexes and F-waves, prolonged distal CMAP duration, and/or temporal dispersion may be seen. Conduction block and slowed velocities may be seen later. Conduction block accounts for most of the initial weakness, but after 2 to 3 weeks, axonal damage may contribute to weakness with EMG evidence of muscle denervation. "Sural sparing" is a particular electrophysiologic finding seen in AIDP. Sural sparing refers to the phenomenon of intact sural sensory responses but absent upper extremity sensory responses, which is atypical for more common length-dependent generalized polyneuropathies.

36. What is the significance of *Campylobacter jejuni* infection in GBS?
    Most patients (75%) with GBS and a preceding *C. jejuni* infection present with AIDP and often the axonal form. Not all patients with serologic evidence of *C. jejuni* have gastrointestinal symptoms before the onset of GBS. Cross-reactivity due to molecular mimicry between antigens from *C. jejuni* and various peripheral nerve gangliosides may explain the pathogenetic connection between the infection and GBS.

37. What are the predictors of severe disease and poorer outcome in patients with GBS?
    • Old age
    • Rapid onset of severe tetraparesis
    • Need for early artificial ventilation
    • Severely decreased CMAPs (<20% of normal)
    • Acute motor-sensory axonal form of the disease
       There are conflicting data as to whether evidence of preceding *C. jejuni* infection or presence of anti-GM1 antibodies is a predictor of disease severity or outcome. Mortality is greatest in the elderly and those with comorbid illnesses. Of the complications occurring during intensive care unit (ICU) admission, one study found that the development of ileus and risk of bowel perforation was most strongly associated with mortality. Recovery in ventilated patients with GBS may be prolonged, and final prognosis may require 2 or more years of follow-up. The Erasmus GBS Outcome Score (EGOS) and modified EGOS (mEGOS) has been developed to provide a better predictor of poor prognosis in patients with GBS. This study found that patients with preceding diarrhea, older age, and low Medical Research Council (MRC) sumscore (a measure of weakness) at presentation had the worst outcomes.

38. What percent of patients with GBS suffer a relapse or second episode?
    Based on several series of GBS patients, the incidence of recurrence lies somewhere between 1% and 6%, and recurrences may occur months to years after the initial episode. A recent study found that patients with Miller–Fisher syndrome, younger age, and milder disease were more likely to suffer a recurrence. There also appeared to be a trend toward shorter intervals between subsequent episodes and a more severe deficit with each recurrence.

39. How is GBS treated?
    Corticosteroids are not indicated in GBS. Plasma exchange (PE) and intravenous immunoglobulin (IVIG) started within 2 weeks of the illness equally improve the degree and rate of recovery. The Quality Standards Subcommittee of the AAN (2003) recommends treatment with PE for non-ambulant patients within 4 weeks of symptom onset; it should also be considered for ambulant patients within 2 weeks of symptom onset. Efficacy of the two treatments appears to be equal

in all subsets of GBS, except perhaps IgG anti-GMI-positive patients, who usually present with AMAN and for whom IVIG may be somewhat superior. Because IVIG offers the advantages of greater ease and convenience as well as greater safety of administration at similar costs, it is now considered the treatment of first choice. There is no added benefit from combining the two treatments. Immunoabsorption is an alternative to PE and obviates the need to use human blood products. Good supportive care is an essential part of GBS management (e.g., monitoring for and management of autonomic dysfunction, respiratory failure, and cardiovascular instability). Forty percent of hospitalized patients with GBS require inpatient rehabilitation, and patients may also require long-term follow-up for lingering symptoms (e.g., severe fatigue or sensory disturbances).

The prognosis in Miller–Fisher syndrome and Bickerstaff brainstem encephalitis is usually excellent, and therefore the role of IVIG or PE in the recovery from these conditions remains uncertain.

CHRONIC IMMUNE-RELATED DEMYELINATING POLYRADICULONEUROPATHY (CIDP) AND OTHER IMMUNE-MEDIATED NEUROPATHIES

40. What are the chronic acquired demyelinating polyneuropathies?
    - CIDP
    - CIDP variants: CIDP with central nervous system (CNS) demyelination, and CIDP in patients with hereditary neuropathy (i.e., CMT disease)
    - Lewis–Sumner syndrome/MADSAM
    - Sensory predominant demyelinating neuropathy
    - Distal acquired demyelinating symmetric neuropathy (DADS)
    - CIDP associated with systemic disorders: hepatitis B and C, inflammatory bowel disease, HIV, bone marrow and organ transplants, collagen vascular disease, thyrotoxicosis, lymphoma, melanoma, nephrotic syndrome, diabetes mellitus

41. What are the cardinal features of CIDP?
    - Progression over longer than 8 weeks or a relapsing course
    - Symmetric proximal and distal weakness in all extremities (legs more than arms)
    - Sensory impairment
    - Hyporeflexia or areflexia in all extremities
    - Elevated cerebrospinal fluid (CSF) protein without pleocytosis (cytoalbuminologic dissociation)
    - Electrodiagnostic evidence of demyelinating neuropathy
    - Pathologic evidence of demyelinating neuropathy on sural nerve biopsy

42. What are the electrodiagnostic findings that suggest a demyelinating neuropathy?
    Findings on nerve conduction studies consistent with a demyelinating neuropathy are prolonged F-wave latency or absent F waves, slowed conduction velocity, prolonged distal latency, and, particularly in acquired demyelinating neuropathies, presence of conduction block and/or temporal dispersion.

43. What immunosuppressive therapies are used in CIDP?
    The most common treatments for CIDP are corticosteroids, PE therapy, and high-dose IVIG. Randomized controlled studies have demonstrated efficacy in CIDP for all three therapies and comparable efficacy has been shown. Retrospective studies have shown that one-fourth of patients who are refractory to the standard treatments (i.e., IVIG, PE, or steroids) respond to another immunosuppressant.

    Other immunosuppressives considered for CIDP include cyclophosphamide, cyclosporine, mycophenolate mofetil, interferon-β, interferon-α, methotrexate, etanercept, rituximab, alemtuzumab, tacrolimus, and azathioprine.

44. What is the role of corticosteroids in the treatment of CIDP?
    Corticosteroids are an effective treatment for CIDP, and a trial of corticosteroids should be considered in all patients with this condition. Most patients who respond to prednisone demonstrate a positive effect within 8 weeks of therapy, but high doses (1 mg/kg/day) may be required. Overall prednisone, prednisolone, or dexamethasone can be used but there is no consensus on whether daily or every other day or intravenous pulse is better.

45. What is the role of PE in CIDP?

The efficacy of PE therapy in CIDP has been confirmed in two double-blind randomized controlled studies. With careful monitoring, benefit usually can be demonstrated within 6 weeks though improvement can be transient. PE is most commonly used in (1) the subgroup of patients with disability requiring treatment with immediate effectiveness while prednisone therapy is initiated; (2) patients with intermittent acute exacerbations; and (3) patients who are refractory or intolerant of other immunosuppressive therapies or in whom such therapies present substantial risks (e.g., diabetic or immunocompromised patients). Approximately 20% to 30% of patients with CIDP become refractory to all other therapies and are dependent on long-term intermittent PE or intravenous immunoglobulin.

46. Discuss the role of IVIG in CIDP.

The usefulness of IVIG in refractory and untreated CIDP has been confirmed by controlled studies. IVIG usually is administered intravenously at a dose of 0.4 g/kg/day for 3 to 5 days or 1 g/kg/day for 2 days. Benefits can be remarkable but are often short-lived (2 to 6 weeks), and stabilization of CIDP has been shown with regularly repeated infusions. The two factors that predict the need for continuing IVIG therapy for more than 2 years are the presence of profound weakness when the therapy is initiated and an incomplete recovery with residual deficits after 6 months of treatment.

47. What distinguishes multifocal motor neuropathy (MMN) with conduction block from CIDP and motor neuron disease?

MMN with conduction block is a presumed immune-mediated, chronic asymmetric motor neuropathy. The presence of weakness, atrophy, and fasciculations with normal sensation and asymmetric hypoactive reflexes identifies it as a lower motor neuron syndrome. Hyperreflexia does not typically occur, and there are no pathologic reflexes. Bulbar involvement is rare. Unlike CIDP, motor deficits usually start and are most prominent in the distal upper limbs. There is also a distinct predilection for more restricted and multifocal involvement of motor nerves. Motor conduction block in at least two nerves outside of the common entrapment sites with normal sensory nerve conduction study in the same segment defines MMN electrophysiologically. Antibodies to the ganglioside GM1 have been reported in about 40% to 50% of affected patients. Effective treatments include high-dose IVIG (first choice) and cyclophosphamide. IVIG may result in fairly rapid, although temporary, improvement in association with partial resolution of conduction block. Corticosteroids and PE are not effective in treating MMN and can sometimes result in worsening of symptoms. There is no correlation between the presence of conduction block and elevated anti-GM1 antibodies titer with responsiveness to IVIG.

48. Where are immune-mediated peripheral neuropathies most likely to cause initial nerve damage?

Immune-mediated peripheral neuropathies are most likely to cause initial nerve damage in areas where the blood–nerve barrier is deficient (i.e., motor roots, dorsal root ganglion, and motor–nerve terminals). The blood–nerve barrier serves to protect nerve fibers and endoneurial content from the vascular compartment. Where this barrier is incomplete, circulating cellular and humoral immune components have access to the nerve.

49. What is POEMS syndrome?

*P*olyneuropathy
*O*rganomegaly
*E*ndocrinopathy
M-protein
*S*kin changes

POEMS syndrome is an expanded variant of osteosclerotic myeloma with peripheral neuropathy. Not all features of the syndrome are required to make the diagnosis. Patients typically have a chronic progressive sensory-motor demyelinating polyneuropathy, monoclonal gammopathy (usually lambda light chain), peripheral edema, ascites, hypertrichosis, diffuse hyperpigmentation and thickening of the skin, hepatomegaly, splenomegaly, lymphadenopathy, gynecomastia, impotence, amenorrhea, and digital clubbing. Increased serum level of vascular endothelial growth factor (VEGF) is frequently observed in POEMS syndrome. Treatment results in a decrease in the level of VEGF, which correlates with symptomatic improvement, though there can be a delayed response in VEGF levels.

50. **How are monoclonal gammopathy and neuropathy associated?**
    Approximately 10% of peripheral neuropathies are associated with serum monoclonal gammopathy (M-protein). Two-thirds of such cases are initially classified as monoclonal gammopathy of uncertain significance (MGUS), but the remaining one-third, in decreasing frequency, are identified as multiple myeloma, amyloidosis, Waldenström macroglobulinemia, lymphoma, and leukemia. Of the patients with MGUS and neuropathy, the risk of ultimately developing an identifiable cause of the paraprotein (e.g., a hematologic malignancy) is 25%. Neuropathies associated with MGUS are a heterogeneous group that includes symmetric polyneuropathy, mononeuritis multiplex, isolated mononeuropathy, and cranial nerve palsies. While IgG forms the most common M-protein (74%) in patients with MGUS, in patients with MGUS and neuropathy, IgM is more common (48% vs 37% IgG and 15% IgA) and the best characterized.

51. **What is distal acquired demyelinating symmetric neuropathy (DADS), and how does it relate to anti-myelin-associated glycoprotein (anti-MAG) neuropathy?**
    DADS is a length-dependent sensory or sensorimotor neuropathy with demyelinating features on electrodiagnostic studies (typically prolonged distal motor latencies) and associated with an IgM paraprotein (usually with a kappa light chain) in about two-thirds of patients. When an IgM paraprotein is present with DADS, several features are typical. Patients are usually men in their 60s or 70s with predominantly large fiber sensory loss in their distal lower extremities. Motor involvement occurs to a lesser extent as the disease progresses. Patients have significant gait ataxia and may manifest hand tremors. In about 50% of patients with DADS and IgM paraprotein, the paraprotein reacts against MAG, which is thought to interfere with Schwann cell–axon interactions. In general, patients with DADS and IgM paraprotein are poorly responsive to immunomodulatory treatments but benefit in some patients given IVIG, rituximab, cyclophosphamide, or fludarabine has been reported. The DADS pattern without an IgM paraprotein is a nonspecific phenotype that can represent many different neuropathies but CIDP should be considered.

OTHER NEUROPATHIES

52. **How are the inherited neuropathies classified?**
    Most neuropathies that are initially labeled as idiopathic, and for which a cause is ultimately found, are inherited. As a group, they are probably underdiagnosed. They may be classified according to the pattern of inheritance (e.g., autosomal dominant: CMT1A–D, CMT2A–E; autosomal recessive: CMT4A–C; X-linked: CMTX); the gene involved (e.g., *PMP22*: CMT1A and HNPP; *MPZ*: CMT1B); the conduction velocity (e.g., demyelinating: CMT1A, CMT1B; axonal: CMT2; or with conduction velocities in the intermediate range: CMTX); or by the type of nerves involved (e.g., motor: HMN; sensory: HSN; autonomic: HAN; or combinations of all three: HMSN, HSAN). In addition, peripheral neuropathy forms part of several of the inherited ataxic syndromes (e.g., Friedreich's ataxia, spinocerebellar ataxias 3, 4, 10, and 18, among others) and accompanies many of the complicated hereditary spastic paraplegias. Finally, there are many inherited multisystem disorders that include peripheral neuropathy as part of the syndrome (e.g., Fabry's disease, Tangier disease, acute intermittent porphyria, and some of the leukodystrophies). The term *hereditary motor and sensory neuropathy* (HMSN) is broadly interchangeable with CMT.

53. **How does one recognize and diagnose hereditary neuropathy with liability to pressure palsies (HNPP)?**
    HNPP, also called recurrent pressure-sensitive neuropathy or tomaculous neuropathy, is readily identified in cases of recurrent compression-induced painless mononeuropathies and in patients with autosomal dominant familial patterns, demyelinative features on electrophysiologic studies, and "sausage-shaped" swellings or tomaculi on nerve biopsy (Fig. 6-4). However, a traumatic or compression-induced mechanism is not always obvious, and the pathologic evidence of numerous tomaculi may be the only diagnostic clue in sporadic cases presenting with a generalized polyneuropathy. Demonstrating *PMP22* gene deletion confirms the diagnosis. The most common nerves affected are the fibular and ulnar nerves. Generally mononeuropathies spontaneously resolve within days or weeks and recovery is complete 50% of the time. Electrophysiologic studies show prolonged distal motor latencies, especially involving the median and fibular nerves. Conduction block and focal motor slowing are noted at entrapment sites during an attack.

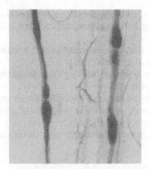

Figure 6-4. Teased nerve fiber preparation. Note focal areas of sausage-like (tomacula) thickening of the myelin sheaths.

54. **What are the causes of trigeminal sensory neuropathy?**
Trigeminal sensory neuropathy, a slowly progressive cranial neuropathy with unilateral or bilateral facial numbness or paresthesia, may be the presenting manifestation of connective tissue disease, especially Sjögren's syndrome. Celiac neuropathy is also prone to cause trigeminal neuropathy.

55. **What nutritional deficiencies can cause myelopathy and neuropathy?**
- Vitamin B12 deficiency
- Copper deficiency
- Vitamin E deficiency
- Folate deficiency

56. **What are the clinical features of copper deficiency?**
The main neurologic symptom of copper deficiency is gait difficulty. Examination shows predominantly large fiber sensory loss in the distal legs, spasticity in the lower extremities, hyperreflexia, and extensor plantar responses. Nerve conduction studies and needle EMG show an axonal sensorimotor neuropathy. Somatosensory evoked potential study shows impairment of central conduction. Anemia is a known associated laboratory finding, but the neurologic symptoms can be present in the absence of hematologic abnormalities. Risk factors include zinc overdose, gastric bypass, surgery, malabsorption syndrome, total parenteral nutrition without adequate copper supplementation, gastrectomy and small bowel resection, as well as nephrotic syndrome.

57. **What are the different types of Lyme neuropathies?**
Lymphocytic meningitis, cranial neuritis, or radiculoneuritis occur in up to 15% of patients with untreated *Borrelia burgdorferi* infection. Meningitis is the most common neurologic abnormality in Lyme disease often with associated cranial nerve involvement. A Guillain–Barré–like illness, a symmetric sensory-motor neuropathy (which may begin 6 months to 8 years after exposure), or radiculitis indistinguishable from a compression-induced radiculopathy is also possible. In endemic areas, Lyme disease accounts for about two-thirds of pediatric cases of facial palsy and as many as one-fourth of adult cases.

58. **How is Lyme disease of the CNS diagnosed and treated?**
Serologic testing is highly accurate after 4 to 6 weeks of infection. In CNS infection, production of anti-*B. burgdorferi* antibody is often demonstrable in CSF. All positive enzyme-linked immunosorbent assay results should be confirmed with Western blots to minimize false positives. Oral or IV antimicrobials are microbiologically curative in virtually all patients, including acute European neuroborreliosis. Some patients report fatigue and cognitive symptoms that do not improve with further antibiotics and are not evidence of continued infection.

59. **Which kinds of peripheral neuropathies are associated with HIV infection?**
Up to 50% of patients with HIV infection develop a peripheral neuropathy, which may take one or a combination of the following forms:
1. Distal symmetric neuropathy (30% to 60%)—Patients normally present with a stocking-glove pattern of numbness and paresthesias, hyporeflexia, and pain/temperature/vibratory loss with minimal

    motor weakness. Autonomic symptoms are often seen. Severity has not been correlated with low CD4 count or high viral load, but is associated with older age, height, statin use, substance abuse, diabetes, and triglyceridemia.

2. Acute inflammatory demyelinating polyneuropathy (AIDP) is associated with acute seroconversion and CIDP is more common in patients with HIV.
3. Mononeuropathy multiplex—early and mild in HIV infection or more severe associated with CMV, varicella, and hepatitis C infections
4. Polyradiculopathy—usually late (associated with CMV, herpes zoster, syphilis, lymphomatous)
5. Cranial and compressive neuropathies similar to the general population
6. Nutritional or vitamin deficiency neuropathy
7. Drug-induced neuropathy (associated with both nucleoside reverse transcription inhibitors and protease inhibitors)

60. What heavy metal exposures result in neuropathies?
    1. **Lead**—In children, lead exposure leads to cognitive problems; however, in adults, exposure is more likely to lead to a neuropathy associated with abdominal pain and anemia. An axonal multifocal motor neuropathy with radial neuropathy is most common though distal symmetric sensory loss can also be seen.
    2. **Arsenic**—Toxicity results in an acute or more chronic axonal sensorimotor neuropathy. Acutely, nausea, vomiting, abdominal pain, psychosis, and seizures are seen while chronic exposure causes Mee's lines, hyperpigmentation, and palmar/solar keratoses.
    3. **Thallium**—Acute toxicity causes a painful sensory neuropathy associated with alopecia. Chronic exposure produces an axonal sensorimotor neuropathy.
    4. **Mercury**—While primarily mercury causes cognitive and behavioral changes as well as ataxia, subacute exposure to the vapors can cause a motor axonal neuropathy and more chronic exposure causes a painful axonal sensorimotor polyneuropathy.

61. What are the most important industrial agents causing peripheral neuropathy?
    Peripheral neuropathy arising from exposure to industrial agents is uncommon in the developed world.
    1. **Organophosphates**—Found in insecticides, petroleum additives, and nerve gases, acute toxicity leads to cholinergic crisis. A length-dependent sensorimotor axonal neuropathy and possibly myelopathy can occur 7 to 10 days after exposure.
    2. **Ethylene oxide**—After exposure to ethylene oxide in antifreeze, paints, or detergents, CNS depression, cardiopulmonary toxicity, and renal toxicity occur early followed by severe axonal distal polyneuropathy.
    3. **Hexacarbons (*n*-hexane, methyl *n*-butyl ketone)**—Exposure to this toxin occurs with industrial use of hexacarbon solvents or inhalant abuse (glue sniffing). High-level exposure, especially in glue sniffers, can result in a subacute motor neuropathy leading to quadriparesis mimicking GBS while chronic exposure normally presents as an axonal sensory neuropathy.
    4. **Acrylamide**—Direct skin exposure or inhalation leads to a length-dependent sensory axonal neuropathy.

62. What are the causes of neuropathy in neoplastic disease?
    - Toxic neuropathy from chemotherapy—platinum salts, vinca alkaloids, taxanes, bortezomib, thalidomide, epothilones, eribulin, etc.
    - Nutritional neuropathy
    - Direct tumor infiltration—plexus involvement or rarely single nerve infiltration
    - Radiation plexopathy
    - Paraneoplastic vasculitic neuropathy or neuronopathy

63. Describe paraneoplastic neuropathies.
    The most common paraneoplastic neuropathy is distal sensorimotor axonal neuropathy indistinguishable from an idiopathic, nonparaneoplastic neuropathy with the same features. A sensory ganglionopathy or neuronopathy, which presents with severe sensory loss with marked sensory ataxia with minimal weakness, is also a paraneoplastic condition that accounts for 20% of cases of sensory ganglionopathies (the remainder being largely idiopathic or associated with Sjögren's syndrome). Subacute autonomic (widespread or limited) neuropathy and vasculitic neuropathy may also represent a paraneoplastic disorder. Lastly, the paraproteinemia-associated sensorimotor neuropathies such as POEMS are paraneoplastic.

Paraneoplastic neuropathies may occur in isolation or as part of a more generalized paraneoplastic neurologic syndrome (e.g., with limbic encephalitis and ataxia). The most common associated antibodies are anti-Hu (ANNA-1) and anti-CV2 (CRMP-5), with less common antibodies including amphiphysin, anti-Ri (ANNA-2), ANNA-3, and N-type calcium channel antibodies. Small-cell lung cancer tends to be the most common tumor associated with these syndromes, but many tumors are potential culprits.

64. Define critical-illness polyneuropathy.
Critical-illness polyneuropathy (CIP) develops in up to 50% of adult ICU patients who have lengthy mechanical ventilation, sepsis, or multiorgan failure. CIP may coexist with critical-illness myopathy in the same patient. Attention typically is brought to the neuropathy by difficulty in weaning the patient from the ventilator as a result of respiratory muscle weakness. Severe cases, with lengthy hospitalization, have limb weakness, sensory loss, and depressed stretch tendon reflexes. Electrophysiologic testing and nerve and muscle biopsies show findings consistent with axonal polyneuropathy and help to distinguish CIP from GBS, disorders of neuromuscular transmission, and myopathy. Most patients who survived their critical illness recover from CIP but recovery may be slow and often incomplete, even after 1 to 2 years.

65. How are the vasculitic neuropathies classified? What is their presentation and how are they treated?
Vasculitic neuropathies can be classified into either systemic vasculitic neuropathies (SVN) or nonsystemic vasculitic neuropathies (NSVN), where the vasculitis is largely restricted to the peripheral nervous system (Fig. 6-5). Vasculitis itself can be primary (e.g., Churg–Strauss syndrome, microscopic polyangitis, polyarteritis nodosa) or secondary (e.g., associated with connective tissue disorders such as rheumatoid arthritis; Sjögren's syndrome; infections such as hepatitis B, CMV, or HIV; or other causes such as medications).

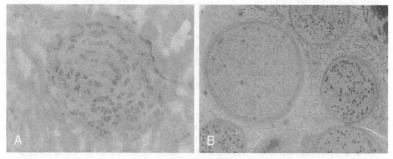

Figure 6-5. A, Modified trichrome. Inflammatory infiltrate with destruction of the blood vessel wall and obliteration of the lumen in a patient with vasculitic neuropathy. **B,** Semithin section. Differential involvement between and within nerve fascicles in a patient with vasculitic neuropathy. In most nonangiopathic/nonischemic neuropathies, involvement is more homogeneous.

The classic presentation from a neuropathy point of view involves acute or subacute painful sensory loss and weakness in the distribution of multiple peripheral nerves (a mononeuritis multiplex pattern). The stepwise progression and asymmetric multifocal involvement may become less evident as affected nerve territories become more confluent. Rare patients do have a distal symmetric sensory or sensorimotor neuropathy, and a plexopathy or polyradiculoneuropathy pattern may also occur. Pain and sensory symptoms are almost always present. In order of frequency, the most common nerves affected are the peroneal, sural, tibial, ulnar, median, radial, femoral, and sciatic. In SVN, there may be constitutional symptoms (fever, weight loss, malaise) that generally are absent in NSVN. Treatment for SVN usually involves induction therapy with steroid and cyclophosphamide (intravenous pulsed or oral daily doses) transitioning after several months to methotrexate or azathioprine to maintain remission. NSVN in contrast to SVN usually runs a more indolent course and may remit without treatment. For vasculitides associated with viral infections, treatment is aimed at the underlying infection (e.g., hepatitis C).

MOTOR NEURON DISEASES

66. **What is amyotrophic lateral sclerosis (ALS)?**

    ALS is the most common adult-onset progressive degenerative disorder of the upper and lower motor neurons. It produces a combination of muscular weakness, spasticity, and hyperreflexia (upper motor neurons) as well as flaccidity, atrophy, fasciculations, and hyporeflexia (lower motor neurons). Onset is bulbar in 20% of patients and in a limb in 80%. The deficits are strictly motor without significant signs of sensory loss, dementia, cerebellar, or extrapyramidal disease. Motor neurons controlling eye movements and sphincter function are usually spared as well. The disease, which usually begins in the sixth decade of life with a range spanning most of adulthood, generally progresses to death within 3 to 5 years from aspiration or respiratory failure.

KEY POINTS: PERIPHERAL NEUROPATHIES

1. The most common causes of peripheral neuropathy are diabetes and alcoholism.
2. The most common motor neuropathy is GBS.
3. Nerve biopsy is seldom necessary for the diagnosis of peripheral neuropathy.
4. Peripheral neuropathy is a common complication of HIV infection.
5. The most often overlooked cause of peripheral neuropathy is genetic.
6. The spinal fluid of patients with GBS has high protein but normal cell counts (cytoalbuminologic dissociation).
7. The most common motor neuron disease is ALS.

---

67. **How is ALS diagnosed?**

    ALS is a clinical diagnosis based on the revised El Escorial criteria. Requirements include signs of upper motor neuron and lower motor neuron dysfunction by exam and/or neurophysiological testing with progressive spread to other regions. Electrodiagnostic testing is required and shows widespread denervation and reinnervation (fibrillation, fasciculations, and polyphasic high-amplitude muscle potentials) without significant sensory abnormalities or demyelination. Craniospinal axis neuroimaging is required to exclude other pathology that may explain symptoms. Underlying structural compromise is important. Although serum creatine kinase levels may be mildly elevated, other laboratory studies are usually normal.

68. **What genetic abnormalities are associated with ALS?**

    The exact cause of ALS is unknown. Approximately 8% to 10% of patients have a family history of the disease, usually in an autosomal dominant pattern. Multiple genes have now been associated with familial as well as sporadic ALS. The first discovered genetic defect, superoxide dismutase type 1 (SOD1), accounts for 15% to 20% of familial ALS and was the basis for the development of the drug riluzole used in treatment. Most importantly, a hexanucleotide repeat expansion (GGGGCC) in the noncoding region of chromosome 9 open reading frame 72 (C9orf72) accounts for 40% to 50% of familial ALS as well as likely many sporadic cases. Other important genes include transactive response DNA binding protein 43 (TARDBP) and fused in sarcoma (FUS), which both account for 5% of familial ALS. C9orf72 and TARDBP mutations clinically overlap with frontotemporal dementia syndromes as well.

69. **What is the differential diagnosis of ALS?**

    The most common condition misdiagnosed as ALS is multifocal motor neuropathy. Other diagnoses to consider include cervical cord/foramen magnum lesions (tumor, syringomyelia, syringobulbia, spondylosis), tropical or hereditary paraparesis, copper or vitamin B12 myelopathy, multiple sclerosis, spinal muscular atrophy, spinal bulbar muscular atrophy, myasthenia gravis, thyrotoxicosis, hyperparathyroidism, paraneoplastic conditions, and hexosaminidase A deficiency.

70. **Are ALS patients cognitively normal?**

    Traditionally, cognition was felt to be spared in patients with ALS. However, up to 50% of patients who have ALS have some cognitive impairment when detailed neuropsychologic evaluations are performed. Frontal executive dysfunction (i.e., verbal fluency and attention) is the most common finding. Other symptoms may range from mild behavioral impairment to up to 15% to 20% having severe cognitive impairment fulfilling the diagnostic criteria for frontotemporal dementia, especially given the genetic association with frontotemporal dementia.

71. **What topics need to be addressed when caring for patients with ALS?**
    - Possible use of disease-modifying drugs (riluzole)
    - Cognitive and behavioral screening
    - Symptomatic treatment of pseudobulbar palsy, sialorrhea, etc.
    - Pulmonary function testing, discussion/use of noninvasive ventilation (bilevel positive airway pressure [BiPAP])
    - Addressing dysphagia, weight loss, and other nutrition. Considering PEG tube placement
    - Considering the need for communication support
    - Discussion of wishes for end-of-life care

72. **What other conditions primarily affect the lower motor neuron (anterior horn cell)?**
    The differential diagnosis of deficits primarily confined to the anterior horn cell (AHC) includes several inherited diseases such as X-linked bulbospinal muscular atrophy and proximal spinal muscular atrophy. Acquired lower motor neuron syndromes including poliomyelitis, postpolio syndrome, progressive muscular atrophy, and AHC degeneration in other conditions (e.g., CJD) also need to be considered.

73. **What causes spinal muscular atrophy (SMA)?**
    SMA is an autosomal recessive disorder most commonly caused by deletions in the survival motor neuron gene 1 (*SMN1*) on chromosome 5q13. The severity of the clinical phenotype for an individual is inversely correlated with the number of *SMN2* copies.

74. **What are the clinical subtypes of SMA?**
    SMA subtypes are usually defined by the highest level of motor function achieved by the patient.
    - SMA type 1 (Werdnig–Hoffmann disease) is the most severe and common phenotype, accounting for 50% of patients diagnosed with SMA. Children with SMA type 1 are never able to sit independently, and most patients die by 2 years of age from respiratory failure. The diagnosis is usually made before 6 months of age.
    - SMA type 2 represents intermediate severity, and the age of onset is between 7 and 18 months. Patients are able to sit but unable to walk independently.
    - SMA type 3 (Kugelberg–Welander disease) is variable in its prognosis for motor function. Some patients require a wheelchair for mobility during childhood, while others are able to ambulate independently and only have minor weakness.
    - SMA type 4 is the mildest form of the disease and patients are diagnosed during the second and third decade of life. These patients have very mild weakness.

75. **What is Kennedy's disease?**
    Kennedy's disease, or X-linked spinal and bulbar muscular atrophy, is caused by an expansion of trinucleotide (CAG) repeats in the androgen receptor gene on chromosome Xq11-12. Affected individuals have more than 40 repeats. Kennedy's disease usually presents with a bulbar-onset lower motor syndrome associated with gynecomastia and prominent early perioral and tongue fasciculations but no dysphagia or dysarthria. EMG shows chronic and acute denervation with NCVs showing motor and sensory conduction abnormalities in the absence of significant sensory findings on exam. Progression is very slow and often does not limit lifespan.

76. **What is primary lateral sclerosis?**
    Primary lateral sclerosis is a rare, adult-onset, slowly progressive acquired motor neuron disease in which only signs of corticospinal tract dysfunction are seen. The diagnosis of primary lateral sclerosis requires the presence of symptoms for more than 4 years and the absence of lower motor neuron findings, family history of similar disorder, and sensory signs on examination. Laboratory evaluation for other causes of myelopathy and craniospinal imaging should be normal. Electrodiagnostic tests show normal nerve conduction study, and the EMG should not satisfy the El Escorial criteria for ALS.

77. **Who was Lou Gehrig?**
    Lou Gehrig, whose name has been given to ALS, played first base for the New York Yankees from 1923 to 1939, usually batting after Babe Ruth in the lineup, and won six World Series Championships. He had a lifetime batting average of 0.340 with 23 grand slams (a record) and was the first

modern player to hit four home runs in one game. He is best known as "Ironman" for his record of playing 2130 consecutive games. In 1939, he was elected to the Baseball Hall of Fame and was the first Major League Baseball player to have his uniform number retired. He died of ALS 2 years after diagnosis in 1941.

Acknowledgments

The authors would like to acknowledge the contributions of Dr. Yadollah Harati who authored this chapter in the previous edition.

 References available online at expertconsult.com.

WEBSITES

http://www.neuro.wustl.edu/neuromuscular
http://www.genetests.org

BIBLIOGRAPHY

1. Aminoff MJ: Electrodiagnosis in Clinical Neurology, Philadelphia, Churchill Livingstone, 2012.
2. Bertorini TE: Clinical Evaluation and Diagnostic Test for Neuromuscular Disorders, Boston, Butterworth-Heinemann, 2002.
3. Dyck PJ, Thomas PK: Peripheral Neuropathy, Philadelphia, Saunders, 2005.
4. Gries FA, Cameron N (eds): Textbook of Diabetic Neuropathy, New York, Thieme, 2003.
5. Harati Y: Peripheral Neuropathies, An Issue of Neurologic Clinics, Philadelphia, Saunders, 2007.
6. Harati Y, Bosch EP: Disorders of peripheral nerves. In Neurology in Clinical Practice, Boston, Butterworth Heinemann, 2007.
7. Mendell JR, Cornblath DR, Kissell JT: Diagnosis and Management of Peripheral Nerve Disorders, Oxford, Oxford University Press, 2001.
8. Mitsumoto H, Przedborski S, Gordon PH: Amyotrophic Lateral Sclerosis (Neurological Disease and Therapy), Oxford, Informa Healthcare, 2005.

CHAPTER 7

RADICULOPATHY AND DEGENERATIVE SPINE DISEASE

Randall Wright

BASIC ANATOMY

1. **Describe the difference between the dorsal and ventral rami of the spinal cord.**
   Nerve roots are attached to each segment of the spinal cord. Those that exit from the posterior lateral sulcus are called the *dorsal roots*, whereas the ventral roots emerge anterior over a wider area. Short mixed spinal nerves are formed when a pair of dorsal roots and ventral roots unites beyond the dorsal root ganglion. This mixed spinal root then divides into the thin dorsal root ramus and the thicker ventral root ramus. The dorsal root rami are the central processes of the unipolar cells located in the dorsal root ganglion. These fibers innervate the paraspinal muscles and overlying skin and also carry sensory information. The ventral root rami are essentially extensions of the anterior horn motor neurons, and innervate the muscles of the cervical, brachial, or lumbosacral plexus. In addition to motor fibers, the ventral ramus also contains axons originating from sensory and sympathetic ganglia (Fig. 7-1).

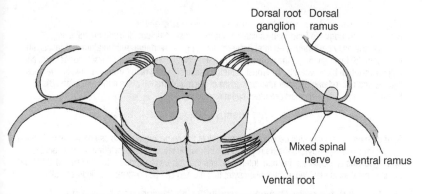

Figure 7-1. Anatomy of the spinal cord and its roots. *(Courtesy Randall J. Wright, MD.)*

2. **How many spinal nerve pairs exit the spinal cord?**
   There are 31 pairs of spinal nerves (8 cervical, 12 thoracic, 5 lumbar, 5 sacral, and 1 coccygeal). Because there are only seven cervical vertebrae, the first seven cervical nerves exit **above** the same numbered cervical vertebrae. The eighth cervical nerve exits above the T1 vertebrae, and the rest of the spinal nerves (T2 to L5) exit below their same numbered vertebrae. Think of it as "the heavenly seven cervical nerves arise above the vertebral body" (Fig. 7-2).

3. **Where do the lumbar nerve roots exit, and which root is most likely to be injured in a disc herniation?**
   The lumbar nerve roots exit beneath the corresponding vertebral pedicle through the respective foramen. For example, the L5 nerve root exits beneath the L5 vertebral pedicle through the L5/S1 foramen. Since most disc herniations occur posterolaterally, the root that is compressed is actually the root that exits the foramen **below** the herniated disc. So, a disc protrusion at L4/L5 will compress the L5 root, and a protrusion at L5/S1 will compress the S1 root. Ninety-five percent of disc herniations occur at the L4/5 or L5/S1 disc spaces. Herniations at higher levels are uncommon.

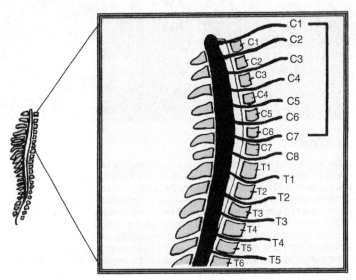

Figure 7-2. The first seven cervical nerves ("heavenly seven") exit above their corresponding vertebral bodies. *(Courtesy Randall J. Wright, MD.)*

4. Which anatomic structures are potential pain generators?
   Back pain may originate from many spinal structures. These structures include the following: (1) the vertebral body periosteum, (2) intervertebral discs, (3) paravertebral musculature and fascia, (4) ligaments, (5) facet joints, (6) the annulus fibrosus, (7) spinal nerve roots, (8) dorsal root ganglia, and (9) paravertebral blood vessels. The most common causes for pain result from musculoligamentous injuries and age-related degenerative processes of the intervertebral discs and facet joints. Disc herniations and spinal stenosis are other common causes.

5. What is the distinction between spondylosis, spondylolisthesis, and spondylolysis?
   Spondylosis is a nonspecific degenerative process of the spine, often due to osteoarthritis with osteophyte formation. **Spondylolisthesis** refers to anterior subluxation of one vertebral body on another. **Spondylolysis** is a defect in the pars interarticularis that allows the vertebra to slip upward. All three of these conditions may cause pain when symptomatic and can be confirmed radiographically.

6. What is the difference between a disc bulge, protrusion, and herniation?
   A **bulging disc** occurs when dehydration leads to gradual flattening of the disc and an increase in the circumference of the intact annular ring, which then extends beyond the margins of the vertebral body. **Disc protrusion** occurs when the gelatinous disc material protrudes focally into tears or fissures within the intact annular shell, causing a focal outpouching of the still intact annular fibers. **Disc herniation** refers to extrusion of nuclear material through the disrupted annular shell.

7. What are the most common causes of spinal stenosis?
   A variety of conditions can cause spinal stenosis. It may result from minor developmental anatomic changes in the diameter of the spinal canal (e.g., shorter than normal pedicles, thickened lamina). These conditions are rarely symptomatic but may predispose to degenerative changes that do become symptomatic. Such changes include degeneration of facets posteriorly and the disc anteriorly. Osteophyte formation may occur, thus narrowing both the nerve root and central canals. Degeneration of the intravertebral disc may also cause narrowing of the nerve root and central canals. Other causes of spinal stenosis include degenerative spondylolisthesis and postoperative spinal stenosis.

8. What are the differences between radicular and referred pain?
   The key feature of **radicular pain** is hot, electric sensations that radiate in the territory of the affected nerve root. The pain will be sharp, shooting, and burning. The pain radiates down the limb but never up. Sensory loss is rarely complete due to overlapping of other roots.

Referred pain is a phenomenon that occurs when irritated or injured tissues (e.g., muscle, facet joint, or periosteum) cause pain that is perceived in a dermatomal distribution. This pain may be shooting but is typically not hot or electrical as in radicular pain.

9. **Which spinal disorders cause both axial pain (back or neck) and disturbances in neurologic function of the limb (leg or arm)?**
   Three syndromes are recognized in which spinal disorders cause both back or neck pain and neurologic dysfunction. The following examples are from the lumbar spine:
   - **Herniated disc causing a single nerve root compression** (leg pain > back pain). Clinical features include positive straight leg-raising test and radicular pain in the limb disproportionate to pain in the spine. Loss of strength, reflex, and sensation occurs in the territory of the compressed root.
   - **Lateral recess syndrome** (leg pain ≥ back pain). Single or multiple nerve roots on one or both sides become compressed. Pain in the limb is usually equal to or greater than that in the spine. Symptoms are brought on by either walking or standing and are relieved with sitting. Testing by straight leg raise may be negative.
   - **Spinal stenosis** (leg pain < back pain). Multiple nerve roots are involved, and the pain in the spine is significantly greater than that in the limb. Symptoms develop with standing or walking. Impairment in bowel and bladder dysfunction as well as sexual dysfunction may occur.

LUMBAR SPINE DISEASE

10. **What are the clinical features of lumbar disc disease?**
    Acute lumbosacral disc herniation may cause a continuum of pain ranging from an isolated dull ache to severe radicular pain due to neurocompression in the foramen or lateral recess. A rare complication is cauda equina syndrome due to a massive central herniation. Pain is often sudden in onset and exacerbated with the Valsalva maneuver. Concomitant paraspinal spasm is often present. Ninety-five percent of disc herniations occur at the L4/5 or L5/S1 disc spaces. Herniations at higher levels are uncommon.

11. **What are the signs of an L4 radiculopathy?**
    Compression of the L4 root produces pain and paresthesias radiating to the hip, anterior thigh, and medial aspects of the knee and calf. Sensation is impaired over the medial calf. Weakness occurs in the quadriceps and hip adductors. The knee jerk is diminished.

12. **What are signs of an L5 radiculopathy?**
    L5 root compression produces pain radiating to the posterolateral buttock, lateral posterior thigh, and lateral leg. Sensory loss is most likely in a triangular wedge involving the great toe, second toe, and adjacent skin on the dorsum of the foot. Weakness occurs in the muscles innervated by the L5 root (gluteus medius, tibialis anterior and posterior, peronei, and extensor hallucis longus). This results in difficulty in ankle dorsiflexion, eversion, inversion, and hip abduction. It is most easily identified by weakness in the extensor hallucis longus (extension of the big toe). The ankle reflex is usually normal.

13. **What are the signs of an S1 radiculopathy?**
    S1 root compression causes pain to radiate to the posterior buttock, posterior calf, and lateral foot (classic sciatica). Sensory loss occurs along the lateral aspect of the foot, especially in the third, fourth, and fifth toes. Weakness may occur in the gluteus maximus (hip flexor) and plantar flexors. The ankle jerk is usually diminished (Fig. 7-3).

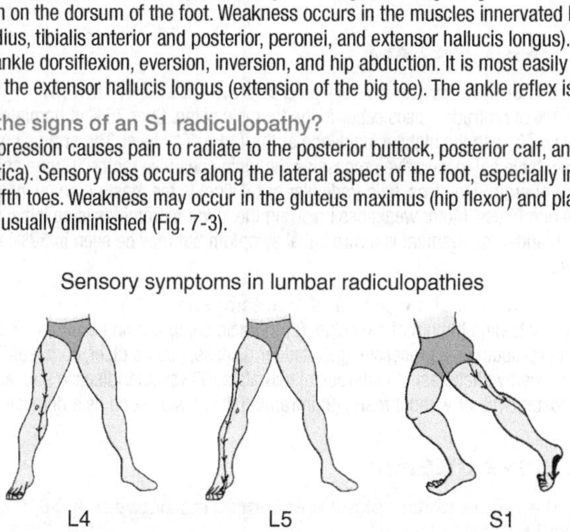

Sensory symptoms in lumbar radiculopathies

L4   L5   S1

Figure 7-3. Pain from L4 compression radiates to the anterior thigh and medial portion of the lower leg. L5 compression causes radiating pain to the lateral aspect of the leg and big toe. S1 compression causes pain in the lateral foot. *(Courtesy Randall J. Wright, MD.)*

14. **What are the clinical features of lumbar stenosis?**

    Most patients are age 50 years and older and have had symptoms referable to lumbar spinal stenosis for more than 1 year. Neurogenic intermittent claudication or pseudoclaudication is the most common presenting and constant symptom in lumbar spinal stenosis. Symptoms are usually bilateral, with one leg more involved than the other, but they may be unilateral. The whole lower extremity is generally affected. Pain is provoked by walking and, in many patients, merely by standing. It is typically dull in character and is quickly relieved by sitting or leaning forward. In some patients, the pain is accompanied by numbness of the affected leg and the feeling that it "may give out" on them.

KEY POINTS: CLINICAL FEATURES OF LUMBAR STENOSIS

1. Presence of intermittent neurogenic claudication (pseudoclaudication).
2. Pain is provoked by walking or standing and is relieved with rest (lying, sitting, or flexing).
3. Symptoms are usually bilateral but may be asymmetric.
4. Often there is no objective sensory loss.
5. Leg weakness and urinary incontinence are seldom present.
6. Unlike vascular claudication, pain may persist if the patient stops walking without flexing the spine.

---

15. **What is the mechanism for neurogenic claudication in lumbar spinal stenosis?**

    Symptoms are related to the increase in lordotic posture provoked by standing or walking. Myelographic studies have shown that in lordosis, the cross-sectional area of the spinal canal narrows because of anterior encroachment by bulging discs, posterior encroachment by shortening and thickening of the ligamentum flavum, and lateral approximation of the articular facets. In flexion (as in sitting), all of these encroachments reverse, with a resultant increase in the cross-sectional area of the spinal canal. This may explain why some patients with neurogenic claudication may be able to ride a stationary bike (in the sitting position), while patients with vascular claudication may still have pain.

16. **What is the differential diagnosis of low back pain?**

    The most common alternate diagnoses include focal hip pathology, vertebral compression fractures, metastasis from malignancy, ankylosing spondylitis, and vertebral osteomyelitis. Rare causes of low back pain include abdominal aortic aneurysm, pelvic disorders, abdominal visceral pathology, and other neuropathic disorders (e.g., inflammatory polyneuropathies or mononeuropathies).

THORACIC SPINE DISEASE

17. **Describe the clinical presentation of a thoracic disc herniation.**

    Fewer than 1% of protruded discs occur in the thoracic spine. Over 75% of herniated thoracic discs develop below T8, with the highest incidence at the T11 to T12 level. The protrusion is usually central. Most patients have a degenerative process as the main causative factor; trauma accounts for only 10% to 20% of protruded discs. Pain (radicular or midline) is the most common initial symptom, followed by numbness. Motor weakness involving the lower extremities is an initial symptom in 28% of patients. Bladder involvement is a rare initial symptom but may be seen in 30% of patients at presentation.

18. **What is the differential diagnosis of thoracic pain?**

    (1) Malignant or benign tumors of the spine, (2) thoracic compression fractures, (3) ankylosing spondylosis, (4) intra-abdominal processes (gallbladder disease, gastric ulcer, pancreatitis), (5) thoracoabdominal neuropathy (diabetes), (6) intercostal neuralgia, (7) vascular disease (i.e., aortic aneurysm), (8) herpes zoster (with or without rash), (9) intramedullary lesion such as a demyelinating process.

CERVICAL SPINE DISEASE

19. **What are the differentiating signs and symptoms between a C6, C7, and C8 radiculopathy?**

    Compression of the cervical roots typically occurs from either osteophyte or disc herniation. Compression of the C6 nerve root results in radicular pain involving the shoulder, upper arm, and lateral side of the forearm and thumb. Weakness may occur in the deltoids, biceps, and pronator teres. Paresthesias may be felt in the thumb and index fingers. The bicep and brachioradialis reflexes may be diminished. Compression of the C7 nerve root results in radicular pain in the shoulder, chest, and forearm, as well as the index and middle fingers. Weakness may occur in the triceps and flexor carpi radialis. Paresthesias may occur in the index and middle fingers. The triceps reflex is typically diminished. C8 nerve root compression causes a similar pattern of pain as C7 radiculopathies, but paresthesias may occur in the fourth and fifth fingers. Weakness may occur in the intrinsic muscles of the hand and finger extensors (Fig. 7-4).

Sensory symptoms in cervical radiculopathies

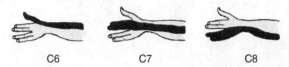

C6   C7   C8

Figure 7-4. Compression of the C6 nerve root causes radicular pain in the lateral side of the forearm and thumb. C7 compression causes pain in the index and middle fingers. C8 compression causes symptoms in the fourth and fifth fingers. *(Courtesy Randall J. Wright, MD.)*

KEY POINTS: SENSORY SYMPTOMS

1. The first seven cervical nerves exit **above** the same numbered cervical vertebrae.
2. L5 radiculopathies cause radiating pain along the posterior thigh to the dorsum of the foot and big toe.
3. Indications for surgery in patients with radiculopathies are intractable pain, progressive motor weakness or sensory deficits, or symptoms refractory to a reasonable period of nonoperative therapy.
4. Neurogenic claudication (pseudoclaudication) presents typically as bilateral, asymmetric, lower extremity pain that is provoked by walking (occasionally standing) and is relieved by rest.
5. Compression of the C6 nerve root causes radicular pain in the lateral side of the forearm and thumb, C7 compression causes pain in the index and middle fingers, and C8 compression causes symptoms in the fourth and fifth fingers.

20. **What is Spurling's sign?**
    Named after the neurosurgeon who popularized the posterior approach for cervical disc surgery, this maneuver is the cervical equivalent to the lumbar straight leg raise. Reproduction of the patient's pain occurs when the examiner exerts downward pressure on the vertex of the head while tilting the head (and occasionally extending it a little) toward the symptomatic side. This causes narrowing of the intervertebral foramen, which is painful.

21. **What is the differential diagnosis for cervical pain?**
    Diseases that most closely mimic cervical disc disease include brachial plexus lesions and shoulder dysfunction due to tendinitis, subacromial bursitis, or rotator cuff disease. Neoplastic or infectious processes also need to be excluded.

DIAGNOSTIC EVALUATION

22. **Which tests are useful in evaluating back pain?**
    - **Plain radiographs** provide information about bony alignment and degenerative changes.
    - **Dynamic flexion/extension films** provide information about osseous instability.
    - **Magnetic resonance imaging (MRI)** is sensitive for identifying intrinsic cord lesions, spinal root compression, spinal cord tumors, infections (abscesses), and herniated discs (Fig. 7-5).
    - **Computed tomography myelography** is especially valuable for evaluating nerve root compression (Fig. 7-6).

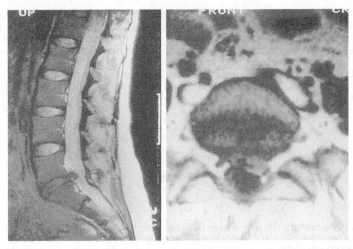

Figure 7-5. Magnetic resonance imaging scan shows a herniated disc at L5 and sagittal (*left*) and axial (*right*) views.

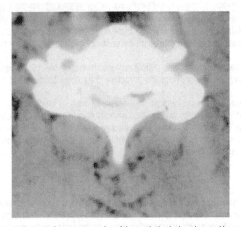

Figure 7-6. Computed tomography scan shows compression of the cervical spinal cord caused by severe cervical spondylosis.

23. Discuss the role of electromyography (EMG) in the evaluation of radiculopathy.

EMG provides neurophysiologic confirmation of the radiographic lesion. EMG evidence of altered innervation suggests significant nerve root compromise. The most widely accepted EMG evidence of radiculopathy is the presence of positive sharp waves and fibrillation potentials. EMG changes are first seen in the muscles closest to the site of nerve injury, underscoring the importance of examination of the paraspinous muscles. A disadvantage of EMG is the delay in the appearance of reliable abnormalities until 7 to 10 days after a root injury. The sequence of EMG changes begins with positive sharp waves in paraspinal muscles between days 7 and 10, followed by paraspinous fibrillation potentials and positive sharp waves in limb muscles between days 17 and 21.

24. What is the role of the H-reflex in an S1 radiculopathy?

The H-reflex is an evoked potential study performed by submaximal electrical stimulation of the S1 root and measuring the nerve conduction velocity proximally. Its absence indicates proximal (root) injury. It is the electrodiagnostic equivalent of the ankle jerk. The H-reflex may demonstrate abnormalities within 1 or 2 days after nerve root injury.

NONOPERATIVE TREATMENT OF SPINAL PAIN

25. **What is the rationale for nonoperative treatment of spine-related pain?**
The natural history of nonspecific spinal pain has been demonstrated to be benign. Approximately 90% of patients experience improvement within 3 months. Recent studies temper these results by suggesting that 75% of patients have one or more relapses, and 72% may still have at least some residual pain at 1 year. Patients with radiculopathy, whether due to soft disc herniation or spondylitic compression, usually improve with time. However, spinal stenosis usually stays stable or worsens with time. About 15% of patients with spinal stenosis improve, 70% remain stable, and 15% worsen after 4 years.

26. **Are bed rest and exercise helpful in treating acute and chronic back pain?**
Studies suggest that empiric bed rest in the acute phase of back pain is not as helpful as we once thought. It has not been found to increase the speed of recovery and in some instances may even delay recovery. However, in patients who report symptomatic relief from bed rest, 1 or 2 days of rest can be recommended. In the acute phase, back exercises have not been found to be helpful, but their role is very important in treating chronic back pain. In general, rapid return to normal activities with neither bed rest nor exercise seems to be the best recommendation for most patients in the acute phase of back pain. However, patients should be told to avoid heavy lifting, twisting of the trunk, and bodily vibrations during the acute phase of their back pain. Chronic back pain responds well to intense exercise programs.

27. **Which categories of medication may be of help during acute phases of pain?**
Nonsteroidal antiinflammatory drugs help relieve pain from mild musculoskeletal inflammation. Severe inflammation or nerve root swelling may be treated with a brief, tapering schedule of glucocorticoids. **Muscle relaxants** have been found helpful in some patients with muscle spasms and in helping to facilitate sleep (due to their sedative side effects). **Antidepressant** drugs (e.g., tricyclics) and **antiepileptic** drugs (e.g., gabapentin) may be helpful in treating neuropathic pain and may also help with sleep. Short-term pain relief with **opiate-based medications** can be beneficial in limited cases. For best results, pain medications should be given on a scheduled basis rather than on an as-needed basis.

OPERATIVE TREATMENT OF THE SPINE

28. **What is the role of surgery to treat cervical radiculopathies?**
Over 95% of patients with cervical radiculopathies due to a herniated disc improve with nonsurgical interventions. Surgery is indicated when symptoms fail to improve or progressive neurologic deficits develop. The goal of surgery for cervical radiculopathy is adequate decompression of the nerve roots, using either an anterior or posterior approach. The anterior approach is recommended for medial or central disc herniation or when fusion is contemplated. A posterior approach is necessitated by a posterolateral disc or osteophytes that are otherwise inaccessible.

KEY POINTS: INDICATIONS FOR SURGERY IN PATIENTS WITH RADICULOPATHIES

1. Intractable pain that has been refractory to conservative therapy
2. Severe or progressive motor weakness or sensory deficits
3. Symptoms refractory to a reasonable period of nonoperative therapy
4. Of note, outcomes are much better when signs and symptoms correlate with radiographic findings.

29. **Which surgical procedures are recommended for cervical radiculopathy?**
- **Anterior cervical discectomy (ACD)** is indicated when patients have minimal neck pain, normal cervical lordosis, and single-level pathology to avoid the potential complications of fusion. There is a 5% risk of laryngeal nerve injury with ACD.
- **Anterior cervical discectomy and fusion (ACDF)** is indicated for patients with symptoms of instability or more than one operative level. It is limited to levels C3 to C7. It allows for safe removal of osteophytes.

- **ACDF with internal fixation:** Plating is recommended for multilevel fusions with documented instability or history of prior fusion failure. It allows early mobilization without bracing.
- **Posterior cervical discectomy:** Usually reserved for either multiple cervical discs or osteophytes, cervical stenosis superimposed on disc herniation, and in situations where the risk of laryngeal nerve injury that is associated with ACD is unacceptable (e.g., professional singers and speakers).
- **Posterior keyhole laminotomy:** Used to decompress only individual nerve roots (not spinal cord). Useful in monoradiculopathy with posterolateral soft disc fragments and in cases in which the anterior approach is either difficult (patients with thick necks) or the risks are unacceptable (professional singers or speakers).

30. **What is the most common postoperative complication of spinal surgery?**
Arachnoiditis is commonly seen in the cauda equina after lumbar surgery, myelography using oil-based dye, and even intrathecal injections. It results in the adhesion and clumping of the nerve roots to each other and in turn results in radicular type pain, paresthesias, weakness, and sphincter dysfunction. MRI may show thickening and clumping of the nerve roots, adherence of roots to the thecal sac with enhancement, and loculations of spinal fluid. Surgical debridement and epidural and intrathecal steroid injections have been attempted as treatment, but none have shown efficacy. In fact, these techniques may even worsen the condition. Thus, treatment is mainly symptomatic.

31. **What are the most common causes of the failed (surgical) back?**
- The diagnosis was wrong. Therefore, even if the surgical treatment was technically flawless, the patient must be regarded as having never been treated for the presenting signs and symptoms and requires a thorough reassessment with generation of a new treatment plan.
- The diagnosis was correct, but the treatment was technically flawed or inappropriate.
- Whether or not the diagnosis was correct, something new has happened—perhaps an immediate or late consequence of treatment or an unrelated but intercurrent complication. This situation usually occurs when two or more pain-generating mechanisms coexist. For example, in disc herniation removal of disc material improves radicular symptoms but fails to address the mechanical pain produced by spinal instability after the herniation.
- A complication of diagnosis or treatment has arisen such as arachnoiditis, injury to a nerve root, or disc space infection.
- No preoperative counseling has been given. Physicians must discuss and in some instances negotiate with patients a plan of postsurgical treatment, stressing patient participation in functional restoration and dispelling unrealistic expectations of complete restoration to normal.

 References available online at expertconsult.com.

WEBSITE

http://www.backandbodycare.com

BIBLIOGRAPHY
1. Daroff RB, Fenichel GM, Jankovic J, Mazziotta JC (eds): Bradley's Neurology in Clinical Practice, 6th ed. Philadelphia, Elsevier, 2012.
2. Deyo R, Weinstein J: Low back pain. N Engl J Med 344:363-370, 2001.
3. Frymoyer JW, Wiesel SW (eds): The Adult and Pediatric Spine, 3rd ed. Philadelphia, Lippincott Williams & Wilkins, 2004.
4. Kaye AH: Essential Neurosurgery, 3rd ed. Malden (MA), Blackwell, 2005.
5. Malanga GA, Nadler SF: Nonoperative treatment of low back pain. Mayo Clin Proc 74:1135-1148, 1999.
6. Narayan P, Haid RW: Treatment of degenerative cervical disc disease. Neurol Clin 19:217-229, 2001.

CHAPTER 8

MYELOPATHIES

John Eatman, Ericka P. Simpson

1. Describe the most important long tracts in the spinal cord, their locations, and their functions.
   See Table 8-1.

2. Draw the anatomic locations of the anterior horn cells, cortical spinal tracts, dorsal column, and spinothalamic tracts.
   See Figure 8-1.

3. Where do the cortical spinal, dorsal column, lateral spinothalamic, and spinocerebellar tracts decussate (cross)?
   The descending cortical spinal tract decussates in the lower medulla, travels down the spinal cord, and innervates muscles contralateral to its motor strip of origin. The dorsal column tracts enter the spinal cord and ascend ipsilateral to their entry point. They then decussate in the lower medulla. The lateral spinothalamic tract enters the spinal cord and immediately decussates one to two levels above their entry points and then ascends in the spinal cord contralateral to their points of entry. The spinocerebellar tracts do not decussate.

4. What are the dermatomes at the umbilicus and the nipple line?
   The umbilicus is at T10. The nipple line is at T4.

5. What is the relationship of the cord segment and its spinal nerves to the vertebral body?
   The spinal cord extends from the medullary cervical junction at the foramen magnum to the level of the body of the first or second lumbar vertebra. The spinal roots exit in relation to their corresponding vertebral body. The first seven cervical nerves exit above the vertebral body, and the eighth exits below C7. The remainder of the spinal roots exit below their corresponding vertebral body.

6. What are signs of the anterior spinal artery syndrome?
   Anterior spinal artery syndrome occurs when the anterior spinal artery is occluded. This artery supplies blood to the anterior two-thirds of the spinal cord. Occlusion results in bilateral loss of pain and temperature below the lesion, accompanied by weakness and bladder dysfunction. The reflexes may be hyperactive below the level of the lesion. Dorsal column functions (position and vibration sense) are spared.

7. What is the artery of Adamkiewicz?
   The artery of Adamkiewicz is the major thoracolumbar radicular artery supplying the spinal cord. The artery is a branch off the aorta and is also known as the great anterior radiculomedullary artery. It's exact origin off the aorta varies widely and enters the cord between T6 and L1, typically on the left side of the body, but it can originate on the right in about one-third. It supplies the lumbar and lower thoracic segments. It forms anastomoses with the anterior spinal artery in the lower thoracic region, where the watershed area of the spinal cord is located.

8. What areas of the spinal cord are supplied by the posterior spinal artery?
   The posterior spinal arteries are paired arteries that run dorsolateral to the spinal cord. They extend the length of the cord and supply the posterior third of the cord through circumflex and penetrating vessels. Occlusion of one of these arteries results in ipsilateral deficits in vibratory and proprioceptive sensation below the site of occlusion.

9. What is a myelopathy?
   A myelopathy is any pathologic process that affects primarily the spinal cord and causes neurologic dysfunction. The most common causes of myelopathies are as follows:
   1. Congenital and developmental defects:
      - Syringomyelia
      - Neural tube formation defects

Table 8-1. Long Tracts in the Spinal Cord

TRACT	LOCATION	FUNCTIONS
Gracile medial	Dorsal column	Proprioception from the leg
Cuneate	Lateral dorsal column	Proprioception from the arm
Spinocerebellar	Superficial lateral column	Muscular position and tone
Pyramidal	Deep lateral column	Motor control
Lateral spinothalamic	Ventrolateral column	Pain and thermal sensation

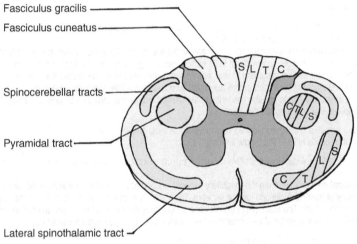

Figure 8-1. Relative location of each tract. The cortical spinal and spinothalamic tracts are laminated so that the most lateral fibers are the sacral fibers and the most medial are the cervical. The opposite is true in the dorsal columns; the most lateral fibers are the cervical and the most medial fibers are the sacral. This becomes important when distinguishing intramedullary from extramedullary lesions. *C*, Cervical; *T*, thoracic; *L*, lumbar; *S*, sacral.

2. Trauma
3. Compromise of the spinal cord:
    - Cervical spondylosis
    - Inflammatory arthritis
    - Acute disc herniation
4. Neoplasms:
    - Primary spinal and paraspinal
5. Physical agents:
    - Decompression sickness
    - Electrical injury
    - Radiation
6. Toxins:
    - Nitrous oxide
    - Triorthocresyl phosphate
7. Metabolic and nutritional disorders:
    - Vitamin B12 deficiency
    - Copper deficiency
    - Chronic liver disease
    - Thiamine deficiency (beri-beri)

8. Paraneoplastic myelitis
9. Arachnoiditis
10. Systemic autoimmune disorders:
    - Lupus
    - Sjögren's syndrome
    - Systemic vasculitis
11. Demyelinating disease:
    - Multiple sclerosis
    - Neuromyelitis optica
12. Epidural infections
13. Primary infections:
    - Human immunodeficiency virus (HIV vacuolar myelopathy)
    - Syphilis (tabes dorsalis)
    - Human T-lymphotropic virus (HTLV)-1,2 (tropical spastic paraparesis)
    - Varicella zoster virus myelopathy
    - Lyme radiculomyelitis
    - Tuberculosis
    - Spinal epidural abscess
14. Vascular causes:
    - Epidural hematoma
    - Atherosclerotic, abdominal aneurysm
    - Spinal dural arteriovenous fistula and other vascular malformations
    - Spinal artery infarction

KEY POINTS: CLINICAL FINDINGS SUGGESTIVE OF A MYELOPATHY

1. Bilateral upper motor neuron weakness of the legs (paraparesis, paraplegia) or legs and arms (quadriparesis, quadriplegia)
2. Bilateral impairment of sensation with a "sensory level" that separates a region of normal sensation from a region of impaired sensation
3. Bowel or bladder sphincter dysfunction

10. What is Lhermitte's sign?

Lhermitte's sign (also known as Lhermitte's phenomenon) is present when the patient reports an electric shock-like sensation down the spine with neck flexion. It is most commonly associated with multiple sclerosis. In patients with multiple sclerosis, the prevalence is thought to be approximately 15%. The symptom is produced by stretching or irritating damaged fibers in the dorsal columns of the cervical cord. In addition to multiple sclerosis, it may also occur in cervical spondylogenic myelopathy, intramedullary lesions, or as part of subacute combined degeneration from vitamin B12 deficiency.

11. What is the anal wink?

Anal wink is a reflex that tests the integrity of S2 to S5 segments. The anal wink reflex is tested by pricking the skin of the perianal region and watching for the external anal sphincter to contract. The absence of this contraction signifies a lesion in the sacral region.

12. What is "saddle anesthesia"?

It is tempting to believe that saddle anesthesia results from prolonged horseback riding. However, this condition describes the sensory loss in the perianal region (saddle) that results from lesions involving the S1 and S2 segments of the spinal cord. It may be accompanied by sensory loss in the medial aspects of the calf and posterior thigh. Symmetric saddle anesthesia may result from lesions in the conus medullaris.

13. What is the superficial abdominal reflex?

The superficial abdominal reflex is elicited by pricking the skin of the abdomen and watching for contraction of the abdominal wall muscles. This reflex is often diminished or absent below the level of a spinal cord lesion. In individuals with excessive adipose tissue in the abdominal region, this reflex may be difficult to observe.

14. **How does the jaw jerk reflex help in localizing lesions in patients with hyperreflexia?**

    The jaw jerk is a reflex that involves the contraction of the masseter and temporalis muscles when the patient's lower jaw is tapped. The afferent limb travels via the mandibular branch of the trigeminal nerve to the mesencephalic nucleus of the trigeminal nerve. The efferent limb arises from the motor nucleus of the trigeminal nerve and also travels via the mandibular branch. The jaw jerk is exaggerated with bilateral lesions above the trigeminal nerve but will not be affected by lesions below it in the spinal cord. This is helpful in patients who have hyperreflexia in all four extremities because an exaggerated jaw jerk reflex suggests that the lesion is above the level of the spinal cord (i.e., high brain stem or above).

15. **What is Brown–Sequard syndrome?**

    Brown–Sequard syndrome is caused by a lateral hemisection of the spinal cord that severs the pyramidal tract (which has already crossed in the medulla), the uncrossed dorsal columns, and the crossed spinothalamic tract. The region ipsilateral and below the level of the lesion demonstrates upper motor neuron weakness (paralysis), loss of tactile discrimination, loss of position sense, and loss of vibratory sense. The ipsilateral deep tendon reflexes become hyperactive with subsequent spasticity, and an extensor plantar response develops. Contralateral to the lesion, there is loss of pain and temperature sensation below the lesion.

16. **What is spinal shock?**

    If the spinal cord is damaged suddenly by mechanical trauma, ischemia, or compression, spinal shock may occur. This is a condition in which there is temporary loss of all spinal reflexes, motor activity, and sensation below the level of the lesion. Flaccid paralysis, hyporeflexia, sensory loss, and loss of bladder tone are cardinal features. There also may be autonomic dysfunction with diffuse sweating and hypotension. Development of upper motor neuron signs may take several weeks.

17. **What is transverse myelitis?**

    Transverse myelitis is an inflammatory process that is localized over several segments of the cord and functionally transects the cord. It may occur as an infectious or parainfectious illness or as a manifestation of multiple sclerosis, neuromyelitis optica, or other autoimmune process. Transverse myelitis is extremely rare with an incidence of 3 cases per 100,000 patient-years. Unfortunately, two-thirds of patients have moderate to severe residual disability. In a significant number of cases (40%), no specific etiology is ever identified (Fig. 8-2).

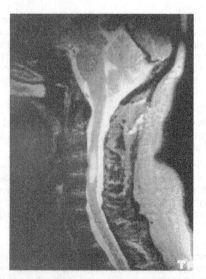

Figure 8-2. Sagittal T2-weighted magnetic resonance imaging (MRI) shows increased signal within the cervical cord caused by acute inflammatory transverse myelitis.

18. **What are the clinical features of acute transverse myelitis?**
The sudden onset of weakness and sensory disturbance in the legs and trunk is the usual present-ing feature. Ultimately, sphincter dysfunction is common. Pain and temperature are usually affected, but proprioception and vibration are often spared. The tendon jerks below the lesion may be initially depressed and then hyperactive. A sensory level indicates the level of the lesion.

19. **What is cervical spondylosis?**
Cervical spondylosis is a condition in which osteophyte proliferation in the cervical region results in narrowing of the spinal canal. These changes may result in cord compression if the canal diameter becomes small enough, and spinal cord circulation may also be compromised. Spon-dylitic changes also may compress the spinal nerves that exit through the foramen. If the spinal cord is compressed, upper motor neuron weakness (paresis, hypertonia, hyperreflexia) may be seen. This may appear before sensory impairment. When sensory loss does develop, dorsal col-umns tend to be more affected than lateral spinothalamic tracts. Bladder and bowel dysfunction is less common.

20. **Summarize the anatomy of masses that compress the spinal cord.**
    1. **Extramedullary extradural lesions** (outside the spinal cord and outside its dural covering). Such lesions include the following:
       • Epidural metastases from a remote primary neoplasm
       • Epidural abscess
       • Epidural hematoma
       • Herniated disc
    2. **Extramedullary intradural lesions** (outside the spinal cord but inside its dural covering). Such lesions include:
       • Neurofibroma and schwannoma
       • Meningioma
    3. **Intramedullary intradural lesions** (inside the cord itself). Such lesions include the following:
       • Primary cord neoplasms
       • Syringomyelia
       • Metastasis or abscess within the substance of the cord (rare)
    See Figure 8-3.

21. **What are the most common neoplasms arising with the spinal cord?**
Most primary spinal cord tumors are astrocytomas, ependymomas, or oligodendrogliomas (Fig. 8-4).

22. **What tumors commonly metastasize to the spinal cord?**
Neoplasms typically metastasize to the vertebral bodies and extend into the epidural space, causing extramedullary extradural compression of the spinal cord. The most common metastatic tumors to the spinal cord are: breast, lung, gastrointestinal (GI) tract, lymphoma/myeloma, and prostate.

23. **Describe the features of extramedullary lesions.**
Extramedullary lesions are lesions that compress the spinal cord from the outside. They can be extra-medullary extradural or extramedullary intradural. Either way, extramedullary lesions cause exterior compression of the spinal cord. Because of the somatotopic organization of the spinal cord, the spino-thalamic tracts and the corticospinal tracts are arranged so that the sacral fibers are the most lateral and the cervical fibers are the most medial. Because of this, external compression of the spinal cord causes the sacral regions to be affected first, followed by the lumbar, then thoracic, and then cervical. Thus, external compression causes ascending deficits starting in the sacral region and traveling up to one or two levels below the actual level of the lesion.

24. **Describe the features of intramedullary lesions.**
Intramedullary lesions are lesions that originate from within the spinal cord. If the lesion starts within one-half of the cord and grows outward, the innermost fibers are affected first. Once again, the somatotopic organization of the spinal cord is responsible for the clinical presentation. If the lesion is high (i.e., cervical cord), the cervical fibers are affected first, followed by thoracic, then lumbar, and finally sacral. So in this case, **intramedullary lesions cause sacral sparing of sensation.** Because the spinothalamic tracts cross the midline, intramedullary lesions cause sensory loss at one to two levels below their location. As the lesion (tumor) expands outward, the sensory deficits appear to descend as they subsequently affect the cervical, thoracic, lumbar, and finally sacral regions (Fig. 8-5).

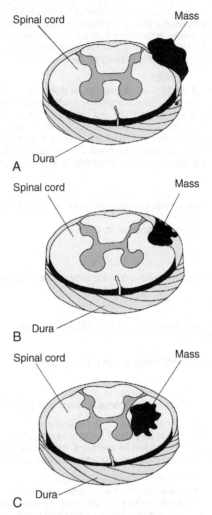

Figure 8-3. Location of spinal masses: **A,** extradural extramedullary; **B,** intradural extramedullary; **C,** intradural intramedullary.

25. Describe the features of lesions in the dorsal columns.

The dorsal columns relay fibers that are involved in proprioception and vibration. These fibers are also arranged somatotopically. However, within the dorsal columns the sacral fibers are medial and the cervical fibers are lateral. Thus, lateral lesions within the dorsal column will damage fibers from the cervical region. And conversely, medially located lesions in the dorsal column will damage sacral fibers. Lesions in the dorsal columns may result in deficits in vibration, proprioception, and two-point discrimination. Lhermitte's sign may also be present.

26. What is syringomyelia?

Syringomyelia is a longitudinal cystic cavity that develops within the substance of the cord. It may extend over a few or many segments of the cord and even into the medulla (syringobulbia). The cavity is irregular and tends to intrude into the anterior horns of the gray matter and the gray matter dorsal to the central canal. This condition may result from a developmental anomaly, trauma (hyperextension injuries of the neck), or ischemia, or it may be part of an intramedullary tumor.

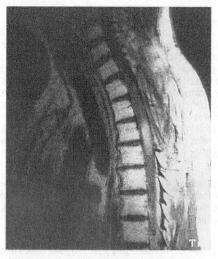

Figure 8-4. Sagittal T1-weighted magnetic resonance imaging (MRI), after gadolinium enhancement, shows an astrocytoma arising within the thoracic spinal cord (an intramedullary, intradural lesion).

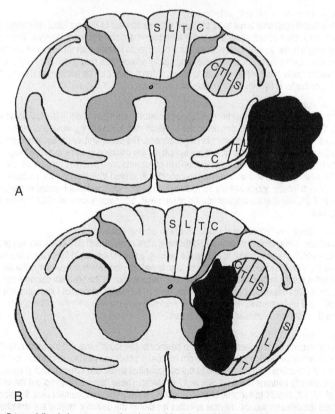

Figure 8-5. Extramedullary lesions compress the spinal cord from the outside **A,** causing the sacral fibers to be affected first. As the lumbar, thoracic, and cervical fibers are compressed, the "level" of injury seems to rise. In intramedullary lesions **B,** the cervical fibers are affected first, thus causing "sacral sparing."

27. What are the clinical features of syringomyelia?

The classic clinical features are dissociated sensory loss (loss of temperature and pain with intact proprioception) and lower motor neuron weakness (flaccid paralysis, atrophy, fasciculations) at the level of the lesion with upper motor neuron weakness below the level of the lesion. These symptoms develop because centrally located lesions initially compromise the decussating fibers of the spino-thalamic tract, which carry pain and temperature information. Because of the lamination of the spinal cord, the cervical and thoracic fibers are affected first (if the lesion is in the cervical region), resulting in a "cape" or "shawl" distribution of sensory loss bilaterally. Dorsal column function is preserved, thus causing the dissociation of sensory loss. With forward extension of the cavity, anterior horn cells are affected, resulting in atrophy, paresis, and areflexia at the level of the lesion. If the lesion extends to involve the corticospinal tract, upper motor neuron weakness and hyperreflexia will develop below the lesion. Lateral extension may also result in an ipsilateral Horner's syndrome. Neurogenic arthropa-thies may also develop (Figs. 8-6 and 8-7).

28. What part of the spinal cord does Friedreich's ataxia involve?

Friedreich's ataxia is an autosomal recessive disorder that arises from triplet expansion of the frataxin gene. It affects the cerebellum, spinal cord, peripheral nerves, and heart. In the spinal cord, the follow-ing tracts are affected: the dorsal columns, lateral corticospinal tracts, and the anterior and posterior spinocerebellar tracts. This condition typically presents with ataxia.

29. What part of the spinal cord is affected in tabes dorsalis?

Tabes dorsalis is one of the many manifestations of neurosyphilis, caused by infections of the brain, meninges, or spinal cord by *Treponema pallidum*. When the spinal cord is infected, degeneration of the dorsal columns occurs. This results in profound loss of joint position sense and fine touch.

30. What is "man-in-a-barrel" syndrome?

Man-in-a-barrel syndrome is not to be confused with vacationers to Niagara Falls! Neurologically, this syndrome refers to individuals who suffer from hyperextension injuries to the neck. This results in quadriplegia in the acute phase, with the arms being much weaker than the legs (like a man with a barrel around his chest). Urinary retention and patchy sensory loss may occur. Recovery of strength may spontaneously occur within minutes to hours, or the deficits may be permanent. Damage to the central gray matter is hypothesized to cause the syndrome.

31. What is tropical spastic paraparesis?

Tropical spastic paraparesis has been recognized clinically for many years in tropical areas and Japan. It is characterized by a chronic course in which mild to severe leg weakness develops with increased muscle tone and extensor plantar responses. The upper limbs may become hyperreflexic, but do not usually show weakness. Urinary symptoms are common such as increased urgency and incontinence due to neurogenic bladder. One-half of patients have posterior column sensory signs, and 15% have optic nerve involvement. The condition is caused by infection with a retrovirus, HTLV-1, which infects approximately 10 to 20 million people worldwide. Of infected individuals, 0.25% to 3.8% will develop tropical spastic paraparesis, otherwise known as HTLV 1-associated myelopathy.

32. What is subacute combined degeneration of the spinal cord?

This condition is the result of vitamin B12 deficiency. Most patients with B12 deficiency will pres-ent with a peripheral neuropathy that causes a burning, painful sensation in their hands and feet. Examination shows a stocking-glove sensory loss as well as vibratory loss. However, if the spinal cord is affected, it results in demyelination and vacuolar degeneration of the posterior columns and cortico-spinal tracts. This results in upper motor neuron signs of weakness, increased tone, hyperreflexia, and Babinski's and Hoffmann's signs. Nitrous oxide exposure may produce a similar pathologic picture. Treatment is with intramuscular B12 replacement.

33. What is the micturition reflex?

The act of voiding is controlled by a delicate balance between reflexive actions and cortical control. Bilateral projections originating from cortical (frontal) and pontine micturition centers descend in the spinal cord just medial to the corticospinal tracts and synapse with preganglionic parasympathetic neurons in the S2, S3, and S4 regions. These fibers then travel out the ventral roots of S2, S3, and S4 to synapse at postganglionic parasympathetic ganglia near the bladder to innervate the detrusor muscle. Muscle spindles located in the detrusor muscle are stretched when the bladder is filled, increasing their firing rate. This signal change increases the firing rate of the

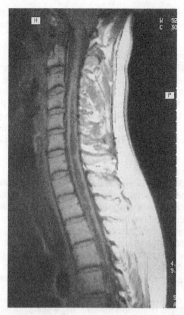

Figure 8-6. Sagittal magnetic resonance imaging (MRI) shows an extensive syrinx cavity in the cervical and thoracic spinal cord. This syrinx is associated with a developmental defect—an Arnold–Chiari malformation at the base of the skull (protrusion of the cerebellar tonsils down through the foramen magnum).

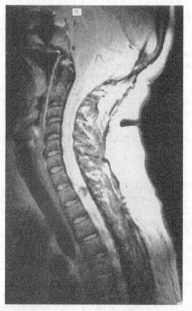

Figure 8-7. Sagittal T2-weighted magnetic resonance imaging (MRI) shows a neurofibroma displacing the thoracic spinal cord (an extramedullary, intradural lesion).

preganglionic parasympathetic fibers of S2, S3, and S4, resulting in detrusor muscle contraction, and thus voiding of the bladder. This reflex is normally under the voluntary control of descending inputs from the cortex.

34. **Describe what happens to micturition in spinal cord injury.**
Following bilateral lesions to the spinal cord, the bladder initially becomes flaccid (acute) and eventually becomes spastic (chronic). This dysfunction occurs because with bilateral cord damage the detrusor muscle of the bladder loses its cortical inputs. Like the deep tendon reflexes, it initially becomes flaccid, resulting in urinary retention. As the bladder fills, overflow incontinence may develop because the bladder cannot hold any more urine. As time passes, the detrusor muscle becomes spastic (just as the deep tendon muscles become hyperactive). Small stretches in the detrusor muscle result in voiding. This spastic bladder results in urinary frequency and urgency.

35. **What is cauda equina syndrome?**
The spinal cord ends around the L1/L2 level. If damage occurs at this level or below, the exiting roots (the cauda equina) may be injured. Cauda equine syndrome is typically caused by a herniated disc in the lumbosacral region. This results in weakness and sensory deficits in the lower extremity (which may be asymmetric). Bowel and bladder functions are affected as well. Because the compression is of the nerve roots, a lower motor neuron pattern of deficits is seen. Patellar and ankle reflexes may be absent. Radicular pain is often very prominent and occurs early in the course. It may be worse at night or in the recumbent position. Asymmetric saddle distribution sensory loss may occur, and urinary incontinence may occur late in the course due to a flaccid bladder. Cauda equina syndrome is reversible if intervention is initiated early in the course, so *this syndrome is a neurosurgical emergency!*

36. **What are the clinical signs of conus medullaris lesions?**
Lesions at the base of the spinal cord result in an autonomous neurogenic bladder and paralysis of the muscles of the pelvic floor. There is loss of voluntary control of the bladder because there is no awareness of fullness. This results in urinary retention and secondary overflow incontinence. Constipation, erectile dysfunction, and symmetric saddle anesthesia may also be present. Pain is not a typical part of this condition (which differentiates it from the cauda equina syndrome) but may occur late in the course.

37. **What is copper deficiency myelopathy (CDM)?**
CDM is a rare treatable form of noncompressive myelopathy due to copper deficiency. Copper is active in several enzymes important for structure and function in the nervous system. CDM is over three times more common in women than men, and zinc overload, upper GI surgery, and celiac disease are important risk factors. In enterocytes, zinc upregulates a chelator metallothionein that preferentially binds copper and causes it to be excreted. A careful history must include denture use as many denture adhesives contain zinc. These denture adhesives can be an important source of nondietary zinc. Malabsorption of copper can be caused by either previous upper GI surgery such as gastric bypass, or celiac disease. Routine blood work may reveal anemia due to copper deficiency's effect on the bone marrow. Clinically it is indistinguishable from subacute combined degeneration secondary to vitamin B12 deficiency, and the spinal magnetic resonance imaging (MRI) may show increased T2 signal in the posterior cord.

KEY POINTS: CAUSES OF MYELOPATHY

1. Intramedullary lesions cause sacral sparing sensory loss and symptoms that appear to descend (as the cervical, thoracic, lumbar, and finally sacral regions are affected).
2. Sudden damage to the spinal cord can cause spinal shock, which results in temporary flaccid paralysis, hyporeflexia, sensory loss, and loss of bladder tone.
3. Occlusion of the artery of Adamkiewicz may result in anterior spinal artery syndrome, causing bilateral weakness, loss of pain and temperature, and hyperreflexia below the lesion with preserved dorsal column functions (position and vibration).
4. Cauda equina syndrome is a neurosurgical emergency that presents with weakness and sensory loss in the lower extremity, prominent radicular pain, saddle anesthesia, and late-occurring urinary incontinence.

38. What are the symptoms of CDM?

CDM usually presents with a progressive gait abnormality due to both dorsal column dysfunction with a sensory level, as well as corticospinal tract dysfunction with spastic para or tetraparesis. The clinical picture can sometimes be confused from a coexisting sensory neuropathy with decreased distal reflexes.

 References available online at expertconsult.com.

WEBSITE

http://www.spinalinjury.net

BIBLIOGRAPHY

1. Daroff RB, Fenichel GM, Jankovic J, Mazziotta JC (eds): Bradley's Neurology in Clinical Practice, 6th ed. Philadelphia, Elsevier, 2012.
2. Ropper AH, Samuels MA, Klein JP: Adams and Victor's Principles of Neurology, 10th ed. New York, McGraw-Hill, 2014.
3. Rowland LP, Pedley TA: Merritt's Neurology, 12th ed. Philadelphia, Lippincott Williams & Wilkins, 2010.
4. Greenberg DA, Aminoff MJ, Simon RP: Clinical Neurology, 8th ed. New York, McGraw-Hill, 2012.

CHAPTER 9

BRAIN STEM DISEASE

Eugene C. Lai

CLINICAL ANATOMY OF THE BRAIN STEM

1. **What is the functional importance of the brain stem?**
   The brain stem is a small, narrow region connecting the spinal cord with the diencephalon and cerebrum. It lies ventral to the cerebellum, which it links via the cerebellar peduncles. Its functions are critical to survival. The brain stem is densely packed with many vital structures such as long ascending and descending pathways that carry sensory and motor information to and from higher brain regions. It contains the nuclei of cranial nerves III through XII and their intramedullary fibers. It also possesses groups of neurons that are the major source of noradrenergic, dopaminergic, and serotonergic inputs to most parts of the brain. In addition, other specific nuclear groups, such as the reticular formation, olivary bodies, and red nucleus, lie within the brain stem. In short, it is a complicated but highly organized structure that controls motor and sensory activities, respiration, cardiovascular functions, and mechanisms related to sleep and consciousness. Consequently, a small lesion in the brain stem can affect contiguous structures and cause disastrous neurologic deficits.

KEY POINTS: MAIN DIVISIONS OF THE BRAIN STEM

1. Medulla
2. Pons
3. Midbrain

---

2. **Describe the function of the medulla.**
   The medulla (bulb) is the direct rostral extension of the spinal cord. It contains the nuclei of the lower cranial nerves (mainly IX, X, XI, and XII) and the inferior olivary nucleus. The dorsal column pathways decussate in its central region to form the medial lemniscus, whereas the corticospinal tracts cross on the ventral side as they descend caudally. Together with the pons, the medulla also participates in vital autonomic functions such as digestion, respiration, and regulation of heart rate and blood pressure (Fig. 9-1).

3. **Describe the function of the pons.**
   The pons (bridge) lies rostral to the medulla and appears as a bulge mounting from the ventral surface of the brain stem. The pons contains nuclei for cranial nerves V, VI, VII, and VIII as well as a large number of neurons that relay information about movement from the frontal cerebral hemispheres to the cerebellum (frontopontocerebellar pathway). Other clinically pertinent pathways in the pons are those for the control of saccadic eye movements (medial longitudinal fasciculus) and the auditory and vestibular connections (Fig. 9-2).

4. **Describe the function of the midbrain.**
   The midbrain, the smallest and most rostral component of the brain stem, plays an important role in the control of eye movements and coordination of visual and auditory reflexes. It contains the nuclei for cranial nerves III and IV. Other important structures are the red nuclei and substantia nigra. The periaqueduct area has an important but poorly understood influence on consciousness and pain perception (Fig. 9-3).

5. **Which cranial nerves are not found in the brain stem?**
   The 12 pairs of cranial nerves are numbered in rostral caudal sequence. The brain stem contains the nuclei of all cranial nerves except two: the optic (II) nerve, which terminates in the thalamus, and the olfactory (I) nerve, which synapses in the olfactory bulb.

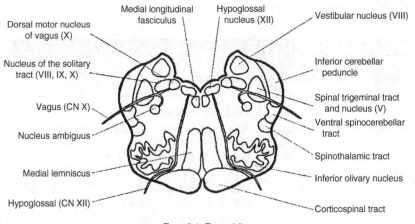

Figure 9-1. The medulla.

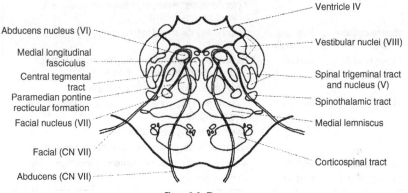

Figure 9-2. The pons.

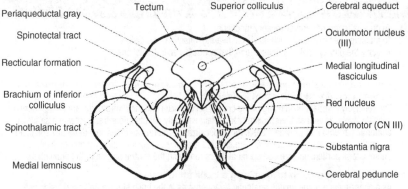

Figure 9-3. The midbrain.

6. **What are the locations and functions of the individual cranial nerves?**
See Table 9-1.

Table 9-1. Location and Function of Cranial Nerves

NERVE	LOCATION OF NUCLEI	FUNCTIONS
Olfactory (I)	Olfactory bulb	*Sensory:* smell and olfactory reflex
Optic (II)	Thalamus	*Sensory:* vision and visual reflexes
Oculomotor (III)	Midbrain	*Motor:* eye movement, eyelids, pupillary constriction, accommodation of lens
Trochlear (IV)	Midbrain	*Motor:* eye movement (superior oblique)
Trigeminal (V)	Midbrain	*Sensory:* proprioception for chewing
	Pons	*Sensory:* from face and cornea
		Motor: to masticatory muscles and tensor tympani muscle
	Medulla	*Sensory:* from face and mouth
Abducens (VI)	Pons	*Motor:* eye movement (lateral rectus)
Facial (VII)	Pons	*Sensory:* from skin of external ear, taste from anterior tongue
		Motor: facial expression, stapedius muscle movement, salivation, and lacrimation
Vestibulocochlear (VIII)	Pons and medulla	*Sensory:* equilibrium and hearing
Glossopharyngeal (IX)	Medulla	*Sensory:* from middle ear, palate, pharynx, and posterior tongue, taste from posterior tongue
		Motor: swallowing, parotid gland salivation
Vagus (X)	Medulla	*Sensory:* from pharynx, larynx, thorax, and abdomen, taste from epiglottis
		Motor: swallowing and phonation
		Autonomic: parasympathetics to thoracic and abdominal viscera
Spinal accessory (XI)	Medulla	*Motor:* sternocleidomastoid and upper trapezius muscles
Hypoglossal (XII)	Medulla	*Motor:* tongue

From Wilson-Pauwels L, Akesson EJ, Stewart PA: Cranial nerves: anatomy and clinical comments. Toronto: B.C. Decker, 1988.

KEY POINTS: MAIN FUNCTIONS OF THE CRANIAL NERVES

1. To provide motor or general sensory functions
2. To mediate special senses such as vision, hearing, olfaction, and taste
3. To carry the parasympathetic innervation that controls visceral functions

7. **How can understanding the anatomy and function of individual cranial nerves assist in localizing brain stem lesions?**
The relatively compact positioning of the cranial nerve nuclei and their intramedullary nerve fibers at specific levels, as well as their proximity to certain vertically directed fiber tracts, create a series of anatomic patterns that provide a basis for the localization of brain stem lesions. Generally speaking, the motor nuclei of the cranial nerves are situated medially, the spinothalamic fibers run along the dorsal lateral portion, and the corticospinal fibers run along the ventral portion of the brain stem.

8. **What is the approach to localizing a brain stem lesion?**
As a consequence of the unique anatomic arrangements in the brain stem, a unilateral lesion within this structure often causes "crossed syndromes," in which ipsilateral dysfunction of one or more

cranial nerves is accompanied by hemiplegia and/or hemisensory loss on the contralateral body. Exquisite localization of a brain stem lesion depends on signs of long-tract (corticospinal and spino-thalamic pathways) dysfunction to identify the lesion in the longitudinal (or sagittal) plane and on signs of cranial nerve dysfunction to establish its position in the cross-sectional (or axial) plane. Localization of disorders of the brain stem can be simplified by summarizing the patient's neurologic deficits to answer the following questions: Is the lesion affecting unilateral or bilateral structures of the brain stem? What is the level of the lesion? If the lesion is unilateral, is it medial or lateral in the brain stem?

9. **What is the approach to localizing an isolated cranial nerve deficit?**
   An isolated cranial nerve defect, especially of VI and VII, is most often due to a peripheral and not a brain stem lesion.

10. **How do the presentations of intra-axial and extra-axial lesions of the brain stem differ?**
    A lesion that directly affects the tissues of the brain stem is called *intra-axial* or *intramedullary*. It usually presents with simultaneous cranial nerve and long-tract symptoms and signs. A lesion outside the brain stem is called *extra-axial*. It affects the brain stem by initially compressing and interfering with the functions of individual cranial nerves. Later, as it enlarges, neighboring structures within the brain stem may be affected, causing additional long-tract signs.

11. **What is the radiographic examination of choice for brain stem lesions?**
    Magnetic resonance imaging (MRI) is the examination of choice for suspected brain stem lesions. It provides a highly sensitive and noninvasive method of evaluating the posterior fossa, unhampered by skull base artifact. Enhancement with gadolinium may be useful to characterize breakdown of the blood–brain barrier. Magnetic resonance angiography also may be helpful to investigate further the major branches of the vertebrobasilar system in brain stem ischemia or infarction.

BRAIN STEM VASCULAR DISEASES

12. **Describe the vascular supply of the medulla.**
    The medulla is supplied by the vertebral arteries and their branches. Its blood supply may be further subdivided into two groups, the **paramedian bulbar** and the **lateral bulbar arteries.** The paramedian bulbar arteries are penetrating branches, mainly from the vertebral artery, that supply the midline structures of the medulla. At the lower medulla, branches from the anterior spinal artery also contribute to this paramedian zone. The lateral portion of the medulla is supplied by the lateral bulbar branches of the vertebral artery or the posterior inferior cerebellar artery.

13. **Describe the vascular supply of the pons.**
    The basilar artery is the principal supplier of the pons. It gives off three types of branches. The **paramedian arteries** supply the medial basal pons, including the pontine nuclei, corticospinal fibers, and medial lemniscus. The **short circumferential arteries** supply the lateral aspect of the pons and the middle and superior cerebellar peduncles. The **long circumferential arteries** together with branches from the anterior inferior cerebellar and superior cerebellar arteries supply the pontine tegmentum and the dorsolateral quadrant of the pons.

14. **Describe the vascular supply of the midbrain.**
    Arteries supplying the midbrain include branches of the superior cerebellar artery, posterior cerebral artery, posterior communicating artery, and anterior choroidal artery. Branches of these arteries, like those of the pons, can be grouped into **paramedian arteries,** which supply the midline structures, and the **long and short circumferential arteries,** which supply the dorsal and lateral midbrain.
    Because the blood supply to the brain stem at each level is divided into several territories (usually medial and lateral), occlusion of specific arteries manifests clinical features that reflect their vascular distribution.

15. **What is the medial medullary syndrome?**
    The medial medullary (Dejerine's) syndrome is caused by occlusion of the anterior spinal artery or its parent vertebral artery, resulting in the following signs:
    - Ipsilateral paresis of the tongue (damage to cranial nerve XII), which deviates toward the lesion
    - Contralateral hemiplegia (damage to corticospinal tract) with sparing of the face
    - Contralateral loss of position and vibratory sensation (damage to medial lemniscus)

16. **What is the consequence of occlusion of a dominant anterior spinal artery?**
   The central medullary area may be supplied by a single dominant anterior spinal artery. Occlusion of this vessel then leads to bilateral infarction of the medial medulla, resulting in quadriplegia (with face sparing), complete paralysis of the tongue, and complete loss of position and vibratory sensation. The patient will be mute although fully conscious.

17. **What is the lateral medullary syndrome?**
   The lateral medullary (Wallenberg's) syndrome is often due to vertebral artery or posterior inferior cerebellar artery occlusion. Vertebral artery dissection can also be a cause. Damage to the dorsolateral medulla and the inferior cerebellar peduncle results in the following signs:
   - Ipsilateral loss of pain and temperature sensation of the face (damage to descending spinal tract and nucleus of cranial nerve V)
   - Ipsilateral paralysis of palate, pharynx, and vocal cord (damage to nuclei or fibers of IX and X) with dysphagia and dysarthria
   - Ipsilateral Horner's syndrome (damage to descending sympathetic fibers)
   - Ipsilateral ataxia and dysmetria (damage to inferior cerebellar peduncle and cerebellum)
   - Contralateral loss of pain and temperature on the body (damage to spinothalamic tract)
   - Vertigo, nausea, vomiting, and nystagmus (damage to vestibular nuclei)
   - Other signs and symptoms may include hiccups, diplopia, or unilateral posterior headache. See Figure 9-4.

18. **What is the ventral pontine syndrome?**
   The ventral pontine (Millard–Gubler) syndrome is caused by paramedian infarction of the pons and results in the following signs:
   - Ipsilateral paresis of the lateral rectus (damage to cranial nerve VI) with diplopia
   - Ipsilateral paresis of the upper and lower face (damage to cranial nerve VII)
   - Contralateral hemiplegia (damage to corticospinal tract) with sparing of the face

19. **What is the lower dorsal pontine syndrome?**
   The lower dorsal pontine (Foville's) syndrome is caused by lesions in the dorsal tegmentum of the lower pons, resulting in the following signs:
   - Ipsilateral paresis of the whole face (damage to nucleus and fibers of VII)
   - Ipsilateral horizontal gaze palsy (damage to paramedian pontine reticular formation and/or VI nucleus)
   - Contralateral hemiplegia (damage to corticospinal tract) with sparing of the face

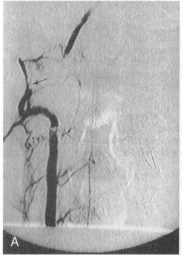 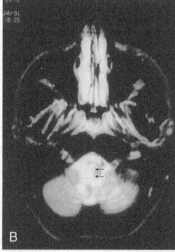

Figure 9-4. Dissection of the right vertebral artery (**A,** *arrow*) causing a lateral medullary infarct (Wallenberg's syndrome), seen as an area of increased signal (**B,** *arrows*) on a T2-weighted magnetic resonance image (MRI) of the brain stem.

20. What is the upper dorsal pontine syndrome?

The upper dorsal pontine (Raymond–Cestan) syndrome is caused by obstruction of the long circumferential branches of the basilar artery and results in:

- Ipsilateral ataxia and coarse intention tremor (damage to the superior and middle cerebellar peduncles)
- Ipsilateral paralysis of muscles of mastication and sensory loss in face (damage to sensory and motor nuclei and tracts of V)
- Contralateral loss of all sensory modalities in the body (damage to medial lemniscus and spinothalamic tract)
- Contralateral hemiparesis of the face and body (damage to corticospinal tract) may occur with ventral extension of the lesion
- Horizontal gaze palsy may occur, as in the lower dorsal pontine syndrome

21. What is the ventral midbrain syndrome?

The ventral midbrain (Weber's) syndrome is caused by occlusion of median and paramedian perforating branches and may result in:

- Ipsilateral oculomotor paresis, ptosis, and dilated pupil (damage to fascicle of cranial nerve III, including parasympathetic fibers)
- Contralateral hemiplegia, including the lower face (damage to corticospinal and corticobulbar tracts)

22. What is the dorsal midbrain syndrome?

The dorsal midbrain (Benedikt's) syndrome results from a lesion in the midbrain tegmentum caused by occlusion of paramedian branches of the basilar or posterior cerebral arteries or both. Its signs are:

- Ipsilateral oculomotor paresis, ptosis, and dilated pupil (damage to fascicle of cranial nerve III, including parasympathetic fibers as in Weber's syndrome).
- Contralateral involuntary movements, such as intention tremor, ataxia, and chorea (damage to red nucleus).
- Contralateral hemiparesis may be present if the lesion extends ventrally.
- Contralateral hemianesthesia may be present if the lesion extends laterally, affecting the spinothalamic tract and medial lemniscus.

23. What is the dorsolateral midbrain syndrome?

The dorsolateral midbrain syndrome is caused by infarction of the circumferential arteries and results in:

- Ipsilateral Horner's syndrome (damage to sympathetic tract).
- Ipsilateral severe tremor that may be present at rest and grossly worsened by attempted movement (damage to superior cerebellar peduncle prior to crossing to the opposite red nucleus). Tremor and ataxia can be present bilaterally, if both the superior cerebellar peduncle and red nucleus are affected.
- Contralateral loss of all sensory modalities (damage to spinothalamic tract and medial lemniscus that now ascend together).

24. What are the symptoms of brain stem transient ischemic attacks?

Transient circulatory insufficiency in the vertebrobasilar distribution causes brief episodes of brain stem dysfunction characterized by a more patchy and variable presentation. The symptoms of the recurrent attacks may be identical or varying in detail. In basilar artery disease, each side of the body may be affected alternately. All of the structures in the same ischemic distribution may be affected simultaneously, or symptoms of brain stem dysfunction may spread from one region to another. The symptoms may then end abruptly or fade gradually. They are often premonitory symptoms of impending brain stem strokes that may result in devastating consequences.

Transient brain stem ischemic attacks affecting the medulla occur particularly often. Vertigo, dysarthria, dysphagia, and tingling around the mouth suggest dysfunction in this region. At pontine levels, frequent symptoms are vertigo; imbalance; hearing abnormalities; tingling, numbness, or weakness of the limbs; and diplopia. Midbrain ischemia may cause diplopia, ataxia, sudden loss of consciousness, and weakness of limbs. Symptoms of brain stem ischemia are usually multiple, and isolated findings (such as vertigo or diplopia) are more often caused by peripheral lesions affecting individual cranial nerves.

25. What is the "top of the basilar" syndrome?

Occlusion of the rostral basilar artery, usually embolic, often results in the "top of the basilar" syndrome caused by infarction of the midbrain, thalamus, and portions of the temporal and occipital lobes. This syndrome should be suspected in a patient with sudden onset of unresponsiveness, confusion, amnesia, abnormal eye movement, and visual defect. The neurologic signs may be variable, but the most common include:

- **Impairments of ocular movements**—unilateral or bilateral vertical (upgaze, downgaze, or complete) gaze palsy, skew deviation, hyperconvergence or convergence spasms causing pseudo-VI nerve palsy, convergence-retraction nystagmus, and retraction of the upper eyelids.
- **Abnormalities in pupils**—small with incomplete light reactivity (diencephalic dysfunction), large or midposition and fixed (midbrain dysfunction), ectopic pupils (corectopia), oval pupils.
- **Alterations of consciousness and behavior**—stupor, somnolence, apathy, lack of attention, memory deficits, agitated delirium.
- **Defects in vision**—homonymous hemianopsia, cortical blindness, Balint's syndrome (impaired visual form discrimination and color dysnomia), and abnormal color vision.
- **Motor weakness, sensory deficits, and reflex abnormalities** are usually variable and subtle and due to the involvement of long tracts at the infarcted region.

This syndrome may be reversible in patients who are younger and do not have significant risks for cerebrovascular disease.

26. What is the locked-in syndrome?

The locked-in syndrome occurs in patients with bilateral ventral pontine lesions. Its most common cause is pontine infarction. Other common causes include pontine hemorrhage, trauma, central pontine myelinolysis, tumor, and encephalitis. The patient is quadriplegic because of bilateral damage to the corticospinal tracts in the ventral pons. He or she is unable to speak and incapable of facial movement because of involvement of the corticobulbar tracts. Horizontal eye movements are also limited by the bilateral involvement of the nuclei and fibers of cranial nerve VI. Consciousness is preserved because the reticular formation is not damaged. The patient has intact vertical eye movements and blinking because the supranuclear ocular motor pathways that run dorsally are spared. The patient is able to communicate by movement of the eyelids, but otherwise is completely immobile. Sometimes an incomplete state of this syndrome may occur when the patient retains some horizontal gaze and facial movement. The locked-in syndrome must be distinguished from the persistent neurovegetative state (such as coma vigil or akinetic mutism), in which the patient appears awake but does not react to environmental stimuli and is unable to communicate in any form (thought to be due to a lesion in the rostral midbrain, basal–medial frontal region, or limbic lobes).

27. What are the common causes of brain stem hemorrhage?

Pontine hemorrhage is usually caused by uncontrolled systemic hypertension, resulting in a sudden loss of consciousness, quadriparesis, and pinpoint pupils. Progressive central herniation from supratentorial mass lesions can compress the brain stem and cause hemorrhage in the midline of the midbrain (Duret hemorrhage), producing coma and bilateral large and fixed pupils. Diencephalic bleeding, such as thalamic hemorrhage, can dissect into the cerebral peduncles and midbrain, producing acute severe headache, hemiparesis, and III nerve palsy. Small petechial hemorrhages occur in the brain stem of patients with head injuries, blood dyscrasias, or hemorrhagic disorders. Ruptured aneurysms or arteriovenous malformations of the vertebrobasilar system may result in subarachnoid hemorrhage that injures the brain stem.

OTHER BRAIN STEM SYNDROMES

28. What is Parinaud's syndrome?

Parinaud's syndrome is also known as the *dorsal midbrain* or *collicular syndrome*. The lesion is in the rostral dorsal midbrain, damaging the superior colliculi and pretectal structures. Patients report difficulty in looking up and blurring of distant vision. The common tetrad of findings is:

- Paralysis of upgaze and accommodation, but sparing of other eye movements
- Normal to large pupils with light-near dissociation (loss of pupillary reflex to light with preservation of pupilloconstriction in response to convergence)
- Eyelid retraction
- Convergence-retraction nystagmus (eyes make convergent and retracting oscillations following an upward saccade)

Causes include tumors of the pineal gland, stroke, hemorrhage, trauma, hydrocephalus, or multiple sclerosis. The upgaze palsy can be mimicked by progressive supranuclear palsy, thyroid ophthalmopathy, myasthenia gravis, Guillain–Barré syndrome, or congenital upgaze limitation.

29. **What is internuclear ophthalmoplegia (INO)?**

INO is a disorder of horizontal ocular movement due to a lesion in the brain stem (usually in the pons, specifically along the medial longitudinal fasciculus between the VI and III nuclei). Horizontal gaze requires the coordinated activity of the lateral rectus muscle of the abducting eye (innervated by the VI nerve) and the medial rectus muscle of the adducting eye (innervated by the III nerve). This integrated function is regulated by the paramedian pontine reticular formation (or pontine gaze center), which receives inputs from the contralateral occipital and frontal eyefields and sends fibers to the ipsilateral abducens (VI) nucleus and the contralateral oculomotor (III) nucleus. Fibers from the pontine gaze center run rostrally together with vestibular and other fibers to make up the medial longitudinal fasciculus (MLF).

The cause is commonly multiple sclerosis in young adults, especially when the syndrome is bilateral. In older people, the syndrome is often unilateral and caused by occlusion of the basilar artery or its paramedian branches. Occasionally INO can be caused by lupus erythematosus and drug overdose (e.g., barbiturates, phenytoin, amitriptyline). Pseudo-INO occurs rarely as a feature of myasthenia gravis, Wernicke's encephalopathy, and Guillain–Barré syndrome.

Many patients with INO have no symptoms, but some have diplopia or blurred vision. On lateral gaze, the signs of INO include:

- Impaired or paralyzed adduction of the eye ipsilateral to the lesion. The deficit can range from complete medial rectus paralysis to slight slowing of an adducting saccade.
- Horizontal nystagmus of the abducting eye contralateral to the lesion.
- Bilateral INO results in defective adduction to the right and left, and nystagmus of the abducting eye on both directions of gaze.
- Convergence is usually preserved. Skew deviation and vertical gaze nystagmus are sometimes present.

30. **What is the "one-and-a-half" syndrome?**

This disorder of horizontal ocular movement is characterized by a lateral gaze palsy on looking toward the side of the lesion and INO on looking in the other direction. The location of the lesion is the paramedian pontine reticular formation or VI nerve nucleus. MLF fibers crossing from the contralateral VI nucleus are also involved, causing INO. The common causes of this syndrome are similar to those of INO (e.g., multiple sclerosis, stroke). Hemorrhage or tumor in the lower pons is also in the differential diagnosis. Pseudo-one-and-a-half syndromes may occur with myasthenia gravis, Wernicke's encephalopathy, or Guillain–Barré syndrome. Clinical signs include:

- Horizontal gaze palsy on looking toward the size of the lesion ("one").
- INO on looking away from the side of the lesion ("half"). This paralyzes adduction and causes nystagmus on abduction. As a result, the ipsilateral eye has no horizontal movement, and the only lateral ocular movement that remains is abduction and nystagmus of the contralateral eye.
- Associated signs include: skew deviation, gaze-invoked nystagmus on vertical gaze, and exotropia of the eye contralateral to the lesion.
- Vertical ocular movements and convergence are usually intact.

31. **What is bulbar palsy?**

The bulb is the medulla, and the term *bulbar palsy* refers to a syndrome of lower motor neuron paralysis, affecting muscles innervated by cranial nerves (mainly IX to XII) that have their nuclei closely approximated in the lower brain stem. Muscles of the face, palate, pharynx, larynx, sternocleidomastoid, upper trapezius, and tongue are usually affected. Patients may present clinically with dysarthria, dysphagia, hoarseness, nasal voice, palatal deviation, diminished gag reflex, or weakness of the sternocleidomastoid, upper trapezius, or tongue. Atrophy and fasciculations may be evident. Bulbar palsy may result from various conditions involving the motor nuclei of the lower brain stem or their intramedullary fibers, the corresponding peripheral nerves, the myoneural junction, or the musculature. Causes of intra-axial lesions include: brain stem infarction, syringobulbia, glioma, poliomyelitis, encephalitis, and motor neuron disease (amyotrophic lateral sclerosis or progressive bulbar palsy). Extra-axial causes are neoplasms (meningioma or neurofibroma), chronic meningitis, aneurysms, neck trauma, and congenital abnormalities (Chiari malformation or basilar impression). Myasthenia gravis, Guillain–Barré syndrome, myositis, and diphtheria also may present with similar signs and symptoms.

32. What is pseudobulbar palsy?

   Pseudobulbar palsy is a syndrome of upper motor neuron paralysis that affects the corticobulbar system above the brain stem bilaterally. Although it presents with most of the signs and symptoms of bulbar palsy, the causative lesion is not in the brain stem. This condition causes dysphagia, dysarthria, and paresis of the tongue (without atrophy or fasciculations). In contrast to bulbar palsy, the reflex movements of the soft palate and pharynx are frequently hyperactive. The jaw jerk is brisk. Frontal signs (grasp, snout, suck, and glabellar reflex) may be present. Emotional incontinence with exaggerated crying (or, less often, laughing), known as *pseudobulbar affect*, is also common and may be due to disruption of frontal efferents subserving emotional expression. Multiple lacunar infarcts or chronic ischemia in the hemispheres affecting bilateral corticobulbar fibers usually causes this syndrome. Other causes are amyotrophic lateral sclerosis (ALS) and multiple sclerosis. In ALS, a combination of upper and lower motor neuron disease often results in coexisting bulbar and pseudobulbar palsies (wasting and fasciculations of the tongue associated with brisk jaw jerk).

KEY POINTS: COMMON SYMPTOMS OF BRAIN STEM LESIONS

Common symptoms of brain stem lesions involve combinations of:
1. Double vision
2. Vertigo
3. Nausea/vomiting
4. Numbness of face
5. Hoarseness
6. Difficulties with swallowing and speaking
7. Incoordination
8. Gait imbalance
9. Altered mental status

KEY POINTS: COMMON SIGNS OF BRAIN STEM LESIONS

Common signs of brain stem lesions involve combinations of:
1. Multiple cranial nerve dysfunctions
2. Gaze palsies
3. Nystagmus
4. Sympathetic dysfunction (Horner's syndrome)
5. Hearing loss
6. Dysphagia
7. Dysarthria
8. Dysphonia
9. Tongue deviation and atrophy
10. Paresis or dysesthesia of the face with contralateral motor or sensory deficits in the body (crossed symptoms)
11. Unilateral hemiparesis with ataxia
12. Decreased responsiveness

KEY POINTS: INTRA-AXIAL BRAIN STEM LESIONS

1. Neoplasm
2. Ischemia/infarction
3. Hemorrhage
4. Vascular malformation
5. Demyelinating disease
6. Inflammatory lesion

KEY POINTS: EXTRA-AXIAL BRAIN STEM LESIONS

1. Schwannoma/acoustic neuroma
2. Meningioma
3. Chordoma
4. Aneurysm
5. Epidermoid
6. Arachnoid cyst

KEY POINTS: COMMON CAUSES OF BRAIN STEM ISCHEMIA

1. Atherosclerotic stenosis of vessels of the vertebrobasilar system
2. Embolization from the heart or ulcerated plaques
3. Recurrent hypotension
4. Vertebral steal syndrome
5. Cervical spondylosis compromising the vertebral circulation

OTHER BRAIN STEM DISEASES

33. What is a brain stem glioma?

Brain stem glioma is the most frequent neoplasm affecting the brain stem. It occurs mostly in children and adolescents and is often associated with neurofibromatosis. The tumor arises in the region of the VI nerve nucleus and gradually enlarges to involve the VI and VII nerves and adjacent vestibular structures. Vestibular, cerebellar, and lower cranial nerve symptoms may be present and slowly progressive over a period of months or years before the diagnosis is made because motor and sensory symptoms in the body are usually absent.

34. What other neoplasms affect the brain stem?

Ependymomas occur in the fourth ventricle and may cause obstruction, resulting in intermittent noncommunicating hydrocephalus accompanied by headache and protracted vomiting from involvement of the chemoreceptor trigger zone on the floor of the fourth ventricle. Metastatic lesions of the brain stem may arise from malignant melanoma or neoplasms of the lung and breast, but are relatively rare.

35. What are the common metabolic causes of brain stem dysfunction?

Extraocular movements and cerebellar pathways are vulnerable to damage by metabolic insults because they are highly metabolically active. These dysfunctions are usually acute and reversible. The common presentations are ataxia, vertigo, nausea, vomiting, dysarthria, nystagmus, and gaze palsies such as INO. Common causes are alcohol intoxication and overdose of sedative drugs (e.g., barbiturates) and anticonvulsants (e.g., phenytoin).

36. How does thiamine deficiency affect the brain stem?

Wernicke's encephalopathy is a complication of alcoholism and malnutrition resulting in thiamine deficiency. It usually presents with characteristic mental changes of gross confusion, ataxia, extraocular movement abnormalities, and other signs of brain stem dysfunction. The brain stem signs can be readily reversed by parenteral thiamine therapy, but the confusional state may resolve more slowly.

37. How does demyelinating disease affect the brain stem?

Multiple sclerosis often results in demyelination of the fast-conducting, heavily myelinated nerve fibers traveling along the brain stem. These include the cerebellar–vestibular pathways, medial longitudinal fasciculus, and pyramidal pathways. Bilateral INO is almost pathognomonic of multiple sclerosis. Another hallmark of brain stem multiple sclerosis is the combination of bilateral cerebellar and pyramidal signs producing ataxia and pathologically brisk reflexes.

38. What is central pontine myelinolysis?

Central pontine myelinolysis, or osmotic demyelination syndrome, is another demyelinating disease that affects the brain stem white matter, mostly in the central pons and occasionally the cerebral hemispheres. It occurs primarily in patients suffering from malnutrition or alcoholism complicated by hyponatremia. Rapid correction of the hyponatremia has been implicated as a cause of the demyelination. This disorder develops as a subacute progressive quadriparesis with lower cranial nerve involvement. It is often fatal, but survival with recovered neurologic function is possible. It can be prevented by correcting the electrolyte disturbance gradually rather than rapidly.

39. What is Bickerstaff's brain stem encephalitis?

This is an inflammatory disorder of the brain stem, probably autoimmune mediated, but without specific etiology. It is characterized by acute progressive cranial nerve dysfunction (such as diplopia, ophthalmoparesis, facial palsy, and bulbar palsy), associated cerebellar ataxia, and altered mental status. Very often it follows an illness, and an association with certain infections, including cytomegalovirus, *Campylobacter jejuni*, typhoid fever, and *Mycoplasma pneumoniae* has been reported. Serum anti-GQ1b IgG antibodies may be present in patients with this condition. Diagnosis is by cerebrospinal fluid analysis showing central nervous system inflammation. Brain magnetic resonance imaging (MRI) scan may show contrast enhanced abnormal signals in the brain stem, but a normal MRI scan does not exclude the diagnosis. Treatments include intravenous steroid, therapeutic plasma exchange, and other immunosuppressive agents. Although the initial presentation may be severe, there is usually a good outcome with full recovery. Occasional recurrent cases may need repeat treatments.

40. What is syringobulbia?

Syringobulbia is characterized by a cerebrospinal fluid filled cavity (syrinx) in the medulla. It is a rare condition often found in association with congenital abnormalities such as Chiari malformations, as well as with neoplasms or as sequelae to spinal cord trauma. It may affect one or more cranial nerves, causing facial palsies, or cause compression and/or interruption of sensory and motor nerves pathways in the brain stem. The symptoms progress from minor sensory changes to weakness and wasting bulbar musculature, to respiratory compromise, and even to death. Surgical treatment involves drainage or decompression of the syrinx cavity with diversion of fluid to the subarachnoid space or peritoneal cavity. Posterior fossa decompression may also be used.

VERTIGO

41. What is vertigo?

Vertigo is a false sense of movement, either of oneself or of the environment. The feeling may involve the whole body or be limited to the head. Vertigo should be distinguished from dizziness or giddiness resulting from near syncope, postural hypotension, hyperventilation, multiple sensory deficits, ataxia, or other etiologies. The spinning or swirling sensations of vertigo are related to disturbances of the vestibular system.

42. What are the common causes of vertigo?

The causes of vertigo are central (due to a brain stem lesion) or peripheral (due to an inner ear or vestibular nerve lesion). Central vertigo is almost always accompanied by other signs of brain stem dysfunction, such as double vision, weakness or numbness of the face, dysarthria, or dysphagia. Peripheral vertigo is usually accompanied by tinnitus or hearing loss but no other neurologic abnormalities (Table 9-2).

Table 9-2. Common Causes of Vertigo

CENTRAL	PERIPHERAL
Brain stem stroke or transient ischemic attack	Vestibular neuronitis
Multiple sclerosis	Benign paroxysmal positional vertigo
Neoplasms	Ménière's disease
Syringobulbia	Local trauma or posttraumatic
Arnold–Chiari deformity	Physiologic (e.g., motion sickness)
Antineoplastics	Drugs/toxins (e.g., antibiotics, diuretics, or anticonvulsants)
Basilar migraine	Posterior fossa tumors/masses (e.g., acoustic neuroma)
Cerebellar hemorrhage	—

43. What signs and symptoms help distinguish central from peripheral vertigo?
    See Table 9-3.

Table 9-3. Central versus Peripheral Vertigo

SIGNS AND SYMPTOMS	CENTRAL VERTIGO	PERIPHERAL VERTIGO
Nystagmus	Often vertical or rotatory, may change with direction of gaze, increase with looking toward side of lesion	Mostly horizontal or sometimes rotatory; unidirectional and conjugate; increases with looking away from side of lesion
Latency of onset and duration of nystagmus	No latency after head motion; persistent and lasts >60 seconds	Latency after head motion; fatigable and lasts <60 seconds
Caloric test	May be normal	Abnormal on side of lesion
Brain stem or cranial nerve signs	Often present	Absent
Hearing loss, tinnitus	Absent	Often present
Nausea and vomiting	Usually absent	Usually present
Vertigo	Usually mild	Severe, often rotational
Falling	Often falls toward side of lesion	Often falls to side opposite nystagmus
Visual fixation or eye closing	No change or increase of symptoms	Inhibits nystagmus and vertigo

44. What is vestibular neuronitis?
    Vestibular neuronitis is a condition affecting primarily young adults causing a sudden attack of vertigo without tinnitus or hearing loss. This benign disorder usually resolves within several days. The etiology is presumed to be a viral infection or inflammation of the vestibular nerve.

45. What is Ménière's disease?
    Ménière's disease causes the symptomatic triad of episodic vertigo, tinnitus, and hearing loss. It is caused by an increased amount of endolymph in the scala media. Pathologically, hair cells degenerate in the macula and vestibule.

46. What is benign paroxysmal positional vertigo (BPPV)? How is it diagnosed?
    BPPV is a disorder characterized by paroxysms of vertigo and nystagmus on assumption of certain positions of the head. Hearing tests are normal. The diagnosis is made by performing head maneuvers that elicit the patient's symptoms and nystagmus. The cause is calcification and dislocation of otoliths, which move freely in the semicircular canal, thus abnormally stimulating the hair cells within the semicircular canals.

47. What are canalith repositioning (Epley) maneuvers?
    Epley maneuvers are performed as a treatment for BPPV. While lying supine, the patient's head is rotated through a series of positions that rolls the otoliths out of the semicircular canals and thus removes the cause of the positional vertigo.

CONSCIOUSNESS

48. What are the functions of the reticular formation in the brain stem?
    The reticular formation is composed of a network of diffuse aggregations of neurons distributed throughout the central parts of the medulla, pons, and midbrain. It fills the spaces between cranial nerve nuclei and olivary bodies and intermixes between ascending and descending fiber tracts. Its neurons receive afferent information from the spinal cord, cranial nerve nuclei, cerebellum, and cerebrum and send efferent impulses to the same structures. Their widespread connections give them extensive influence over many neuronal activities. The main functions of the reticular formation are:
    - Activation of the brain for behavioral arousal and different levels of awareness
    - Modulation of segmental stretch reflexes and muscle tone for control of motor function
    - Coordination of autonomic functions, such as control of breathing and cardiovascular activities
    - Modulation of the perception of pain

49. **How do you examine for brain stem dysfunction in a comatose patient?**

    When examining a comatose patient, one should be aware of signs and symptoms indicating that the coma is due to brain stem (reticular formation) dysfunction. This is especially true of impending brain stem failure from increased intracranial pressure causing herniation into the posterior fossa. This dysfunction travels in a rostral caudal direction, ending in death with medullary involvement. Emergency management to reduce the intracranial pressure should be implemented immediately. The following observations are used to monitor the patient's condition:
    - Mental status
    - Oculovestibular test of gaze response to ice-water calorics
    - Breathing pattern
    - Pupillary size and light response
    - Motor response to supraorbital nerve pressure (noxious stimulus)
    - Spontaneous eye movement or deviation
    - Oculocephalic reflex on head turning (doll's eye movement)
    - Presence of other brain stem reflexes (corneal, gag, and ciliospinal)

50. **How does the clinical examination localize the level of brain stem dysfunction in a comatose patient?**

    See Table 9-4.

Table 9-4. Location of Level of Brain stem Dysfunction

SYMPTOMS AND SIGNS	SUBCORTICAL	MIDBRAIN	PONS	MEDULLA
Consciousness	Lethargy or stupor	Coma	Coma	Coma
Breathing	Cheynes–Stokes	Central hyperventilation	Apneustic or cluster	Ataxic
Pupils	Small and reactive	Midposition and fixed (III nucleus); unilateral dilated and fixed (III nerve); large and fixed (pretectal)	Pinpoint	Midposition and fixed, often irregular in shape
Oculocephalic and oculovestibular responses	Present	Absent or abnormal	Absent or abnormal	Absent
Motor response to stimulation	Decortication	Decerebration	Decerebration or no response	No response

51. **How do you test for irreversible loss of brain stem function?**

    Brain death is a clinical diagnosis of irreversible cessation of all cerebral and brain stem function due to a major intracerebral catastrophe (trauma, anoxia, mass lesion, infection, hemorrhage, etc.). Complete loss of brain stem function begins with apneic coma. On examination, all brain stem reflexes (corneal, pupillary, gag, ciliospinal) are absent. The pupils are midposition or large and fixed. Oculocephalic and oculovestibular reflexes are absent. Muscle tone is flaccid, with no spontaneous facial movement and no motor response to noxious stimuli. This condition should be present for 6 to 24 hours in adults. Metabolic causes (hypothermia, hypotension) and drug effects (neuromuscular blockers, sedative drugs) need to be ruled out. Many local institutions have developed their own, slightly modified criteria for brain death.

52. **What is the apnea test?**

    The apnea test is an essential test for the cessation of brain stem function. It stimulates the respiratory centers in the brain stem by inducing hypercarbia. One technique requires ventilating the patient with 100% oxygen for 10 to 30 minutes (depending on the severity of any underlying lung injury) followed by disconnection from the respirator and administration of 100% oxygen through a catheter in the trachea or via a T-piece at a flow rate of 6 L/min. Absence of spontaneous respiratory effort with a $PaCO_2$ of above 60 mm Hg or >20 mm above baseline confirms clinical apnea. Arterial blood gas should be checked before and after the withdrawal of ventilation. Sometimes the test cannot be completed because of ventricular arrhythmias or hypotension. In that situation, the diagnosis of irreversible brain stem dysfunction is made by cerebral blood flow test or other appropriate confirmatory test. The American Academy of Neurology has published an evidence-based practice guideline for determining brain death in adults that provides additional important information.

 References available online at expertconsult.com.

WEBSITES

www.patient.co.uk/leaflets/brain stem_disorders.htm
www.nlm.nih.gov/medlineplus/dizzinessandvertigo.html

BIBLIOGRAPHY

1. Baloh RW: Dizziness, Hearing Loss, and Tinnitus, Philadelphia, F.A. Davis, 1998.
2. Kandel ER, Schwartz JH, Jessell TM: Principles of Neural Science, 5th ed. New York, McGraw-Hill, 2012.
3. Leigh RJ, Zee DS: The Neurology of Eye Movements, 4th ed. Oxford, Oxford University Press, 2006.
4. Posner JB, Saper CB, Schiff N, et al.: Plum and Posner's Diagnosis of Stupor and Coma, 4th ed. Oxford, Oxford University Press, 2007.
5. Ropper AH, Samuels MA, Klein JP: Adams and Victor's Principles of Neurology, 10th ed. New York, McGraw-Hill, 2014.

CHAPTER 10

CEREBELLAR DISEASE

Joohi Jimenez-Shahed

1. **What is the function of the cerebellum?**
   The cerebellum coordinates movement and maintains equilibrium and muscle tone. It compares what you thought you were going to do (according to motor cortex) with what is actually happening in the limbs (according to proprioceptive feedback) and corrects the movement if there is a problem through a complex regulatory feedback system. It receives somatosensory input from the spinal cord, motor information from the cerebral cortex, and balance input from the vestibular organs. It integrates all this information and aids in organizing the range, velocity, direction, and force of muscular contractions to produce steady volitional movements and posture. It does so by constantly screening its sensory inputs and modulating its motor outputs.

2. **What is the functional anatomy of the cerebellum?**
   - **Three sagittal divisions:** the left and right hemispheres and vermis. This segregation helps describe cerebellar syndromes (Table 10-1).
   - **Three transverse divisions** correspond to major lobes, separated by fissures: the anterior, posterior, and flocculonodular lobes (Fig. 10-1).
   - **Three pairs of midline nuclei** organized from medial to lateral are the fastigial, nucleus interpositus (containing the emboliform and globose nuclei), and the dentate nucleus.
   - **Three paired cerebellar peduncles** contain the information flow to and from the cerebellum: the superior (a.k.a. brachium conjunctivum, SCP), the middle (a.k.a. the brachium pontis, MCP) and the inferior cerebellar peduncles (a.k.a. restiform body, ICP).

3. **What are the major input pathways to the cerebellum?**
   Cerebellar inputs include corticopontine fibers (related to planning and initiation of movement), fibers from the inferior olivary nucleus (for motor learning and motor timing), and spinocerebellar pathways (containing proprioceptive information).
   The SCP primarily contains efferent fibers from the cerebellar nuclei, as well as some afferents from the spinocerebellar tract. The MCP primarily contains afferents from the pontine nuclei. The ICP primarily contains afferent fibers from the medulla, as well as efferents to the vestibular nuclei.

4. **How does the cerebellum process movement and somatosensory information?**
   There are three major cellular layers of the cerebellar cortex: the molecular, Purkinje, and granule cell layers. Corticopontine fibers synapse in the pons, cross, and project to the contralateral cerebellar cortex via the MCP (mossy fibers). Information from the inferior olives (climbing fibers) and spinocerebellar tract (also mossy fibers) are received via the ICP.
   Climbing fibers reach the Purkinje layer directly while mossy fibers synapse on granule cells, which then send long parallel fibers that in turn synapse on Purkinje cells. Purkinje cells organize the main output of the cerebellar cortex by sending axons to the deep cerebellar nuclei. The fastigial nuclei connect to the reticular formation, the interposed nuclei to the red nucleus, and the dentate nucleus to the thalamus.

5. **What are the major output targets of the cerebellum?**
   The major output targets are the red nucleus, vestibular nuclei, superior colliculus, reticular formation, and thalamus. The cerebellum therefore influences motor activity via both cortical and spinal projections. Fibers leave via the SCP, projecting first to the ventral lateral and ventral intermediate nuclei of the thalamus, then through thalamocortical projections to modify cerebrocortical motor neurons. Cerebellar projections to the reticulospinal, vestibulospinal, and rubrospinal tracts modify spinal cord alpha and gamma motor neurons.

6. **What is the blood supply to the cerebellum?**
   The vertebral and basilar arteries give off three paired branches to the cerebellum: the superior, the anterior inferior, and the posterior inferior cerebellar arteries, which are interconnected by anastomoses. The superior cerebellar artery runs over the superior surface of the cerebellum, while the other arteries supply the inferior surface.

Table 10-1. Cerebellar Syndromes

CLINICAL SYNDROME	REGION(S) INVOLVED	DISTRIBUTION OF DEFICITS	COMMON CAUSES	OTHER FEATURES
Rostral vermis	Anterior and superior vermis, includes fastigial nucleus	Wide-based stance Gait ataxia with little ataxia on heel to shin Normal or only slightly impaired arm coordination	Alcoholism (affects Purkinje cells) Thiamine deficiency	Infrequent presence of hypotonia, nystagmus, and dysarthria
Caudal vermis	Superior vermis and flocculo-nodular lobe	Axial disequilibrium, ataxic gait, and little or no limb ataxia	Neoplasm (e.g., medulloblas-toma, especially in children)	Sometimes spontaneous nystagmus and rotated postures of the head
Lateral zone	Cerebellar hemi-sphere	Ipsilateral dysfunction: Dysmetria Dysdiadochokinesia Hypotonia Dysarthria Excessive rebound Ocular movement abnormalities	Lesions (e.g., infarct, neoplasm, abscess)	Tremor if dentate nucleus involved No balance or gait disorder
Pancerebellar	All areas	Bilateral signs of cerebellar dysfunction	Infectious/parain-fectious causes, toxic/metabolic, paraneoplastic cerebellar syn-dromes, hereditary cerebellar degen-erations	—

7. **What are the signs and symptoms of cerebellar dysfunction?**
   - **Dysmetria**—movements that fall short of or go past the intended target. Hypometria = premature arrest; hypermetria = failure to arrest movements. Dysmetria is examined by the finger-to-nose test or great toe-to-examiner's finger test (using only hip movement).
   - **Dysdiadochokinesia**—a disturbance in rapid alternating movements, tested by rapid supination/pronation of the forearm on a tabletop or the lap to evaluate the rate, range, force, and accuracy of voluntary movements. This should not be confused with bradykinesia.
   - **Dysarthria**—ataxic speech has an irregular pattern, caused by interference from articulation, respiration, and phonation. Also: *adiodochokinesis* (slow and deliberate speech), explosive-hesitant speech (syllables can be explosive and produced at incorrect points of emphasis), or scanning speech (stretching of the syllables, which also sharply cut off).
   - **Hypotonia**—decreased resistance to passive limb manipulation. There may be a greater than normal range of motion in the first 7 to 10 days after cerebellar injury.
   - **Oculomotor signs**—nystagmus (gaze-evoked, rebound, downbeat, or positional), skew deviation, saccadic dysmetria, impaired smooth pursuit, and impaired optokinetic nystagmus.
   - **Gait ataxia**—wide-based and staggering steps, possibly stiff-legged due to disturbed postural reflexes. Impaired tandem gait and truncal swaying may be present. Patients generally fall to the side of the lesion. Ataxia does not significantly worsen when visual input is removed (e.g., Romberg test is negative) whereas in sensory ataxia, a patient may compensate for proprioceptive defects by visual guidance (positive Romberg).

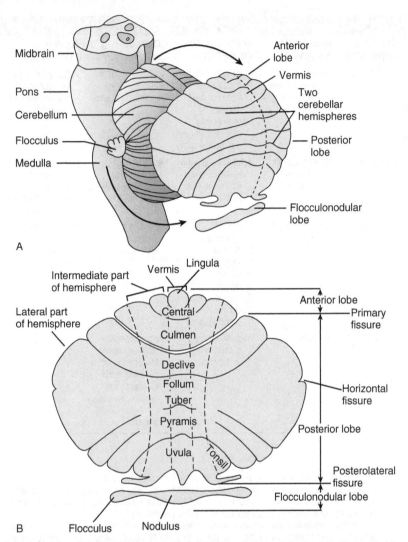

Figure 10-1. The cerebellum is divided into anatomically distinct lobes. **A,** The cerebellum is unfolded to reveal the lobes normally hidden from view. **B,** The main body of the cerebellum is divided by the primary fissure into anterior and posterior lobes. The posterolateral fissure separates the flocculonodular lobe. Shallower fissures divide the anterior and posterior lobes into nine lobules. The cerebellum has three functional regions: the central vermis and the lateral and intermediate zones in each hemisphere. *(From Ghez C: The cerebellum. In Kandel ER, et al. (eds): Principles of neural science. New York: Elsevier, 1991.)*

- **Tremor**—worsens as the target is approached ("intention tremor") during finger-to-nose testing. A "static tremor," manifested as titubation of the head or trunk, can be observed while holding the arms or legs parallel to the floor and observing rhythmic movements at the shoulder or hip. A Holmes or rubral tremor is a combination of rest, postural, and action tremors of 3 to 4 Hz, often due to midbrain lesions in the vicinity of the red nucleus. Large amplitude proximal tremors (tested in the wing-beating position) are characteristic, enhanced with posture and aggravated with movement.

8. What are the general principles in localizing a cerebellar lesion?
   - Lesions of the midline impair coordination involving stance and gait.
   - Lateral lesions impair the limbs ipsilateral to the cerebellar lesion.
   - Lesions of the cerebellar hemisphere impair movement ipsilaterally due to three major decussations. With movement initiation, corticopontine fibers synapse in the pons→cross in the MCP (first decussation) via the pontocerebellar fibers→cerebellum→cross back to the red nucleus via the SCP decussation (second)→cerebral cortex. With movement execution, the corticospinal tracts cross at the decussation of the pyramids (third) in the medullocervical junction. Hence, a left cerebellar hemispheric lesion causes a deficit in the left hemibody by influencing movement(s) originating in the right cerebral cortex.
   - Lesions of the afferent or efferent pathways may also cause cerebellar signs.
   - Lesions of the SCP and the deep nuclei usually produce the most severe disturbances.

9. What are the major cerebellar syndromes?
   The four major cerebellar syndromes are described in detail in Table 10-1 and include the rostral vermis, caudal vermis (flocculonodular lobe), lateral/hemispheric, and pancerebellar syndromes. They are distinguished by their presentations and the anatomic regions affected. Recognition of these syndromes may help to narrow the differential diagnosis of cerebellar lesions.

10. What are the classic cerebellar stroke syndromes?
    The cerebellar stroke syndromes are described in Table 10-2 and are suggested by abrupt onset, nausea, and vomiting in the absence of other localizing symptoms (or disproportionate to amount of dizziness or vertigo), sudden/severe/sustained headache particularly with other neurologic symptoms, persistent dizziness (>24 hours) especially in association with sudden hearing loss, or cranial nerve dysfunction. Physical examination features that should suggest cerebellar stroke include normal vestibulo-ocular reflexes, spontaneous nystagmus, skew deviation, severe difficulty or inability to stand or walk, or other localizing neurologic findings.

Table 10-2. Cerebellar Stroke Syndromes

	POSTERIOR INFERIOR CEREBELLAR ARTERY	ANTERIOR INFERIOR CEREBELLAR ARTERY	SUPERIOR CEREBELLAR ARTERY
Origin	Vertebral artery	Proximal or midbasilar artery	Distal basilar artery
Key brain stem structures affected	Posterolateral medulla Inferior cerebellar peduncle	Posterolateral pons Middle cerebellar peduncle	Posterolateral midbrain Superior cerebellar peduncle
Key cerebellar structures affected	Posteroinferior cerebellum	Anteroinferior cerebellum Inner ear (labyrinth, cochlea)	Superior cerebellum
Major features	Isolated acute vestibular syndrome without auditory symptoms	Isolated acute vestibular syndrome with auditory symptoms	Acute gait or trunk instability with dysarthria, nausea, vomiting
Neurologic signs	*Lateral medullary syndrome* (unilateral absent gag reflex; palatal palsy; vocal cord palsy; Horner's syndrome; body hemianalgesia; limb hemiataxia; dysmetria)	*Lateral pontine syndrome* (hemifacial sensory loss; lower motor neuron facial palsy; Horner's syndrome; body hemianalgesia limb hemiataxia; dysmetria)	*Lateral midbrain syndrome* (hemifacial sensory loss; Horner's syndrome; body hemisensory loss; limb hemiataxia; dysmetria)

11. **What are potential complications of a cerebellar stroke or hemorrhage?**
Edema from a cerebellar infarction or expanding hematoma can mimic a mass lesion and cause brain stem compression and obstructive hydrocephalus. These effects are most likely to peak on the third day after the stroke. New onset of gaze palsy, progressive decline in level of consciousness, new hemiparesis, and irregular breathing are indicators of hydrocephalus and constitute a neurologic and neurosurgical emergency. In such cases, 85% of patients may die without surgical intervention such as placement of a ventriculostomy or craniectomy.

12. **How can cerebellar disorders be classified?**
    - **Congenital/developmental** (Joubert syndrome, Dandy–Walker syndrome, Chiari malformations [Table 10-3])
    - **Acquired:**
      1. *Vascular* (infarction [thrombotic > embolic] or ischemia; hemorrhage [from hypertension, vascular malformation, or tumor]; vertebral dissection; basilar migraine; vascular malformation; systemic vasculitides)
      2. *Neoplasms* (see later section)
      3. *Infections* (acute cerebellar ataxia of childhood [possibly viral]; tuberculosis or tuberculoma; cysticercosis; bacterial infection/abscess [extension of mastoid infection]; chronic panencephalitis of congenital rubella; viral encephalitis [involving cerebellum or brainstem]; Whipple's disease)
      4. *Inflammatory/autoimmune* (multiple sclerosis, acute postinfectious cerebellitis, acute disseminated encephalomyelitis, Miller–Fisher variant of acute inflammatory polyneuropathy, anti-GAD-associated cerebellar ataxia, celiac and gluten ataxia)
      5. *Paraneoplastic* (paraneoplastic cerebellar degeneration [see later section]; opsoclonus–myoclonus [secondary to neuroblastoma])
      6. *Metabolic* (hypothyroidism, hyperthermia, hypoxia, deficiencies of thiamine [in those with alcoholic abuse], niacin [pellagra], vitamin E, essential amino acids, zinc)
      7. *Drugs/toxins* (antiepileptic drugs [phenytoin, carbamazepine, barbiturates]; chemotherapeutic agents [5-fluorouracil, cytosine arabinoside]; heavy metals [thallium, lead, organic mercury])
      8. *Trauma* (postconcussion syndrome, intracranial hematoma, brain contusion)
    - **Degenerative** (multiple systems atrophy [cerebellar type], Creutzfeld–Jakob disease)
    - **Inherited/genetic** (autosomal dominant, autosomal recessive, episodic mutations)

Table 10-3. Chiari Malformations

TYPE	CHARACTERISTICS
I	Extension of tonsils into foramen magnum without brain stem involvement
	May be asymptomatic
II	Extension of tonsils and brain stem into foramen magnum, vermis may be partially complete or absent
	Myelomeningocele is present
III	Cerebellum and brain stem herniate through foramen magnum and into spinal canal
	Can have occipital encephalocele with severe neurologic deficits
IV	Incomplete or underdeveloped cerebellum

13. **What are features of autosomal dominant ataxias?**
Also referred to as *spinocerebellar ataxias* (SCAs), these disorders have common core features of cerebellar and brainstem signs and symptoms and dysfunction of associated pathways and connections (Table 10-4). Over 30 types are identified and grouped by shared mechanisms: polyglutamine expansions, ion-channel dysfunction, mutations in signal transduction molecules, and disease associated with noncoding repeats. Although family history with an autosomal dominant inheritance pattern should heighten suspicion for an SCA, individual SCAs are difficult to distinguish based on clinical grounds. Phenotypes may include pure cerebellar ataxia or ataxia with various comorbidities. Anticipation, where subsequent generations manifest symptoms at an earlier age, is seen in polyglutamine expansions. SCA3 is the most common worldwide. SCAs 1, 2, 3, 6, and 7 account for 50% of all dominant ataxias. With onset >50 years, SCA6 and fragile X tremor/ataxia syndrome (FXTAS) are most frequent.

Table 10-4. Select Autosomal Dominant Spinocerebellar Ataxias

TYPE	MUTATION AND FUNCTION	FEATURES
SCA1	Ataxin 1 CAG repeats 41-81 Gene transcription and RNA splicing	Pyramidal signs Amyotrophy Extrapyramidal signs Ophthalmoparesis
SCA2	Ataxin 2 CAG repeats 35-59 RNA processing	Slow saccades Extrapyramidal signs Dementia (rarely) Ophthalmoplegia Peripheral neuropathy Pyramidal signs
SCA3 (Machado–Joseph disease)	Ataxin 3 CAG repeats 62-82 Deubiquinating enzyme	Pyramidal signs Amyotrophy Exophthalmos Extrapyramidal signs Ophthalmoparesis
SCA6	Cav2.1 CAG repeats 21-30 Calcium channel	Pure cerebellar ataxia Late onset, usual >50 years old
SCA7	Ataxin 7 CAG repeats 38-130 Gene transcription	Pigmentary macular degeneration Ophthalmoplegia Pyramidal signs
SCA17 (HDL4)	TATA box-binding protein CAG repeats 46-63 Gene transcription	Chorea Dementia Extrapyramidal features Hyperreflexia Psychiatric symptoms
DRPLA	Atrophin 1 CAG repeats 49-75 Transcriptional coregulator	Myoclonic epilepsy Choreoathetosis Dementia

FXTAS	FMR1 (gene for fragile X
	   syndrome)
	Premutation: CAG repeats
	   55-200
		Gait ataxia
		Action > resting tremors
		Frontal/dysexecutive syndrome
		Peripheral neuropathy
		Increased T2 signal in MCP

FXTAS, Fragile X-associated tremor/ataxia syndrome; DRPLA, dentatorubral-pallidoluysian atrophy; SCA, spinocerebellar ataxia; HDL4, Huntington's disease-like 4; MCP, middle cerebellar peduncle.

14. **What are the most common autosomal recessive ataxias?**
   Autosomal recessive cerebellar ataxias are heterogeneous, often multisystem neurodegenerative diseases that tend to manifest in children and young adults, and should be suspected in anyone under the age of 30 with insidious and progressive ataxia, hypotonia, or clumsiness.
   - **Friedreich's ataxia (FA):** FA is the most frequent and presents between 7 and 25 years of age. A repeat expansion in frataxin, a mitochondrial protein involved in cellular iron homeostasis, leads to dysfunction in the respiratory chain and Krebs cycle. FA manifests with progressive gait and limb ataxia, dysarthria, sensory neuropathy, and pyramidal signs. Patients are generally areflexic but exhibit extensor plantar responses. Scoliosis, square wave jerks, left ventricular hypertrophy (60% of patients), and diabetes mellitus (15%) or carbohydrate intolerance (25%) may also be present. Nystagmus and cerebellar atrophy are not prominent. Progression includes significant difficulties with activities of daily living, loss of ambulation, dysarthria, and dysphagia.
   - **Ataxia-telangiectasia (AT):** AT is the second most frequent and often starts before age 5 years. Progressive hypotonia and clumsiness are accompanied by conjunctival telangiectasias, oculomotor apraxia, dysarthria, chorea ± dystonia, and sensorimotor axonal neuropathy. Mutations of the

ATM gene, a member of the phosphatidylinositol-3 kinase family of proteins involved in repair of DNA damage, cause a predilection for lymphoid malignancies and recurrent infections. Loss of ambulation occurs within 10 years. Severe cerebellar atrophy develops over time. Elevated serum alpha-fetoprotein levels can assist with diagnosis.

15. What are the features of the episodic ataxias?
These autosomal dominant conditions include attacks of acute recurrent ataxia that can be treatable. In type 1 (EA1), patients have brief (1- to 2-minute) episodes of ataxia triggered by exercise, emotionality, or startle and interictally have myokymia of the face or hand muscles. EA1 is caused by mutations in a voltage-gated potassium channel (*KCNA1*). Episodic ataxia type 2 (EA2) consists of longer attacks (hours to days) triggered by stress, exercise, phenytoin, and caffeine. Interictal nystagmus may be present. EA2 is caused by mutations in the calcium channel alpha 1 subunit (*CACN1A4*), the same gene responsible for familial hemiplegic migraine and SCA6. Slowly progressive ataxia, dysarthria, and vermian atrophy may occur. Response to acetazolamide is quite dramatic in EA2, less so in EA1.

16. What is paraneoplastic cerebellar degeneration (PCD)?
PCD is the most common remote effect of neoplasm affecting the brain, associated with lung (especially small-cell), ovarian, and breast neoplasms as well as Hodgkin's disease. A prodrome (a viral-like illness, dizziness, nausea, or vomiting) may be followed by rapid development and progression of gait unsteadiness, ataxia, diplopia, dysarthria, and dysphagia over a few weeks to months. Pathology reveals extensive loss of Purkinje cells and inflammatory infiltrates. Neuroimaging is typically normal early, with delayed progressive cerebellar atrophy. Associated antibodies include (1) anti-Hu or ANNA1 (found predominantly in small-cell lung cancer); (2) anti-Yo or PCA1 (ovarian and breast cancers); and (3) anti-Tr (Hodgkin's lymphoma). Treatment includes steroids, plasmapheresis, intravenous immunoglobulin, tacrolimus, and rituximab, with varying success, or complete removal of the underlying malignancy.

17. How do posterior fossa tumors differ between adults and children?
Posterior fossa tumors are more common in children (approximately 50% to 70% of all brain tumors) than in adults. Pediatric tumors include medulloblastoma, pineoblastoma, ependymomas, primitive neuroectodermal tumors (PNETs), and astrocytomas of the cerebellum and brain stem. Cerebellar astrocytoma presents as a laterally located cyst with a well-defined solid component, either in the vermis or cerebellar hemisphere. Low-grade brainstem gliomas may also occur. PNETs originate from undifferentiated cells in the subependymal region in the fetal brain. Medulloblastomas often fill the fourth ventricular space and infiltrate surrounding tissue.
     In adults, extra-axial tumors are more common and include vestibular schwannomas (the most common cerebellopontine angle mass), meningiomas, choroid plexus papillomas, solitary fibrous tumors, and epidermoid cysts. Schwannomas are associated with neurofibromatosis type 2, and bilateral vestibular schwannomas are diagnostic of this condition. Intra-axial tumors include hemangioblastomas (the most common adult primary intra-axial posterior fossa mass), lymphoma, ganglioglioma, Lhermitte–Duclos disease, and metastases.

18. What are the clinical features and causes of the cerebellopontine angle syndrome?
Lesions at the space between the cerebellum and the pons often compress and interfere with the functions of the nearby cranial nerves V, VII, and VIII. Symptoms may include depression or absence of the ipsilateral corneal reflex, facial numbness, and weakness of the mastication muscles (cranial nerve V); facial myokymia or ipsilateral lower motor neuron paralysis (cranial nerve VII); and hearing loss, tinnitus, and vertigo (cranial nerve VIII). Enlarging lesions may distort the brain stem, producing long-tract signs or obstruction of the aqueduct to cause hydrocephalus and increased intracranial pressure. Compression of the cerebellar hemisphere adjacent to the cerebellopontine angle presents with ipsilateral limb ataxia and intention tremor or nystagmus.
     Vestibular schwannoma (also called *acoustic neuroma*) is the most common extra-axial cause. It originates from Schwann cells in the sheath of cranial nerve VIII, close to its attachment to the brain stem. Early cranial nerve VIII involvement is characteristic, while cranial nerve VII is spared until much later. Early cranial nerve VII involvement should suggest other lesions, such as meningioma, epidermoidoma, craniopharyngioma, glomus jugulare tumor, and aneurysm of the basilar artery. Intra-axial masses of the brain stem and cerebellum also may cause the syndrome if they are sufficiently large and extend into the cerebellopontine space (Fig. 10-2).

19. What are the clinical features of the cerebellar herniation syndromes?
Mass lesions, particularly neoplasms and hematomas, often present as nonspecific symptoms such as headache. As they enlarge, the increased pressure causes herniation of the cerebellum.

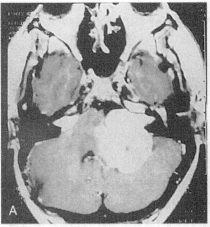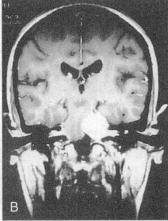

Figure 10-2. Gadolinium-enhanced T1-weighted magnetic resonance images (MRIs) show bilateral acoustic neuromas (especially large on the left) in a patient with neurofibromatosis. **A,** Axial view. **B,** Coronal view.

With downward herniation, the cerebellar tonsils are pushed through the foramen magnum and compress the medulla (tonsillar herniation), causing progressive vomiting, stiff neck, skew deviation of the eyes, coma, ataxic breathing, apnea, and death if not anticipated and prevented.

In upward herniation, the cerebellum and upper brain stem are pushed through the tentorial opening (uncal herniation), leading to progressive compression of the pons and midbrain. The patient is usually obtunded or comatose with small pupils (reactive at first) or anisocoria. Oculocephalic and oculovestibular responses are abnormal. Hemiparesis may progress to quadriparesis and decorticate posturing.

20. **What is the treatment for cerebellar herniation?**
    Osmotic agents and hyperventilation may provide temporary relief, but definitive treatment for cerebellar herniations consists of surgical decompression and removal of the mass, if possible.

KEY POINTS

1. Cerebellar organization allows for simultaneous processing of motor and sensory information to coordinate movements:
   - The three major inputs to the cerebellum are from corticopontine fibers, fibers from the inferior olivary nucleus, and spinocerebellar pathways.
   - The superior cerebellar peduncle relays most cerebellar efferents.
   - The cerebellum influences motor activity via both cortical and spinal projections.
   - Cerebellar disease generally produces effects ipsilateral to the lesion.
2. Cerebellar signs and symptoms represent a unique constellation of findings:
   - Dysmetria
   - Dysdiadochokinesia (to be differentiated from bradykinesia)
   - Dysarthria
   - Hypotonia
   - Oculomotor signs
   - Gait ataxia (to be differentiated from sensory ataxia)
   - Tremor (including Holmes/rubral tremor)
3. Identification of cerebellar syndromes based on anatomy can help generate a differential diagnosis:
   - Rostral vermis syndrome is most classically related to alcoholism.
   - Caudal vermis syndrome is often due to a neoplasm.
   - Lateral zone syndrome is due to a lesion of the cerebellar hemisphere (e.g., infarct, neoplasm, or abscess).
   - Pancerebellar syndromes are most often due to infections, paraneoplastic syndromes, or hereditary conditions.

Acknowledgment

The author would like to acknowledge the contributions of Eugene C. Lai, MD, PhD, who was the author of this chapter in the previous edition.

 References available online at expertconsult.com.

WEBSITE

National Ataxia Foundation: www.ataxia.org.

BIBLIOGRAPHY

1. Brazis PW, Masdeu JC, Biller J (eds): Localization in Clinical Neurology, 6th ed. Philadelphia, Lippincott Williams & Wilkins, 2011.
2. Fahn S, Jankovic J, Hallet M (eds): Principles and Practice of Movement Disorders, 2nd ed. Philadelphia, Saunders, 2011.
3. Jankovic J, Tolosa E (eds): Parkinson's Disease and Movement Disorders, Philadelphia, Lippincott Williams & Wilkins, 2007.
4. Purves D, Augustine GJ, Fitzpatrick D, Katz LC, LaMantia A, McNamara JO, Williams SM (eds): Neuroscience, 2nd ed. Sunderland (MA), Sinauer Associates, 2001.
5. Ropper AH, Samules MA, Klein JP (eds): Adams and Victor's Principles of Neurology, 10th ed. New York, McGraw-Hill, 2014.

CHAPTER 11

BASAL GANGLIA DISORDERS

Subhashie Wijemanne, Philip A. Hanna, Joseph Jankovic

ANATOMY AND PHYSIOLOGY

1. **What are the components of the basal ganglia?**

    The basal ganglia are a group of nuclei situated in the deep part of the cerebrum and upper part of the brain stem. Included among these nuclei are the *striatum,* which is composed of the **caudate, putamen,** and **nucleus accumbens** (ventral striatum); the *pallidum,* composed of the internal (medial) and external (lateral) parts of the **globus pallidus** (GP); the **subthalamic nucleus** (STN); and the **substantia nigra** (SN), composed of the pars compacta (SNc) and pars reticulata (SNr). The putamen and GP are combined to form the lenticular (or lentiform) nucleus because of their lens-like appearance. These interrelated structures are primarily responsible for control of motor functions (Fig. 11-1).

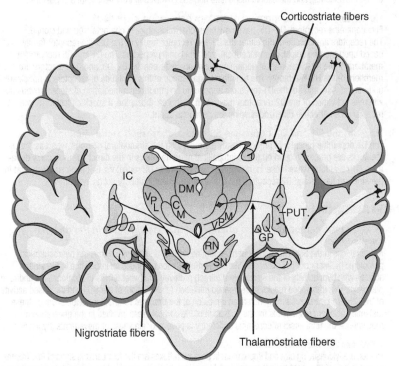

Figure 11-1. The basal ganglia and thalamus. *PUT,* Putamen; *GP,* globus pallidus; *SN,* substantia nigra; *RN,* red nucleus; *IC,* internal capsule; *VPL,* ventral posterior lateral nucleus; *VPM,* ventral posterior medial nucleus; *CM,* centromedian nucleus; *DM,* dorsomedian nucleus.

2. **How are the basal ganglia organized?**

    There are three levels of organization within the basal ganglia. The first level consists of the two major striatal outputs: (1) the indirect pathway to the external segment of the GP (GPe) and (2) the direct pathway to the SNr and internal segment of the GP (GPi). The second level of organization consists of pathways from the cerebral cortex (sublaminae of layer V) to the patch (striosome) and matrix compartments of the striatum (which are organized in a mosaic pattern). The third level of organization is related to the topography of cortical projections to other regions of the striatum.

3. What are the neurotransmitters of the two major striatal output pathways?
Medium spiny neurons (MSN), the principal neurons of the striatum, are GABAergic and project to the GPe, GPi, and SNr. Approximately 50% of MSN also contain substance P and dynorphin and project to the SNr and GPi. The other half of the neurons expresses enkephalin and projects their axons to the GPe. These pathways are, respectively, called striatonigral or **direct pathway** and striatopallidal or **indirect pathway**. The direct and indirect pathways are thought to have opposing actions: direct pathway activation may inhibit GPi/SNr activity, thereby disinhibiting thalamocortical interactions, while indirect pathway activates thalamocortical interactions.

4. What is the source of the major output of the basal ganglia?
The primary basal ganglia output arises from GPi and SNr. The GPi and SNr bear many similarities and are often regarded as a functional unit separated during development by the internal capsule. The output neurons from the GPi and SNr to the thalamus are mainly GABAergic and innervate the mediodorsal and ventral tier thalamic nuclei (which provide feedback to the frontal cortex), the intralaminar thalamic nuclei (which provide feedback to the striatum), the superior colliculus (important in the control of the ocular movements), and the pedunculopontine nucleus (involved in the maintenance of posture).

5. How many types of dopamine receptors have been identified?
Five dopamine receptors, D1–D5, have now been pharmacologically characterized and cloned. The receptors are classified into either the D1-like receptor family or the D2-like receptor family, based upon morphological, pharmaceutical, and functional properties. The D1 and D5 receptors are members of the D1-like family of dopamine receptors, whereas the D2, D3, and D4 receptors are members of the D2-like family. The functional significance of this multitude of receptors is not clearly understood. Activation of the D1 receptors appears to be important in mediating dystonic movements, whereas activation of the D2 receptors may result in chorea. Clozapine, a specific blocker for the D4 receptor, is an effective dibenzodiazepine antipsychotic agent.

6. How are the D1 and D2 dopamine receptors expressed in the striatum?
The D1 dopamine receptor is predominantly expressed on the striatonigral neurons, whereas the D2 receptors are primarily found on the striatopallidal neurons. MSNs in the direct pathway carry dopamine D1 receptors, while those in the indirect pathway carry D2 receptors. Evidence suggests that in the striatum the D1 and D2 receptors have an excitatory and inhibitory action, respectively.

PARKINSONISM

7. What are the neurophysiologic changes in the basal ganglia in Parkinson's disease (PD)?
Neuronal loss in the SNc with consequent dopamine depletion in the striatum is the neurochemical–pathologic hallmark of PD. This dopaminergic deafferentation produces an imbalance in the striatal activity, with hypoactivity of the striatonigral (direct) pathway and hyperactivity of striatopallidal (indirect) pathways. This imbalance results in decreased inhibition (disinhibition) of the STN and increased activity of the GPi/SNr neurons, causing increased inhibition of the thalamic ventral tier nuclei. Because these thalamic nuclei are responsible for the activation of the cortical areas involved in the generation of movements, the final effect of dopamine deficiency is poverty or slowness of movements (hypokinesia).

8. What are the cardinal signs of PD?
Tremor, bradykinesia, rigidity, and impairment in postural reflexes are the four cardinal signs of PD. **Tremor** at rest is one of the most typical signs of parkinsonism. It is characterized by an oscillatory pronation–supination at a 3- to 5-Hz frequency. In addition to the hands, where it assumes an appearance of pill rolling, this type of tremor is commonly observed in the facial musculature (lips and chin) as well as in the legs. Head tremor, however, is rare in parkinsonism, and its presence should suggest the diagnosis of essential tremor (ET). The term **bradykinesia** is used to describe slowness of movements that often causes difficulties for the patients in getting dressed, feeding, and maintaining personal hygiene. Bradykinesia is evident when a patient performs rapid alternating movements, such as pronation and supination of the forearms. **Rigidity**, often associated with the cogwheel phenomenon, is another hallmark of parkinsonism. **Impairment of the postural reflexes** is responsible for the falls that are frequently experienced by parkinsonian patients. Parkinsonian gait often reflects a combination of bradykinesia, rigidity, and postural instability.

9. **What are the most common causes of parkinsonism?**
In a highly selected population, such as that attending a movement disorders clinic, PD is responsible for 77.7% of the cases of parkinsonism. The other most frequent causes are parkinsonism-plus syndrome (12.2%), secondary parkinsonism (8.2%), and inherited neredodegenerative parkinsonism (0.6%) (Table 11-1).

Table 11-1. Causes of Parkinsonism

I. Idiopathic Parkinsonism
Parkinson's disease
    Sporadic form
    Familial form

II. Secondary Parkinsonism
Drug induced
    Dopamine receptor blockers (neuroleptics, antiemetics such as metoclopramide)
    Dopamine depleters (reserpine, tetrabenazine)
    Calcium channel blockers (flunarizine, cinnarizine, diltiazem)
    Lithium
    Methyldopa
Hemiparkinsonism–hemiatrophy syndrome
Hydrocephalus
    Normal pressure hydrocephalus
    Noncommunicating hydrocephalus
Hypoxia
Infectious diseases
    Postencephalitic parkinsonism
    Acquired immunodeficiency syndrome
    Intracytoplasmic hyaline inclusion disease
    Creutzfeldt–Jakob disease
    Subacute sclerosing panencephalitis
Metabolic
    Acquired hepatocerebral degeneration (chronic liver insufficiency)
    Hypocalcemic parkinsonism
Paraneoplastic parkinsonism
Syringomesencephalia
Toxin
    Carbon disulfide
    Ethanol
    Carbon monoxide
    Manganese
    Cyanide
    Methanol
    Disulfiram
    MPTP
Trauma
Tumor
Vascular
    Multi-infarcts
    Binswanger's disease
    Lower body parkinsonism

III. Parkinsonism-Plus Syndromes
Diffuse Lewy body disease
Progressive supranuclear palsy

Continued on following page

Table 11-1. Causes of Parkinsonism *(Continued)*

Corticobasal degeneration
MSA
   MSA with predominant parkinsonism (MSA-P)
   MSA with predominant cerebellar ataxia (MSA-C)
Alzheimer's disease–parkinsonism
Parkinsonism–dementia–amyotrophic lateral sclerosis
Progressive pallidal atrophy
IV. Heredodegenerative Diseases
Ceroid lipofuscinosis
X-linked dystonia–parkinsonism
Gerstmann–Strausler–Scheinker disease
Disinhibition–dementia–parkinsonism
Familial OPCA amyotrophy complex
Neurodegeneration with brain iron accumulation
Autosomal dominant Lewy body disease
Huntington's disease
Hereditary ceruloplasmin deficiency
Dopa-responsive dystonia
Familial progressive subcortical gliosis
Familial basal ganglia calcification
Machado–Joseph disease
Familial parkinsonism with peripheral neuropathy
Mitochondrial cytopathies with striatal necrosis
Parkinsonian–pyramidal syndrome
Neuroacanthocytosis
Wilson's disease

MPTP, 1-Methyl-4-phenyl-1,2,3,6-tetrahydropyridine; *OPCA*, olivopontocerebellar atrophy; *MSA*, multiple system atrophy.

10. **What causes PD?**

Although PD was first described by James Parkinson in 1817, its cause is still unknown. The recognition that 1-methyl-4-phenyl-1,2,3,6-tetrahydropyridine (MPTP) can produce in humans and nonhuman primates a parkinsonian syndrome very similar to PD led to the hypothesis that an MPTP-like substance in the environment could cause PD. One of the theories about the cause of PD is that, as a result of a defective antioxidant system and increased formation of highly reactive and toxic-free oxygen radicals (oxidative stress), abnormally folded proteins accumulate in the affected neurons and overwhelm the ubiquitin–proteasome system. When the compensatory autophagic mechanisms fail, intracytoplasmic neuronal inclusions called Lewy bodies form, and the neuron eventually dies. A growing body of evidence supports the role of genetics in the etiology of PD. Families with an autosomal dominant and recessive transmission of otherwise typical PD have been described, as have monozygotic twins concordant for the disease. In addition to several monogenetic causes of PD, such as mutations in genes that code for alpha-synuclein, leucine-rich repeat kinase 2, Parkin, and others, there are other genetic abnormalities that increase vulnerability to cell death, including glucocerebrosidase, particularly common in people of Jewish and Middle Eastern origin. The etiology of PD is still speculative, but a combination of environmental factors may be associated with a genetic predisposition. In addition, there is growing evidence that PD pathology, particularly accumulation and aggregation of toxic alpha-synuclein, originates in the peripheral system and then spreads from the caudal brainstem rostrally via a prion-like mechanism.

11. **What are the clinical and pathologic hallmarks of PD?**

Patients with PD may have several combinations of parkinsonian symptoms. Typically, the onset is insidious in the sixth decade of life, and the symptoms usually begin unilaterally or predominate on one side of the body. It is possible to recognize two clinical types of PD: a **tremor-dominant** form with earlier age of onset, slower progression, and relatively preserved cognition and **a postural instability and gait difficulty** form with more bradykinesia, more rapid progression, and dementia. Furthermore, ET is more likely to coexist in the tremor-dominant form. Pathologically, there is loss of dopaminergic neurons in the SNc, and the surviving neurons contain Lewy bodies. Although to a lesser degree than the SNc, other pigmented nuclei of the brain stem, such as the locus ceruleus and tegmental ventral area, are also involved by a similar process. A recent clinicopathologic study showed that the presence of a resting tremor is more likely to be associated with Lewy bodies at autopsy. Lewy bodies have also been demonstrated in nondopaminergic nuclei of the brain stem, the olfactory system, and the spinal cord. This distribution of Lewy bodies appears to correlate with the nonmotor, "preclinical" manifestations of PD. In addition to a deficiency of dopamine, nondopaminergic abnormalities are increasingly recognized in PD. These nondopaminergic abnormalities may be responsible for some of the symptoms that are resistant to dopaminergic therapy such as freezing, depression, cognitive decline, and dysautonomia.

12. **How specific is the clinical diagnosis of PD?**
   In one clinical–pathological study using the data from the Arizona Study of Aging and Neurodegenerative Disorders, only 80 of 97 (82%) cases diagnosed at first visit with probable PD had neuropathologically confirmed PD (Adler et al., 2014). Furthermore, only 8 of 15 (53%) diagnosed with probable PD with less than 5 years of disease duration had the diagnosis confirmed at autopsy, whereas 72 of 82 (88%) with ≥5 years of disease duration had pathologically confirmed PD. Thus, clinical diagnosis of PD identifies patients who will have pathologically confirmed PD with a sensitivity of 88% and specificity of 68%. Although the presence of rest tremor, bradykinesia, and rigidity has been thought in the past to be highly predictive of the correct diagnosis, this study found that response to dopaminergic drugs and levodopa-related motor complications were most helpful in making an accurate diagnosis of PD. Furthermore, only 20% to 26% of untreated cases who would be considered candidates for drug trials had accurate diagnosis of PD. These studies show that patients with typical symptoms may have variable pathologic findings; conversely, typical pathologic findings can be expressed by dissimilar signs. Findings of asymmetric onset, no evidence for other causes of parkinsonism, and no atypical features of PD increase the specificity of the clinical diagnosis.

13. **What is the role of DaTSCAN in the diagnosis of PD?**
   Reduction of DaT radiotracer uptake correlates with the loss of presynaptic nigrostriatal neurons and is more sensitive than clinical examination to detect nigrostriatal defects.
   Striatal dopamine transporter imaging using ^{123}I-FP-CIT single photon emission tomography (DaTSCAN) can reliably distinguish patients with PD and other parkinsonian syndromes (i.e., multiple system atrophy, progressive supranuclear palsy, and corticobasal degeneration) from controls or patients with ET, but it cannot differentiate PD and the other parkinsonian syndromes from one another.

14. **What is the role of monoamine oxidase (MAO)-B inhibitors in PD?**
   MAO-B inhibitors include selegiline and rasagiline, which help to block the breakdown of dopamine in the brain, thus making more dopamine available. These are modestly effective as symptomatic treatment for PD and may have neuroprotective properties. MAO-B inhibitors are usually used as early monotherapy or as an add-on medication to drugs such as levodopa in more advanced PD to decrease "off" time.

15. **What is the role of anticholinergic drugs and amantadine in the treatment of PD?**
   In the early stages of PD, anticholinergic drugs, combined with rasagiline or selegiline, may be used as the primary treatment. With progression of disease, most patients require the addition of levodopa. Tremor is occasionally resistant to dopaminergic therapy and may be better controlled in combination with anticholinergic medication such as trihexyphenidyl. Amantadine, a drug that has mild anticholinergic effects and increases the release of dopamine, also improves rigidity and bradykinesia. Furthermore, studies have revealed the utility of amantadine in reducing levodopa-induced dyskinesias (LID).
   The anticholinergic medications must be used cautiously because, in addition to causing dryness of the mouth and bladder retention, they may produce disorientation, confusion, and memory loss, particularly in the elderly. Amantadine in some patients also may cause cognitive side effects as well as livedo reticularis, hallucinations, ankle swelling, and worsening of congestive heart failure.

16. **When should levodopa therapy be started in the treatment of PD?**
   The mainstay in the treatment of PD is the replacement of dopamine. This therapy was introduced in the 1960s. Instead of using dopamine, which does not cross the blood–brain barrier, the current approach consists of combining levodopa and carbidopa. Levodopa is transformed into dopamine, and

carbidopa is a peripheral inhibitor of the enzyme dopa-decarboxylase. The inhibition of this enzyme in the periphery, but not in the brain, decreases substantially the required levodopa dosage and the occurrence of gastrointestinal side effects (nausea and vomiting). In Europe and other countries, benserazide is available as an inhibitor of dopa-decarboxylase.

The effectiveness of levodopa may be limited by early motor fluctuations and dyskinesia attributed to nonphysiological stimulation of dopamine receptors by multiple and higher cumulative levodopa doses. This effect is believed to occur more in younger PD patients.

A rational strategy is to start levodopa when the parkinsonian symptoms begin to impair activities of daily living or to interfere with social and occupational functioning. A typical starting dose for carbidopa/levodopa is 25/100 mg tab, 1-2 tabs 2 or 3 times/day. Maintenance doses of 200 to 600 mg/day of levodopa may be needed in patients with moderately advanced PD. Although some PD experts believe that delaying levodopa therapy is a prudent approach, longitudinal studies show no difference between patients who started on levodopa versus those who started on a dopamine agonist. Several recent studies have suggested that motor fluctuations and dyskinesias are not associated with the duration of levodopa therapy but rather with longer disease duration and higher levodopa daily dose. These studies show that patients who were started on levodopa relatively early in the course of the disease have very similar long-term outcomes as those with levodopa-sparing therapies. The approach to early therapy must be individualized, and generally those patients who require symptomatic therapy in order to maintain a satisfactory level of functioning at home and at work are started on levodopa early, whereas those whose symptoms are not troublesome may be started on dopamine agonists.

17. **What are the most common peripheral side effects of levodopa therapy, and how are they managed?**
Nausea and vomiting are common side effects in the beginning of the use of levodopa. Most of the patients overcome this difficulty by taking the medication after meals. In some patients, extra amounts of carbidopa (typically, one 25-mg tablet with each dose of carbidopa/levodopa) may be necessary. A small proportion of patients have nausea and vomiting despite these measures. Treatment of the gastrointestinal (GI) side effects should not include dopamine blockers, such as metoclopramide, because they may cause worsening of PD. Hydroxyzine, trimethobenzamide, diphenidol, cyclizine, or domperidone are useful alternatives. The most common cardiovascular side effect is orthostatic hypotension. The management of this complication involves adding salt to the diet, wearing elastic stockings, and using medications such as fludrocortisone, midodrine, or droxidopa.

18. **What clinical fluctuations are recognized in PD?**
Although the most dramatic fluctuations in patients with PD are related to levodopa therapy, some who have not been previously treated with dopaminergic drugs exhibit fluctuations in severity of their symptoms and signs. Fluctuations are not exclusively motor phenomena. The nonmotor fluctuations (NMF) are classified into three categories: dysautonomic, psychiatric, and sensory. Anxiety, drenching sweat, mental slowing, fatigue, akathesia, and dyspnea are some common NMF described in PD. They may occur during "on" or "off" periods and are associated with higher doses of levodopa. Significant improvements in such fluctuations have been reported following chronic subthalamic nucleus stimulation. Mood and autonomic functions also fluctuate. For example, some patients display depression when they are "off" and euphoria when they are "on." Fatigue and stress usually make these symptoms more prominent. The most dramatic example of spontaneous fluctuations is paradoxical dyskinesia: under extreme stress, patients completely immobilized by parkinsonism are suddenly able to stand up and run (Table 11-2).

19. **What are some of the strategies useful in the management of fluctuations in PD?**
The concept of continuous dopaminergic stimulation has been used as a guiding principle in the prevention and treatment of motor fluctuations. Strategies designed to achieve this goal include the use of catechol-O-methyltransferase (COMT) inhibitors, such as entacapone, MAO inhibitors such as selegiline and rasagiline, dopamine agonists, and STN deep brain stimulation (DBS).

20. **What are the most common types of LID and how are they treated?**
After 3 years of treatment, approximately 50% of patients with PD display some degree of involuntary movements related to levodopa. Phenomenologically, LID may be classified into three main categories:
- Peak-dose dyskinesias (improvement–dyskinesia–improvement, or I–D–I) coincide with the time of maximal clinical improvement and usually consist of choreiform movements. Such dyskinesias may improve with levodopa dose reduction.

Table 11-2. Clinical Fluctuations in Parkinson's Disease

FLUCTUATION	MANAGEMENT
End-of-dose deterioration ("wearing off")	COMT inhibitors Increase frequency of levodopa doses Dopamine agonists Rasalgiline/Selegiline Amantadine Infusions of levodopa or dopamine agonists
Delayed onset of response	Give before meals Reduce protein Infusions of levodopa or dopamine agonists
Drug-resistant "offs"	Increase levodopa dose and frequency Give before meals Infusions of levodopa or dopamine agonists
Random oscillation ("on-off")	Dopamine agonists Selegiline Infusions of levodopa or dopamine agonists Levodopa withdrawal
Freezing*	Increase dose Dopamine agonists Atomoxetine

COMT, Catechol-O-methyltransferase.
*May not be related to levodopa therapy.

- Diphasic dyskinesias (dyskinesia–improvement–dyskinesia, or D–I–D) occur at the onset and/or at the end of the "on" period during rising and falling levels of levodopa blood levels and usually consist of dystonia and repetitive stereotypic movements of the legs. Some patients display a combination of the two types and have dyskinesia the entire "on" period (square-wave dyskinesias). Such dyskinesias may improve with dose increments.
- "Off" dyskinesias, typically painful dystonias, coincide with the period of decreased mobility. The most common example is early morning dystonia. Dopaminergic stimulation increases "on" dyskinesias and decreases the other two types. Conversely, antidopaminergic drugs improve all forms of LID, although they worsen the PD. Dystonia induced by levodopa may improve significantly with either the use of baclofen, an agonist of gamma-aminobutyric acid (GABA) receptors, or local intramuscular injection of botulinum toxin (Table 11-3). Amantadine may reduce dyskinesia without worsening PD symptoms possibly via N-methyl-D-aspartate receptor inhibition. Finally, STN or GPi DBS may be used to smooth out motor fluctuations and reduce dyskinesias.

21. **What is the role of dopamine agonists in the treatment of PD?**
Dopamine agonists directly stimulate dopamine receptors and, in contrast to levodopa, do not require enzymatic transformation into metabolites. Because dopamine agonists bypass the presynaptic elements of the nigrostriatal system, they have some advantages in relation to levodopa. For example, they cause dyskinesias and clinical fluctuations less frequently and usually have a levodopa-sparing effect. The most established use of dopamine agonists is as an adjunct to levodopa, especially in patients with clinical fluctuations and dyskinesias. Evidence indicates that early introduction of dopamine agonists delays the development of complications of levodopa therapy, such as motor fluctuations and dyskinesias, although this benefit may not be sustained. After 10 years, there is no observable difference between patients initially treated with levodopa or a dopamine agonist with respect to levodopa-induced motor complications.

22. **What dopamine agonists are available to treat PD, and what are their most common side effects?**
Until 1997, only two dopamine agonists (bromocriptine and pergolide) were clinically used in PD. Since then, pramipexole, ropinirole, apomorphine, and rotigotine have become commercially available.

Table 11-3. Levodopa-Induced Dyskinesias

PATTERN	PHENOMENON	MANAGEMENT
Peak dose (I–D–I)	Chorea	Reduce each dose of levodopa
		Add dopamine agonists
	Dystonia	Reduce each dose of levodopa
		Clonazepam
		Baclofen
		Anticholinergics
	Pharyngeal dystonia	Reduce each dose of levodopa
		Add anticholinergics
	Respiratory dyskinesia	Reduce each dose of levodopa
		Add dopamine agonists
	Myoclonus	Clonazepam
	Akathisia*	Anxiolytics
		Propranolol
		Opioids
Diphasic (D–I–D)	Dystonia	Increase each dose of levodopa
		Baclofen
		Sinemet CR
	Stereotypies	Increase each dose of levodopa
		Baclofen
Off dyskinesia	Dystonia	Baclofen
		Dopamine agonists
		Anticholinergics
		Sinemet CR
		Tricyclics
		Botulinum toxin
	Akathisia*	Anxiolytics
		Propranolol
		Opioids
Striatal posture*	Dystonia	Increase levodopa
		Anticholinergics
		Thalamotomy
		Botulinum toxin

I–D–I, Improvement–dyskinesia–improvement; D–I–D, dyskinesia–improvement–dyskinesia.
*May be unrelated to levodopa therapy.

Both bromocriptine and pergolide are ergot derivatives and have the risk of complications such as vasoconstriction (with acroparesthesias and angina), exacerbation of peptic ulcer disease, erythromelalgia, and valvular, pulmonary, and retroperitoneal fibrosis. Pramipexole, ropinirole, and rotigotine are nonergoline agonists and have a lower risk of such complications. Although dopamine agonists display fewer motor complications than levodopa, they may exacerbate peak-dose dyskinesias and other undesired dopaminergic effects, such as nausea, vomiting, anorexia, drowsiness, sudden sleep attacks, malaise, orthostatic hypotension, confusion, and hallucinations, may occur. Furthermore, dopamine agonists have been linked to the dopamine dysregulation syndrome, including impulse control disorders as well as hypersexuality, pathological gambling, compulsive shopping, and other impulsive and compulsive behaviors.

23. **What is the role of surgery in the treatment of PD?**
DBS of the ventralis intermedius of the thalamus (VIM) has been shown to be of marked benefit, primarily for tremor, and is able to suppress dyskinesias. DBS involves implanting an electrode in the VIM and delivering high-frequency chronic stimulation via an implantable pulse generator located subcutaneously in the subclavicular area. Patients can turn the device on and off via an external

magnet. DBS can be done bilaterally with a lower risk of dysarthria than thalamotomy. The recognition that PD is associated with hyperactivity of the STN led to a successful treatment of MPTP monkeys by subthalamotomy. Some human patients, inadvertently treated with subthalamotomy instead of thala-motomy, noted improvement not only in tremor but also in bradykinesia. STN DBS has demonstrated in numerous studies to provide benefit for contralateral bradykinesia, dyskinesia, and other parkinso-nian signs. This was demonstrated by the improvement in off-period motor symptoms and activities of daily living in a recent meta-analysis. Patients most likely to benefit had severe off-period symptoms, long disease duration, and a history of good presurgical response to levodopa. The pallidum, particu-larly the posteroventral part of the GPi, is also a surgical target in PD. The main benefit of pallidotomy is the marked reduction of contralateral LID, with some ipsilateral benefit. Tremor, bradykinesia, and rigidity are also reduced but more variably. After pallidotomy, patients typically have a lower levodopa requirement. DBS into the GPi is receiving increased attention as a treatment for LID as well as other hyperkinesias, including dystonia and tics.

24. **Is there any relationship between Alzheimer's disease (AD) and PD?**
Currently available data do not support the existence of a common etiology for AD and PD. However, approximately 20% of patients with PD have troublesome dementia. AD accounts for an unknown proportion of these cases. Unlike AD, the pattern of dementia in PD is characterized by lack of cortical signs, such as aphasia and apraxia, and the presence of forgetfulness, bradyphrenia, and depression. In a longitudinal study clinical features that differentiated dementia in PD were cognitive fluctuations, auditory/visual hallucinations, sleep disturbance, and depression. The different patterns suggest that different mechanisms are responsible for cognitive dysfunction in the two diseases, and pathologic studies support this distinction. PD is characterized by relative sparing of the cortex and by neuronal loss in the SN and other subcortical structures, such as the locus ceruleus. Lewy bodies are found in the remaining cells. On the other hand, the cerebral cortex is primarily involved in AD; neurofibrillary tangles and deposits of amyloid are the most important lesions. However, a recent study shows that over 50% of patients with AD display parkinsonism and myoclonus during the course of the disease.

25. **What are the main clinical features of progressive supranuclear palsy (PSP)?**
PSP is the second most common cause of idiopathic parkinsonism. Typically, the onset is in the seventh decade, with no family history. Patients have ophthalmoparesis of downgaze, parkinsonism, pseudobulbar palsy, and frontal lobe signs. Eyelid abnormalities are common. For example, patients with eyelid freezing have difficulty with either opening or closing the eyes due to inhibition of levator palpebrae or orbicularis oculi muscles, respectively. The prevalence of dystonia in patients with patho-logically proven PSP is about 13%.

26. **What is the cause of PSP?**
The cause of PSP is unknown. Radiologic and pathologic evidence indicates that a multi-infarct state can cause a picture identical to PSP. Idiopathic PSP is pathologically characterized by marked neuronal cell loss in subcortical structures, such as the nucleus basalis of Meynert, palli-dum, STN, SN, locus ceruleus, and superior colliculi. Other pathologic features include neurofibril-lary tangles, granulovacuolar degeneration, and gliosis. Atrophy, generalized or focal (midbrain or cerebellum), is the most common neuroradiologic finding in idiopathic PSP. Because of disproportion-ate atrophy of the dorsal midbrain compared to the pons, the sagittal view of magnetic resonance imaging (MRI) often gives the appearance of a "penguin" or "hummingbird," and these "birds of PSP" are characteristic radiological features. However, up to 25% of the patients with PSP have no abnormality on computed tomography and/or MRI of the brain. Growing evidence suggests linkage disequilibrium between a PSP gene and allelic variants of the tau gene. PSP is classified as a form of tauopathy.

27. **How can PSP be distinguished from PD?**
The most distinctive feature of PSP is the supranuclear downgaze palsy, which is not found in PD, the most common misdiagnosis of PSP. The differentiation is particularly difficult when the characteris-tic supranuclear ophthalmoparesis is not evident, as may be the case in early stages of PSP. Some patients who never develop this finding are found at autopsy to have PSP. The difficulty in establish-ing the diagnosis of PSP is suggested by an average delay in making the diagnosis of 3.6 years after onset of symptoms. The measurement of midbrain atrophy ratio on MRI as well as the use of comput-erized posturography to analyze gait and posture are useful tools in reliably differentiating early PSP from PD and age-matched controls (Table 11-4).

Table 11-4. Differential Diagnosis of Progressive Supranuclear Palsy and Parkinson's Disease

CLINICAL FEATURES	PSP	PD
Age at onset (decade)	7th	6th
Initial symptoms	Postural and gait disorder	Tremor and bradykinesia
Family history	−	±
Multi-infarct state	±	−
Dementia	± (visual/motor)	±
Downgaze ophthalmoparesis	+	−
Eyelid abnormalities	+	±
Pseudobulbar palsy	+	±
Gait	Wide, stiff, unsteady	Slow, shuffling, narrow, festinating
Rigidity	Axial (neck)	Generalized
Facial expression	Astonished, worried	Hypomimia
Tremor at rest	−	+
Dystonia	+	±
Corticobulbospinal signs	±	−
Symmetry of findings	+	−
Weight loss	−	+
Improvement with dopamine drugs	−	+
Levodopa-induced dyskinesias	−	+

+, Yes or present; −, no or absent; ±, may be present or absent; *PSP*, progressive supranuclear palsy; *PD*, Parkinson's disease.

28. **What is the treatment for PSP?**
    Levodopa and dopamine agonists are the most frequently used agents in the treatment of PSP. However, even with high doses, they usually provide only a transient and slight improvement of parkinsonian symptoms. The loss of dopamine receptors in the striatum and the presence of extensive lesions involving other neurotransmitters, such as acetylcholine, probably account for the failure of pharmacologic therapy. Currently, no drug provides sustained relief in patients with PSP. With progression of disease, patients usually become bedridden, unable to swallow and talk. Gastrostomy is necessary in advanced stages. Death, usually related to respiratory complications, occurs after a mean disease duration of 7 to 8 years.

29. **What are the most important characteristics of vascular parkinsonism?**
    Multiple vascular lesions in the basal ganglia may be associated with parkinsonism. Tremor at rest is not a common finding, and bradykinesia and rigidity tend to be more significant in the legs. In some patients, the findings are virtually limited to the lower extremities; hence the designation of vascular parkinsonism as "lower body" parkinsonism. Unlike PD, the gait in patients with vascular parkinsonism is characterized by a broad base. Some patients show stepwise progression. Associated findings, such as dementia, spasticity, weakness, and Babinski's signs, are commonly observed. Neuroradiologic studies, especially MRI, show a multi-infarct state. The response to dopaminergic therapy is usually poor.

30. **Is it possible to distinguish drug-induced parkinsonism from PD on clinical grounds?**
    Drugs are one of the most common causes of parkinsonism in the general population. Drugs that block postsynaptic dopamine receptors and/or deplete presynaptic dopamine may cause parkinsonism. Clinical studies indicate that drug-induced parkinsonism is indistinguishable from PD. Discontinuation of the offending drug promotes remission of the syndrome in most cases, although sometimes

the parkinsonism persists. Such patients may have subclinical PD and require dopaminergic therapy. DaTSCAN is a useful tool to differentiate between PD and drug-induced parkinsonism.

31. **What is multiple system atrophy (MSA)?**
MSA was once considered to be three separate clinicopathological disorders termed *olivopontocerebellar atrophy* (OPCA), *striatonigral degeneration* (SND), and *Shy–Drager syndrome* (SDS). Currently the motor phenotype of MSA is clinically stratified into those with predominant parkinsonism (MSA-P) or cerebellar ataxia (MSA-C). MSA-P is characterized by parkinsonism, which occasionally responds to dopaminergic therapy, and dysautonomia. Although cerebellar findings dominate in MSA-C, mild parkinsonism and pyramidal signs are also usually recognized. Patients with MSA-P, typically have parkinsonism and pyramidal signs with laryngeal stridor, although in some cases, MSA-P, is indistinguishable from PD. The division of MSA into SDS, OPCA, and SND is controversial, with some authorities grouping the spectrum into the prominence of either cerebellar or parkinsonisms designated as MSA-C, or MSA-P, respectively. Although usually clinically distinct at onset, with progression symptoms overlap substantially. The two syndromes have a common pathologic substratum consisting of cell loss and gliosis in the striatum, SN, locus ceruleus, inferior olive, pontine nuclei, dorsal vagal nuclei, cerebellar Purkinje cells, and intermediolateral cell columns of the spinal cord. The characteristic histologic marker—glial cytoplasmic inclusions, which are seen particularly in oligodendrocytes—has helped to distinguish MSA as a clinicopathologic entity. The presence of autonomic dysfunction early on is thought to predict a poor prognosis.

32. **What is the treatment for MSA?**
Dopaminergic drugs are the mainstay of the treatment of MSA. However, despite the use of high doses of levodopa, no significant improvement is usually observed. The loss of cells in the striatum and widespread lesions of other neurotransmitters probably accounts for the failure of treatment. The use of midodrine, fludrocortisone, droxidopa, and pyridostigmine may assist in the symptomatic management and control of orthostatic hypotension from autonomic dysfunction.

33. **What is corticobasal degeneration (CBD)?**
Patients with CBD display a combination of cortical (pyramidal signs, myoclonus, progressive aphasia, and apraxia) and subcortical findings (rigidity and dystonia) as well as a distinctive alien limb sign. CBD is virtually the only disease that causes this constellation of symptoms and signs, although there appears to be an overlap of CBD, progressive aphasia, and frontotemporal dementia. Until late stages of the disease, patients do not experience cognitive decline or dysautonomia. Convergence disturbances and oculomotor apraxia are common neuro-ophthalmic signs. The neuropathologic hallmarks are swollen achromatic neurons, neuronal loss, gliosis in the cerebral cortex, SN, lateral nuclei of the thalamus, striatum, locus ceruleus, and Purkinje layer of the cerebellum. The cause is entirely obscure. No familial forms have been reported. The disease progresses relentlessly until death, usually within 10 years after onset. Response to dopaminergic therapy is usually poor.

KEY POINTS: BASAL GANGLIA DISORDERS

1. Loss of pigmented dopaminergic neurons in the SN is the pathologic hallmark of PD.
2. Levodopa remains the most valuable therapy for PD.

 References available online at expertconsult.com.

WEBSITES

http://www.apdaparkinson.org
http://www.psp.org
https://www.michaeljfox.org/
www.parkinson.org
http://medlink.com

BIBLIOGRAPHY

1. Fahn S, Jankovic J, Hallett M: Principles and Practice of Movement Disorders, Philadelphia, Churchill Livingstone, 2011, pp 1-548.
2. Jankovic J, Lang AE: Diagnosis and assessment of Parkinson's disease and other movement disorders. In Daroff RB, Jankovic J, Maziotta J, Pomeroy S (eds): Bradley's Neurology in Clinical Practice, 7th ed. Philadelphia, Elsevier, 2015 (in press).
3. Jankovic J: Parkinson's disease and other movement disorders. In Daroff RB, Jankovic J, Maziotta J, Pomeroy S (eds): Bradley's Neurology in Clinical Practice, 7th ed. Philadelphia, Elsevier, 2015 (in press).
4. Jankovic J, Tolosa E (eds): Parkinson's Disease and Movement Disorders, 6th ed. Baltimore, Lippincott Williams & Wilkins, 2015.
5. Jankovic J (ed): Neurologic Clinics: Movement Disorders (33). 2015, pp 1-314.
6. Jankovic J: Etiology and pathogenesis of Parkinson's disease. In UpToDate in Neurology, Wellesley, MA: Annual updates 2008–2015.

CHAPTER 12

MOVEMENT DISORDERS

Subhashie Wijemanne, Philip A. Hanna, Joseph Jankovic

TREMORS

1. **What is essential tremor (ET)?**

   ET is a neurologic disease characterized by action tremor of the hands in the absence of any identifiable causes, such as drugs or toxins. Other types of tremors, such as isolated head and voice tremors, are also expressions of ET. It is estimated that ET affects at least 5 million Americans. Characterized by action-postural tremor of the hands and arms, ET may be asymmetric at onset and have a kinetic component. Patients with severe forms of ET may display tremor at rest. ET is presumably transmitted by an autosomal dominant gene with variable expression.

2. **How can enhanced physiologic tremor be differentiated from ET?**

   Physiologic tremor is a rhythmic oscillation with a frequency of 8 to 12 Hz, determined largely by the mechanical properties of the oscillating limb. Under several circumstances, the tremor may be enhanced and appears identical to ET. Enhanced physiologic tremor is the most common cause of postural tremor. However, unlike ET, mass loading can reduce its frequency (Table 12-1).

Table 12-1. Causes of Enhanced Physiologic Tremor
Stress induced
Anxiety
Emotion
Exercise
Fatigue
Fever
Endocrine
Adrenocorticosteroids
Pheochromocytoma
Thyrotoxicosis
Hypoglycemia
Drugs
Beta agonists (e.g., theophylline, terbutaline, epinephrine)
Cyclosporine
Dopaminergic drugs (levodopa, dopamine agonists)
Methylxanthines (coffee, tea)
Psychiatric drugs (lithium, neuroleptics, tricyclics)
Stimulants (amphetamines, cocaine)
Valproic acid
Toxins (arsenic, bismuth, bromine, ethanol withdrawal, mercury, lead)

3. **What pathophysiologic mechanisms underlie ET?**

   The pathological findings in several series have suggested a heterogeneous pathology in ET with the majority showing cerebellar Purkinje cell loss and gliosis. The abnormal pathology appears to be supported by functional imaging studies. Only 14 patients with ET have had a thorough pathologic examination, and no specific abnormality was found. It has been suggested that the postural tremor of ET arises from spontaneous firing of the inferior olivary nucleus, which drives the cerebellum and its outflow pathways via the thalamus to the cerebral cortex and then to the spinal cord. Functional magnetic resonance imaging (fMRI) studies have demonstrated increased activation of the cerebellum and red nucleus in ET. Most positron emission tomography (PET) and fMRI evidence indicates that the inferior olive is not likely to be the tremor generator in ET; instead, the generator is probably in the cerebellum. This theory is supported by bilateral overactivity of cerebellar connections by PET in patients with primary writing and primary orthostatic tremor. Clinical data also support a cerebellar role in the pathogenesis of ET: over 50% of patients with ET have difficulty in performing tandem gait, which is considered an indicator of cerebellar function, and hemispheric cerebellar stroke may abolish ipsilateral ET.

4. Is there an association between ET and Parkinson's disease (PD)?
   According to different sources, the prevalence of ET in patients with PD ranges from 3% to 8.5%. The prevalence of PD in ET is debated (4.5% to 21.8%). The relatively high frequency of familial tremor (15% to 23%) among patients with PD supports the existence of an etiologic link between PD and ET. An additional ET marker was mapped to chromosome 4p14-16.3 in an autosomal dominant PD family. Furthermore, an allele (263_bp) of the nonamyloid component of plaques-Rep1 polymorphism has been associated with sporadic PD in a German and more recently in an American population of patients with PD. The authors conclude that the association of this allele with PD and ET "suggests a possible etiologic link between these two conditions." In addition, Lewy body pathology has been demonstrated in several pathological series in brains of patients with ET. Further epidemiologic and genetic studies are needed before the controversy about the relationship between PD and ET can be resolved.

5. What is the relationship between ET and dystonia?
   Although tremor is frequently found in patients with dystonia, it is not always clear whether the oscillatory movement is a form of dystonia (hence, a dystonic tremor) or whether it represents coexistent ET. Postural hand tremor, phenomenologically identical to ET, may either precede or be the initial manifestation of dystonia. The lack of demographic and other differences between patients with ET and ET–dystonia supports the notion that ET is a single disease entity with a clinical spectrum that often includes dystonia. Some investigators argue, however, that the postural tremor in patients with dystonia has different clinical characteristics—such as irregularity and a broader range of frequencies, asymmetry of contractions, and associated myoclonus—that distinguish it from ET.

6. What is orthostatic tremor (OT)?
   OT is a relatively rare but frequently misdiagnosed disorder. It is more common in women, and the onset is typically in the sixth decade. It consists of a rapid (13 to 14 Hz) tremor of the legs triggered by standing. Postural tremor of the hands and a family history of ET are frequent features, suggesting that OT is a variant of ET. Transcranial magnetic stimulation of the cortex motor area has suggested a supraspinal generator of OT. Clonazepam is the treatment of choice; other less effective options are propranolol, primidone, gabapentin, and phenobarbital.

7. What other tremors are variants of ET?
   Besides OT, other types of tremors are also considered to be variants of ET. However, some authors argue that the pharmacologic differences between these tremors and ET support the notion that they represent distinct entities. There is evidence, for example, that some isolated site (head tremor) and task-specific tremors, such as primary handwriting tremor, actually represent forms of dystonic tremors. This controversy will not be settled until biologic markers for ET and dystonia are available (Table 12-2).

8. How is ET treated?
   Propranolol remains the most effective medication for ET, although other beta-blockers also have an antitremor activity. Daily doses of up to 360 mg may be necessary to control tremor. Primidone, an anticonvulsant medication, also has been shown to be highly effective for the treatment of ET in both open and controlled studies. It should be started at low doses (25 mg at bedtime) to avoid the occasional acute idiosyncratic toxic reaction characterized by severe nausea, vomiting, sedation, confusion, and ataxia.
   Less effective but occasionally useful medications are lorazepam, clonazepam, diazepam, alprazolam, gabapentin, and topiramate. A double-blind, placebo-controlled trial revealed mild to moderate benefit of botulinum toxin injections in the treatment of severe hand tremor. Alcohol, although effective in approximately two-thirds of patients with ET, is not recommended because of the possibility of addiction, although ET does not appear to increase the risk of alcoholism. For intractable ET, contralateral thalamotomy is effective and well tolerated. The current main surgical treatment for ET is high-frequency thalamic stimulation (deep brain stimulation [DBS]). Gamma knife thalamotomy has also been shown to suppress completely disabling ET.

Table 12-2. Variants of Essential Tremor

VARIANT	TREATMENT
Chin tremor	Propranolol, primidone
Facial tremor	Clonazepam, propranolol, primidone
Head tremor	Clonazepam, primidone, propranolol, trihexyphenidyl
Orthostatic tremor	Clonazepam, propranolol, primidone, phenobarbital
Shuddering attacks (childhood)	Propranolol
Task-specific tremor (writing)	Propranolol, primidone, trihexyphenidyl, botulinum toxin
Tongue tremor	Propranolol, primidone
Truncal tremor	Clonazepam, propranolol, primidone
Voice tremor	Propranolol, ethanol, botulinum toxin

9. **What are the characteristics and most common causes of kinetic tremor?**

   Kinetic tremors result from lesions of the cerebellar outflow pathways. The tremor has a 3- to 4-Hz frequency and is typically observed on the finger-to-nose test. In patients with cerebellar lesions, titubation (anterior/posterior oscillation of the trunk and head) and postural tremor of the hands are often seen in addition to the kinetic tremor. Patients who have lesions in the midbrain involving the superior cerebellar peduncle and nigrostriatal system also display tremor at rest (midbrain tremor). Multiple sclerosis, trauma, stroke, Wilson's disease, phenytoin intoxication, acute alcoholic intoxication, cerebellar parenchymatous alcoholic degeneration, and tumor are the most important causes of kinetic tremor. The treatment of kinetic tremors remains unsatisfactory. Drugs useful in the treatment of ET, such as propranolol and primidone, are ineffective in the treatment of kinetic tremors. Isoniazid, carbamazepine, and glutethimide may control kinetic tremor in some patients. Attaching weights to the wrist also may be modestly helpful. Injections of botulinum toxin or thalamotomy may benefit selected patients. Buspirone has been reported to help some patients with mild cerebellar tremor.

10. **What is the relationship between tremor and peripheral trauma?**

    The occurrence of tremor and other movement disorders, especially dystonia and myoclonus, after peripheral trauma is well established. Typically, peripherally induced tremors have rest and action components. Some patients develop a typical picture of parkinsonism, with rest tremor, bradykinesia, hypomimia, and response to levodopa. The physiopathology of this movement disorder is unknown. Although conventional neurophysiologic studies show abnormalities of the peripheral nerves in less than one-half of patients, it is reasonable to speculate that damage to the peripheral nervous system causes sustained changes in the central nervous system connectivity and in motor unit-sensory reflex feedbacks, which account for the movement disorders. The common association with reflex sympathetic dystrophy suggests that dysautonomia plays a role in the generation of posttraumatic movement disorders. About 60% of patients have predisposing factors such as personal and family history of ET and exposure to neuroleptics. Treatment is difficult. Anticholinergic agents and antitremor medications, such as propranolol and primidone, are usually ineffective. Clonazepam may provide moderate relief in some patients. Some authors have successfully used injections of botulinum toxin into the affected musculature to control posttraumatic movement disorders. Surgical treatment is another consideration when pharmacological treatment fails.

DYSTONIA

11. **What is torsion dystonia and how is dystonia classified?**

    Dystonia is characterized by sustained or intermittent muscle contractions causing abnormal, often repetitive movements, postures, or both (Fig. 12-1). Dystonic movements are typically patterned, twisting, and may be tremulous, are often initiated or worsened by voluntary action, and are associated with overflow muscle activation. Because there is no biochemical, pathologic, or radiologic marker for dystonia, the diagnosis is based on the recognition of clinical features. A characteristic feature of dystonia that helps to differentiate it from other hyperkinetic movement disorders is that dystonic movements are repetitive and patterned. For reasons that are poorly

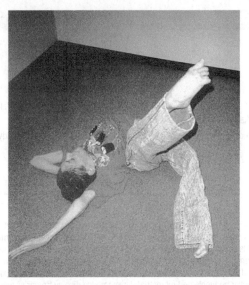

Figure 12-1. Patient with childhood-onset generalized dystonia.

understood, patients with dystonia have the ability to either suppress or decrease the involuntary movements by gently touching the affected area (alleviating maneuvers, sensory trick, or geste antagonistique). Stress and fatigue make dystonia worse, whereas sleep and relaxation improve it (Table 12-3).

Dystonia may be classified according to age of onset, genetics, topographical distribution, or etiology (see Table 12-3). A new classification of dystonia was recently published based on an axis system (axis I and axis II). Axis I includes clinical characteristics such as age of onset, body distribution, temporal pattern, and whether dystonia is isolated or combined. Axis II includes etiology. Usually there is temporal progression of focal to generalized dystonia in early-onset primary dystonia as compared to late-onset dystonia, which will usually remain localized or segmental. The advancement in identifying several dystonia loci of genes, with various modes of inheritance and penetrance, has aided genetic counseling in families with dystonia.

12. **What features suggest the diagnosis of secondary dystonia?**
Secondary forms of dystonia, which account for 25% of cases, are suspected in patients with a history of head trauma, peripheral trauma, encephalitis, toxin exposure, drug exposure, perinatal anoxia, kernicterus, and seizures. Abnormal findings such as dementia, ocular motility abnormalities, ataxia, spasticity, weakness, or amyotrophy are often present in patients with secondary dystonia. Furthermore, onset of dystonia at rest instead of with action, early onset of speech involvement, hemidystonia, abnormal laboratory tests, and abnormal brain imaging suggest the diagnosis of secondary dystonia. The list of causes of secondary dystonia is long, but it is important to try to identify those that are potentially treatable, especially Wilson's disease and tardive dystonia (Table 12-4).

13. **What are the most common types of idiopathic dystonias?**
The classic primary torsion dystonia (DYT1) is much more common among Ashkenazi Jews and is transmitted by an autosomal dominant gene whose expression is extremely variable. Patients with DYT1 dystonia often start in early childhood with distal dystonia, such as dystonic writer's cramp or foot inversion. Over several subsequent years the dystonia becomes more proximal and generalized (see Fig. 12-1). In severe cases, the dystonia may cause not only abnormal postures but also the intense contractions of muscles resulting in muscle breakdown and myoglobinuria. This severe, life-threatening dystonia is referred to as either *dystonic storm* or *status dystonicus*.

Dopa-responsive dystonia (DRD) comprises a clinically and genetically heterogeneous group of disorders, manifested typically by generalized dystonia, with or without diurnal fluctuation, but with

Table 12-3. Classification of Dystonia

Axis I: Clinical Characteristics
Age at Onset
Infancy (0-2 years)
Childhood (3-12 years)
Adolescence (13-20 years)
Early adulthood (21-40 years)
Late adulthood (>40 years)

Distribution

Focal	Single body part
Segmental	One or more contiguous body parts
Multifocal	Two or more noncontiguous body parts
Generalized	Segmental crural dystonia and dystonia in at least one additional body part
Hemidystonia	One-half of the body

Temporal Pattern
By disease course
    Static or progressive
By variability
    Diurnal
    Task specific
    Paroxysmal
Dystonia is Isolated or Combined

Axis II: Etiology
Pathology
Evidence of degeneration
Evidence of structural lesions, often static lesions
Neither of above
Inherited
Autosomal dominant
Autosomal recessive
X-linked.
Mitochondrial
Acquired
Perinatal-dystonic CP, delayed-onset dystonia
Infection, drugs, toxin, vascular, neoplastic, brain injury, psychogenic
Idiopathic:
Sporadic or familial

a robust improvement with levodopa. Autosomal dominant GTP cyclohydrolase-1 deficiency, also known as Segawa disease, is the most studied form of DRD, but deficiencies in tyrosine hydroxylase, sepiapterin reductase, and other genetic abnormalities can interfere with the biosynthetic pathway of dopamine and result in the DRD phenotype.

Paroxysmal dystonia encompasses a heterogeneous and relatively rare group of conditions. One type is psychogenic dystonia. The organic forms, whether sporadic or autosomal dominant, can be categorized as either kinesiogenic or nonkinesiogenic. Mutations in the *PRRT2* gene on chromosome 16 were recently identified in multiple families of different ethnicities affected by paroxysmal kinesiogenic dyskinesia with or without infantile convulsions. Sudden movements precipitate attacks of kinesiogenic dystonia. These attacks typically last less than 5 minutes and recur up to 100 times per day. Anticonvulsants such as carbamazepine and phenytoin are usually effective in preventing the episodes.

Three distinct mutations in the *PNKD* gene, previously referred to as the *myofibrillogenesis regulator gene (MR-1)*, have been identified as the causes of paroxysmal nonkinesiogenic dystonia. In the nonkinesiogenic paroxysmal dystonia, the attacks are less frequent (three per day), last longer (minutes to hours), and often are triggered by alcohol, coffee, and fatigue.

Table 12-4. Causes of Secondary Dystonia

METABOLIC DISORDERS	MISCELLANEOUS
Aminoacid disorders	Arteriovenous malformation
Glutaric aciduria	Atlantoaxial dislocation or subluxation
Hartnup's disease	Brain tumor
Homocystinuria	Cerebellar ectopia and syringomyelia
Methylmalonic acidemia	Central pontine myelinolysis
Tyrosinosis	Cerebral vascular or ischemic injury
Lipid disorders	Drugs
Ceroid lipofuscinosis	Anticonvulsants
GM1-gangliosidose	Antipsychotics
GM2-gangliosidose	Bromocriptine
Metachromatic leukodystrophy	Ergot
Miscellaneous metabolic disorders	Fenfluramine
Leber's disease	Levodopa
Leigh's disease	Metoclopramide
Lesch–Nyhan syndrome	Head trauma
Mitochondrial encephalopathies	Infection
Triosephosphate isomerase deficiency	Acute infectious torticollis
Vitamin E deficiency	AIDS
Neurodegenerative disorders	Creutzfeldt–Jakob disease
Ataxia telangiectasia	Encephalitis lethargica
Azorean heredoataxia	Reye's syndrome
Machado–Joseph disease	Subacute sclerosing panencephalitis
Familial basal ganglia calcifications	Syphilis
NIBA	Tuberculosis
Huntington's disease	Paraneoplastic brain stem encephalitis
Infantile bilateral striatal necrosis	Perinatal cerebral injury and kernicterus
Intraneuronal inclusion disease	Peripheral trauma
Multiple sclerosis	Plagiocephaly
Neuroacanthocytosis	Psychogenic dystonia
Parkinson's disease	Toxins
Progressive pallidal degeneration	Carbon monoxide
Progressive supranuclear palsy	Carbon disulfide
Rett syndrome	Methane
Wilson's disease	Wasp sting

NIBA, Neurodegeneration with brain iron accumulation.

14. Where is the gene for classical dystonia located?

    Molecular genetic techniques link the dystonia (*DYT1*) gene to chromosome 9 (9q34). The mutation in the *DYT1* gene has been characterized as a GAG deletion in the carboxy terminal of the gene that codes for an adenosine triphosphate-binding protein called torsin-A.

15. What is the most common form of focal dystonia?

    The cervical region is the area most frequently affected by dystonia. Among 1000 patients with dystonia at the Baylor College of Medicine Parkinson's Disease Center and Movement Disorders

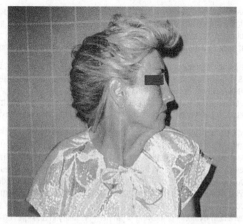

Figure 12-2. Patient with cervical dystonia manifested chiefly by torticollis to the left and marked contraction and hypertrophy of the right sternocleidomastoid muscle.

Clinic, 76% have cervical dystonia either alone (33% patients) or associated with involvement of other areas. It is slightly more common in women (61%). Depending on the muscles involved, different types of postures are observed. Most patients with cervical dystonia have a combination of abnormal postures, such as torticollis, laterocollis, and anterocollis. Pain is a feature in about 70% of the patients with neck dystonia, whereas tremor, either dystonic or essential type, is observed in 60% (Fig. 12-2).

16. **What are the other forms of focal dystonias?**
Blepharospasm, either isolated (11%) or combined with oromandibular dystonia (23%), is the second most common form of focal dystonia. It is defined as an involuntary, bilateral eye closure produced by dystonic contractions of the orbicularis oculi muscles. Blepharospasm is three times more common in women than men. Onset is usually gradual. Often, before the onset of sustained eyelid closure, patients experience excessive blinking triggered by bright light, wind, and stress. With progression, most patients develop dystonia involving other facial muscles as well as the masticatory and cervical musculature. Sensory tricks (alleviating maneuvers) that help to maintain the eyes open include pulling on the upper eyelids, talking, and yawning. Up to 15% of patients with blepharospasm become legally blind because of an inability to keep their eyes open.

Dystonic writer's cramp is a form of task-specific dystonia associated with handwriting. Although able to use their hands for performing daily chores, after a few seconds or minutes of writing patients develop dystonic, usually painful, spasms of the forearm musculature, which prevent them from writing further. With progression of disease, the dystonia becomes less task specific, occurs during other activities, and may spread to involve more proximal muscles. Approximately 50% of patients develop similar symptoms contralaterally. Other task-specific dystonias occur among musicians (piano player's cramp, guitar player's cramp) and others whose recreational or occupational activities require fine motor coordination. The actual prevalence of these task-specific dystonias is unknown because only a few patients seek medical attention.

17. **What are the most effective medications for the treatment of generalized or segmental dystonias?**
Levodopa, effective in about 10% of children with dystonia, should be tried in all childhood-onset dystonias. If there is no significant improvement in 2 months, levodopa is replaced by anticholinergics. The initial dose of trihexyphenidyl (Artane) is 2 mg twice daily. High doses, sometimes up to 100 mg/day, may be necessary. The benefits may not be appreciated for 3 to 4 months after initiation of therapy. Moderate to dramatic improvement is observed in up to 70% of patients, but efficacy may decrease with chronic use. The usefulness of these medications, especially in adults, is limited by the occurrence of peripheral (dry mouth and blurred vision) and central (forgetfulness, confusion, hallucinations) side effects. Other drugs that can be tried are baclofen, benzodiazepines, and tetrabenazine. Levodopa (in children) and anticholinergics (in adults) are the first options among the systemic drugs. Clonazepam is

occasionally highly effective in blepharospasm, whereas baclofen may be particularly useful in cranial dystonia. Systemic treatment of focal dystonias is disappointing, however. If oral medications are ineffective, local injections of botulinum toxin should be considered in patients with focal dystonia. Injections of botulinum toxin into the affected musculature are now considered the first choice of treatment.

18. **What surgical procedures are available for the treatment of dystonia?**
    DBS of the globus pallidus internus is an effective treatment option for generalized dystonia as well as cervical dystonia. Ablative procedures, such as thalamotomy and pallidotomy, have largely been replaced by DBS. Other procedures include peripheral denervation surgery and myectomy. Intrathecal baclofen infusions have been used for patients with predominantly lower limb dystonia and spasticity.

19. **What is the role of botulinum toxin in the treatment of dystonia?**
    Botulinum toxin, one of the most lethal biologic toxins, is produced by the bacteria *Clostridium botulinum*. It acts at the neuromuscular junction, where it binds to the presynaptic cholinergic terminal and inhibits the release of acetylcholine. This functional denervation causes weakness and atrophy. After 3 to 4 months, sprouting and regrowth of the nerve terminals occur. Botulinum toxin has been found to be effective in 95% of patients with blepharospasm, 90% of patients with spasmodic dysphonia, 85% of patients with cervical dystonia, and a majority of patients with oromandibular and hand dystonia. Patients with generalized dystonia displaying prominent disability in a single region may benefit from application of botulinum toxin to the involved area. The complications of botulinum toxin treatment are limited to local weakness; different consequences depend on the area. For example, patients with blepharospasm may have ptosis, whereas dysphagia is a potential complication of treatment for cervical dystonia. Most complications, however, resolve spontaneously after 2 to 4 weeks. A small percentage (3% to 5% in some series) of patients develop antibodies directed against botulinum toxin.

20. **What other conditions may be treated with botulinum toxin?**
    Conditions other than dystonia also have been successfully treated with botulinum toxin. Strabismus was the first disease to be treated with botulinum toxin. Ninety percent of patients with hemifacial spasm, a form of segmental myoclonus, improve with injections of the toxin. Over 50% of patients with tremor of the hand and/or head improve with botulinum toxin. Reports also describe efficacy of this treatment in patients with various disorders associated with abnormal or inappropriate muscle contractions, including tics.

TIC DISORDERS

21. **What are tics?**
    Tics are relatively brief, sudden, rapid, and intermittent movements (motor tics) or sounds (vocal tics). They may be repetitive and stereotypic. Tics are usually abrupt in onset and brief (clonic tics) but may be slow and sustained (dystonic tics). Examples of even more prolonged tics (tonic tics) include abdominal or limb tensing. Simple tics are caused by contractions of only one group of muscles and result in a brief, jerk-like movement or single, meaningless sound. Motor tics may also be complex, consisting of coordinated sequenced movements that resemble normal motor acts but are inappropriately intense and timed. Complex vocal tics include linguistically meaningful utterances and verbalizations. Tics, especially if dystonic, are associated with premonitory feelings that are relieved by performing the tics. Unlike other hyperkinetic dyskinesias, tics may be temporarily suppressed, leading some authors to suggest that in many patients they are purposefully, albeit irresistibly, performed (Table 12-5).

22. **What are the most common causes of tic disorders?**
    Tourette syndrome and related disorders are the most important and common causes of tics. However, these dyskinesias may accompany other hereditary disorders or follow acquired diseases (Table 12-6).

23. **What features are necessary to make the diagnosis of Tourette syndrome (TS)?**
    According to currently established criteria, the diagnosis of TS requires all of the following features: onset before age 21, multiple motor tics, one or more vocal tics, fluctuating course, and presence of tics for more than 1 year. Tics that last less than 1 year are categorized as transient tic disorder (TTD). TTD is estimated to occur in 5% to 24% of school children; there is no accurate way to predict whether TTD will evolve into TS. Chronic motor tic disorder (CMTD) or chronic phonic tic disorder (CPTD) have the same criteria as TS, but patients only display either motor or phonic (vocal) tics.

    TS, defined by the motor manifestations, is three times more frequent in males, but when obsessive compulsive disorder (OCD) is included, the male preponderance becomes much less significant.

Table 12-5. Phenomenologic Classification of Tics

MOTOR TICS	VOCAL TICS
Simple tics	Simple tics
Clonic tics	Blowing
Blinking	Coughing
Head jerking	Grunting
Nose twitching	Screaming
Dystonic tics	Sneezing
Abdominal tensing	Squeaking
Blepharospasm	Sucking
Bruxism	Throat clearing
Oculogyric movements	Complex tics
Shoulder rotation	Coprolalia (shouting of obscenities)
Sustained mouth opening	Echolalia (repetition of someone else's phrases)
Torticollis	Palilalia (repetition of one's own utterances, complex tics, or phrases)
Complex tics	
Copropraxia (obscene gestures)	
Echopraxia (imitating gestures)	
Head shaking	
Hitting	
Jumping	
Kicking	
Throwing	
Touching	

The onset is around age 7 years for facial tics with gradual progression in a rostrocaudal fashion. The diagnosis is often delayed because of a tendency to misinterpret or not recognize the tics or behavioral problems as abnormal. Behavioral problems usually precede the onset of tics by 2 to 3 years.

24. **What is the clinical spectrum of tic disorders and TS?**
    A growing body of evidence supports the notion that primary tic disorders represent a clinical spectrum, ranging from the mild TTD to TS. Several studies show that TTD, CMTD, CPTD, and TS are transmitted as inherited traits in the same families, suggesting that they may represent an expression of the same genetic defect. One problem with the current criteria of TS is that they do not take into account the extensive range of psychopathology and academic problems. For example, OCD is encountered in at least 50% of patients and is related to the same gene responsible for the expression of tics. Attention-deficit hyperactivity disorder (ADHD) is also quite frequent (50% to 60%) among patients with TS, but the genetic association between the two conditions is less well understood. Other behavioral disturbances frequently observed in TS are aggressiveness, anxiety, conduct disorders, depression, learning difficulties, panic attacks, and sleep abnormalities.

25. **How is TS genetically transmitted?**
    Tourette syndrome displays a sex-influenced, autosomal dominant mode of inheritance with variable expressivity as TS, CMTD, or OCD. A frameshift mutation in the slit and Trk-like1 (*SLITRK1*) gene located on chromosome 13q31.1 was also reported.

26. **How is TS treated?**
    Tics require treatment when they are socially embarrassing, painful (dystonic tics often cause pain), and severe enough to interfere with functioning. Medications such as topiramate, dopamine blockers

Table 12-6. Etiologic Classification of Tics

Physiologic Tics
Mannerisms
Gestures

Pathologic Tics
Primary
Transient tic disorder
Chronic tic disorder
    Chronic motor tic disorder
    Chronic phonic tic disorder
    Tourette syndrome
Neuroacanthocytosis
Huntington's disease
Torsion dystonia

Secondary
Chromosomal abnormalities
    Down syndrome
    Fragile X syndrome
    XYY syndrome
    XXX 9p mosaicism
Drugs
    Anticonvulsants
    Dopamine receptor-blocking drugs
    Levodopa
    Stimulants
      Amphetamine
      Cocaine
      Methylphenidate
      Pemoline
Head trauma
Infections
    Creutzfeldt–Jakob disease
    Encephalitis
    Postencephalitic parkinsonism
Sydenham's chorea
Pervasive developmental disorders
Autism
Rett's syndrome
Others
    Carbon monoxide poisoning
    Schizophrenia
    Head trauma
    Stroke
    Rubella syndrome
    Static encephalopathy

such as fluphenazine, or dopamine depletors such as tetrabenazine are used. Tetrabenazine has the added advantage, unlike neuroleptics, of not causing tardive dyskinesia (TD). The behavioral problems present in TS usually can be more disabling than tics. For ADHD, currently three classes of drugs are used: alpha-agonists (clonidine and guanfacine), stimulants (amphetamine enantiomers, methylphenidate enantiomers, or slow release preparation), and a selective norepinephrine reuptake inhibitor (atomoxetine). For management of bothersome OCD, cognitive-behavioral therapy, selective serotonin reuptake inhibitors such as fluvoxamine, sertraline, and fluoxetine or tricyclincs such as clomipramine, or imipramine, may be useful. Carbamazepine and lithium are sometimes used in patients with impulse control problems (Table 12-7). Deep brain stimulation can be effective in medically refractory patients.

Table 12-7. Guidelines for the Treatment of Tourette Syndrome

FEATURE	TREATMENT
Tics	Topamax
	Fluphenazine
	Tetrabenazine
	Botox
ADHD	Clonidine
	Methylphenidate
	Dextroamphetamine
OCD	Fluvoxamine
	Sertraline
	Clomipramine
	Imipramine
Low impulse control	Carbamazepine
	Lithium

ADHD, Attention deficit hyperactivity disorder; *OCD*, obsessive compulsive disorder.

CHOREA

27. **What is Huntington's disease (HD)?**
    HD is clinically characterized by the presence of a triad composed of chorea, cognitive decline, and a positive family history. Chorea consists of involuntary, continuous, abrupt, rapid, brief, unsustained, irregular movements that flow randomly from one body part to another. Patients can suppress chorea partially and temporarily and frequently incorporate movements into semipurposeful activities (parakinesia). Affected patients have a peculiar, irregular gait. Besides chorea, other motor symptoms include dysarthria, dysphagia, postural instability, ataxia, myoclonus, and dystonia. Motor impersistence is the inability to maintain constant voluntary muscle contraction such as in the characteristic milkmaid's grip during a handshake. The tone is decreased, and the deep reflexes are often hung up and pendular. All patients eventually develop dementia, mainly characterized by loss of recent memory, impairment of judgment, concentration, and acquisition. Neurobehavioral disturbances occasionally precede motor symptoms and consist of personality changes, apathy, social withdrawal, agitation, impulsiveness, depression, mania, paranoia, delusions, hostility, hallucinations, and psychosis.
    Virtually all patients have a family history of a similar condition transmitted in an autosomal dominant fashion. Caudate and putamen atrophy on neuroimaging studies is another feature supportive of the diagnosis of HD.

28. **What is the Westphal variant?**
    In 10% of cases of HD, the onset is before age 20 (juvenile or Westphal variant). The disease is then characterized by the combination of progressive parkinsonism, dementia, ataxia, and seizures.

29. **What are other common causes of chorea?**
    It is probable that levodopa-induced chorea in parkinsonism is the most common cause of chorea. Usually this diagnosis is not difficult once the history is available. The combination of chorea and psychiatric symptoms can be found in Wilson's disease. However, the diagnosis is easily made by finding a Kayser–Fleischer ring, low-plasma ceruloplasmin, and evidence of hepatic dysfunction. Sydenham's chorea is a form of autoimmune chorea, preceded by a group A streptococcal infection. Rarely encountered in the United States, this condition is one of the most common causes of chorea in underdeveloped areas. Systemic lupus erythematosus and primary antiphospholipid antibody syndrome are other causes of autoimmune chorea. Senile chorea is a condition in which chorea is the only feature; no family history of HD is present.

30. **How is genetic diagnosis of HD confirmed?**
    The HD gene (designated *IT15*) has been identified near the tip of the short arm of chromosome 4 (4p16.3). An unstable expansion of the CAG repeat sequence is present at the 5′ end of this large

(210 kb) gene. The HD gene encodes a 348-kDa protein called huntingtin. Aggregation of mutant huntingtin may be part of the pathogenesis of HD. With 40 or more repeats, a person develops HD with 100% certainty, but with repeats of 36 to 39, there is incomplete penetrance. The intermediate range, from 27 to 35 repeats, does not cause HD, with a few reported exceptions. All alleles of 27 repeats and higher are unstable and prone to expand in future generations, particularly when transmitted by a male parent. HD families also display "anticipation," or progressively earlier onset of disease in successive generations, typically with increasing CAG repeat size. Such findings allow genetic testing of at-risk individuals before the onset of symptoms. However, until effective treatment is available for HD, many ethical and legal dilemmas associated with genetic testing remain to be solved.

31. **What are the neuropathologic findings in HD?**
The most important pathologic findings in HD are neuronal loss and gliosis in the cortex and striatum, particularly the caudate nucleus. Chorea seems to be primarily related to loss of medium spiny striatal neurons projecting to the lateral pallidum. This results in functional hypoactivity of the STN with consequent hyperactivity of the thalamic tier. Cortical thinning in various parts such as sensorimotor, parietal, occipital, and inferior temporal lobes is now being recognized in HD and has been associated with earlier cognitive symptoms.

32. **What is the treatment for HD?**
Unfortunately, to date no therapeutic intervention has been capable of halting the relentless progression of HD. In the adult form, death occurs after a mean duration of 15 years, whereas in the juvenile variant the mean survival is 9 years. In both observational and randomized controlled trials tetrabenazine has been shown to reduce HD chorea significantly. Tetrabenazine is now considered the treatment of choice for chorea associated with HD as well as other choreas. Other treatments include neuroleptics, which temporarily relieve both chorea and psychosis by interfering with dopaminergic transmission. However, these drugs cause several side effects, including TD. Selective serotonin reuptake inhibitors are the first-choice class of drugs for the treatment of depression in HD and also have been reported to be effective in the treatment of irritability and obsessive-compulsive behaviors.

DRUG-INDUCED MOVEMENT DISORDERS

33. **What is an acute dystonic reaction (ADR)?**
ADR is an abrupt, drug-induced dystonia, especially of the head and neck. About 2.5% of patients treated with neuroleptics develop ADR within the first 48 hours of treatment. Although it is one of the first described neuroleptic-induced movement disorders, the pathophysiology of ADR remains unknown. Because it follows the use of dopamine receptor-blocking drugs and improves with anticholinergics, it is presumed that changes in the striatal dopamine and acetylcholine are important in the genesis of ADR.

34. **What is TD?**
TD is a hyperkinetic movement disorder caused by dopamine receptor-blocking drugs. According to current criteria, it is possible to make the diagnosis of TD when the hyperkinesia develops during treatment with neuroleptics or within 6 months of their discontinuation and persists for at least 1 month after stopping all neuroleptic agents. It is estimated that 20% of patients exposed to neuroleptics develop TD, but the values range from 13% to 49%. Severe TD seems to be more common in young males and elderly females.

KEY POINTS: BASAL GANGLIA AND MOVEMENT DISORDERS

1. ET is the most common cause of nonparkinsonian tremor.
2. Cervical dystonia (torticollis) is the most common form of focal dystonia.
3. Botulinum toxin is the treatment of choice for most focal dystonias.
4. TD is a serious side effect of many neuroleptic drugs.

35. **What is the importance of recognizing stereotypy in an adult patient?**
Stereotypy is defined as a seemingly purposeful, coordinated, but involuntary, repetitive, ritualistic gesture, mannerism, posture, or utterance. Examples of stereotypies include repetitive grimacing, lip smacking, tongue protruding, and chewing movements. The tongue also may move laterally in the mouth ("bon-bon sign"). In addition, patients with TDs, the most common form of adult-onset stereotypy, often exhibit head bobbing, body rocking, leg crossing and uncrossing, picking at clothing,

shifting weight, and marching in place. Stereotypy is the most common form of TD (78% of cases). The second most common form of TD is dystonia (75% of patients). The presence of stereotypies in an adult without mental retardation or untreated schizophrenia strongly suggests the diagnosis of TD, especially in association with other movement disorders commonly present in TD (akathisia, tremor, myoclonus, chorea, and tics) (Fig. 12-3).

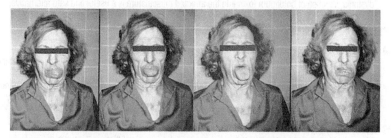

Figure 12-3. Patient with tardive dyskinesias (TDs) manifesting stereotypic orolingual movements.

36. **What is the pathogenesis of TD?**
Because medications that cause TD block the dopamine receptors, dysfunction of striatal dopaminergic systems has been implicated in the pathogenesis. However, the mechanism of production of TD is still not understood. Clinical and experimental evidence suggests that TD and levodopa-induced dyskinesias share a common pathogenetic mechanism. These studies suggest that TD ultimately results from disruption of the lateral pallidal–subthalamic GABAergic projection, leading to inhibition of the STN. Recent evidence supports the notion that dopamine receptor-blocking drugs exert a neurotoxic effect, resulting in neuronal damage. There is no explanation, however, for the diversity of movement disorders in TD. The relatively specific pharmacologic profile of each of these dyskinesias suggests that different mechanisms are involved in their generation (Fig. 12-4).

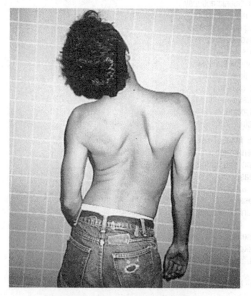

Figure 12-4. Patient with axial tardive dystonia.

37. How is TD treated?

The first step in the treatment of TD is to stop the offending drug, which results in spontaneous remission in approximately 60% of cases. Drugs that deplete dopamine, such as tetrabenazine, are the most effective agents for treatment of TD. Tardive dystonia has a less satisfactory response to systemic treatment than other forms of TD. TD may improve with anticholinergic agents, whereas the other types, including stereotypy, may worsen. In patients with focal forms of dystonia, such as cranial and cervical dystonia, injection of botulinum toxin into the affected musculature is a useful and safe alternative.

OTHER MOVEMENT DISORDERS

38. How can myoclonus be distinguished from chorea and tics?

Myoclonus is defined as a brief, sudden, shock-like jerk that may be caused not only by active muscle contractions (positive myoclonus) but also by lapses of muscle contraction (negative myoclonus). Many of the individual movements of chorea are myoclonic, but, unlike myoclonus, they are continuous, occurring in a constant flow. Tics may resemble myoclonus, but they are usually preceded by premonitory feelings, and patients usually have some degree of control over them.

39. How is myoclonus classified?

Myoclonus may be classified by etiology, pathophysiology, and distribution (Table 12-8).

Table 12-8. Classification of Myoclonus

Physiologic Myoclonus
Anxiety
Benign infantile myoclonus with feeding
Exercise
Hiccup
Nocturnal myoclonus

Essential Myoclonus
Autosomal dominant
Sporadic

Epileptic Myoclonus
Benign familial myoclonic epilepsy
Childhood myoclonic epilepsies
  Infantile myoclonic encephalopathy
  Cryptogenic myoclonus epilepsy
  Infantile spasms
  Juvenile myoclonus epilepsy
  Myoclonic astatic epilepsy
Epilepsia partialis continua
Myoclonic absences in petit mal
Photosensitive myoclonus
Progressive myoclonus epilepsy

Symptomatic Myoclonus
Corticobasal degeneration
Neurodegeneration with brain iron accumulation
Huntington's disease
Myoclonic dystonia
Parkinson's disease
Progressive supranuclear palsy
Dementias
  Alzheimer's disease
  Creutzfeldt–Jakob disease
  Gerstmann–Sträussler–Scheinker syndrome
Focal lesions
  Dentato-olivary lesions
  Stroke

Table 12-8. Classification of Myoclonus *(Continued)*

    Thalamotomy
    Trauma (central nervous system or peripheral nervous system)
    Tumor
Metabolic and toxic encephalopathies
    Biotin deficiency
    Bismuth
    Dichlorodiphenyltrichloroethane
    Drugs, including levodopa
    Dialysis syndrome
    Heavy metal poisoning
    Hepatic failure
    Hypoglycemia
    Hyponatremia
    Methyl bromide
    Mitochondrial encephalopathy
    Multiple carboxylase deficiency
    Nonketotic hyperglycemia
Physical encephalopathies
    Decompression injury
    Electric shock
    Heat stroke
    Post hypoxia
Spinocerebellar degeneration
Storage disease
    Ceroid lipofuscinosis
    Lafora body disease
    GM1-gangliosidosis
    GM2-gangliosidosis
    Krabbe's disease
    Tay–Sachs disease
Viral encephalopathies
    Arbor virus encephalitis
    Herpes simplex encephalitis
    Postinfectious encephalitis
    Subacute sclerosing panencephalitis

Pathophysiology
Clinical Presentation
Spontaneous
Action
Reflex

Distribution
Focal
Segmental
Multifocal
Axial
Generalized
Neurophysiologic origin
Cortical
Subcortical
Brain stem
    Hyperekplexia
    Brain stem reticular myoclonus
    Palatal myoclonus
Spinal
    Propriospinal

Continued on following page

Table 12-8. Classification of Myoclonus *(Continued)*

Etiology
Physiologic
Essential
Symptomatic

40. **How is myoclonus treated?**
    Recognition of the different types of myoclonus has practical implications because each of the categories has a unique pathophysiologic mechanism and specific treatment. Myoclonus related to metabolic encephalopathies improves with treatment of the metabolic disturbance. Epileptic myoclonus is initially treated with sodium valproate. If toxic reactions occur or the patient is still symptomatic, either clonazepam or primidone may be added. Clonazepam is the first choice in myoclonus arising from the brain stem, but 5-hydroxytryptophan, clomipramine, and fluoxetine are useful alternatives. Spinal and other segmental myoclonus also may respond to clonazepam or drugs that enhance serotoninergic transmission, but injections of botulinum toxin in the affected musculature has been the most useful treatment. Recent studies with levetiracetam for the treatment of cortical myoclonus have shown some promising results as an antimyoclonic agent.

41. **What is asterixis?**
    Asterixis is a form of negative myoclonus mainly associated with metabolic encephalopathies; electrophysiologically, it is characterized by the presence of brief silences of electric muscular activity. Although originally described in patients with hepatic encephalopathy, asterixis may be caused by many other conditions. The early stages of metabolic dysfunction assume a rhythmic aspect, resembling tremor. With progression of the underlying cause, when patients hold their arms outstretched, the wrists display a characteristic flexion (caused by electric silence in the antigravity muscles) (Table 12-9).

Table 12-9. Causes of Asterixis

Hepatic failure
Respiratory failure
Renal failure
Cardiac failure
Chronic hemodialysis
Polycythemia

Drugs
    Anticonvulsants
    Salicylates
    Levodopa

Lesions in the central nervous system
    Medial frontal cortex
    Parietal lobe
    Internal capsule
    Thalamus
    Rostral midbrain

42. **What is the stiff person syndrome (SPS)?**
    Patients with this rare disorder have progressive, usually symmetric, rigidity of the axial muscles that may fluctuate in intensity. Motion, tactile stimulation, emotion, and startle are common triggering factors of the spasms. Electromyography shows continuous normal motor unit potentials in the affected muscles despite the patient's attempts to relax. The diagnosis is supported by relief of the rigidity with general and spinal anesthesia, peripheral nerve blocks, and diazepam, which is still the first-line

treatment of SPS. In refractory cases propofol, rituximab, and intravenous immunoglobulin have been reported to be of benefit. It should be noted that use of general anesthesia in patients with SPS carries a risk of postoperative hypotonia especially with concomitant use with muscle relaxants. An insight into the pathophysiology of SPS was provided by the finding that 20 of 33 patients had autoantibodies against glutamic acid dehydroxylase. The hypothesis of an autoimmune etiology of SPS is further supported by the presence of other autoantibodies (to islet cells and gastric parietal cells, for example), coexistent autoimmune diseases such as insulin-dependent diabetes mellitus, vitiligo, thyroid disease, family history of presumed autoimmune conditions, and improvement with plasmapheresis and corticosteroid drugs.

43. **What is Wilson's disease?**

Wilson's disease is an autosomal recessive disease; the gene is linked to markers located in the q14–21 region on chromosome 13. The prevalence of the disease is estimated to be 1 in 30,000. It is associated with impaired incorporation of copper into ceruloplasmin as well as impaired biliary excretion of copper. The result is copper overloading in the liver, cornea, and brain, particularly in the basal ganglia. Virtually all patients display laboratory and/or clinical evidence of liver insufficiency. The most useful laboratory-screening test is plasma ceruloplasmin, which usually is less than 20 mg/dL (normal: 24 to 45 mg/dL). The most common neurologic findings are parkinsonism, bulbar signs (e.g., dysarthria and dysphagia), dystonia, postural tremor, and ataxia. Psychiatric symptoms, such as depression and psychosis, are particularly common among adults.

MRI of the head may display either decreased or increased signal intensity in the striatum on T2-weighted images. MRI of the midbrain may show a specific "face of a giant panda" appearance, which is produced by reversal of the normal hypointensity of the substantia nigra, midbrain tegmentum, and hypointensity in the superior colliculi.

44. **What is the treatment for Wilson's disease?**

Early diagnosis is essential because treatment with copper-chelating agents often completely reverses the neurologic and hepatic symptoms. All siblings and cousins should be screened because presymptomatic patients require treatment to prevent development of symptoms. D-Penicillamine is the drug of choice for Wilson's disease; the typical dose is 250 mg four times/day given in combination with pyridoxine (25 mg/day). Side effects are initial exacerbation of symptoms, rash, optic neuritis, thrombocytopenia, leukopenia, and nephrotoxicity. Other options to decrease copper overload are triethylene tetramine dihydrochloride, zinc sulfate, and tetrathiomolybdate. Symptomatic treatment of neurologic symptoms includes levodopa, anticholinergics, and injections of botulinum toxin. Liver transplant may be necessary in terminal cases of hepatic insufficiency.

45. **What are the paraneoplastic movement disorders?**

Opsoclonus–myoclonus designates a combination of rapid, erratic, involuntary movements of the eyes, with multifocal myoclonus (dancing eyes–dancing feet syndrome). Most cases occur between ages 6 and 18 months. Fifty percent of cases are related to an underlying neoplasm, especially neuroblastoma. This syndrome also occurs in adults with brain stem encephalitis, either paraneoplastic or infectious (Whipple's disease). Steroids dramatically improve this form of myoclonus. A few cases have been reported in patients with SPS, breast cancer, and autoantibodies against amphiphysin. Ataxia is another well-established paraneoplastic movement disorder. The mechanism is cerebellar degeneration related to anti-Purkinje cell antibodies. There are also reports of parkinsonism, chorea, dystonia, segmental rigidity, and action and segmental myoclonus as remote effects of neoplasm.

46. **What is restless legs syndrome (RLS)?**

RLS, also referred to as Willis–Ekbom disease, is a chronic neurological disorder manifested by an urge or a need to move the limbs to stop unpleasant sensations in the evening or while at rest. Periodic limb movements of sleep are seen in over 80% to 90% of RLS patients. Primary RLS is characterized by high familial aggregation suggesting a genetic component. Approximately 63% of patients report having at least one first-degree relative with the condition.

47. **How do you diagnose RLS?**

The diagnosis is clinical and is based on the 2012 revised International Restless Legs Syndrome Study Group diagnostic criteria. Compared to 2003 criteria, the 2012 version includes a fifth criterion to rule out RLS mimickers, and in addition, all the essential diagnostic criteria have to be met: (1) the urge to move the legs, usually but not always accompanied by or felt to be caused by uncomfortable and unpleasant sensations in the legs; (2) the urge to move the legs and any accompanying unpleasant sensations begin or worsen during periods of rest or inactivity such as lying down or sitting; (3) the urge to move the legs and any accompanying unpleasant sensations are partially or totally relived by movement, such as walking or stretching, at least as long as the activity continues; (4) the urge to move and any accompanying unpleasant sensations during rest or inactivity only occur or are worse in the evening or night than during the day; and (5) the above features are not solely accounted for by other medical or behavioral conditions, such as myalgias, venous stasis, leg edema, arthritis, leg cramps, positional discomfort, habitual foot tapping, and other nocturnal sensory-motor symptoms.

48. What is the pathogenesis of RLS?

Brain iron dysregulation is considered to play a key role in the pathogenesis of RLS. There is dysregulation of iron transport across the blood–brain barrier, which is considered the chief mechanism of the low brain iron. The circadian change in brain iron status also plays an important role in RLS.

49. What treatment options are available for RLS?

Several categories of medications are used in the management of RLS, such as calcium channel alpha-2-delta ligands, which include gabapentin, gabapentin enacarbil, and pregabalin, and dopamine agonists, which include ropinirole, pramipexole, and rotigotine. Opioids also help. If the serum ferritin is <75 ng/mL, iron replacement therapy is recommended.

50. What is augmentation?

This is an important therapy-related complication of RLS seen in those patients chronically treated with dopaminergic drugs, such as dopamine agonist and carbidopa/levodopa. Augmentation is characterized by progressively earlier onset of RLS symptoms associated with increased intensity of symptoms, shorter latency after rest, an expansion of symptoms to the upper limbs and the trunk, and a shorter duration of the effect of the medication. Patients with augmentation typically describe their RLS symptoms as being worse than those before treatment. A US community-based study estimated prevalence of augmentation in all patients treated with a dopaminergic medication to be 76%, with a yearly growth rate of 8%.

 References available online at expertconsult.com.

WEBSITES

http://tourette.org/
http://www.hdsa.org/
https://www.dystonia-foundation.org/
http://www.rls.org/

BIBLIOGRAPHY

1. Fahn S, Jankovic J, Hallett M: Principles and Practice of Movement Disorders, 2nd ed. Edinburgh, Elsevier, 2011.
2. Jankovic J, Tolosa E (eds): Parkinson's Disease and Movement Disorders, 6th ed. Baltimore, Lippincott Williams & Wilkins, 2015.
3. Singer HS, Mink JW, Gilbert DL, Jankovic J: Movement Disorders in Childhood, 2nd ed. Philadelphia, Elsevier, 2015 (in press).
4. Jankovic J (ed): MedLink Neurology. http://medlink.com.
5. Jankovic J: Hypokinetic movement disorders. In: UpToDate in Pediatrics. Wellesley, MA, Wolters Kluwer. http://www.uptodateonline.com, annual updates 2001–2015.
6. Jankovic J: Hyperkinetic movement disorders. In: UpToDate in Pediatrics, Wellesley, MA: Wolters Kluwer. http://www.uptodateonline.com, annual updates 2001–2015.
7. Jankovic J: Etiology and pathogenesis of Parkinson's disease. In: UpToDate in Neurology, Wellesley, MA: Wolters Kluwer, annual updates 2008–2015.

CHAPTER 13

AUTONOMIC NERVOUS SYSTEM

Shahram Izadyar

1. What are the physiologic responses to stimulation of the sympathetic and parasympathetic systems?

Sympathetic Stimulation	Parasympathetic Stimulation
Tachycardia	Bradycardia
Increased heart contractility	Decreased heart contractility
Bronchodilation	Bronchoconstriction
Decreased peristalsis	Increased peristalsis
Mydriasis	Miosis
Ciliary muscle relaxation (far vision)	Ciliary muscle contraction (near vision)
Bladder internal sphincter contraction	Bladder internal sphincter relaxation
Detrusor relaxation	Detrusor contraction
Ejaculation	Penile erection
Decreased kidney output	Increased exocrine gland secretion (salivary, lacrimal)
Vasoconstriction	Vasodilation
Piloerection	
Increased sweating	
Glycogenolysis, gluconeogenesis	
Lipolysis	

2. What features of the history must be explored in all patients with suspected autonomic dysfunction?

Some cardinal symptoms of autonomic dysfunction may be drug induced or have a psychogenic etiology. With this caveat in mind, special attention to symptoms involving the following systems is essential when obtaining a history:

- **Cardiovascular**—Orthostatic lightheadedness, dizziness, blurred vision, syncope or near-syncope, fatigue, weakness (especially in the legs on standing), headache, and neck ache after prolonged standing (coat hanger phenomenon), postprandial or postexercise lightheadedness or angina pectoris, fainting after alcohol ingestion or insulin injection, palpitations, resting tachycardia, orthostatic cerebral transient ischemic attack symptoms, angina pectoris.
- **Sudomotor and vasomotor**—Partial or complete loss of sweating, heat intolerance, excessive sweating (partial or total), facial and upper trunk gustatory sweating (especially when food incites salivation or with ingestion of cheese), nocturnal sweating, skin cracks on distal extremities, dry and shiny skin, unusually cold or warm feet, reduced skin wrinkling, peripheral edema.
- **Secretomotor**—Dry mouth and eyes, increased saliva production.
- **Genitourinary**—History of urinary tract infections, lengthened interval between micturitions, increased volume of first morning void, need for straining to initiate and maintain voiding, weakness of stream, postvoid dribbling, sensation of incomplete emptying of bladder, overflow incontinence, frequency and urgency with or without dysuria (with superimposed infection), difficulty in initiating and/or maintaining erection, reduced or absent waking erection, diminished libido, decreased volume of ejaculation, inability to ejaculate, retrograde ejaculation, reduced vaginal lubrication.
- **Respiratory**—Irregular breathing or apnea during sleep.
- **Gastrointestinal**—Dysphagia, retrosternal discomfort, heartburn, anorexia, epigastric fullness during or after meals, recurrent episodes of nausea and vomiting (fasting and/or postprandial) associated with upper abdominal pain, constipation, diarrhea (especially nocturnal), fecal incontinence (especially at night), weight loss. Note that explosive diarrhea and severe constipation may alternate.

- **Ocular**—Blurring of vision, trouble focusing, photophobia, difficulty seeing at night, drooping of eyelids.
- **Factors aggravating symptoms**—Alcohol, continued standing, hot temperature (environmental, hot bath, fever), exercise, bed rest, food ingestion, and hyperventilation.

3. What physical examination must be performed in all patients with suspected autonomic dysfunction?
   - **Eye**—With attention to the symmetry, shape and size of the pupils, and eyelids (ptosis). Examples of abnormal findings are Horner's syndrome (asymmetry in pupil size due to ipsilateral dysfunction of sympathetic dilatory pathways) or Adie's tonic pupil (dilated pupil that constricts poorly to light, and reacts better to accommodation, due to parasympathetic denervation)
   - **Cardiovascular**—Measurement of supine blood pressure and heart rate after 5 to 10 minutes of rest followed by measurement after standing for 3 minutes. Orthostatic hypotension is defined as a drop in systolic blood pressure of ≥20 mm Hg or diastolic blood pressure of ≥10 mm Hg with only modest increase in heart rate.
   - **Skin**—A careful examination of the skin provides valuable clues to the presence of autonomic dysfunction. Particular attention should be given to acral vasomotor and trophic changes of the skin, abnormal temperature and sweating patterns (a dry and warm skin may imply impaired sympathetic output, whereas a cold and sweaty skin may imply overactivity of sympathetic output).

4. What are the major anatomic differences between the sympathetic and parasympathetic nervous systems?
   The sympathetic neurons are located in the interomediolateral (IML) and interomediomedial (IMM) columns of the thoracic and upper lumbar spinal cord. Axons of these neurons make synaptic contact with ganglionic neurons in the bilateral paravertebral or largely unpaired prevertebral ganglia. The parasympathetic neurons lie in the brainstem and the intermediate zone of the sacral spinal cord. The parasympathetic relay ganglia are located near or in the wall of the effector organs (Fig. 13-1).

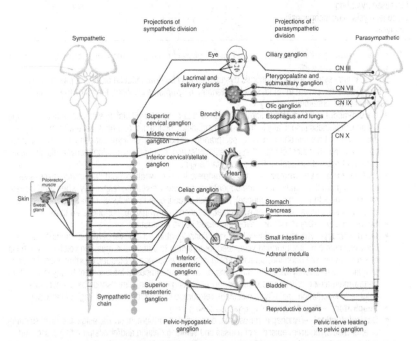

Figure 13-1. Sympathetic and parasympathetic nervous systems. *(From Nadeau SE, Ferguson TS, Valenstein E, et al.: Medical Neuroscience. Philadelphia, Saunders, 2004, p 504.)*

Because of the close proximity of sympathetic ganglia to the primary efferent sympathetic neurons (IML and IMM columns), the sympathetic preganglionic fibers are short, whereas the postganglionic fibers may extend a long way to their target organs. The parasympathetic preganglionic axons, on the other hand, are relatively long myelinated fibers that synapse with parasympathetic relay ganglia located near or within the wall of individual innervated organs. The postganglionic parasympathetic fibers are, therefore, short (1 mm to several centimeters).

The number of postganglionic neurons is very close to the number of preganglionic neurons in the parasympathetic system. On the other hand, the high ratio of postganglionic to preganglionic neurons in the sympathetic system explains the massive sympathetic outflow and the wide range of autonomic effects that occur during strenuous and stressful situations.

5. Name the four hierarchical levels of the central nervous system (CNS) that play a role in control of the autonomic nervous system.
Forebrain level, pontomesencephalic or upper brain stem level, bulbopontine or lower brain stem level, and spinal level.

6. What are the components of the forebrain level of the central autonomic network? Briefly describe the role of each component.
Insular cortex integrates the interoceptive inputs with emotional and cognitive processing and also controls the sympathetic and parasympathetic outputs.
Anterior cingulate cortex controls sympathetic and parasympathetic functions through extensive connections with insula, amygdala, hypothalamus, prefrontal cortex, and brain stem.
Amygdala, a complex structure that adds emotional and affective value to the incoming sensory information.
Hypothalamus is the location where the autonomic and endocrine responses are integrated and controlled.

7. What are the components of the brain stem level of the central autonomic network?
Periaqueductal gray matter in the midbrain, parabrachial nucleus, nucleus of the solitary tract (NTS), ventrolateral reticular formation of the medulla and medullary raphe.

8. What is the role of the NTS in the central autonomic network?
This important nucleus, located at the dorsomedial medulla (Fig. 13-2), serves as an integration station for the autonomic and somatic information and plays a vital role in the maintenance of body homeostasis. NTS receives inputs from neocortical regions and from nuclei of the forebrain, higher brain stem, and diencephalon. The visceral afferents, which convey information important to the reflexive regulation of cardiac rhythm and motility, peripheral vascular tone, respiration, and gastrointestinal (GI) motility and secretion, terminate at different parts of this nucleus. Most efferent fibers from the NTS terminate in the parabrachial nucleus, which in turn project to higher brain stem sites, hypothalamus, basal forebrain, and cerebral cortex. Efferent fibers from the NTS also end on the

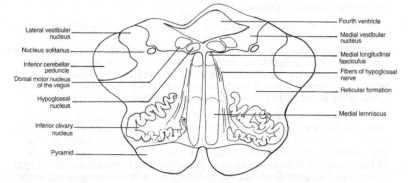

Figure 13-2. Transverse section through the rostral medulla, showing the nucleus solitarius or nucleus solitarii. *(From Crossman AR, Neary D: Neuroanatomy, An Illustrated Colour Text. Edinburgh, Churchill Livingstone, 2000, p 94.)*

neurons of the reticular formation of the ventrolateral medulla, which in turn project to the IML cell column of the lateral horn of the spinal cord. In addition, the NTS also receives somatic afferents from the spinal cord (dorsolateral horn) and spinal trigeminal lemniscus.

Note: *Nucleus tracti solitarii* is the correct Latin term for this nucleus. Nucleus tractus solitarius or nucleus tracti solitarius are distorted but commonly used terms.

9. Discuss the major neurotransmitters and their receptors in the autonomic nervous system.

Acetylcholine (ACh) is the neurotransmitter for all preganglionic and for the parasympathetic postganglionic neurons. ACh receptors in the autonomic nervous system are divided into nicotinic and muscarinic types. Nicotinic receptors, of which multiple subtypes are found mainly in the ganglia, are ligand-gated sodium channels that mediate fast responses. Muscarinic receptors mediate slower responses and are found mostly throughout autonomic effector tissues. Five subtypes of muscarinic receptors (M_1 to M_5) have been identified.

Norepinephrine (NE) is the neurotransmitter for most sympathetic postganglionic fibers. Adrenergic receptors are divided into alpha (α_1 and α_2) and beta (β_1, β_2, and β_3) types and are localized in various autonomic effector tissues.

Sweat glands are innervated by sympathetic cholinergic nerves.

10. What other neurotransmitters play a role in the autonomic nervous system?

Nonadrenergic noncholinergic (NANC) autonomic transmitters can act as either cotransmitters in both sympathetic and parasympathetic systems or as presynaptic or postsynaptic modulators of release and action of the major neurotransmitters. Examples of NANC neurotransmitters include neuropeptides such as substance P, neuropeptide Y, calcitonin gene-related peptide, somatostatin, vasoactive intestinal peptide; adenosine triphosphate and other nucleotides; serotonin; and nitric oxide.

11. What are the catecholamines that can be detected in human plasma?

There are six detectable catecholamines in human plasma: the three main catecholamines of the body (epinephrine, NE, and dopamine [DA]), their precursor (L-3,4-dihydroxyphenylalanine [DOPA; levodopa]), and the metabolites of NE (dihydroxyphenylglycol [DHPG]) and DA (dihydroxyphenylacetic acid).

12. How useful is measurement of plasma NE in the evaluation of dysautonomia?

The main source of plasma NE is the sympathetic network around blood vessels. However, most of the released NE is metabolized before spilling over to the plasma, and only a small proportion enters the bloodstream unchanged. An elevated plasma NE level could suggest either a high rate of sympathetic activity or a decreased rate of clearance from plasma. Measurement of both NE and its metabolite DHPG levels can provide further information about the mechanism involved: an increased plasma level of NE mediated by increased sympathetic activity is associated with elevated DHPG. On the other hand, if the diminished NE reuptake is the cause of increased NE level, an increase in plasma DHPG would not be observed.

In normal subjects, the plasma level of NE is 150 to 170 pg/mL after 30 minutes in the supine position; it increases 50% to 100% above supine values after 5 minutes of standing and remains constant after 10 minutes of standing.

13. What are the confounding factors to consider when interpreting NE measurement in plasma?

The plasma NE level must be interpreted with caution as various processes such as emotion, exercise, eating, smoking, caffeine, medications, time of day, blood volume, hypoglycemia, and pathologic states such as cardiac ischemia affect the release, reuptake, metabolism, and removal of this hormone. In addition, the plasma NE value must be corrected for age. The level of NE increases with increasing age, and the mechanisms involved are both reduced clearance and increased release.

14. Can catecholamine measurements localize the site of autonomic dysfunction?

Patients with a neuropathy causing a primarily postganglionic autonomic abnormality (such as pure autonomic failure) have a subnormal plasma level of NE in the supine position that fails to increase during standing. In patients with intact postganglionic neurons (such as multiple system atrophy) the plasma level of NE in the supine position remains within normal limits but fails to increase upon standing, similar to postganglionic abnormalities. Because of considerable overlap between preganglionic and postganglionic abnormalities in individual patients with autonomic dysfunction, plasma NE values alone are usually not sufficiently diagnostic for the site of the lesion.

KEY POINTS: AUTONOMIC NERVOUS SYSTEM ANATOMY AND PHYSIOLOGY

1. ACh is the neurotransmitter for all preganglionic and for the parasympathetic postganglionic neurons.
2. NE is the neurotransmitter for most sympathetic postganglionic fibers.
3. Sweat glands are innervated by sympathetic cholinergic nerves.

15. **What are the most common causes of acquired autonomic failure?**
   Chronic and progressive autonomic neuropathy can occur in the setting of a more diffuse peripheral neuropathy such as diabetic neuropathy.
   Chronic dysautonomia may occur without sensorimotor neuropathy. This category is referred to as *pure autonomic failure* (PAF) and encompasses several disorders with different etiologies including chronic immune-mediated autonomic failure.
   Most disorders of autonomic failure with subacute course, defined as less than 3 months from onset to peak deficit, are of autoimmune etiology. These can be subdivided into dysautonomia associated with acute inflammatory neuropathies such as Guillain–Barré syndrome (GBS), paraneoplastic autoimmune autonomic neuropathy, or idiopathic autoimmune autonomic ganglionopathy (AAG).
   Acute autonomic neuropathy can be related to toxic, metabolic, or autoimmune causes.

16. **What are the most important peripheral neuropathies associated with autonomic dysfunction?**
   See Table 13-1.

17. **What autonomic dysfunction is seen in GBS?**
   About two-thirds of patients with GBS have some degree of dysautonomia. In fact, dysautonomia is an important cause of death in patients with severe GBS. During the acute phase of the disease overactivity of the sympathetic system manifesting as episodes of hypertension, tachycardia, and hyperhidrosis is usually seen. Failure of the parasympathetic system mostly occurs in the recovery phase. Episodes of severe hypertension can alternate with episodes of hypotension. Sinus tachycardia, severe bradyarrhythmias, orthostatic hypotension, and cardiac arrest are also seen.
   Other less common symptoms of autonomic dysfunction include episodes of flushing, urinary incontinence or retention, constipation, fecal incontinence, gastroparesis, sudomotor dysfunction, and pupillary abnormalities.

18. **Is there a difference in autonomic involvement between different subtypes of GBS?**
   There are two major subtypes of GBS: demyelinating, or acute inflammatory demyelinating neuropathy (AIDP), and axonal, or acute motor axonal neuropathy (AMAN). They differ in pathogenesis, clinical course, and response to treatment. They also differ in the extent of autonomic involvement. AIDP patients show the more serious manifestations of cardiosympathetic hyperactivity. Some authors suggest that the long, myelinated, preganglionic neurons of the vagal fibers are vulnerable to demyelinating processes, which eventually leads to the predominance of the sympathetic system involvement in AIDP patients. Others postulate that demyelination of both afferent and efferent limbs of the baroreflex loop are the leading cause of tachycardia in these patients. On the other hand, autonomic manifestations in AMAN patients are limited to hypoactivity of sudomotor and skin vasomotor function.

19. **Describe the appropriate management for the blood pressure fluctuations seen in GBS.**
   Blood pressure fluctuations in GBS are best monitored in a medical intensive care unit (ICU) setting. Generally, it is recommended that spontaneous fluctuations in the blood pressure be treated only if symptoms are present or the target organs are at risk. Treatment of the triggering factors, such as pain, is important.
   Simple measures such as putting the patient in the Trendelenburg position and administration of intravenous (IV) fluids can be taken when hypotension is symptomatic. Use of vasopressor drugs may be necessary, with extreme caution, because hypersensitivity responses are common. If needed, use of short-acting agents such as dopamine or phenylephrine is recommended.

Table 13-1. Peripheral Neuropathies Associated with Autonomic Dysfunction	
Inherited Peripheral Neuropathies with Dysautonomia	
• HSAN I, II, III* (Riley-Day syndrome), IV, and V	• Amyloidosis* (familial amyloid polyneuropathy
• HMSN I and II	types I, II, and III)
• Fabry's disease*	• Porphyria*
• MEN 2b	• Some spinocerebellar degenerations
Infectious, Parainfectious, and Immune-Mediated Peripheral Neuropathies with Dysautonomia	
• Leprosy	• Rheumatoid arthritis
• AIDS	• Mixed connective tissue disease
• Chagas' disease	• GBS*
• Diphtheria	• Inflammatory bowel disease
• Systemic lupus erythematosus	• Chronic inflammatory neuropathy
• Systemic sclerosis	• Acute pandysautonomia*
• Sjögren syndrome	• Pure cholinergic dysautonomia*

Autonomic Neuropathies Associated with Systemic Metabolic Disease		
• Diabetes*	• Nonalcoholic liver disease	• Paraneoplastic syndrome
• Chronic renal failure	• Vitamin B12 deficiency	• Primary amyloidosis*
• Alcoholism		

Autonomic Neuropathies Associated with Industrial Agents, Metals, Toxins, and Drugs		
• Organic solvents	• Botulism*	• Vincristine*
• Organophosphates	• Amiodarone	• Cisplatinum
• Acrylamide	• Pentamidine	• Paclitaxel
• Vacor	• Doxorubicin	• Cisplatinum
• Heavy metals		

AIDS, acquired immunodeficiency syndrome; *GBS*, Guillain-Barré syndrome; *HMSN*, hereditary motor-sensory neuropathy; *HSAN*, hereditary sensory and autonomic neuropathy; *MEN 2bn*, multiple endocrine neoplasia type 2b.
*Autonomic dysfunction is prominent and clinically important.

Treatment of hypertension also should be done with caution as there is a risk of exaggerated response due to innervation hypersensitivity and baroreflex failure. If antihypertensive agents are used, it is best to use a low dose of hydralazine or angiotensin converting enzyme inhibitors in less severe cases and nicardipine or nitroprusside, with caution, in more severe cases.

20. Describe the appropriate management for the arrhythmias seen in GBS.
    Bradyarrhythmias leading to serious events such as atrioventricular block and asystole can be treated with atropine or pacemaker. Sinus tachycardia is usually temporary and does not need treatment other than in the elderly with coronary artery disease. Atrial and ventricular tachycardias are also often temporary and need treatment only in life-threatening situations. These situations are best managed by ICU experts, but if beta-blockers are used, they must have a rapid onset and offset of action.

21. What is the appropriate management for the other dysautonomias seen in GBS?
    Adynamic ileus and atonic bladder may occur. Adynamic ileus requires upper GI tract decompression via a nasogastric tube and maintenance of nil per os (NPO; Latin, nothing by mouth) status. Urinary retention is treated with an indwelling catheter while the patient is on IV fluids; if present in the rehabilitation phase of GBS, it is treated with sterile intermittent catheterization.

22. Describe the clinical features of AAG.
    AAG (formerly known as acute pandysautonomia or idiopathic subacute autonomic neuropathy) is an acute and acquired immune-mediated involvement of both sympathetic and parasympathetic components of the autonomic nervous system, with relative or complete sparing of the somatic nerve fibers. Antibodies against ganglionic nicotinic acetylcholine receptors (AchR) are found in about 50% of patients. The typical patient has symptoms related to sympathetic failure (orthostatic hypotension, anhidrosis) or parasympathetic failure (reduced lacrimation and salivation, disturbances of the

GI motility [such as ileus, diarrhea, and constipation], bladder atony, impotence, fixed heart rate, and fixed pupils). The progression of symptoms is rapid in the majority of cases, while some patients have a more insidious onset of disease. Treatment of AAG primarily consists of supportive care for orthostatic hypotension and bowel and bladder symptoms. A number of studies have supported the use of intravenous immunoglobulin (IVIG), plasma exchange, and immunomodulatory medications such as prednisone, azathioprine, and rituximab, alone or in combination.

23. **What are the autonomic abnormalities seen in primary Sjögren's syndrome?**
    This chronic autoimmune disorder, which affects women nine times as frequently as men, is characterized by highly specific autoantibodies, Ro (SS-A) and La (SS-B), directed against low-molecular-weight ribonuclear proteins. Signs of all forms of peripheral neuropathy (sensory neuropathy, sensorimotor neuropathy, multiple mononeuropathies, sensory neuronopathy, cranial neuropathy, and entrapment syndromes) may be seen in 5% to 20% of patients with Sjögren's syndrome. Autonomic dysfunction, including Adie's pupil, anhidrosis, urinary retention, orthostatic hypotension, and impaired cardiac parasympathetic function, may be superimposed on a generalized neuropathy. It is hypothesized that antibodies to M3-receptors and antibodies to nicotinic ganglionic acetylcholine receptors may play a role in some autonomic manifestations in primary Sjögren's syndrome.

24. **Name the four main categories of paraneoplastic autonomic dysfunction.**
    1. Diseases involving the CNS—such as limbic encephalitis
    2. Diseases that involve both central and peripheral nervous system—subacute sensory neuronopathy and enteric neuronopathy fall within this category.
    3. Diseases involving the peripheral nervous system—widespread autonomic neuropathy is an example within this category.
    4. Disease involving the neuromuscular junction—such as Lambert–Eaton myasthenic syndrome (LEMS)

25. **What is limbic encephalitis?**
    Several antibodies such as anti-Hu, anti-Ma2, voltage-gated potassium channel antibodies, and N-methyl-D-aspartate receptor antibodies involve the limbic system and cause symptoms such as hallucinations, short-term memory loss, seizures, and mood changes. Some patients may manifest autonomic instability symptoms such as episodic mydriasis, tachycardia, diaphoresis, and hypertension.

26. **What is LEMS?**
    LEMS is an antibody-mediated autoimmune disease. The target of the aberrant immune response is the presynaptic P/Q voltage-gated calcium channel (VGCC) at the neuromuscular junction. The cardinal symptom of LEMS is weakness, usually in the proximal muscles and more prominent in the lower extremities. In about 50% to 60% of cases, the syndrome is paraneoplastic, associated mostly with small-cell lung cancer. Onset of symptoms may precede detection of tumor by 1 to 4 years. LEMS is frequently associated with autonomic symptoms, including dry mouth, impotence, and constipation. Less common symptoms include orthostatic hypotension, micturition difficulties, dry eyes, and impaired sweating. Variations in heart rate and blood pressure may occur with the Valsalva maneuver or deep breathing, and sweat tests also may be abnormal.

27. **How is LEMS treated?**
    When an underlying neoplasm is identified, removal or treatment of the tumor usually results in substantial improvement in all symptoms, including those of autonomic dysfunction. In patients who do not have an underlying malignancy, the treatment is directed toward the enhancement of cholinergic function and immunosuppression. The first treatment of choice is 3,4-diaminopyridine. Previously, it was thought that blocking voltage-gated potassium channels, resulting in prolongation of action potential at the motor nerve junctions and lengthening the opening time of the VGCC, mediates this agent's effect. Recent studies show that it may also target the VGCC β-subunit directly and result in potentiating neuromuscular transmission. In cases when this agent is not available, guanidine or pyridostigmine may provide benefit. When the symptoms persist, immunosuppression with corticosteroids, azathioprine, or IVIG may be needed.

28. **What is paraneoplastic subacute sensory neuronopathy (SSN)?**
    Sudden onset and rapid progression of dysesthesia, paresthesia, and lancinating pain and numbness in all limbs and occasionally the trunk and face are the characteristics of SSN. Almost 75% of these patients have small-cell lung carcinoma, but other malignancies such as prostate cancer,

neuroblastoma, and seminoma have also been associated with SSN. Some patients with this syndrome may have one or several of the following autonomic dysfunctions: orthostatic hypotension, tonic pupils, hypohidrosis, dry mouth, diminished lacrimation, impotence, urinary retention, and constipation. Serum and cerebrospinal fluid of patients with this syndrome frequently contain antineuronal nuclear antibody (ANNA-1 or anti-Hu). Treatment of the underlying tumor may result in the partial alleviation of autonomic and somatic symptoms.

29. **What is paraneoplastic autonomic neuropathy?**
Some patients with small-cell lung cancer, pancreatic adenocarcinoma, prostate cancer, or Hodgkin's lymphoma may develop autonomic symptoms (orthostatic dizziness, impotence, dry mouth, urinary retention, or GI symptoms) with either no or minimal somatic involvement that may improve with treatment of the tumor. In these patients, the autonomic neuropathy may be part of a generalized paraneoplastic syndrome that variably includes sensory neuronopathy, limbic and brain stem encephalitis, cerebellar degeneration, and a sensorimotor neuropathy. Approximately 40% of patients have antibodies directed against the nicotinic ACh receptors in the autonomic ganglia. The list of antibodies in paraneoplastic autonomic neuropathies has been constantly expanding and includes antineuronal nuclear antibodies, Purkinje cell cytoplasmic autoantibody (PCA), and collapsin response-mediated protein 5 (CRMP-5). The presentation of autonomic neuropathy may either precede or follow the diagnosis of malignancy.

30. **What is paraneoplastic enteric neuropathy?**
Enteric neuropathy of the GI tract, with or without other symptoms of autonomic dysfunction, may be seen in association with small-cell lung cancer, pulmonary carcinoid, undifferentiated epithelioma, and breast cancer. Based on the segment of the GI tract involved, the neuropathy can clinically present as achalasia, gastroparesis, intestinal pseudo-obstruction, or megacolon. Patients may subsequently develop other dysautonomic symptoms. The motility disorder may resolve with the treatment of the underlying tumor. Some patients have elevated titers of antineuronal nuclear antibody (ANNA-1 or anti-Hu), which reacts with antigens shared by the tumor cells and the myenteric plexus neurons.

31. **What cardiac arrhythmias are associated with CNS disease?**
A number of CNS disorders, including subarachnoid hemorrhage, cerebral infarction and hemorrhage, brain tumors, and head injury, may cause a variety of supraventricular and ventricular arrhythmias unrelated to the any underlying cardiac disease. The incidence of cardiac arrhythmias increases if there is more than one infarction site and is highest in subarachnoid hemorrhage. The most common arrhythmia following stroke is atrial fibrillation, whereas in intracranial hemorrhage the incidence of ventricular tachycardia is high. The occurrence of arrhythmias may further compromise the prognosis of the CNS disease: 4% to 5% of sudden deaths in patients with subarachnoid hemorrhage are attributed to arrhythmias. Arrhythmias occur because of an imbalance between sympathetic and parasympathetic influences on the heart, presumably from an enhanced release of peripheral catecholamines triggered by the central lesion.

32. **What is the nature of the myocardial injury associated with CNS disease?**
CNS lesions, particularly intracerebral and subarachnoid hemorrhage, may cause a number of electrocardiogram (ECG) abnormalities suggestive of myocardial ischemia. These changes may closely resemble myocardial infarction and include prolongation of the QT interval, ST segment depression, flattening or inversion of T waves, and the appearance of U waves. With the exception of QT interval prolongation and the U waves, these changes usually revert to normal within 2 weeks after the CNS event. Other less frequently observed ECG changes are increased amplitude of the P wave, development of Q waves, ST segment elevation, and T wave elevation, notching, or peaking. Differentiation between a centrally induced ECG abnormality and a true myocardial infarction may be difficult, but the patient must be cared for in a monitored setting until a "true" myocardial infarction is excluded. The ECG changes are thought to be due to a neurogenically mediated excessive release of catecholamines upon cardiac myocytes, resulting in myonecrotic changes. In fact, a higher level of serum catecholamines correlates with a poor outcome in patients with subarachnoid hemorrhage (Fig. 13-3).

33. **What is the relationship of changes in blood pressure to CNS disease?**
Lesions of the hypothalamus and medulla oblongata or tumors of the posterior fossa may cause arterial hypertension. Ischemic, degenerative, or destructive lesions of the NTS in the medulla may result in chronic lability of blood pressure. Cushing's response of hypertension, bradycardia, and apnea, an important sign of increased intracranial pressure and potential herniation, also may develop after

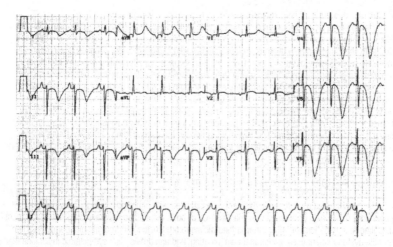

Figure 13-3. Electrocardiogram of a 41-year-old woman showing typical central nervous system (CNS) changes of prolonged QT interval and deep, inverted, peaked T waves.

ischemic lesions of the dorsal medullary reticular formation along the floor of the fourth ventricle. Hypertension caused by posterior fossa tumors is due to the compression of the pressor center at the rostral ventrolateral medulla (RVLM). Such an increase in blood pressure may present as malignant hypertension and may be indistinguishable from a pheochromocytoma. Patients with normal pressure hydrocephalus also may have chronic hypertension. Decreased blood pressure is rare with CNS disease, but orthostatic hypotension may accompany brain stem tumors, although the exact mechanism and the specific nuclei involved are not clear.

34. **Which autonomic dysfunctions occur following heart transplantation?**
Either heart or heart–lung transplantation results in afferent and efferent denervation (i.e., loss of autonomic control) of the transplanted organ with a relative resting tachycardia, little or no rise in heart rate after standing, and a delayed increase in heart rate in response to exercise. Also, there are no changes in heart rate with the Valsalva maneuver or carotid sinus massage. In general, the heart rate response in such patients depends on the circulating catecholamines. The resting tachycardia seen in severe autonomic neuropathies (e.g., diabetes) resembles that seen in a denervated, transplanted heart.

35. **Which neurologic conditions cause hypothermia?**
Experimental studies suggest that lesions of the anterior hypothalamus cause hyperthermia, lesions of the posterior hypothalamus cause hypothermia, and lesions of the suprachiasmatic nucleus cause alteration in the circadian rhythm of temperature. Tumors and degenerative and inflammatory processes involving the hypothalamus may produce hypothermia (core body temperature below 35° C).

   Wernicke's encephalopathy, by damaging the posterolateral hypothalamus and the floor of the fourth ventricle, may present with continuous hypothermia. Prompt treatment with thiamine results in normalization of temperature.

   Paroxysmal hypothermia with hyperhidrosis (PHH) is a syndrome manifested as episodic hypothermia, lasting between 30 minutes and 2 hours, associated with excessive sweating. PHH is probably caused by a low core temperature set in the hypothalamus and is mostly seen in a Shapiro's syndrome (agenesis of the corpus callosum). The underlying mechanism of this syndrome is largely unknown, but disturbances in the function of ion channels may play a role in its pathogenesis. Cyproheptadine, clonidine, chlorpromazine, and peripheral muscarinic agents such as oxybutynin or oxypyrrolate may control hypothermia and diaphoresis.

   Episodic spontaneous hypothermia is a rare periodic childhood syndrome with no known systemic cause or underlying brain lesion. Manifestations include episodic hypothermia (<35° C), marked facial pallor, and absent shivering. Some patients may have bradycardia and hypertension. It is believed that this childhood periodic syndrome is related to migraines.

36. What are the autonomic manifestations that accompany severe brain injury?

    In the initial phase of severe traumatic brain injury, dysautonomic manifestations are frequent. The main features of this syndrome include marked agitation, diaphoresis, hyperthermia, hypertension, tachycardia, tachypnea, and dystonia of limbs. Various names have been given to this complex of symptoms, including paroxysmal sympathetic storm, diencephalic seizures, hypothalamic-midbrain dysregulation syndrome, paroxysmal sympathetic hyperactivity, and paroxysmal autonomic instability with dystonia.

    The pathophysiology of this syndrome seems to be related to the dysfunction of autonomic centers in the diencephalon (thalamus and hypothalamus) or their connections to cortical, subcortical, and brain stem loci that mediate autonomic function. It has been suggested that a disinhibition phenomenon occurs, with loss of cortical and subcortical control of vegetative functions, including blood pressure and temperature. First-line treatment options in the acute setting of the syndrome include opioids, gabapentin, benzodiazepines, centrally acting α-agonists and β-antagonists, and in refractory cases intrathecal baclofen.

37. What are the major differences between the syndrome of PAF and multiple-system atrophy (MSA)?

    MSA is characterized by autonomic dysfunction associated with either poor levodopa-responsive parkinsonism (MSA-P) or cerebellar ataxia (MSA-C), or both. Orthostatic hypotension is one of the most disabling manifestations of MSA. Other autonomic symptoms include neurogenic bladder dysfunction, erectile dysfunction, nausea, abdominal pain, bloating, and anhidrosis. Glial cytoplasmic inclusions that contain deposits of α-synuclein are found in oligodendroglia and some neurons of patients with MSA.

    PAF, previously called idiopathic orthostatic hypotension, is a sporadic disorder characterized by orthostatic hypotension, usually accompanied by evidence of more widespread autonomic failure. There are no other neurologic signs, and the natural history is slow progression over 10 to 15 years. PAF now is considered to be part of the spectrum of "Lewy body synucleinopathies," where the intracytoplasmic eosinophilic inclusions are found in neurons of autonomic ganglia and postganglionic nerves. After a few years, it is not uncommon that a patient presumed to have PAF develops symptoms and signs similar to MSA or less frequently Parkinson's disease or dementia with Lewy bodies. Accordingly, the diagnosis of PAF cannot be made with certainty until prolonged follow-up has been established.

38. Which autonomic dysfunctions occur in Parkinson's disease (PD)?

    In the classic forms of PD, disturbances in salivation, sweating, bladder and bowel functions, and erection may be seen. Some patients may have orthostatic or postprandial dizziness; however, one should not overlook the possibility that orthostatic symptoms may result from dopaminergic agents used in treatment. The cardiovascular reflexes are generally preserved, although responses may be somewhat reduced. The resting recumbent levels of plasma NE and DHPG are lower in patients with orthostatic hypotension than in patients without orthostatic hypotension. These subtle autonomic disturbances in PD are thought to be due to a central rather than a peripheral lesion. Of interest, however, is that Lewy bodies may be present in the sympathetic ganglia of patients with PD.

KEY POINTS: ACQUIRED AUTONOMIC FAILURE

1. Cardinal symptoms of autonomic insufficiency include orthostatic hypotension, bowel and bladder dysfunction, impotence, and sweating abnormalities.
2. Diabetic neuropathy is one of the most common causes of acquired autonomic dysfunction.
3. Autonomic dysfunction can be seen in up to one-third of patients with GBS and can be severe or life threatening.
4. LEMS resembles myasthenia gravis, with autonomic dysfunction, and arises from an autoimmune attack on presynaptic VGCCs.

39. What are the most important genetic causes of autonomic failure?

    - Dopamine/beta-hydroxylase deficiency
    - Familial dysautonomia
    - Fabry's disease
    - Familial amyloidosis
    - Multiple endocrine neoplasia type 2b
    - Porphyria

40. What is dopamine beta-hydroxylase deficiency? What is the best treatment for this disease?

Beta-hydroxylase is the last enzyme in the synthesis pathway of NE, and the encoding gene is located on chromosome 9. Several recessively inherited mutations of this gene have been detected, resulting in undetectable levels of NE in the circulation and tissues. Patients with this very rare disorder present with severe orthostatic hypotension, episodic hypoglycemia, and hypothermia. Dihydroxyphenylserine (DOPS), a precursor of NE, has effectively treated these patients.

41. What is familial dysautonomia?

Familial dysautonomia (Riley–Day syndrome, hereditary sensory and autonomic neuropathy type III) is an autosomal recessive disorder affecting primarily people of Ashkenazi Jewish descent. It affects the development and survival of sensory, sympathetic, and some parasympathetic neurons. The genetic abnormality responsible for the disease has been identified as the splicing mutation in the *IKBKAP* (IKB kinase-associated protein) gene on the distal long arm of chromosome 9. The cardinal clinical features include alacrima (absence of tears), absent fungiform papillae of the tongue, depressed patellar reflexes, and absent skin response to scratch and histamine injection. Autonomic features result primarily from sympathetic system dysfunction and include transient and emotionally induced erythematous skin blotching, orthostatic hypotension, hyperhidrosis or erratic sweating, and esophageal and GI transit dysfunction. Dysautonomic crisis is a constellation of symptoms including vomiting, tachycardia, excessive sweating, blotching of the skin, piloerection, ileus, and dilation of the pupils that may occur in response to physiologic or psychologic stress.

42. What is Fabry's disease?

This X-linked recessive metabolic disease, also known as angiokeratoma corporis diffusum, is due to a deficiency of the lysosomal enzyme alpha-galactosidase, with resulting cell storage of the glycolipid ceramide trihexoside in several organs, including the skin (corpora angiokeratomas), kidneys, cardiovascular and pulmonary systems, blood vessels, and central and peripheral nervous systems in the dorsal root and peripheral autonomic ganglia. The most common clinical presentation includes bouts of severe painful burning sensation in hands and feet, angiokeratoma, hypohidrosis, heat intolerance, and lenticular and corneal opacities.

The clinical presentation of autonomic dysfunction includes diminished sweating (which may be due to lipid accumulation in sweat glands rather than neuropathy), absent skin wrinkling after immersion in warm water, reduced cutaneous flare response, reduced tear and saliva production, disturbed intestinal motility, abnormal cardiovascular responses, and abnormal pupillary response to pilocarpine.

Regular intravenous infusions of recombinant human alpha-galactosidase A have been used as an enzyme replacement therapy (ERT) in patients with Fabry's disease. ERT appears to improve neuropathic pain, renal function, and glomerular pathology and may also improve the overall prognosis of the disease.

43. What is familial amyloid polyneuropathy?

Transthyretin (TTR) is an amyloidogenic protein with more than 120 TTR gene mutations that can lead to a heterogeneous group of disorders characterized by accumulation of polypeptide amyloid fibrils. One of the most common mutations is Val30Met mutation, responsible for familial amyloid polyneuropathy. Patients with Val30Met mutation are classified into two groups, early onset and late onset. Early-onset patients have marked autonomic dysfunction, including orthostatic hypotension, impotence, disturbance in the bladder contraction and bowel movements, and cardiac conduction blocks. The late-onset variant presents with mild autonomic dysfunction.

The only treatment for familial amyloidosis is liver transplantation. When performed early in the course of the disease, it may stop clinical progression and modestly improve symptoms.

44. What is multiple endocrine neoplasia type 2b (MEN 2b)?

MEN 2b, an autosomal dominant inherited disorder, is characterized by multiple mucosal neuromas (conjunctiva, oral cavity, tongue, pharynx, and larynx), medullary thyroid carcinoma, pheochromocytoma, ganglioneuromatosis, bony deformities, marfanoid appearance, muscle underdevelopment, and hypotonia. Gross and microscopic abnormalities of the peripheral autonomic nervous system affect both sympathetic and parasympathetic systems. Patients have disorganized hypertrophy and proliferation of autonomic nerves and ganglia (ganglioneuromatosis). Neural proliferation of the alimentary tract (Auerbach and Meissner's plexi), upper respiratory tract, bladder, prostate, and skin also may be seen. The clinical autonomic manifestations include impaired lacrimation, orthostatic hypotension, impaired reflex vasodilation of the skin, and parasympathetic denervation supersensitivity of pupils, with intact sweating and salivary gland function. Nerve biopsy shows degeneration and regeneration of unmyelinated fibers. A few point mutations in the *RET* proto-oncogene located on chromosome 10 have been associated with the disease. Genetic testing is critical for detection of young carriers, who can undergo regular screening for medullary thyroid cancer.

45. **What is porphyria?**
Acute hepatic porphyrias (acute intermittent porphyria, variegate porphyria, and hereditary coproporphyria) are autosomal dominant hereditary disorders that manifest as acute or subacute, severe, life-threatening neuropathy. The basic genetic defect is a 50% reduction in porphobilinogen deaminase activity (acute intermittent porphyria), protoporphyrinogen-IX oxidase (variegate porphyria), and coproporphyrinogen oxidase (coproporphyria), resulting in abnormalities of heme biosynthesis. In the presence of sufficient endogenous or exogenous stimuli (e.g., drugs, hormones, menstruation, starvation), this partial deficiency may lead to clinical manifestations, including peripheral neuropathy, autonomic dysfunction, skin symptoms, and CNS abnormalities.

    Pathologic involvement of the autonomic nervous system (degeneration of the vagus nerve and sympathetic trunk) may explain certain features of acute attacks, including abdominal pain, severe vomiting, constipation, intestinal dilatation and stasis, persistent sinus tachycardia (100 to 160 minutes), labile hypertension, postural hypotension, hyperhidrosis, and sphincteric bladder problems.

46. **What are the most important factors in the maintenance of normal blood pressure?**
    - Blood volume
    - Vascular reflexes (e.g., reflex arteriolar-venous constriction, baroreflex-induced tachycardia)
    - Hormonal mechanisms (e.g., increased plasma catecholamines, renin–angiotensin–aldosterone system, arginine, vasopressin, atrial natriuretic factor)

47. **Which age-related physiologic changes predispose to hypotension?**
Decreased baroreflex sensitivity, impaired neuroendocrine response to changes of intravascular volume (e.g., reduced secretion of renin, angiotensin, and aldosterone), and impaired early cardiac ventricular filling (diastolic dysfunction).

48. **What are the baroreceptors? What is their significance?**
Baroreceptors are spray-type nerve endings in the walls of blood vessels and heart that are stimulated by the absolute level of, and changes in, arterial pressure. They are extremely abundant in the wall of carotid sinus and aortic arch. The primary site of termination of baroreceptor afferent fibers is the NTS.

    The function of the baroreceptors is to maintain systemic blood pressure at a relatively constant level, especially during a change in body position. Intact baroreceptors are extremely effective in preventing rapid changes in blood pressure from moment to moment or hour to hour, but because of their adaptability to prolonged changes of blood pressure (>2 or 3 days), the system is incapable of long-term regulation of arterial pressure.

    Stretching of the baroreceptors as a result of increased blood pressure causes an increase in the activity of the vagal nerve by projection to the nucleus ambiguus. It also causes inhibition of the sympathetic outflow from the RVLM, ultimately leading to decreased heart rate and blood pressure. Conversely, decreased blood pressure results in decreased signal output from the baroreceptors, leading to disinhibition of the central sympathetic control sites and decreased parasympathetic activity. The final effect is an increase in blood pressure.

49. **What are the clinical features of baroreceptor failure?**
Baroreflex failure is a heterogeneous entity that can result from abnormalities in vascular baroreceptors, cranial nerve IX or X abnormalities, or brain stem abnormalities that involve the baroreflex control centers such as NTS. As a result of impairment in the baroreflex, these patients have volatile blood pressures and heart rates. The clinical presentation can resemble pheochromocytoma. The ability of clonidine to inhibit neurons of RVLM and therefore to profoundly reduce the blood pressure differentiates these patients from patients with pheochromocytoma.

50. Why do patients with orthostatic hypotension have diurnal variation in blood pressure?

Many patients with orthostatic hypotension have supine hypertension, even before they are treated with fludrocortisone or other medications. The reason for supine hypertension remains to be determined; however, it seems that baroreflex dysfunction may play a role. Prolonged supine position at night may lead to natriuresis and diuresis and eventually contracture of intravascular volume. These events cause the orthostatic hypotension to become more severe in the morning.

51. What is the difference in orthostatic hypotension caused by autonomic dysfunction and that caused by hypovolemia during a tilt table test?

In most autonomic neuropathies associated with orthostatic hypotension, failure of vascular reflexes to increase sympathetic outflow to splanchnic and muscular vasculature results in a drop in both systolic and diastolic pressures. However, there is no increase in plasma NE (hypoadrenergic response). Conversely, in orthostatic hypotension secondary to hypovolemia, plasma NE increases excessively in response to standing (hyperadrenergic response).

In orthostatic hypotension secondary to generalized sympathetic failure, a drop in systolic blood pressure is not associated with reflex tachycardia, whereas in orthostatic hypotension secondary to hypovolemia or deconditioning, with intact sympathetic nerves, reflex tachycardia is prominent. A fall in systolic pressure alone is most likely caused by a non-neurologic disturbance (e.g., hypovolemia).

52. What are the three main mechanisms of syncope?

- **Orthostatic hypotension** may be due to a reduction in vascular resistance, hypovolemia, drugs, chronic baroreflex failure, or a neurally mediated mechanism (vasovagal syncope triggered by pain or fear). Reflex syncope and vasodepressor syncope are synonymous with vasovagal syncope.
- **Fall in cardiac output** may be due to cardiac arrhythmias, obstructions to flow, or myocardial infarction.
- **Increased cerebrovascular resistance** may be due to hyperventilation or increased intracranial pressure.

53. What general advice should you give to a patient with orthostatic hypotension secondary to dysautonomia?

- Avoid straining, which results in the Valsalva maneuver, by treating and preventing constipation with a high-fiber diet.
- Avoid severe diurnal variation, particularly morning postural hypotension, by head-up tilt or sleeping in a sitting position at night, sitting for several minutes at the edge of the bed before standing and shaving while sitting.
- When presyncopal symptoms occur immediately assume a squatting position, cross the legs, bend forward and place the head between the knees, or place one foot on a chair.
- Avoid exposure to a warm environment to prevent uncompensated vasodilation (e.g., travel to warm countries, hot baths).
- Avoid postprandial aggravation of orthostatic hypotension by eating smaller and more frequent meals with reduced carbohydrate content.
- Avoid a low-sodium diet by increasing the food sodium content to at least 150 mEq.
- Avoid dehydration by increasing fluid intake to 2.0 to 2.5 L/day.
- Avoid vigorous exercise; moderate isotonic exercises are preferable to isometrics.
- Avoid prolonged recumbency.
- Avoid vasodilators such as alcohol.
- Avoid drugs known to cause vasodilation and/or bradycardia (nitroglycerin or beta-blockers).

54. What are the most common pharmacologic agents used for the treatment of orthostatic hypotension secondary to autonomic failure?

Fludrocortisone, a potent mineralocorticoid, is the most common agent in use. Its mechanism of action is increasing of the blood volume by retention of sodium from the kidneys. Usually 1 to 2 weeks is required to see the effect.

The α_1-agonist midodrine stimulates both arterial and venous systems without directly affecting the CNS or heart. This drug is converted to the active agent desglymidodrine and is best used to elevate the daytime blood pressure. Up to one-fourth of patients may develop supine hypertension, which can best be prevented by taking the last dose at least a few hours before bed time.

A precursor of NE (L-threo-3,4-dihydroxyphenylserine [L-DOPS]) can be converted to NE outside of the CNS and improve orthostatic tolerance.

α_2-Agonists such as clonidine are sometimes used as an adjunctive therapy, but their use is limited by supine hypertension.

55. **What is postural tachycardia syndrome (POTS)? How is it treated?**
This increasingly recognized condition, often observed in females aged 15 to 50 years, is defined as a syndrome of consistent orthostatic symptoms associated with an excessive heart rate of equal to or greater than 120 beats/min or an increase in the heart rate of 30 beats/min or greater within 5 minutes of standing or tilt-up. There is only a minimal or no drop in blood pressure after standing, but the patient feels many of the orthostatic symptoms, including dizziness, fatigue, tremulousness, palpitations, nausea, vasomotor skin changes, hyperhidrosis, or chest wall pain. Some patients with the diagnosis of chronic fatigue syndrome or anxiety or panic disorder may instead have POTS, especially if their symptoms are consistently reproduced after standing and cease after assuming a recumbent position. Patients with orthostatic headaches but no evidence of cerebrospinal fluid leak should also be investigated for POTS.

POTS has heterogeneous etiologies, and based on the postulated pathophysiologic mechanisms, has been divided into neuropathic and hyperadrenergic POTS. In another classification based on the measurement of leg venous pressure and calf blood flow, it has been divided into low flow, normal flow, and high flow POTS.

Treatment options include increased intake of fluids and salt (to increase blood volume), fludrocortisone, desmopressin, midodrine (an α_1-adrenergic agonist that induces vasoconstriction), propranolol, pyridostigmine, and measures to reduce blood pooling in the legs.

56. **What cardiovascular autonomic changes are seen during rapid eye movement (REM) sleep?**
During REM sleep, sympathetic activity of the splanchnic and renal circulation is decreased, but activity by skeletal muscles is increased. Whereas the slow phases of sleep are accompanied by hypotension and bradycardia, which become increasingly more pronounced with the progression of sleep from stage 1 to stage 4, REM sleep is associated with large, transient increases in blood pressure, reversing the hypotension of slow-wave sleep. Direct recording of sympathetic nerve traffic to the skeletal muscle vascular bed by microneurography shows more than a 50% reduction in sympathetic activity during the slow phases of sleep but a significant increase to the level of wakefulness during REM. This finding may suggest that slow-wave sleep provides a protective effect on the cardiovascular and cerebrovascular systems; during REM sleep or immediately afterward, such protective effects may disappear. This phenomenon may explain why cardiovascular and cerebrovascular events occur more frequently in the early morning hours after awakening.

57. **There is a higher incidence of sudomotor and vasomotor disturbances of the arm with injuries to the lower trunk of the brachial plexus than with injuries to the upper trunk. Why?**
There is a higher density of postganglionic sympathetic fibers in the medial cord of the brachial plexus and the median and ulnar nerves.

KEY POINTS: ACQUIRED AUTONOMIC FAILURE

1. Syncope can be caused by orthostatic hypotension, decrease in cardiac output, or increase in cerebrovascular resistance.
2. Nonpharmacological measures can be effective in managing symptomatic orthostatic hypotension.
3. Some patients with diagnosis of chronic fatigue syndrome, panic attack, or anxiety in fact may be suffering from POTS.

58. **What are the most common tests to quantitatively evaluate the autonomic nervous system?**
Quantitative sudomotor axon reflex test (QSART) is used to evaluate the sympathetic cholinergic nerves that innervate the sweat glands.

Variability of heart rate to deep breathing and Valsalva maneuver are used to assess the cardiovagal component of the autonomic nervous system.

Beat-to-beat changes of blood pressure during Valsalva maneuver and tilt-up test screen the adrenergic component of the autonomic nervous system.

59. Why does skin turn red (flare) after it is scratched?

The normal skin axon-reflex vasodilation (flare) follows skin stimulation from a simple scratch. The scratch causes activation of unmyelinated sensory nerve terminals (C fibers). The impulse generated by this stimulus travels antidromically, reaches a branch point, and then orthodromically arrives at a skin blood vessel, releasing one or more vasodilating peptides or adenosine triphosphate. The released substance leads to further histamine release, activating other sensory terminals, creating a cascade of spreading flare response. Released histamine also causes itching. Antihistamines may reduce both the flare response and the itching. The absence of a flare response provides evidence of dysfunction of unmyelinated sensory fibers in peripheral neuropathies.

60. What is the sudomotor axon reflex?

The sudomotor axon reflex employs the same mechanism as the skin axon-reflex flare, but the neural pathway consists of an axon reflex mediated by the postganglionic sympathetic axon (C fibers) that innervates sweat glands. The axon terminals of these fibers are activated by the local injection of ACh: the generated impulse travels to a branch point where it is deflected and then travels orthodromically to activate a different sweat gland, releasing ACh, which binds to M3 muscarinic receptors. In other words, in the sudomotor axon reflex, the activation of sweat glands results in the reflex activation of another population of nearby glands, the sweat output of which can be quantitatively measured. The QSART is, therefore, a sensitive and reproducible test of the integrity of the postganglionic sympathetic sudomotor axon.

61. What is the basis for the heart rate variability to deep breathing test?

Usually, inspiration increases and expiration decreases the heart rate (sinus arrhythmia). This phenomenon is mediated primarily by the vagus nerve. Pulmonary stretch receptors and cardiac mechanoreceptors, as well as baroreceptors, contribute to its generation. This test is easy to perform with a commercial ECG machine. While supine with the head elevated to 30 degrees, the patient breathes deeply at six respirations per minute (5 seconds' inspiration followed by 5 seconds' expiration, usually for eight cycles), and minimal and maximal heart rate within each respiratory cycle is measured. The simplest index is the heart rate variability defined as maximum heart rate minus minimum heart rate. Another index, the E/I (excitation and inhibition) ratio, is determined by the longest R–R interval on the ECG divided by the shortest R–R interval. An abnormal test indicates parasympathetic dysfunction.

62. What are the confounding factors that influence the heart rate variability to deep breathing?

Heart rate variability to deep breathing decreases with advancing age (about 3 to 5 beats per minute every 10 years). Rate and depth of breathing, position of the subject, obesity, and medications such as cholinergic agents influence the test results.

63. What are the four phases of blood pressure variation during a Valsalva maneuver in a person with intact autonomic nervous system?

During phase I, increased intra-abdominal and intrathoracic pressure results in compression of the large vessels and aorta and therefore transient increase in the blood pressure, accompanied by a reflex bradycardia. Shortly after, reduction in the venous return to the heart leads to reduced stroke volume and blood pressure (early phase II). This decline in blood pressure triggers the sympathetic nervous system with resultant increase in NE level, peripheral vascular resistance, and blood pressure (late phase II). When the Valsalva maneuver is released, the sudden decline in intrathoracic pressure causes a concomitant decrease in blood pressure and tachycardia (phase III). Finally, in phase IV in normal subjects, despite the return of the venous return and cardiac output to the baseline values, blood pressure continues to rise as a result of the persistent high peripheral vascular resistance (residual from late phase II). Therefore, blood pressure usually overshoots the baseline in this phase (Fig. 13-4).

64. What are the changes seen in the blood pressure variation during a Valsalva maneuver in a patient with adrenergic failure?

In patients with inadequate response of the adrenergic system, the blood pressure fails to increase in late phase II. By the same token, the blood pressure fails to overshoot the baseline level in phase IV (Fig. 13-5).

65. What is the Valsalva ratio? What component of the autonomic nervous system is assessed by this ratio?

The valsalva ratio is the ratio of maximum heart rate during the Valsalva maneuver divided by the minimum heart rate occurring within 30 seconds of the maximum rate. This ratio is another quantitative value that reflects the integrity of the cardiovagal component of the autonomic nervous system.

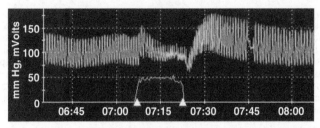

Figure 13-4. Blood pressure variation during Valsalva maneuver in a person with intact autonomic nervous system.

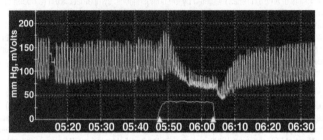

Figure 13-5. Blood pressure variation during Valsalva maneuver in a person with adrenergic failure.

66. How is a tilt table test performed?

The patient rests on a tilt table in a supine position for 20 minutes. Then the table is tilted to 70 degrees within 10 to 20 seconds. The blood pressure is measured at 1 and 5 minutes, although different labs employ different protocols. In normal individuals, there is a transient reduction in systolic, mean, and diastolic blood pressure following tilt, followed by recovery in 1 minute. Orthostatic hypotension is defined as a drop in systolic blood pressure of ≥20 mm Hg or diastolic blood pressure of ≥10 mm Hg within 3 minutes of tilt-up with only a modest increase in the heart rate.

KEY POINTS: ACQUIRED AUTONOMIC FAILURE

1. QSART is used to evaluate the sympathetic cholinergic nerves that innervate the sweat glands.
2. Variability of heart rate to deep breathing and Valsalva maneuver are used to assess the cardiovagal component of the autonomic nervous system.
3. Beat-to-beat changes of blood pressure during Valsalva maneuver and tilt-up test screens the adrenergic component of the autonomic nervous system.

67. During examination of the external ear canal with an otoscope, the patient developed dry cough and became dizzy. Why?

The second branch of the vagus nerve, the auricular nerve, which originates after the vagus nerve has exited from the jugular foramen, is a somatic afferent nerve that provides the sensory fibers for the posterior wall and floor of the external acoustic meatus and the outer surface of the tympanic membrane. Irritation of the external auditory canal and the tympanic membrane by instruments, cerumen, or syringing may, therefore, cause abnormal vagal reflexes, resulting in coughing, vomiting, slow heart rate, or even cardiac inhibition.

68. What is the syndrome of autonomic dysreflexia observed in tetraplegics? What is the best management?

Traumatic spinal cord lesions result in markedly abnormal cardiovascular, thermoregulatory, bladder, bowel, and sexual function. In a recently injured tetraplegic in spinal shock, tactile or painful stimuli originating below the level of the lesion induce no change in blood pressure or heart rate. In the chronic stages of spinal cord injury at the level of T6 and above, however, there is an exaggerated rise in the systolic and diastolic blood pressure, accompanied by bradycardia. Transient tachycardia may precede the drop in heart rate. The plasma NE levels are only marginally elevated. The marked hypertension may lead to neurologic complications, including seizures, visual defects, and cerebral hemorrhage. This uncommon but potentially life-threatening phenomenon, called *autonomic dysreflexia,* is caused by the increased activity of target organs below the lesion supplied by sympathetic and parasympathetic nerves lacking supraspinal modulation. Other clinical manifestations of autonomic dysreflexia include headache, chest tightness and dyspnea, pupillary dilation, cold limbs, flushing of face and neck, excessive sweating of the head, penile erection and discharge of seminal fluid, and contraction of bladder and bowel.

The prolonged episodes of this syndrome may be prevented if the precipitating cause (e.g., painful tactile or visceral urinary and rectal stimuli) is corrected. It is important that the bladder be emptied before performing any procedure on tetraplegic patients. Blood pressure can often be decreased by elevating the head of the bed.

69. **What are the pathologic causes of hyperhidrosis? How is it treated?**
Spinal cord damage or lesions of the peripheral sympathetic nerves may cause localized hyperhidrosis. Generalized and episodic hyperhidrosis may occur in patients with infectious diseases (night sweats), malignancies, hypoglycemia, thyrotoxicosis, pheochromocytomas, carcinoid syndrome, acromegaly, or diencephalic epilepsy and in patients receiving cholinergic agents.

Primary or essential hyperhidrosis usually involves limited areas of the body, particularly the axilla, palms, and plantar regions. Essential hyperhidrosis is, however, usually self-limiting by the fourth or fifth decade of life. Up to one-half of patients have a family history of a similar condition. The cause of this condition seems to be centrally initiated excessive sympathetic output to the sweat glands.

The treatment of essential generalized hyperhidrosis is difficult and requires systemic pharmacotherapy (anticholinergics, clonidine), topical agents (aluminum chloride), excision of axillary sweat glands, botulinum toxin injections, and sympathectomy as the last resort.

70. **How may mastocytosis be confused with autonomic dysfunction?**
Mastocytosis, or abnormal proliferation of tissue mast cells, may be confused with autonomic dysfunction because of symptoms of flushing, palpitation, dyspnea, chest discomfort, headache, lightheadedness and dizziness, fall in blood pressure, nausea, abdominal cramps, and diarrhea, which occur episodically. Some patients may have an elevation of blood pressure. Each attack is followed by profound lethargy and fatigue. Episodes may be brief, lasting several minutes, or protracted, lasting 2 to 3 hours. Exposure to heat or emotional or physical stress may precipitate an attack. Flushing and warm sensations are the most important clues differentiating this syndrome from syndromes of orthostatic intolerance.

71. **When your attending physician pimps you on rounds, why do you get sweaty palms but not sweaty armpits?**
Anxiety and emotional stress primarily aggravate the hyperhidrosis of the palms and soles but not of the axilla. The eccrine sweat glands of the palms and soles, as well as those of the forehead, respond to emotional, mental, or sensory stimuli, whereas the axillary glands respond primarily to thermal stimuli.

Acknowledgments

The author would like to acknowledge the contributions of Dr. Yadollah Harati who authored this chapter in the previous edition.

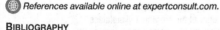 *References available online at expertconsult.com.*

BIBLIOGRAPHY

1. Freeman R, Chapleau MW: Testing the autonomic nervous system. Handb Clin Neurol 115:115, 2013.
2. Goldstein DS: Catecholamines 101. Clin Auton Res 20:331, 2010.
3. Low PA, Benarroch EE: Clinical Autonomic Disorders, 3rd ed. Philadelphia, Lippincott Williams & Wilkins, 2008.
4. Mathias CJ: Autonomic Failure: A Textbook of Clinical Disorders of the Autonomic Nervous System, 5th ed. Oxford, Oxford University Press, 2013.
5. Robertson D, Biaggioni I, Burnstock G, Low PA, Paton JFR: Primer on the Autonomic Nervous System, 3rd ed. San Diego, Academic Press, 2012.
6. Saklani P, Krahn A, Klein G: Syncope. Circulation 127:1330, 2013.

CHAPTER 14

DEMYELINATING AND AUTOIMMUNE DISEASES

Loren A. Rolak

DISEASES OF MYELIN

1. **What is myelin?**
   Myelin is the proteolipid membrane that ensheathes and surrounds nerve axons to improve their ability to conduct electrical action potentials. Oligodendrocytes make central nervous system myelin and wrap the myelin around axons, leaving gaps called *nodes of Ranvier*, where membrane ionic channels are heavily concentrated and powerful action potentials can thus be generated.

2. **How does demyelination cause symptoms?**
   When myelin is stripped away from the axon, the underlying membrane does not contain a high enough concentration of sodium, potassium, and other ionic channels to permit a sufficient flow of ions to cause depolarization. The membrane thus becomes inert. The loss of myelin makes it impossible to depolarize the membrane to conduct an action potential, so the nerve is rendered useless.

3. **What is multiple sclerosis (MS)?**
   MS is the most common condition that destroys myelin in the central nervous system. It affects approximately 250,000 Americans, mostly between the ages of 20 and 40, making it the leading disabling neurologic disease of young people.

4. **How does MS cause demyelination?**
   The demyelination is largely an inflammatory process. Lymphocytes, macrophages, and other immunocompetent cells accumulate around venules focally in the central nervous system and exit into the brain, attacking and destroying the local myelin, in what appears to be an autoimmune process. In many patients with MS, a more degenerative (and poorly understood) pathology appears, with less inflammation and more generalized atrophy.

5. **Are there other demyelinating diseases?**
   Yes, but they are rare. MS is the only common demyelinating disease in adults. Other rare conditions include:
   - **Central pontine myelinolysis**, a syndrome of myelin destruction in the pons, associated with rapid correction of hyponatremia.
   - **Progressive multifocal leukoencephalopathy**, an opportunistic infection of oligodendrocytes by the John Cunningham (JC) virus, seen most often in patients with acquired immunodeficiency syndrome or other immunosuppression.
   - **Acute disseminated encephalomyelitis**, a monophasic, acute, autoimmune demyelination producing encephalopathy, especially in childhood.
   - **Inborn errors of myelin metabolism**, usually presenting in childhood:
     - Metachromatic leukodystrophy, a deficiency of the enzyme aryl sulfatase
     - Adrenoleukodystrophy, a defect in metabolism of very long chain fatty acids
     - Krabbe's globoid leukodystrophy, a deficiency of the enzyme galactosylceramidase
   - **Neuromyelitis optica or Devic's disease**, an autoimmune disease predominantly affecting the optic nerves and spinal cord. Patients have relapses, usually every few years, causing primarily visual and spinal cord deficits. Severe disability often results. Patients have antibodies to aquaporin-4, regulating a water channel on astrocytes, leading to inflammation and secondary demyelination.

CLINICAL FEATURES OF MULTIPLE SCLEROSIS

6. What are the most common symptoms of MS?
   - Pyramidal weakness—45%
   - Visual loss—40%
   - Sensory loss—35%
   - Brain stem dysfunction—30%
   - Cerebellar ataxia and tremor—25%
   - Sphincter disturbances—20%

7. Are there any symptoms that MS does not cause?
   Not many. Virtually every neurologic problem has been described in MS, at least as a case report. However, because MS is predominantly a disease of myelin (white matter), it only rarely causes neuronal (gray matter) symptoms, such as aphasia, seizures, and movement disorders.

8. What is the clinical course of MS?
   MS usually follows one of a few distinctive patterns, classified largely on the timing of the symptoms:
   - Clinically isolated syndrome
   - Relapsing–remitting
   - Primary progressive
   - Secondary progressive

9. What is a clinically isolated syndrome (CIS)?
   A CIS is the first presentation of signs and symptoms that show characteristics of inflammatory demyelination that could be MS but is only a single monophasic event (not disseminated in time). An example of a CIS would be an episode of either optic neuritis or transverse myelitis or other single isolated event. If such patients have abnormal magnetic resonance imaging (MRI) showing other (asymptomatic) lesions characteristic of MS, it is highly likely that a CIS is actually the initial attack of MS.

10. What is relapsing–remitting MS?
    Relapsing–remitting MS is the most common pattern, accounting for about 80% of all MS. Patients have the sudden onset (over hours or days) of neurologic symptoms that usually last several weeks and then resolve, often leaving few or no deficits. On average these attacks/relapses/exacerbations occur every 3 months.

11. What is progressive MS?
    Some patients develop symptoms slowly and gradually, progressive over 6 to 12 months or more. If this gradual worsening develops after an initial relapsing–remitting disease course, it is referred to as *secondary progressive MS*. Approximately 10% to 15% of all MS patients never experience a CIS or a relapse but rather have chronic progressive symptoms from the onset. This is referred to as *primary progressive MS*. The only distinction between these progressive forms is the presence (secondary progression) or absence (primary progression) of relapses prior to the appearance of the progressive symptoms. There are otherwise no known pathophysiological differences between the two forms.

12. What is the prognosis of MS?
    MS varies greatly, not only in its symptoms and clinical course but also in its prognosis. Although not a fatal disease, MS is associated with a slight statistical shortening of lifespan as a result of secondary complications that may afflict severe cases, such as aspiration pneumonia, decubitus ulcers, urinary tract infections, and falls. As a general rule, approximately one-third of patients with MS do well throughout their life, without accumulating significant disability. Another one-third accumulate neurologic deficits sufficient to impair activities but not serious enough to prevent them from leading a normal life—holding a job, raising a family. The final third of people with MS become disabled, requiring a walker, wheelchair, or even total care.

13. What factors help to predict the course of MS?
    The variability of MS makes accurate prediction fallible, but a few factors may portend a good prognosis:
    - Early age of onset (first symptoms before age 40)
    - Sensory symptoms at onset (as opposed to weakness, ataxia, or other motor abnormalities)

- A relapsing–remitting course (vs a primary progressive symptom at onset)
- Female gender: women do better than men.

14. **What is the Expanded Disability Status Score (EDSS)?**
The EDSS is a number that rates a patient's degree of disability from MS on a scale of 0 to 10. Deficits are determined in various functional systems (motor, sensory, cerebellar, etc.). A patient with a score of 6 requires a cane to walk and with a score of 8 is confined to a wheelchair. The EDSS is widely used as a standard method of evaluating MS patients.

DIAGNOSIS

15. **Given the great variability in the signs, symptoms, and clinical course of MS, how can it be accurately diagnosed?**
The diagnosis of MS can be one of the most difficult in neurology. Nevertheless, certain clinical criteria usually identify MS (Table 14-1).

Table 14-1. Clinical Criteria for Definite Multiple Sclerosis (MS)

- Two separate central nervous system symptoms—lesions disseminated in space
- Two separate attacks at least 1 month apart—lesions disseminated in time
- Symptoms must involve the white matter
- Age 10-50 years (although usually 20-40 years)
- Objective deficits are present on the neurologic examination
- No other medical problem can be found to explain the patient's condition

---

16. **How can MRI be used to diagnose MS?**
Because of its sensitivity and noninvasive nature, MRI is the best test to confirm the diagnosis of MS. The inflammatory demyelinated lesions, or plaques, are visualized quite well on MRI. The drawback to MRI is its lack of specificity. The scattered subcortical periventricular white matter abnormalities that characterize MS may occur in various other settings, including cerebrovascular disease, vasculitis, migraine, hypertension, and in some subjects who appear to be normal. For this reason, reliance strictly on MRI may lead to overdiagnosis of MS (Fig. 14-1).

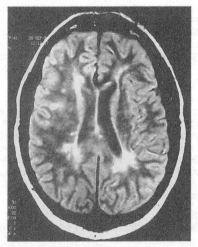

Figure 14-1. Axial flair magnetic resonance imaging (MRI) of the brain shows typical confluent, deep white matter signal intensities characteristic of multiple sclerosis (MS).

17. **What are the McDonald criteria for the diagnosis of MS?**
    The McDonald criteria incorporate features of MRI, to confirm dissemination in time and in space. This can allow MRI to make an accurate diagnosis in patients who do not meet all the clinical criteria. For example, one clinical lesion and a separate MRI lesion confirm dissemination in space.

18. **Can MS be diagnosed after only one attack of symptoms?**
    MS may begin in some patients as a clinically isolated syndrome such as a single, monophasic episode of optic neuritis or transverse myelitis. If this patient has an MRI showing dissemination in space (i.e., subclinical disease in another location in the central nervous system), and the lesions are disseminated in time (i.e., some enhance and some do not), then a diagnosis of MS can be made.

19. **How can the cerebrospinal fluid be used to diagnose MS?**
    Immunoglobulins are increased in the central nervous system in patients with MS. When the immunoglobulin G (IgG) is examined by electrophoresis, it may concentrate into specific bands. The finding of multiple bands in the IgG region, called *oligoclonal bands*, is reasonably sensitive and specific for MS. However, it remains unclear how or why oligoclonal bands are produced or exactly what they represent.

20. **Do other diseases have oligoclonal bands?**
    Yes, especially inflammatory and infectious conditions such as syphilis, meningoencephalitis, subacute sclerosing panencephalitis (a latent measles infection), and Guillain–Barré syndrome. However, these are unlikely to be confused with MS.

21. **What is the differential diagnosis of MS?**
    Although MS is an inflammatory white matter disease, conditions mistaken for MS are usually not other inflammatory or white matter diseases. The differential instead comprises other common conditions that produce neurologic symptoms in young people: migraine, vascular disease, neuropathy, and anxiety.

ETIOLOGY

22. **How does the epidemiology of MS provide clues to its cause?**
    Some unusual features characterize the epidemiology of MS. MS is more common the farther one moves away from the equator. It is more common in women than men. It primarily strikes people of northern European ancestry and is almost unknown in other racial groups such as Eskimos and Gypsies, a finding that may be related to specific human leukocyte antigen type (i.e., immune functions) and genetic predisposition.
    The chance of developing MS seems to be set by approximately age 15 years. A person born in a high-risk area (such as Scandinavia) who leaves for a low-risk area (in the tropics) after age 15 years will carry the high risk for developing MS. A person who emigrates before age 15 years acquires the low risk of the new home. In short, the risk of MS is determined before age 15 years, even though the disease itself does not appear, on average, until age 30 years.
    Unfortunately, none of these tantalizing epidemiologic findings has yet led to a coherent hypothesis for the etiology of MS. The cause of MS is still unknown.

23. **Is MS all one disease?**
    This is not clear. Clinically, it is quite heterogeneous, and pathologically this heterogeneity may prove true. New immunopathologic techniques suggest that there may be different patterns of demyelination and immune activation among different patients. Several distinct pathologic mechanisms may thus underlie the condition we now call MS, but this remains to be proven.

TREATMENT

24. **What is the role of steroids in MS?**
    A number of studies have suggested superiority of steroids over placebo for alleviating relapses of MS. Symptoms resolve more quickly, although it is not clear if treatment of attacks ultimately prevents disability or mitigates the final outcome of the disease. There remains much controversy about the most appropriate steroid preparation, dosage, route of administration, and duration of treatment. A popular therapy employs intravenous methylprednisolone (Solu-Medrol) in a dose of 500 to 1000 mg daily for 3 to 7 days. Sometimes oral prednisone is used, at 60 mg daily for 5 to 7 days.

25. What is the role of immunosuppressants in MS?

Many immune-altering regimens have been used in MS, but prospective, randomized, blinded, controlled, multicentered trials have been few and disappointing. Nevertheless, treatments such as plasmapheresis, cyclophosphamide, azathioprine, methotrexate, mitoxantrone, rituximab, and intravenous immunoglobulin still are occasionally used, more for their theoretical benefits than for any proof of efficacy.

26. What prophylactic drugs are available to decrease attacks of MS?

There is no cure for MS, but several drugs have been approved in the United States as long-term maintenance therapy to reduce the rate of attacks in relapsing–remitting MS. These drugs are indicated for relapsing–remitting disease or clinically isolated syndromes and are probably powerless against any of the progressive, degenerative aspects of MS (Table 14-2).

Table 14-2. Common Prophylactic Drugs for Multiple Sclerosis (MS)

1. Interferons
2. Glatiramer acetate
3. Monoclonal antibodies
4. Oral agents

27. Discuss the role of interferons for the treatment of MS.

These medications are given by self-injection. Some patients do not tolerate interferons because of their flu-like side effects. From 2% to 20% of patients produce neutralizing antibodies against these drugs as well. Interferons may work by altering T cells so they are less active in the inflammatory process. The approved preparations are:
- Beta-interferon-1b (Betaseron—subcutaneous QOD)
- Beta-interferon-1a (Avonex—intramuscular; once weekly)
- Beta-interferon-1a (Rebif—subcutaneous; 3 times per week)
- Beta-interferon-1a glycosylated (Plegridy—subcutaneous every 14 days)

28. Discuss the role of glatiramer acetate (Copaxone) for the treatment of MS.

Copaxone is a synthetic polypeptide resembling a fragment of the myelin basic protein molecule, and it may work by preventing activation and differentiation of myelin-targeting T cells. It has few systemic side effects, and the daily subcutaneous injections are usually well tolerated.

29. Discuss the role of monoclonal antibodies for the treatment of MS.

Nataluzimab (Tysabri) is a monoclonal antibody given by monthly intravenous infusions. It is directed against alpha-1-integrin on the blood–brain barrier and prevents T cells from leaving the circulation and entering the central nervous system, thus reducing attacks on the myelin. Because it also reduces T-cell immune surveillance in the brain, the rate of opportunistic infections is increased, especially from progressive multifocal leukoencephalopathy. Patients are thus carefully screened (with JC virus antibodies and MRI scans) and followed before and during treatment. Alemtuzumab (Lemtrada) is a monoclonal antibody directed against CD52 receptors on monocytes that effectively depletes circulating lymphocytes. It is given intravenously over 5 consecutive days and then repeated for 3 days 1 year later. Its potentially serious toxicity includes development of other autoimmune disorders such as thyroid disease and thrombocytopenia.

30. Discuss the role of oral agents for the treatment of MS.

Only recently have oral agents been approved to reduce relapses in MS. These include:
- Fingolimod (Gilenya)—A sphingosine-1-phosphate receptor modulator that inhibits migration of T cells from lymphoid tissue into the circulation. It has potentially serious cardiac, macular, and other toxicities.
- Teriflunomide (Aubagio)—Interferes with the syntheses of pyrimidines and thus blocks rapidly dividing cells. Because it is an antimetabolite it has potential toxicity from immune suppression and is contraindicated in patients considering childbearing.
- Dimethyl fumarate (Tecfidera)—An antiinflammatory molecule with an unknown mechanism of action. It can cause flushing and diarrhea, with rare reports of opportunistic infections.

31. **What is the best drug to prevent attacks of MS?**

There is no consensus about which of the drugs is superior or even which patients with MS should be treated at all or for how long. Comparison data about efficacy and toxicity do not yet permit definitive recommendations regarding either the initiation of therapy or the indication for switching agents. Thus, the choice of therapy depends largely on personal preferences of doctors and patients. Although these drugs have all been shown to reduce relapse rates by approximately 30% to 50%, none has yet been proven to prevent disability, which may depend more on the chronic degenerative process than on relapses.

KEY POINTS: DEMYELINATING DISEASE

1. Traditionally, the diagnosis of MS requires two separate symptoms at two separate times or lesions disseminated in space and in time.
2. The most common symptoms of MS are weakness, numbness, and visual changes.
3. A patient's prognosis and response to treatment depends upon what pattern of MS he/she has. Relapsing–remitting disease has a better prognosis and response to therapy. No drugs alter the course of progressive MS.
4. No treatment has yet been shown to prevent ultimate disability in MS.
5. Fatigue is a common symptom of MS, but it does not respond well to any medications.
6. Neuromyelitis optica mimics MS but is due to antibodies against aquaporin-4 and requires B-cell immune suppression.
7. The differential diagnosis of MS includes other common conditions affecting young people: migraines, neuropathies, and anxiety.

SYMPTOMATIC TREATMENT

32. **What is the role of symptomatic treatments for MS?**

If MS were cured today, the many sufferers from the disease would still have neurologic deficits. Management of these deficits is an important part of the treatment of MS. The most disabling symptoms reported by patients are fatigue, motor deficits, and sphincter disturbance.

33. **What is the best treatment for fatigue in MS?**

Although fatigue seems to be a vague and subjective symptom, it is one of the leading reasons why victims of MS are unable to work. No drugs are very useful for this symptom, but some are still prescribed. Amantadine may reduce fatigue, usually in doses of 100 mg twice daily. Modafinil and selective serotonin reuptake inhibitors such as fluoxetine also are prescribed. Simple commonsense measures may be more useful, such as resting during the day and reorganizing the home and workplace for better efficiency.

34. **What is the best treatment for motor deficits in MS?**

Unfortunately, little can be done to restore muscle strength. However, spasticity often improves with the use of baclofen (Lioresal) in doses of 60 mg/day (20 mg 3 times/day) or more. Tizanidine (Zanaflex), given up to 8 mg 4 times/day, produces similarly potent muscle relaxation. Benzodiazepines are sometimes useful antispasticity agents, especially at night when their sedating effects are less problematic. For example, clonazepam (Klonopin) may help in a dose of 0.5 mg once or twice daily. Physical therapy can also minimize spasticity. Therapy for cerebellar motor deficits is frustrating—these are among the most difficult symptoms to alleviate. Sometimes simple mechanical measures are helpful, such as attaching weights to the ankles or wrists.

35. **What is the best treatment for urologic problems in MS?**

Urologic consultation is often useful to manage the neurogenic bladder. The most common problem is a hyperreflexic bladder with a small capacity, early detrusor contraction, urinary frequency, and urgency. It can be managed with medications such as oxybutynin (Ditropan), tolterodine (Detrol), or hyoscyamine (Levsinex). A flaccid bladder (more rare) may require self-catheterization. When sphincter–detrusor dyssynergia appears, medications to relax the sphincter, such as the alpha-adrenergic blocking agent prazosin (Minipress), may be useful.

References available online at expertconsult.com.

WEBSITE

http://www.nationalmssociety.org

BIBLIOGRAPHY

1. Giesser BS (ed): Primer on Multiple Sclerosis, 2nd ed. Oxford, Oxford University Press, 2015.
2. Fox RJ, Rae-Grant AD: Multiple sclerosis. Continuum 19(4):899-1157, 2013.
3. Compston A (ed): McAlpine's Multiple Sclerosis, Philadelphia, Churchill Livingstone, 2006.

ALZHEIMER'S DISEASE AND MILD COGNITIVE IMPAIRMENT

Rachelle S. Doody

CHAPTER 15

GENERAL CONSIDERATIONS

1. **How is dementia defined? How do definitions vary?**

   Dementia is generally regarded as an acquired loss of cognitive function due to an abnormal brain condition. The National Institutes of Health criteria (formerly the National Institute of Neurological and Communicative Diseases and Stroke-Alzheimer's Disease and Related Disorders Association or NINCDS-ADRDA criteria) for the diagnosis of Alzheimer's disease (AD) stressed that there must be **progressive** loss of cognitive function, including but not limited to memory loss. A recent revision of these criteria puts less emphasis on memory impairment. The DSM-IV general criteria for dementia included the requirement of **functional decline** that interferes with work or usual social activities in addition to cognitive decline. DSM-5 now calls this *major neurocognitive disorder* instead of *dementia*.

2. **What is senility? Is it normal?**

   Senility is an outdated term. It used to mean cognitive impairment due to aging, which was assumed to be normal. Although memory, learning, and thinking change with age in subtle ways, memory loss and cognitive impairment are not features of normal aging.

3. **What is pseudodementia?**

   Pseudodementia has many meanings. It refers to depressed patients who are cognitively impaired and often have psychomotor slowing but do not have one of the well-defined dementia syndromes. The term does not mean that the patient is consciously simulating dementia (malingering) or is cognitively intact but believes himself or herself to be demented (Ganser's syndrome). Some researchers believe that pseudodementia may be a precursor to dementia.

4. **What features are characteristic of pseudodementia associated with depression?**

   Patients with pseudodementia may or may not have a history of depressive or vegetative symptoms. They tend to have flat affect, to give up easily when mental status is examined, or to say that they cannot perform a task without even trying it. They often respond surprisingly well when given extra time and encouragement, but they may deny their success. Results of mental status examination are inconsistent; for example, they may fail a simple task but perform a similar, more difficult one correctly. Or they may have variable strengths and weaknesses over repeated testing sessions.

5. **What is Ganser's syndrome?**

   Ganser's syndrome is an involuntary and unconscious simulation of altered mental status (confusion or dementia) in a patient who is not malingering and believes in the validity of his or her symptoms.

6. **What is delirium?**

   Delirium is an acute confusional state.

7. **What features distinguish delirium from dementia?**

   Although this distinction cannot always be made with certainty, several features are helpful. Sudden onset suggests delirium, as do findings of altered consciousness, marked problems with attention and concentration out of proportion to other deficits, cognitive fluctuations (e.g., lucid intervals), psychomotor and/or autonomic overactivity, fragmented speech, and marked hallucinations (especially auditory or tactile). Chronically demented patients may develop delirium in addition to dementia, which will change the clinical picture.

8. **Do all patients with dementia develop psychotic features?**

   No. Psychosis is a variable finding in all types of dementias and is not even clearly related to the stage or severity of dementia.

9. Which screening instruments are commonly used in detecting dementia?

The Folstein Mini-Mental Status Examination (MMSE), Short Blessed Dementia Scale, and Mattis Dementia Rating Scale are commonly used clinically and in experimental studies to screen for dementia and to rate severity of dementia. Recently, the AD8 and Mini-Cog have also been suggested, especially in primary care practices conducting the Annual Wellness Examination.

10. What are the limitations of the MMSE in the assessment of dementia?

Besides the fact that it has both false-positive (usually depression) and false-negative (usually early dementia in highly functioning patients) results, the MMSE also has limitations based on its lack of comprehensiveness.

11. At what point is a patient too demented to require an evaluation?

No patient is too demented to be evaluated. The need to rule out reversible causes and structural lesions always remains. Neurologic and psychometric examinations can be tailored to the level of even the most profoundly demented patients. Further, even severely demented patients may respond to treatments.

12. What are the most common causes of dementia or conditions resembling dementia?

AD is the most common form of dementia in adults (>80% in most series). Depression with pseudodementia is a frequent cause of cognitive loss and must be ruled out in all patients. Other important causes include multi-infarct or vascular dementia, dementia with Lewy bodies, frontotemporal dementia, and dementia-like syndromes due to alcohol or chronic use of certain prescription drugs.

13. What uncommon causes of dementia must be considered in the differential diagnosis of every patient with dementia?

- Toxins (lead, organic mercury)
- Vitamin deficiencies (B12, B1, and B6, in particular)
- Endocrine disturbances (hypothyroidism or hyperthyroidism, hyperparathyroidism, Cushing's disease, and Addison's disease)
- Chronic metabolic conditions (hyponatremia, hypercalcemia, chronic hepatic failure, and renal failure)
- Vasculopathies affecting the brain
- Structural abnormalities (chronic subdural hematomas, normal pressure hydrocephalus, and slow-growing tumors)
- Central nervous system (CNS) infections (including human immunodeficiency virus [HIV]), Creutzfeldt–Jakob disease, and cryptococcal or tuberculous meningitis

14. How often is a Wernicke's diagnosis missed and what are the consequences?

Wernicke's encephalopathy is correctly diagnosed in 1 of 22 patients. The classic features of confusion due to encephalopathy, variable ophthalmoplegia, and ataxia may be complete, or only one or two of the features may be present. Untreated, patients can become comatose and death can result.

15. Which dementia syndromes are associated with alcohol?

The DSM-IV includes alcohol amnestic syndrome (Korsakoff's syndrome), in which the amnestic disorder predominates, as well as a more generalized dementia associated with alcoholism. Both are associated with some degree of visuospatial impairment; neither includes aphasia. Patients with or without dementia may experience an acute, alcohol-related delirium known as *Wernicke's encephalopathy* (usually with confusion, eye movement abnormalities, and ataxia).

ALZHEIMER'S DISEASE

16. How is AD diagnosed?

First, the presence of dementia must be established clearly by clinical criteria and confirmed by neuropsychological testing. The clinical manifestations usually include impairment of memory and at least one other area of cognition. There must be no evidence of other systemic or brain disease sufficient to cause the dementia, and the National Institutes of Health criteria suggest basic laboratory studies (which are not all-inclusive) to exclude other disease. The diagnosis is both a diagnosis of exclusion and a diagnosis based on the establishment of certain characteristic features.

17. **How are the alcohol-related dementias differentiated from AD?**
    No absolute features distinguish these conditions. If the patient has a systemic disorder (such as alcoholism) that, in the clinician's opinion, is sufficient to cause dementia, the diagnosis should *not* be probable AD. Possible AD may be used if underlying AD is suspected in an actively drinking patient. The patient should stop drinking with the help of appropriate rehabilitative services. If the dementia improves and the improvement continues or persists for 1 year or more, the diagnosis is not likely to be AD.

18. **Which blood tests are typically ordered in a patient with suspected AD to rule out other causes or contributing factors?**
    - Comprehensive metabolic panel (including sodium, blood sugar, calcium, liver enzymes, and renal function)
    - Complete blood count with differential
    - Thyroid function tests
    - Rapid plasma reagin or equivalent test for syphilis
    - Vitamin B12
    - Antinuclear antibody (extractable nuclear antigen panel, if positive)
    - Sedimentation rate

    Additional tests:
    Folate
    Serum homocysteine
    Serum methylmalonic acid
    Serum arterial ammonia
    Parathyroid hormone
    Serum protein electrophoresis
    Cortisol levels
    Serum (and urine) drug screens
    Hexosaminidase levels
    HIV

19. **What blood tests can be done to assess the risk for AD?**
    Glucose, cholesterol, and homocysteine elevations are risk factors for developing AD, as is an apolipo-protein E4 (ApoE4) genotype.

20. **Which ancillary studies (in addition to blood tests) are useful to evaluate patients with suspected AD?**
    A structural imaging study (magnetic resonance imaging [MRI] or computed tomography [CT] with contrast) and neuropsychological testing to confirm dementia are necessary. Electroencephalography (EEG), single-photon emission CT (SPECT), or positron emission tomography (FDG-PET and/or amyloid imaging PET) studies and lumbar puncture (LP) may be useful or even necessary. Also consider an electrocardiogram (to look for evidence of cardiovascular disease) and chest radiograph.

21. **When is LP necessary in the diagnostic workup?**
    When symptoms are of short duration (<6 months) or have atypical features, such as rapid progression or severe confusion, an LP should be performed early. It also should be done if clinical or laboratory features suggest a specific etiology that is an indication for LP, such as meningitis or CNS vasculitis. Cerebrospinal fluid levels of amyloid beta protein (low) and tau proteins (high) can support a diagnosis of AD in the prodromal and clinical stages.

22. **What are typical symptoms of early AD?**
    Early symptoms of AD include forgetfulness for recent events or newly acquired information, often causing the patient to repeat himself or herself. Other early features are disorientation, especially to time, and difficulty with complex cognitive functions such as mathematical calculations or organization of activities that require several steps.

23. **What are typical symptoms of moderately advanced AD?**
    Advanced AD includes a history of progression of pervasive memory loss sufficient to impair everyday activities, disorientation to place and/or aspects of person (e.g., age), inability to keep track of time, and problems with personal care (such as forgetting to change clothes). Behavioral changes, such as depression, paranoia, or aggressiveness, are more likely in these stages.

24. **Does progression of AD follow a consistent pattern?**
Definitely not. Salient symptoms and rates of progression vary tremendously.

25. **What language disturbances do patients with AD experience?**
Early in the disease, most patients have word-finding difficulties that may cause pauses in spontaneous speech or may be detected by asking the patient to name objects (particularly objects with low frequency in the language). As AD progresses, most patients develop problems with comprehension with intact repetition (similar to transcortical sensory aphasia); then repetition becomes affected while speech remains fluent (similar to Wernicke's aphasia). Ultimately, some patients develop expressive speech problems in addition to the above symptoms, or they may just stop talking secondary to inanition and apparent lack of anything to say.

26. **Does the presence or absence of insight differentiate AD from other dementias?**
Lack of insight into their memory disorder (or anosognosia) occurs in some patients with AD as well as in patients with other dementing disorders. It does not appear to correlate with disease severity and is not useful in differential diagnosis.

27. **What motor features may be associated with AD? What is their significance?**
Rigidity, bradykinesia, and parkinsonian gait may be associated with more rapid progression of disease (both cognitive decline and activities of daily living). Tremor is rare, differentiating patients with AD from patients with Parkinson's disease to some extent. Myoclonus may occur, and recent evidence suggests its association with a younger age of onset of AD. In very severe AD, patients may have gait apraxia.

28. **What is the genetic defect in early-onset familial AD?**
Some families show a mutation in the gene that encodes amyloid precursor protein on chromosome 21. Other families show mutations on chromosome 14 (in the gene for presenilin 1) or chromosome 1 (in the gene for presenilin 2). It is likely that other genes will be linked to the early-onset familial form of AD. These mutations are rare and account for less than 5% of AD cases.

29. **Is there a genetic link to late-onset AD?**
The risk for late-onset familial AD is linked to chromosome 19. It has been demonstrated that the particular inherited form of apolipoprotein E (ApoE) (coded by a gene on chromosome 19) determines the age-dependent risk and age of onset of AD in some patients. Patients who inherit one or more E4 alleles are at greater risk, but only about 50% of AD patients have E4. Other families have been linked to variant forms of TOMM40, a mitochondrial transport protein on chromosome 19. These gene associations likely represent inherited risk factors rather than genetic forms of AD.

30. **Is there a genetic component to all cases of AD?**
The answer is not clear. Patients with a family history of AD in even one primary relative appear to be at increased risk, and the risk is higher (up to 10-fold higher) if both parents have AD. Cases that seem to be sporadic are common, although the ApoE genotype is a clear risk factor for both sporadic and late-onset familial cases. Multiple genetic factors probably account for a predisposition for AD.

31. **What is ApoE? What is its importance?**
ApoE is a cholesterol-carrying blood protein that comes in three forms: ApoE2, E3, and E4. We inherit one ApoE allele from each parent, and people with one or more E4 alleles have an increased risk for developing AD.

32. **What other disorders have been associated with AD in epidemiologic surveys?**
Patients with Down syndrome are at high risk for AD. Whether families of patients with AD have a higher incidence of Down syndrome remains controversial. Parkinson's disease and a history of head trauma have been associated with AD in some large studies but not in others.

33. **What are the risk factors for AD?**
The presence of ApoE4 and serious head injury in ApoE4-positive people, aging, postmenopausal estrogen deficiency, positive family history (independent of ApoE genotype), elevated serum homocysteine levels, elevated blood glucose and/or cholesterol, and low education level (especially early in development) may be risk factors. Aluminum exposure is frequently cited, but no sound evidence supports the association.

34. What factors reduce the risk for AD?

    Although definite proof is lacking, perimenopausal/estrogen replacement (but not later in life), antiin-flammatory drugs (including nonsteroidal agents), antioxidants, and the use of statin drugs have been proposed and are under study.

35. What are the classic neuropathologic changes in AD?

    Senile plaques, neurofibrillary tangles, granulovacuolar degeneration, loss of synapses, and amyloid in blood vessels and plaques are classic changes. Plaques and tangles also may be seen in normal brains but are far less numerous; in normal subjects, tangles outside the hippocampus are rare.

36. Which neuropathologic changes correlate best with the severity of dementia due to AD?

    Both amyloid plaques and neurofibrillary tangles correlate with the overall severity of dementia, but specific cognitive deficits correlate best with neurofibrillary tangles in the expected brain regions that underlie those cognitive functions. Synaptic density has been shown to have an inverse correlation with severity of dementia, at least in some brain regions. Because education seems to increase synaptic density, some have suggested that education may have a protective effect against the manifestation of AD cognitive changes.

37. Which neuropathologic entities overlap with AD?

    Besides normal aging, dementia with Lewy bodies, Parkinson's dementia, progressive supranuclear palsy, and vascular dementias are sometimes difficult to distinguish from AD because plaques and tangles may occur with other pathologic changes. Clinical correlations are extremely important in such cases.

38. Which neuropathologically distinct entities may be clinically indistinguishable from AD?

    Vascular dementias (without plaques and tangles), dementia with Lewy bodies, Pick's disease, dementia lacking distinctive histology, and other frontal lobe dementia syndromes may be impossible to distinguish from AD on clinical grounds alone.

39. What is the clinical picture of frontotemporal dementia?

    This designation includes a group of entities with variable neuropathologic findings and similar clinical features. Patients have early personality changes, particularly impulsivity and Klüver–Bucy-type symptoms (including hyperorality) or withdrawal and depression, but they may present with a semantic dementia (loss of appreciation for word meaning) or progressive nonfluent aphasia. Psychiatric symptoms may precede dementia by several years. Memory and frontal executive tasks (e.g., planning, set-shifting, and set maintenance) are much more impaired than attention, language, and visuospatial skills. SPECT or PET studies may show hypofrontality. Neuropathology includes Pick's disease or primary degeneration at multiple brain sites (dementia lacking distinctive histology), usually with gliosis and often with protein inclusions such as tau, TDP-43, or ubiquitin. Many of these cases have been linked to genetic mutations in the tau protein on chromosome 17 or to mutations in progranulin on chromosome. Many of these cases have been linked to genetic mutations in either the tau protein or the progranulin gene, both located on chromosome 17.

40. What is the cholinergic hypothesis?

    The cholinergic hypothesis attempts to explain many of the cognitive deficits in AD (particularly memory disturbance) by a deficiency of cholinergic neurotransmission. Evidence includes the fact that poor memory can be induced in normal people by anticholinergic drugs. Loss of cholinergic projection neurons in the nucleus basalis of Meynert and loss of choline acetyltransferase activity throughout the cortex of patients with AD correlate with the severity of memory loss.

41. Besides acetylcholine, which transmitters are affected by AD?

    Norepinephrine, somatostatin, dopamine, serotonin, and neuropeptide Y are decreased. Glutamate dysfunction (overproduction or dysregulation) also may play a role in AD.

42. What is the role of amyloid in AD?

    Clearly AD is associated with abnormal accumulation of a breakdown product of the amyloid precursor protein known as beta-amyloid or Aβ-amyloid, especially in the insoluble form. Amyloid appears to be toxic to cells in vitro, and abnormal accumulation may actually cause cell loss. No one knows why the Aβ-amyloid accumulates, but accumulation may be secondary to abnormal processing within neurons, as well as to problems with clearance of amyloid from the brain.

43. **What is the role of tau protein in AD?**

Tau protein is part of the cytoskeleton of neuronal cells. In damaged cells (e.g., after heat shock), its expression is increased. Tau protein is found in the neurofibrillary tangles of patients with AD. Tau appears to be hyperphosphorylated in cells destined to develop neurofibrillary tangles. It may be an early marker of cells with abnormal cytoskeletal function and abnormal metabolism.

44. **What famous people probably had AD?**
    - Ronald Reagan—US president
    - Charlton Heston—actor
    - Rita Hayworth—actress
    - Immanuel Kant—philosopher
    - Ralph Waldo Emerson—writer
    - Maurice Ravel—composer
    - John James Audubon—painter

45. **What is the treatment for the noncognitive secondary behavioral effects of AD?**

Behavioral symptoms, such as disturbed sleep, depression, anxiety, psychotic features, agitation, and aggressiveness, are amenable to treatment. Behavioral modification, such as entraining sleep–wake cycles and increasing daytime activity, should be tried first for **sleep disorders**.

Depression, particularly early in the disease, may respond to low doses of antidepressants, but drugs with anticholinergic side effects should be avoided. Drugs that act on the serotonergic system may be better tolerated (fluoxetine, paroxetine, citalopram, sertraline), although controlled studies are lacking for patients with AD.

Anxiety and agitation frequently respond to behavioral interventions, such as day center participation, that engage the patient and reduce caregiver stress. Other respite interventions for caregivers may help to reduce patient stress. If symptoms are infrequent, anxiety or agitation may be treated with low doses of anxiolytics as needed. Chronic anxiolytics are not indicated for AD, but short-term therapy with buspirone or lorazepam may be justified during periods of transition or change.

Environmental triggers and pain should always be ruled out as causes of agitation before using drugs. **Severe agitation, aggressiveness, and psychotic features** that disturb the patient should be treated with atypical antipsychotics such as olanzapine, risperidone, and quetiapine, in the lowest doses possible, because these drugs further impair cognition (and sometimes motor performance). Antipsychotics have black box warnings for dementia patients on their labeling. Psychotic features that do not disturb the patient or disrupt the household need not be treated.

46. **What treatments exist for the primary process of AD?**

The Food and Drug Administration (FDA) has approved five treatments specifically for AD. Donepezil, rivastigmine, and galantamine are cholinesterase inhibitors, and memantine is an N-methyl-D-aspartate receptor antagonist. Studies of estrogen as a treatment for AD have been negative. Many patients can qualify for experimental studies of potential new AD treatments and should be referred to AD research centers that test medications if they are interested. Available drugs and sites can be identified by calling the National Alzheimer's Disease Association in Chicago or searching ClinTrials.Gov.

47. **Are there any agents besides prescription drugs that improve cognition or slow functional loss in AD?**

Two large-scale double-blind studies support the benefits of vitamin E (1000 IU twice daily) for slowing the time to significant worsening. Vitamin E is well tolerated.

48. **What is respite care?**

Respite care is any caretaking arrangement for the patient that temporarily relieves the primary caregiver. It may be as informal as a friend or relative who comes to the home to care for the patient, a part-time in-home aide, or a few days per week at a day center. It also may apply to short-term stays in residential facilities.

49. **What are the responsibilities of physicians and health care workers with respect to respite care?**

The physician or health care worker must introduce the concept of respite care and assure every primary caregiver that he or she will need it sooner or later. Even early in the disease process, activities that are directed toward patients (such as day centers) help promote their autonomy and provide supervision while providing respite to caregivers. Many caregivers feel guilty about not being able to care for the patient alone every day and night. They need to know that all affected families require help in caregiving.

VASCULAR DEMENTIAS

50. **What entities constitute the vascular dementias?**
    - Multiple large infarctions, which usually involve cortical and subcortical tissue
    - Single or multiple smaller infarctions that involve critical brain regions

    It is less clear whether diffuse, chronic vascular processes such as Binswanger's disease, leukoaraiosis, or diffuse changes in white matter due to microinfarcts also cause dementia.

51. **Can vascular dementia be diagnosed by CT or MRI alone?**
    No. Patients who have changes in white matter on scans or even multiple, definite infarctions may be clinically normal. It is not known how many infarcts or how much change in white matter on a scan translates into dementia for patients who suffer cognitive impairments. Many white matter signal changes, especially on MRI, do not represent strokes.

KEY POINTS: DEMENTIA

1. Dementia must be differentiated from delirium and depression.
2. Dementia is a category, not a diagnosis. The clinician must determine the cause of the dementia.
3. AD is rarely caused by inheriting an abnormal genetic mutation (familial AD). On the other hand, patients may inherit risk factors that predispose them to developing AD, such as ApoE4.
4. Both cognitive and behavioral symptoms of dementia can be treated, and long-term therapy may slow decline and help maintain function.
5. Vascular dementia cannot be diagnosed by MRI or CT scan alone.

---

52. **Can dementia occur after a single stroke?**
    One prospective study of patients after acute stroke showed that the risk of dementia was 9 to 10 times greater than for matched controls without stroke. A single stroke also can lead to dementia by making apparent underlying AD that has not yet become symptomatic.

53. **Can neuropsychologic testing differentiate vascular dementia from AD?**
    Not absolutely. Patchy performances across tests, unilateral motor impairments (e.g., reaction times or finger tapping), and improvements in some but not all areas of cognition over time are typically seen in vascular dementias. Asymmetric finger tapping, however, is also common in AD.

54. **What basic workup should be done when vascular dementia is suspected?**
    The workup should begin with imaging studies and psychometric testing in addition to the history and physical examination. In most cases, all tests recommended for the diagnosis of AD should be pursued to rule out additional conditions that may cause or contribute to the dementia, including a lipid profile and blood homocysteine levels, which are risk factors for both AD and vascular dementia. Some patients, especially those with clear-cut strokes, may benefit from imaging of the carotid arteries, especially when high-grade stenosis or ulcerated plaques are suspected. An echocardiogram is indicated in patients who have a cardiac history or appear to have had embolic strokes. Patients who have had strokes or transient ischemic attacks should be considered for antiplatelet therapies.

55. **What ancillary tests may be useful in diagnosing vascular dementia?**
    The EEG may show multiple slow-wave foci, and SPECT or PET scans may show multiple areas of decreased flow or altered metabolism. These tests have not been adequately studied to assess their utility for differentiating the various forms of vascular dementias.

56. **Can vascular dementia be diagnosed in patients with aphasia due to a left hemisphere infarct?**
    Patients should not be tested for dementia in the acute phase of stroke, whether aphasic or otherwise. Although most tests for cognitive functioning rely heavily on language abilities, tests of nonverbal memory and reasoning help to support the diagnosis of dementia in an aphasic patient. A history of functional decline not related to language-based tasks is also helpful.

57. **What is the treatment of vascular dementia?**
    The FDA has not yet approved any drugs to treat vascular dementia, but research studies suggest that cholinesterase inhibitors and memantine may be helpful. As for AD, noncognitive behavioral effects of

dementia are amenable to therapy, and respite care should be introduced early. In addition, it is advisable to control vascular risk factors as much as possible (blood pressure, blood glucose, cholesterol, and hypertension). Prophylactic antiplatelet therapy (aspirin, clopidogrel, or ticlopidine), although not of proven benefit for dementia, may be helpful by reducing the risk of future strokes.

SUBCORTICAL DEMENTIAS

58. What are the characteristics of subcortical dementias?

Subcortical dementias lack cortical features, such as aphasia, apraxia, and acalculia. Recall memory is impaired worse than recognition memory. Visuospatial skills are often impaired. Frontal executive deficits, bradyphrenia, anomia, personality changes, and psychomotor slowing are prominent. Dysarthria, abnormal posture and coordination, and adventitious movements may be present.

59. How do the general features of subcortical dementias differ from cortical dementias?

The cortical dementias, such as AD, usually involve language and calculations and may involve apraxia and cortical sensory disturbances (e.g., astereognosis, graphesthesia), whereas subcortical dementias do not. Both recall and recognition memory are usually impaired in cortical dementia, whereas recognition memory is relatively preserved in subcortical dementia. Frontal executive functions are lost in proportion to the overall dementia in cortical processes but are prominently affected in subcortical dementia. Bradykinesia and bradyphrenia, as well as other motor features, are usually absent or late findings in cortical dementias but occur early in subcortical dementias. Personality changes are variable in both types but are said to be more prominent early in the course of subcortical dementia.

60. In what ways do the specific memory disturbances of subcortical dementias differ from those of cortical dementias?

Problems with short-term spontaneous recall occur in both types, but strategies to enhance encoding and recognition cuing are mainly helpful in subcortical dementias. Incidental memory (details not related to the task at hand, such as what the examiner was wearing) is better in subcortical dementias. Procedural memory (memory involved in learning tasks) is better preserved in cortical dementias. Remote memory usually shows a temporal gradient in cortical dementias but not in subcortical dementias.

61. Is there a rigid anatomic or functional distinction between cortical and subcortical dementia?

No. So-called subcortical dementias may give rise to or be associated with cortical changes and vice versa. Huntington's dementia, like most subcortical dementias, causes disturbances of cortical frontal lobe functioning. Patients with (subcortical) Parkinson's disease may show atrophy of cortical cells. Patients with AD have subcortical changes in deep nuclei, such as the nucleus basalis of Meynert and locus ceruleus.

62. What disorders or clinical syndromes are typically associated with subcortical dementia?

- Parkinson's disease
- Huntington's disease
- Progressive supranuclear palsy
- Idiopathic basal ganglia calcification
- Multiple sclerosis
- Inflammatory conditions involving the basal ganglia and/or thalamus
- HIV
- Corticobasal syndrome
- Some forms of spinocerebellar ataxia

63. What are the clinical features of Parkinson's dementia?

This dementia occurs in well-established Parkinson's disease. Typically bradyphrenia, dysnomia, and frontal executive dysfunction are present, and depression is common. There may be visuospatial abnormalities, especially on formal testing.

64. **What are the clinical features of Huntington's dementia?**
Psychiatric symptoms or dementia may occur before or after the features of Huntington's disease (e.g., chorea) are well established. Psychiatric features include personality changes, depression, and psychosis. The memory disorder is typically of the subcortical pattern. Language and speech disorders, including dysarthria, reduced spontaneous speech, impaired syntactic complexity, and impaired comprehension, are common, as are visuospatial abnormalities.

65. **What are the clinical features of the dementia associated with progressive supranuclear palsy (PSP)?**
PSP is a syndrome characterized by supranuclear gaze palsy, dystonic rigidity of axial musculature, dysarthria, and pseudobulbar palsy. The dementia is not clearly present in all patients and is difficult to characterize because the associated visual scanning disorder interferes with testing. Memory impairments tend to be mild relative to frontal executive functions.

66. **What is dementia with Lewy bodies?**
A spectrum of disorders probably makes up Lewy body disease, ranging from Parkinson's disease (with Lewy bodies primarily in the subcortical and brain stem regions) to diffuse Lewy body disease, in which Lewy bodies are present throughout the cortex, subcortex, and brain stem. Some authorities describe an intermediate form of Lewy body dementia (senile dementia of the Lewy body type), which is associated with many Lewy bodies in the brain stem and subcortical regions, fewer in the hippocampus, and fewer still in the neocortical region. When Lewy bodies occur in AD brains, the condition may be called *Lewy body variant of AD*.

67. **What are the clinical characteristics of dementia with Lewy bodies?**
Patients typically exhibit fluctuating confusion and dementia, usually with vivid visual hallucinations and extrapyramidal features. The neuropsychological deficits are not well characterized, and little is known about the natural history of the disorder. A rapid eye movement sleep disorder is not uncommon.

68. **What other disorders are in the differential diagnosis of dementia (not necessarily subcortical) with extrapyramidal features?**
- AD
- Parkinson's disease plus dementia
- Creutzfeldt–Jakob disease
- Binswanger's disease
- Multi-infarct or vascular dementia
- Normal pressure hydrocephalus
- Frontotemporal dementia—parkinsonism associated with chromosome 17
- Corticobasal syndrome
- HIV dementia
- Pantothenate kinase-associated neurodegeneration or neurodegeneration with brain iron accumulation 1 (formerly Hallervorden–Spatz syndrome)
- Neuronal intranuclear inclusion disease
- GM1 gangliosidosis type III
- MSA-P (multiple system atrophy with predominant parkinsonism)

69. **How do patients with corticobasal syndrome present?**
Patients tend to present either with an alien limb phenomenon and associated motor features (tremor, rigidity, grasp reflex, apraxia, and myoclonus) or with an akinetic-rigid syndrome similar to Parkinson's disease. Dementia frequently develops over time and affects cognitive function pervasively. The neuropsychological deficits are typical of subcortical dementia.

 References available online at expertconsult.com.

BIBLIOGRAPHY

1. Behatar M: Analytic Neurology, Boston, Butterworth-Heinemann, 2003.
2. Doody RS (ed): Alzheimer's Dementia, Delray Beach, FL, Carma Publishing, 2008.
3. Growdon JH, Rossor MN (eds): The Dementias, Boston, Butterworth-Heinemann, 1998.
4. Noseworthy JH (ed): Neurological Therapeutics: Principles and Practice, 2nd ed. London, CRC Press, 2006.
5. Trimble MR, Cummings JL: Contemporary Behavioral Neurology, Boston, Butterworth-Heinemann, 1997.
6. Trojanowski J, Clark C (eds): Neurodegenerative Dementias, New York, McGraw-Hill, 1998.

CHAPTER 16

NON-ALZHEIMER'S DEMENTIAS

George R. Jackson

1. **Are there variant forms of Alzheimer's (AD) disease that present with an atypical clinical picture?**
   Yes; these include:
   - **Posterior cortical atrophy:** presents with visuospatial and visual perceptual impairments (e.g., Balint's syndrome: simultanagnosia, optic ataxia, and ocular apraxia); can also be associated with dementia with Lewy bodies, corticobasal (CB) syndrome, etc., rather than just Alzheimer's pathology)
   - **Limbic predominant AD:** relatively selective memory impairment; tends to present later that typical AD; many similarities with primary age-related tauopathy (PART; formerly known as *tangle predominant dementia*)
   - **Hippocampal-sparing AD:** memory spared but with aphasia, apraxia, and/or visual perceptual impairment

2. **How does frontotemporal dementia (FTD) present?**
   Either as a behavioral variant or primary progressive aphasia.

3. **What are the three classical frontal lobe syndromes?**
   - **Orbitofrontal:** disinhibition
   - **Dorsolateral prefrontal:** impaired attention, executive function and motor programming, with poor strategies, impaired set shifting, and environmental dependency
   - **Anterior cingulate:** apathy

4. **Do FTDs respond to cholinesterase inhibitors?**
   Probably not.

5. **How do subcortical dementias differ from cortical?**
   - Subcortical dementias tend to respond better to cueing (e.g., categorical cues or multiple choice) during memory testing, as the deficit tends to be one of retrieval rather than encoding.
   - They also tend to be more associated with psychomotor slowing, depression, and more executive dysfunction.
   - They tend to be more associated with early motor abnormalities, such as paratonic rigidity/gegenhalten, as opposed to cortical dementias in which motor abnormalities tend to be a later phenomenon.

6. **What are some of the prototypic subcortical dementias?**
   - Huntington's disease
   - Parkinson's disease

7. **How are the three types of primary progressive aphasias differentiated?**
   - Agrammatic/nonfluent aphasia is a disorder of word *order* and *production*.

Fluency	Impaired
Naming	Some anomia
Repetition	Impaired
Comprehension	Intact (simple items)
Reading	Intact (short pieces)

- Logopenic progressive aphasia is a disorder of word *finding*.

Fluency	OK
Naming	Anomia
Repetition	OK
Comprehension	Intact (simple items)
Reading	Intact (short pieces)

- Semantic dementia is a disorder of word *understanding*.

Fluency	OK
Naming	Some anomia
Repetition	OK
Comprehension	Impaired, even for single words
Reading	Surface dyslexia (literally phonetic reading such that individuals are unable to pronounce irregular nouns)

8. What mutations can cause inherited FTD?
   Most cases are accounted for by mutations in the following genes:
   - MAPT/Tau
   - *CHMP2B* (involved in vacuolar sorting)
   - Progranulin (a neurotrophin-like factor)
   - TDP-43 (TAR DNA-binding protein of 43 kDa)
   - VCP (valosin-containing protein) and other more recently discovered mutations that comprise the multisystem proteinopathies consisting of FTD, Paget's disease of bone, and inclusion body myopathy)
   - FUS (fused in sarcoma)
   - *C9ORF72* (an intronic expanded hexanucleotide repeat)

9. Is there a relationship between amyotrophic lateral sclerosis (ALS) and FTD?
   There is considerable phenotypic overlap, and many of the mutations associated with familial FTD also cause familial ALS, especially the *C9ORF72* mutation.

10. Are the subtypes of primary progressive aphasia associated with different pathology?
    This is an area in which understanding is evolving rapidly, and although there are exceptions and overlap, agrammatic tends to be associated with tau, logopenic with amyloid-beta, and semantic with TDP-43 pathology.

11. What famous American neurologist died of primary progressive aphasia?
    Fred Plum of *Stupor and Coma* fame.

12. In what dementia syndromes does tau pathology coexist with other types of pathologies?
    Examples include:
    - AD (senile plaques, alpha-synuclein, and TDP-43)
    - Down syndrome (senile plaques)

13. Apart from FTD, what other dementias are associated with tau pathology?
    Many! These include:
    - ALS of Guam
    - Parkinsonism–dementia complex of Guam
    - Argyrophilic grain disease
    - Chronic traumatic encephalopathy
    - CB syndrome
    - Down syndrome
    - Gerstmann–Straussler–Scheinker disease (a familial prion disease)
    - Niemann–Pick disease type C
    - Pick's disease
    - Postencephalitic parkinsonism

- Progressive supranuclear palsy (PSP)
- PART
- White matter tauopathy with globular glial inclusions

14. **What is repeat-associated non-AUG (RAN) translation?**
Instead of synthesizing protein based on the canonical AUG start codon, expanded repeats allow protein expression from what would normally be an intron of other noncoding region.

15. **In what dementing disorders does RAN translation occur?**
FTD associated with *C9ORF72* (but also spinocerebellar ataxia 8, mytotonic dystrophy type I, and fragile X tremor–ataxia syndrome).

16. **What is tau?**
MAPT (microtubule-associated protein tau) is a protein that regulates microtubule-based transport and is a major constituent of neurofibrillary tangles in AD and related dementias.

17. **Do the different forms of tau have pathological significance?**
- **Phosphorylation:** some pathological forms of tau are hyperphosphorylated, which is thought to dislodge tau from microtubules and contribute to its aggregation.
- **Microtubule binding repeat number:** due to alternative splicing and the inclusion or exclusion of exon 10, all isoforms of tau have either 4 or 3 microtubule binding repeats.

18. **Are different tau isoforms associated with different diseases?**
Most tauopathies are a mixture of 3 and 4 repeats with the following exceptions:
- 4 repeat (mostly): PSP and CB syndrome
- 3 repeat (mostly): Pick's disease

19. **Is Pick's disease still a valid diagnosis in the modern world of FTDs?**
Yes, but it is made based upon pathologic criteria (widespread 3-repeat tau-containing spherical cytoplasmic inclusions [Pick bodies]).

20. **What is dementia with Lewy bodies?**
A cognitive disorder that features:
- Fluctuating cognition
- Visual hallucinations
- Parkinsonism developing *within a year of* cognitive decline
- Rapid eye movement (REM) behavior disorder
- Worsens when treated with neuroleptics
- May also have orthostatic hypotension, delusions, and depression

21. **What is Parkinson's disease-associated dementia?**
- Cognitive decline developing after typical motor symptoms of Parkinson's disease (resting tremor, bradykinesia, rigidity, and postural instability)
- May be associated with apathy, depression, anxiety, hallucinations, delusions, REM behavior disorder, and excessive daytime somnolence

22. **What are the characteristics of Huntington's disease-associated dementia?**
- Associated with Huntington's motor abnormalities, e.g., chorea, though the dementia may precede them
- Executive dysfunction with slowed processing, poor strategies, and planning observed early rather than learning and memory problems
- Associated with depression, irritability, obsessive-compulsive behavior, or apathy; more rarely, psychosis

23. **What cognitive features are associated with PSP?**
Although the general view of PSP as a disorder consisting of relatively L-DOPA-resistant parkinsonism, eye movement abnormalities, prominent axial rigidity, and prominent frontal dysfunction is useful, PSP phenotypes can range from a pure akinesia/gait freezing variant, through classic Richardson's syndrome with full-blown eye movement abnormalities, a behavioral variant FTD or primary progressive aphasia, to a CB syndrome, depending upon the distribution of tau aggregates (going from brain stem to cortically predominant in the previous list).

24. In what cell types do tau aggregates (4 repeat primarily) accumulate in PSP?
    - Neurons (globose neurofibrillary tangles)
    - Astrocytes (tufted astrocytes)
    - Oligodendrocytes (coiled bodies)

25. What are the cognitive features of CB syndrome?
    Along with a typically asymmetric parkinsonian syndrome with alien limb phenomenon, poor L-DOPA sensitivity, dystonia, and myoclonus, CB syndrome patients can have prominent cortical sensory loss, ideomotor apraxia, and features of FTD, such as disinhibition or progressive aphasia.

26. What are the histologic features of CB syndrome?
    4-repeat tau in:
    - Ballooned neurons
    - Astrocytic plaques
    - Neuropil threads

27. What is primary progressive apraxia of speech?
    A recently described syndrome associated with selective atrophy of the lateral superior premotor cortex and supplementary motor area; patients tend also to develop extrapyramidal signs that can evolve into a PSP-like syndrome.

28. What disorders with adolescent or early adult onset can then present with dementia at a later age?
    These include:
    - **Sphingolipidoses:**
        - Adult GM2 gangliosidosis/Tay–Sachs disease
        - Adult GM1 gangliosidosis
        - Adult (type 3) Gaucher's disease
        - Adult Fabry's disease
    - Adult neuronal ceroid lipofuscinosis/Kuf's disease
    - Adult Leigh's disease
    - Late-onset globoid cell leukodystrophy/Krabbe's disease
    - Adrenoleukodystrophy

29. What are the main infectious causes of dementia?
    Chronic meningitis of fungal (cryptococcus, histoplasma), parasitic (neurocysticercosis, toxoplasma), bacterial (tuberculosis, syphilis, Lyme disease), viral (human immunodeficiency virus [HIV], subacute sclerosing panencephalitis, progressive multifocal encephalopathy, as well as post herpes encephalitis), and prions.

30. What are the features of prion-associated dementia?
    - Generally rapid progression
    - May have motor features, e.g., myoclonus, dystonia, chorea, or ataxia
    - Biomarkers include CSF 14-3-3 protein
    - Stage-dependent electroencephalogram findings include periodic sharp wave complexes
    - Magnetic resonance imaging findings (diffusion-weighted imaging) of multifocal cortical and subcortical hyperintensities

31. How has HIV-associated dementia changed in the era of combination antiretroviral therapy?
    The prevalence of severe stages characterized by impaired attention and memory with slowed processing has declined, and more subtle impairments in learning, memory, and executive function have become more prevalent.

32. What entities constitute the vascular dementias?
    - Large vessel disease (multiple small infarcts with cortical and subcortical involvement)
    - Small vessel disease
    - Strategic infarcts (e.g., angular gyrus syndrome with agraphia, alexia, right/left disorientation, finger agnosia, apraxia, anomia, and verbal amnesia)

33. What are the manifestations of cerebral amyloid angiopathy (CAA) as it relates to dementia?
    - Lobar macrohemorrhages
    - Cortical microhemorrhages
    - Cortical superficial siderosis/focal convexity subarachnoid hemorrhages

34. Are there inherited forms of CAA?
    Many; these include specific amyloid precursor protein mutations (e.g., Dutch and Flemish), as well as cystatin C mutation (Icelandic).

35. Can CAA present as a rapidly progressive dementia?
    Yes. It may also present with seizures and is responsive to immunosuppressive therapies.

36. Can amyloid positron emission tomography (PET) be used to diagnose CAA-related dementia?
    The technique cannot distinguish vascular from parenchymal amyloid, but a negative amyloid PET scan rules out CAA with good sensitivity.

KEY POINTS: NON-ALZHEIMER'S DEMENTIAS

1. FTD can present with behavioral symptoms or primary progressive aphasia.
2. Familial forms of FTD are associated with mutations in tau, progranulin, and *C9ORF72*.
3. Dementia with Lewy bodies is characterized by hallucinations, cognitive fluctuations, and REM behavior disorder.
4. PSP and CB syndrome are parkinsonian disorders associated with dementia and tau aggregation.
5. Cerebral amyloid angiopathy can cause dementia and has manifestations apart from classic lobar hemorrhage.

 References available online at expertconsult.com.

WEBSITE

http://www.nlm.nih.gov/medlineplus/dementia.html

BIBLIOGRAPHY

1. Growdon JH, Rossor MN (eds): The Dementias, Boston, Butterworth-Heinemann, 1998.
2. Trojanowski J, Clark C (eds): Neurodegenerative Dementias, New York, McGraw-Hill, 1998.

CHAPTER 17

NEUROPSYCHIATRY AND BEHAVIORAL NEUROLOGY

Garima Arora, Paul E. Schulz

MEMORY AND AMNESIA

1. **What are the different stages of fact-based memory storage, such as recalling a list of words?**

   Clinically, memory can be conceptualized in a three-stage model. Registration (sensory) memory holds large amounts of incoming information briefly in sensory stores, such as the visual or auditory cortex. This information is then transferred to "working memory," also called *short-term memory,* in the dorsolateral prefrontal cortex, which holds memory from seconds until we change our "train of thought." Working memory functions by holding information, internalizing it, and using it to guide behavior. It can be tested with instruments such as the digit span. It remains intact in pure amnesia, such as early Alzheimer's disease (AD). Short-term memory is then converted to long-term memory, in the process of "consolidation," which sends memory to the cortex for long-term storage.

2. **What is *declarative memory* and how does it differ from *nondeclarative* memory?**

   Declarative or explicit memories are facts and events that are available to consciousness. They require awareness, allow conscious recollection, utilize the hippocampal system, and are the type of memory damaged in amnesia. Declarative memory can be either semantic or episodic.

   Semantic memory refers to fund of knowledge information, language usage, and practical knowledge, whereas *episodic memory* refers to memories that are localizable in time and space. Autobiographical memories stored within the past few hours to few months are clinically termed as *recent memory,* whereas older memories dating from early childhood are termed as *remote memory.* Interestingly, source (contextual) memory is the knowledge of where and when something was learned and is a subtype of declarative memory. Prospective (capacity for remembering to remember) memory and future episodic memory (creation of scenarios requiring drawing upon past experiences to guide what might happen in the future) are other subtypes of declarative memory.

   Nondeclarative or implicit memories are passively acquired. They do not require the hippocampal circuitry and are not consciously accessible. One is unaware of them, they are inflexible, and they remain intact in amnesia. Examples are motor skill learning, such as learning to play golf through repetition, conditioning, priming, cognitive skill learning, and habit learning. This system requires the cerebellum, basal ganglia, and association cortices.

   In healthy individuals, both systems work together. In amnesia, implicit or nondeclarative learning remains intact; this fact can be utilized for rehabilitation. Even patients with AD, for example, can learn through this system—the repetition of facts, rather than single presentations, may allow their storage.

3. **Which areas are responsible for encoding, storage, and retrieval of declarative information?**

   The hippocampal system is concerned with encoding and consolidating information.

   Long-term storage generally occurs in the temporoparietal cortices. The left hemisphere stores primarily verbal or general knowledge (i.e., semantic/lexical information), and the right stores nonverbal and autobiographical information.

   Retrieval uses prefrontal and distributed temporoparietal networks; the role of the hippocampal system in retrieval is time limited.

4. **What is *amnesia* and injury to which areas can cause an amnestic syndrome?**

   Amnesia is a severe, isolated disturbance of declarative memory in the absence of other forms of cognitive dysfunction. Patients are unable to acquire new memories (anterograde amnesia) or recall recent memories (retrograde amnesia). Other memories remain intact, including remote memory, working memory, and semantic memory.

Bilateral lesions of the Papez circuit and related areas can cause an amnestic syndrome, while unilateral lesions can produce a milder, but often clinically relevant, memory deficit. The Papez circuit includes the medial temporal lobes (hippocampus and entorhinal cortex), the diencephalon (fornix and mammillary bodies; dorsomedial and anterior nuclei of the thalamus), and the basal forebrain cholinergic nuclei (medial septal nuclei and the diagonal band of Broca).

The isolated reduced ability to learn new information is referred to as *amnestic mild cognitive impairment* (aMCI). Many patients with aMCI develop Alzheimer's dementia over the next 5 years.

5. What are the most common etiologies for amnestic syndromes?
   The etiologies for amnestic syndromes can be divided according to their anatomic location:
   - Medial temporal lobes—hypoxia, herpes simplex encephalitis, early AD, posterior cortical atrophy (PCA), strokes (thalamic and temporal lobe), surgery
   - Diencephalon—Korsakoff's syndrome (thiamine deficiency), thalamic strokes, surgery
   - Basal forebrain—anterior communicating artery aneurysm bleed or clipping (with damage to the small perforating arteries)
   - Substances—alcohol, benzodiazepines (transient, not permanent)

6. What are the clinical characteristics of *transient global amnesia*?
   Patients develop a sudden, isolated amnestic syndrome without structural brain abnormalities (anterograde and retrograde amnesia), which usually has a duration of 12 to 24 hours. Afterward, patients will not remember the episode because they are unable to encode new memories during it. Working memory is normal during the episode. On positron emission tomography (PET) or single-photon emission computed tomography (SPECT), bilateral temporal hypoperfusion can be demonstrated. The cause of this benign syndrome remains unknown. However, because it occurs more often in migraineurs, it could be a migraine equivalent. It is also more likely in those with epilepsy, patients at risk for transient ischemic attack, and during exercise. Risk of recurrence is low but higher than in the general population.

7. What are the features of *psychogenic amnesia*?
   In most cases of psychogenic amnesia, patients exhibit biologically unlikely patterns of impairment. Commonly, autobiographical memory is disproportionately affected, sparing memories of political and entertainment events. Patients often exhibit deficits in remote memories, which are normally very resistant to damage. New learning (anterograde memory) is often spared. Nevertheless, reversible abnormalities on PET with temporal hypometabolism have been found in some of these patients.

8. What types of memory difficulties occur with *frontal lobe lesions*?
   Frontal lobe damage can lead to important cognitive, emotional, and social dysfunction. The frontal lobes are organized into three basic subdivisions: precentral, premotor, and prefrontal.

   The *prefrontal division* is crucial for higher order functions like planning, judgment, reasoning, decision making, emotional regulation, and social conduct. It can be further subdivided into ventromedial prefrontal cortex, dorsolateral prefrontal cortex, and superior medial prefrontal cortex.

   The *dorsolateral prefrontal cortex* is important for *working memory* and "metamemory," which has executive control over the memory apparatus. For example, it decides whether a retrieved memory is plausible for a given context, does strategic searching of the memory store, and temporally orders memories. Working memory holds about 7 to 10 bits of information as long as they are constantly repeated. Prefrontal damage and difficulty with working memory may manifest as interference with learning and impairment in performing tasks requiring delayed responses.

   An impairment of declarative memory in conjunction with frontal lobe dysfunction may cause *confabulation*, which is the inability to distinguish a true memory from a false memory or from a memory inappropriate for the context. Confabulations are a common occurrence in alcoholic Korsakoff's syndrome.

   Frontal cortical lesions can also cause disorders of one or more functions that facilitate memory, such as *learning strategies*, *retrieval strategies*, and *learning efficiency*.

APHASIAS

9. What is the definition of *aphasia* and how does it differ from *dysarthria*?
   Aphasia is an acquired disturbance of language whereas dysarthria is an acquired disorder of speech production. An example of dysarthria is what happens after having anesthesia for dental work and then being unable to enunciate words.

10. **Which are the *nonfluent* aphasias and which are the *fluent* aphasias?**
    The anterior aphasias are nonfluent and include Broca's, global, and mixed transcortical and transcortical motor. The posterior aphasias are fluent, including Wernicke's, transcortical sensory, and usually thalamic (Table 17-1).

11. **Which aphasias spare repetition and which have impaired repetition?**
    Repetition is spared in those *outside the perisylvian fissure area*, including transcortical motor, transcortical sensory, and thalamic aphasias. Repetition is impaired in the *perisylvian aphasias*, including Broca's, Wernicke's, conduction aphasia, and pure word deafness.

12. **What are the clinical characteristics of *nonfluent aphasia*?**
    Impaired articulation, impaired melodic production, reduced phrase length (five or fewer words per phrase), and decreased grammatical complexity. The production of fewer than 15 words per minute is used to define nonfluent aphasias.

13. **What are the clinical features of *Broca's aphasia* and where is the lesion responsible for it?**
    Speech is nonfluent, effortful, agrammatic, and telegraphic, with poor ability to name, semantic and phonemic paraphasic errors, impaired repetition, and relatively spared comprehension. The lesion is in Broca's area (the frontal operculum, Brodmann areas 44 and 45), inferior left frontal gyrus, the surrounding frontal areas, and the underlying white matter and subjacent basal ganglia.

14. **What are the clinical features of *aphemia* and where is the lesion that underlies it?**
    Aphemia refers to poor speech output with sparing of comprehension and writing. Speech output can be slow and halting. Aphemia has been reported with lesions of the lower motor strip (cortical dysarthria), supplementary motor cortex, and several other areas.

15. **What are the clinical features of *anomic aphasia*, and where is the lesion that underlies it?**
    Persons with anomic aphasia have isolated deficits in word finding. Otherwise, their speech is fluent with good comprehension and good repetition. Lesions producing this aphasia localize less specifically than other aphasias. They may be in the temporo-parieto-occipital association area. This is also a common chronic residual syndrome for other acute aphasias after rehabilitation.

16. **What are the clinical features of *conduction aphasia* and where is the lesion that produces it?**
    Conduction aphasia is a fluent aphasia, with good comprehension, poor repetition, paragrammatic errors, anomia, paraphasic errors, good recitation, and good reading aloud. While any type of paraphasia may be seen, the vast majority of substitutions involves phonemes resulting in literal (phonemic) paraphasic errors. The lesion usually involves the left inferior parietal lobule, especially the anterior supramarginal gyrus. Often the lesion is in the subcortical white matter, deep to the inferior parietal cortex, involving the arcuate fasciculus or the extreme capsule immediately below it. Both structures are connected to the temporal and frontal cortex.

17. **What are the clinical features of *Wernicke's aphasia* and where is the lesion responsible for it?**
    Wernicke's aphasia is characterized by fluent speech, good articulation, good or sometimes exaggerated prosody (the expressivity of language), impaired naming, phonemic and semantic paraphasias, poor auditory and reading comprehension, impaired repetition, and fluent but empty writing. It is usually caused by damage to the posterior sector of the left auditory association cortex, Brodmann area 22. Often there is involvement of Brodmann areas 37, 39, and 40, or all three.

18. **What are the clinical features of *transcortical motor aphasia* and where are the lesions responsible for it?**
    Spontaneous speech is nonfluent, with good repetition and good comprehension, delayed initiation of output, brief utterances, semantic paraphasic errors, and echolalia. Lesions around Broca's area in the supplementary motor area or its connections to Broca's area are responsible.

19. **What are the clinical features of *transcortical sensory aphasia* and where is the lesion responsible for it?**
    Spontaneous speech is fluent, with good repetition, echolalia, impaired auditory and reading comprehension, right visual field deficits, and rare motor and sensory deficits. Lesions outside of Wernicke's area in the surrounding temporoparietal area are responsible.

Table 17-1. The Aphasias

	FLUENCY	REPETITION	NAMING/WORD FINDING	COMPREHENSION	READING	WRITING	PARAPHASIC ERRORS	LESION LOCATION
Transcortical motor	NF	Gd		Gd			Semantic	Supplementary motor
Mixed transcortical	NF	Gd		↓				Watershed distribution
Aphemia	NF			Nl		Nl		Lower motor strip, SMA
Anterior subcortical (basal ganglia)	Dysarthria, decreased fluency	Mild ↓		Mild ↓				Basal ganglia—putamen and caudate
Global	NF	↓	↓	↓	↓	↓		Broca's and Wernicke's
Broca's	NF	↓	Poor	Relatively nl	↓	↓	Semantic and phonemic	Frontal operculum/Brodmann 44 and 45
Conduction	F	↓	Anomia	Nl			Phonemic	Arcuate fasciculus
Wernicke's	F	↓	↓	↓		↓	Semantic and phonemic	Posterior temporal/Brodmann 22, 37, 39, or 40
Transcortical sensory	F	Gd	↓	↓			Semantic	Temporoparietal
Anomic	F	Gd	↓	Nl				Temporal–parietal–occipital Association
Thalamic	F	Gd—fairly	Severe	↓	↓	Nl		Ant, VA, DL, VL, Ant DM nuclei
Alexia w/o agraphia	F	Gd	Gd	Nl	↓			Left occipital plus posterior corpus callosum
Alexia w/ agraphia	F	Gd	Gd	Nl	↓	↓		Angular gyrus

NF, Nonfluent; *F,* fluent; *Gd,* good; *Nl,* normal; *SMA,* supplementary motor area; *Ant,* Anterior nucleus; *VA,* Ventral anterior nucleus; *DL,* Lateral dorsal nucleus; *VL,* Lateral ventral nucleus; *Ant DM,* Anterior part of the medial dorsal nucleus.

20. What are the clinical features of *mixed transcortical aphasia*, where is the lesion responsible for it, and what is its vascular territory?

   There is absent spontaneous speech, impaired comprehension, and intact repetition. Stock phrases, such as "you know" and "the thing is," and echolalia are produced. The lesion includes the areas that cause transcortical motor and sensory aphasias: the dorsolateral frontal region anterior to the motor cortex and the temporal–parietal–occipital junction. This lesion may be caused by hypoperfusion in the distribution of the left internal carotid artery, which produces a watershed stroke.

21. What are the clinical features of *global aphasia* and where are the lesions that produce it?

   Spontaneous speech is nonfluent, with poor repetition and poor comprehension. The output is restricted to meaningless speech sounds or stereotypes. These lesions involve Broca's and Wernicke's area. They may be combined cortical–subcortical or purely subcortical.

22. What is *alexia* and how does it differ from *dyslexia*?

   Alexia is an acquired disorder of written language comprehension, i.e., difficulty in reading. Dyslexia refers to developmental difficulties with reading.

23. What is *alexia without agraphia* and where is the lesion responsible for it?

   Alexia without agraphia (pure word blindness or acquired pure alexia) is the inability to read despite preserved ability to write. It is associated with a lesion in the dominant occipital lobe (frequently producing a homonymous hemianopia), and a disconnection of the nondominant occipital lobe from the dominant parietal lobe via a lesion of the inferior splenium of the corpus callosum. Alternately, it can occur with lesions of the dominant lateral geniculate body and splenium of the corpus callosum or with a single lesion of the dominant occipitotemporal periventricular white matter behind, beneath, and beside the occipital horn of the lateral ventricle. It is most often associated with infarction in the distribution of the dominant hemispheric posterior cerebral artery.

24. Where is the lesion responsible for *alexia with agraphia*?

   Alexia with agraphia is usually associated with a lesion of the angular gyrus.

25. What percentage of people are *left handed*?

   Fewer than 5% of people use their left hands for all skilled tasks. Sixty percent are strongly right handed and 35% have a mixed hand preference.

APRAXIAS

26. What is *apraxia*?

   Apraxia is the loss of the ability to perform a learned, familiar, purposeful motor act despite having the desire and the physical ability to perform the movements. This occurs in the absence of a primary disturbance in attention, comprehension, motivation, coordination, or sensation that would preclude that act.

27. What are the features of *ideational apraxia* and where is the responsible lesion?

   Ideational apraxia is the inability to perform a sequence of learned acts. These are multistep acts such as making coffee, preparing a meal, or mailing a letter. It is usually seen with either diffuse brain injury, delirium, and dementia or with frontal lobe lesions. It is thought to represent a primary disturbance of attention and executive function that interferes with the coherence of sequenced motor output. See Table 17-2 for a comparison of the types of apraxias.

28. What is *ideomotor apraxia* and where is the lesion responsible for it?

   Ideomotor apraxia is the inability to perform learned familiar movements to command. The lesion usually includes the dominant inferior parietal area (and/or the arcuate fasciculus), which is believed to contain spatiotemporal representations of learned skilled movements ("praxicons"). These are then translated into motor output through the mediation of the premotor cortex.

29. What is *sympathetic apraxia* and where is the lesion underlying it?

   Sympathetic apraxia is an ideomotor apraxia of the left hand, commonly associated with a right hemiparesis and a Broca's aphasia. It is caused by left frontal lesions disconnecting the left inferior parietal lobe from the right premotor cortex so that "praxicons" for the left hand cannot reach the hand area of the right frontal lobe.

Table 17-2. Forms of Apraxia

	POOR ACTIONS	LESION LOCATION	ASSOCIATED CONDITIONS/ FEATURES
Ideational apraxia	Sequence of learned acts	Diffuse or frontal	Dementia, delirium
Ideomotor apraxia	Learned familiar movements to command	Dominant inferior parietal	
Sympathetic apraxia	Left-hand ideomotor apraxia	Left frontal	Right HP, Broca's aphasia
Anterior callosal apraxia	Left-hand ideomotor	Corpus callosum	None
Limb-kinetic apraxia	Distal limb reduced dexterity and coordination	Contralateral SMA	

HP, Hemiparesis; *SMA,* supplementary motor area.

30. **What are the features of *anterior callosal apraxia*?**
An anterior callosal lesion disconnects the right premotor cortex (left hand) from the left hemisphere (left inferior parietal lobe), yielding an apraxia to verbal commands confined to the left hand (left ideomotor apraxia). Sympathetic and anterior callosal apraxias are essentially the same syndrome due to interruption of the same pathway, but the lesion in sympathetic apraxia is much larger, causing other deficits (e.g., aphasia and hemiparesis).

31. **What is *limb-kinetic apraxia* and where is the lesion that produces it?**
Limb-kinetic apraxia is a loss of dexterity and coordination of fine distal limb movements. The lesion producing it usually includes the contralateral supplementary motor cortex.

32. **What is *dressing apraxia* and where is the lesion that produces it?**
Dressing apraxia is not a true apraxia. The difficulty in dressing is a result of the inability to align the body axis with the axis of the garment, a complex visuospatial task. Dressing apraxia is a nondominant parietal lobe symptom that is often associated with left visual field deficits and other deficits of visuospatial integration and construction (drawing).
Lesions in the right parietal–occipital–temporal region cause problems with complex perceptual–spatial actions, such as route finding and navigating the body with respect to solid objects such as beds and chairs.
Another problem arising from this region is *hemineglect* in which one-half of the body is neither clothed nor groomed, and attention to one-half of the patient's extrapersonal space is severely diminished.

33. **What is *constructional apraxia* and where is the lesion underlying it?**
Constructional apraxia involves difficulty in copying figures and designs (drawing) but is not caused by a true apraxia. It is also associated with right parietal lobe lesions.

PERCEPTUAL DISORDERS AND AGNOSIAS

34. **What is *agnosia*?**
Agnosia is the inability to recognize objects despite adequate perception in the modality in which the object is presented. See Table 17-3 for a comparison of the types of agnosias as discussed below.

35. **What is *topographagnosia* and where is the lesion responsible for it?**
Topographagnosia is the inability to navigate complex spatial layouts, such as a city, a building, or even one's home, and to describe verbally or with a map how to get to a specific place or room. This difficulty is often combined with some degree of unilateral neglect. It can be seen in right occipitoparietal damage or in bilateral temporoparietal lesions, damaging the "parahippocampal place area (PPA)." Spatial orientation can also be disturbed in memory disorders and bilateral lesions of the visual system.

Table 17-3. Forms of Agnosia or Neglect

	DEFINITION	ASSOCIATED FEATURES	ANATOMIC LOCALIZATION
Topographagnosia	Inability to navigate complex layouts	Often unilateral neglect	Right occipitoparietal or bilateral temporo-parietal
Anosagnosia	Unawareness of impairment	Often left HP	Right parietal
Anosodiaphoria	Recognizes deficits, but is indifferent to them	Often an HP or hemisensory deficit	Right hemisphere
Prosopagnosia	Inability to recognize familiar faces	Inability to identify other specific members of a class, such as car brands; visual field defects	Bilateral inferior occipito-temporal
Simultanagnosia	Inability to interpret complex visual scenes		High occipitoparietal (e.g., posterior watershed)
Achromatopsia	Lack of color vision	Quadrantanopia	Occipital cortex below the calcarine sulcus; inferotemporal
Hemineglect	Lack of attention to one-half of space		Posterior right parietal; then left frontal or left parietal

HP, Hemiparesis.

36. **What is** *anosagnosia* **and where is the lesion responsible for it?**
   Anosagnosia is the unawareness of illness or impairment, such as hemiparesis or blindness, and is most commonly observed with right parietal lesions.

37. **What is** *anosodiaphoria* **and where is the lesion that produces it?**
   Anosodiaphoria is a disorder in which patients recognize a deficit, such as a hemiparesis and/or a hemisensory deficit, but are indifferent to it. It may be seen with right hemisphere lesions.

38. **What is** *prosopagnosia* **and where is the lesion responsible for it?**
   Prosopagnosia (face blindness) is the inability to recognize familiar faces. Patients can perform a *generic recognition*—"it is a face"—and are able to tell age, gender, and emotional expression but are unable to identify the *specific* person. They rely on voice, posture, clothing, etc., to make the identification. Commonly, patients are also unable to identify other specific members of a general class, e.g., car brands or birds. The disorder is commonly associated with unilateral or bilateral visual field defects. It is often associated with achromatopsia because of involvement of the fibers projecting from the inferior lip of the occipital lobe.
   Prosopagnosia is associated with bilateral inferior occipitotemporal lesions affecting both fusiform gyri. The posterior fusiform gyri contain an area called the *fusiform face area* that is specialized in facial processing and identification. Adjacent areas are specialized in identifying individual members of other general classes of objects (birds, cars, buildings, etc.).

39. **What is** *simultanagnosia* **and where is the lesion underlying it?**
   Simultanagnosia is a disorder of visual perception and attention characterized by the inability to interpret complex visual arrays despite preserved recognition of single objects.
   Simultanagnosia occurs predominantly in patients with high occipitoparietal lobe disease such as bilateral infarcts in the posterior watershed region, venous infarcts due to sagittal sinus thrombosis, and in some patients with AD.

40. **What is cerebral** *achromatopsia* **and where is the lesion responsible for it?**
   Achromatopsia is an acquired lack of color vision. Lesions of the occipital cortex below the calcarine sulcus produce upper quadrantanopia and achromatopsia in the preserved inferior visual field. Hemiachromatopsia can result from contralateral inferotemporal lesions of the fusiform and lingual gyri.

41. What is *neglect* and where are the lesions that produce it?

    Neglect, compared in Table 17-3 to agnosias, is a lack of attention to events and actions in one part of one's personal and extrapersonal space. *Hemineglect* is the term used to describe neglect of one-half of one's space, usually on the left in right handers. This inattention to stimuli from that space can involve all modalities, as well as motor acts and motivation.

    The posterior parietal cortex is believed to be critical for spatial attention in that it integrates distributed spatial information across all sensory modalities.

    Although neglect is classically attributed to right parietal lesions, it can be seen with damage to many other cortical and subcortical areas. The most profound neglect is seen with right parietal lesions, followed by left frontal and then left parietal lesions.

NEUROBEHAVIORAL SYNDROMES

42. What are the behavioral alterations observed with lesions of the *orbitofrontal cortex*?

    Impulsive and antisocial behavior (disinhibition, hypersexuality, excessive eating, breaking of social conventions, compulsions, hoarding, and cluttering), high-risk behavior (inability to foresee or learn from negative consequences), unstable mood (lability, irritability, hypomania, mania), inappropriate jocularity (*Witzelsucht, Moria*), and impaired olfactory recognition. These behaviors may be seen with lesions of the orbitofrontal cortex, ventral caudate, globus pallidus, and mediodorsal thalamus. During the exam, patients are often stimulus bound and show utilization behavior.

43. What is utilization behavior and what does it mean to be "stimulus bound"?

    Utilization behavior refers to a patient's inability to suppress the urge to manipulate or use an object in a correct way but in an unacceptable context—for example, drinking from the examiner's cup or writing with the examiner's pen. A patient who is stimulus bound is attracted to each new stimulus, unable to ignore stimuli that are not relevant to the current task. The patient is thus unable to maintain the attention required to pursue one task to full completion.

44. What are the behavioral alterations associated with lesions of the *medial frontal cortex*?

    Medial frontal lesions are associated with impoverished speech and apathy, which can be to the extreme of akinetic mutism, lack of motivation and drive, poor initiation, lack of goal formation, loss of planning, paucity of thought, and profound psychomotor (cognitive) slowing. These changes may occur with lesions of the medial frontal cortex, anterior cingulate cortex, nucleus accumbens, globus pallidus, and mediodorsal/ventral anterior thalamus.

45. What are the behavioral alterations noted with lesions of the *dorsolateral prefrontal cortex*?

    Dorsolateral prefrontal lesions are associated with depression and apathy, reduced verbal fluency (dominant side), reduced nonverbal fluency (nondominant side), psychomotor slowing, poor set shifting, impaired abstraction and logical thinking, inability to understand humor, poor judgment, poor response inhibition, impaired free recall and intact recognition memory, poor memory organization, poor temporal sequencing of events, poor visual construction strategies, poor working memory, reduced divided attention, reduced sustained attention, perseveration on sequential motor tasks, and environmental dependency. *Verbal dysdecorum* is disinhibited, poorly monitored verbal output that is socially unacceptable and is seen most frequently following damage on the right. These behaviors occur after lesions of the dorsolateral prefrontal cortex, head of the caudate, globus pallidus, and mediodorsal/ventral anterior thalamus.

46. What is the *alien hand syndrome*, where is the lesion that produces it, and what is the vascular territory of lesions that can produce it?

    With this syndrome, an individual's nonparalyzed hand appears to carry out activities that cannot be controlled by the individual. It can include behaviors like inappropriate grasping, taking off one's glasses, and throwing off one's covers.

    It is a disconnection syndrome caused by damage to the corpus callosum that can be seen with occlusion of the anterior cerebral artery. It can also be observed in corticobasal degeneration.

47. What are the features of *Gerstmann's syndrome* and where is the lesion responsible for it?

    Gerstmann's syndrome is characterized by four primary symptoms: acalculia, agraphia or dysgraphia, an inability to identify fingers (finger agnosia), and right–left confusion. These occur in the absence of additional language deficits.

The underlying lesion includes the *angular gyrus* in the dominant hemisphere. A pure Gerstmann's syndrome is rare: more commonly, it is associated with aphasia and/or other parietal lobe symptoms.

48. What is *Geschwind's syndrome* and where is the responsible lesion?
Geschwind's syndrome includes a cluster of personality traits: circumstantiality (excessive verbal output, stickiness, hypergraphia), altered sexuality (loss or alteration of sexual interests and a craving for overly close interpersonal relationships), and intensified mental life (deepening of many emotions, often resulting in religious or philosophical preoccupations; a strong moralistic sense).

These personality traits have been attributed to temporal lobe epilepsy and are hypothesized to result from chronic epileptic activation or "kindling" within the amygdala. The specificity of these features for temporal lobe epilepsy is poor.

49. What is *Ganser syndrome*?
Ganser syndrome is sometimes known as the *syndrome of approximate answers* or *pseudostupidity*. It is most often observed in a forensic setting or where marked psychosocial stress is present. The key features are approximate answers (referred to as *vorbeireden*), clouding of consciousness, memory or personal identity loss, somatic conversion symptoms, and hallucinations. Duration of symptoms is brief, and patients usually have amnesia for the episode upon resolution. Most often seen in psychiatric disorders, it has also been reported following neurologic conditions such as head trauma, neurosyphilis, or even imprisonment. There is some controversy as to whether the syndrome is due to a true dissociative disorder, a factitious disorder, or malingering.

50. What is *Balint's syndrome* and where is the responsible lesion?
Balint's syndrome includes misreaching under visual guidance (optic ataxia), failure to scan and integrate an entire visual scene or picture (simultanagnosia), and ocular apraxia ("sticky fixation"). Patients with these symptoms usually have bilateral lesions of the occipitoparietal junctions.

51. What is *Anton's syndrome* and where are the lesions associated with it?
Anton's syndrome is the combination of cortical blindness and denial of blindness. It is typically associated with bilateral posterior cerebral artery infarctions producing "cortical" blindness plus memory impairment.

52. What are the features of *Klüver–Bucy syndrome* and where is the lesion associated with it?
Docility, placidity, hypersexuality, hyperorality, and visual agnosia may be seen as part of the Klüver–Bucy syndrome. Hypermetamorphosis (a desire to explore everything) is also associated. This syndrome is seen in monkeys with experimental bilateral temporal lobectomies.

Occasionally, aspects of the syndrome are seen in human patients with bilateral lesions of anterior temporal lobes, including the amygdala. Herpes simplex encephalitis is one cause of this syndrome in humans.

53. What is *Charles Bonnet syndrome* and when does it occur?
Vivid, well-formed visual hallucinations in the setting of poor vision occurring in mentally healthy, most often elderly, individuals. Severe macular degeneration and glaucoma are common etiologies, but optic nerve damage can also predispose to the disorder. Hallucinations are usually of people, animals, or objects, often "Lilliputian," and perceived as pleasurable by many patients.

NEUROCOGNITIVE DISORDERS

54. What are neurocognitive disorders (NCDs)?
NCDs are syndromes where the core symptom is cognitive impairment affecting at least one domain (complex attention, executive function, learning and memory, language, perceptual-motor, or social cognition), based on the concern of an individual, a knowledgeable informant, or the clinician, leading to a persistent decline in level of functioning as evidenced by performance on an objective assessment (like standardized neuropsychological testing or quantified clinical assessment). The underlying pathology of NCD is usually acquired and not neurodevelopmental, and its etiology can frequently be determined.

The new nomenclature was developed for DSM-5. It further classifies NCDs as *major* or *mild*, according to cognitive and functional impairment. They are also distinguished by level of impairment, i.e., substantial versus modest, and degree of independence in everyday activities.

Both major and mild NCDs are further specified by etiology, i.e., likely due to AD, frontotemporal lobar degeneration (FTLD), Lewy body disease, vascular disease, traumatic brain injury, substance/medication use, human immunodeficiency virus infection, prion disease, Parkinson's disease, Huntington's disease, or another medical condition or stemming from multiple etiologies.

Major NCD corresponds closely to the conditions referred to as *dementia* in the DSM-IV but is broader than the older term. Mild cognitive disorder on the other hand is substantially congruent with the condition of mild cognitive impairment.

55. What is *delirium*?

Delirium is a disturbance in awareness, attention, and cognition developing over a short period of time and represents a decline from baseline. Delirium tends to fluctuate in severity temporally and is a result of another medical condition, or withdrawal, or exposure to toxins, as evidenced by history, physical examination, or laboratory findings. The differential diagnosis of delirium can include infections, withdrawal from drugs of abuse, acute metabolic disorder (like electrolyte imbalance or hepatic or renal failure), trauma, central nervous system pathology (like stroke, hemorrhage, tumor, seizure disorder), hypoxia, vitamin or mineral deficiencies, endocrine dysfunction, acute vascular injury (shock, hypertensive encephalopathy), toxins (including drugs of abuse and medications like anesthetics, narcotics, anticholinergics, steroids, etc.), or heavy metal poisoning or can be due to multiple etiologies. Characteristically delirium cannot be explained by either a preexisting or evolving NCD. However, patients with an underlying NCD are more vulnerable to delirium because of their baseline impaired brain function. Sleep–wake cycle disturbances and emotional lability could also be associated with delirium, but there are no known psychiatric illnesses where the initial presentation is a delirium-like state. Another important distinction between delirium and dementia is the acute onset and temporal fluctuations characteristic of delirium in contrast to the chronic nature of dementia.

56. What is *mild cognitive impairment (MCI)*?

MCI is defined as cognitive dysfunction greater than expected for age and education in either a single cognitive domain or in multiple domains without impairment in activities of daily living (ADLs). In the new classification of NCDs, memory impairment with preserved nonmemory cognition has been referred to as *amnestic MCI*, and episodic memory is the most common initially affected type of memory. Alternately, patients can also present with another area of cognitive dysfunction, including visuospatial, processing speed, verbal ability, attention, and executive function. Such patients have nonamnestic MCI.

MCI is also viewed as a predementia state as the conversion to dementia is quite high. Amnestic MCI, for example, is associated with a 10% to 15% per year conversion to AD. Many researchers view amnestic MCI as the earliest clinical phase of AD, and the utility of distinguishing it from AD has been questioned.

Nonamnestic MCI, on the other hand, has been shown to be associated with other neurodegenerative disorders (FTLD, dementia of Lewy bodies, vascular dementia, etc.).

57. How is a differential diagnosis of NCD made?

The diagnosis is usually made through careful history and examination. Each etiopathology leading to cognitive impairment has a characteristic neurobehavioral pattern, which usually starts focally and then spreads to adjacent brain areas. A careful history and neuropsychological evaluation (by formal testing or quantified clinical assessment) will reveal which cognitive domains are affected. Structural (MRI) and functional imaging (PET or SPECT) scan can also be helpful in determining affected brain regions. Amyloid PET scans have revolutionized our ability to delineate the diagnosis of AD from other causes of cognitive impairment.

58. What are the neurobehavioral characteristics of *AD*?

AD is the most common neurodegenerative dementia in the elderly. In typical cases, the disease process starts in the medial temporal lobe, mainly hippocampus and entorhinal cortex, so the cardinal symptom is progressive memory impairment. Pathology then spreads to involve adjacent lateral temporal and parietal areas, causing visuospatial impairment and difficulties with naming and semantic knowledge. Select frontal functions can be impaired early, such as set shifting. Later in the disease course, there is global decline in cognitive skills and functional status. There are well-described atypical variants of AD, such as PCA characterized by progressive visuospatial dysfunction, and a language variant called *logopenic primary progressive aphasia*.

59. What are the neurobehavioral characteristics of *dementia with Lewy bodies* (DLB)?

    DLB is the second most common progressive neurodegenerative dementia. The clinical findings can be much more variable than are those in AD. The core feature of DLB is a dementia with a predominant dysexecutive syndrome (frontal lobe involvement). Memory impairment is usually milder than it is in AD. Associated features are fluctuations in cognition, early visual hallucinations, and parkinsonian features. Unlike other dementias, visual hallucinations are usually early and recurrent, complex and well formed, and often consist of people and animals. Sensitivity to neuroleptic medications and rapid eye movement sleep behavior disorder are supportive of the diagnosis. DLB can be associated with occipital lobe hypometabolism on PET scan, usually in conjunction with frontal and basal ganglia changes, which can help to distinguish it from AD. Microscopically, it is associated with aggregates of alpha-synuclein called *Lewy bodies* in cortical, subcortical, and limbic regions. DLB is also often accompanied by AD pathology and symptoms.

60. What are the neurobehavioral characteristics of *FTLD*?

    FTLD is a heterogeneous group of disorders that is variable in clinical presentation and has several different associated pathologic findings. FTLD is typically divided into three clinical syndromes: *behavioral variant frontotemporal dementia* (bvFTD), *semantic dementia* (SD), and *progressive nonfluent aphasia* (PNFA or PPA).

    BvFTD typically has a behavioral onset, which can be primarily orbitofrontal (disinhibited), primarily dysexecutive, or primarily medial dorsal (psychomotor retardation and apathy) in character. SD and PNFA have language onsets (see below). All three have an earlier age of onset (average 55 years), a more rapid progression, and a higher genetic susceptibility (40% familial) than AD. In early-onset dementia, its frequency is equal to AD.

    Corticobasal syndrome and progressive supranuclear palsy are two related diseases that are not classified as FTD but often share some symptoms with FTD. They can also be due to mutations in the same genes as FTD. FTD can also occur in conjunction with amyotrophic lateral sclerosis (ALS) (FTD/ALS).

    Pathologically, FTD is associated with several different findings in limbic, paralimbic, temporal, and anterior frontal regions: neurofibrillary tangles (tau pathology), Pick bodies (tau pathology), fused in sarcoma inclusions (FUS), Tar DNA binding protein-43 inclusions (TDP-43), and rarely changes without distinctive histopathology. It is somewhat difficult to correlate a specific clinical syndrome with the underlying pathology, but FTD/ALS and SD are both highly associated with ubiquitin and TDP-43 inclusions.

    Five genetic mutations have thus far been identified in familial FTD. The most common are mutations in the tau (*MAPT*) and progranulin (*PGRN*) genes on chromosome 17.

61. What is PNFA? What is SD?

    Both disorders are characterized under the rubric of primary progressive aphasia and are considered in the family of FTLD. They involve the gradual and relatively isolated dissolution of language function. Language impairment is usually the only factor that compromises ADLs for at least the first 2 years of the disease, but difficulties eventually progress to include other cognitive domains. Both disorders are more commonly seen as variants of frontotemporal dementia, and less commonly in AD or Creutzfeld–Jakob disease (CJD).

    The PNFA variant of primary progressive aphasia presents as a progressive disorder of expressive language. There is effortful speech production, phonologic and grammatical errors, and word retrieval difficulties. These persons are clinically similar to persons with Broca's aphasia, except that the onset is not abrupt as it would be when Broca's is due to stroke. There may be associated acalculia or ideomotor apraxia. Some patients with PNFA develop Parkinson-like motor changes. Twenty percent are associated with tauopathies, 60% are ubiquitinopathies, and 20% are due to AD. Rarely, it can be the presenting feature of CJD.

    The SD variant of primary progressive aphasia is characterized by a severe naming and word comprehension impairment in the context of fluent, effortless, and grammatical speech output as well as the gradual deterioration of knowledge about the world. Overall, speech output in SD is most similar to Wernicke's aphasia. The person can speak but has lost the connection of words to meaning. If patients cannot think of a word with a certain meaning, they may substitute related words from the same category—for example, eventually calling all animals "dog." They also lose information about other aspects of things, such as the use, color, and detailed appearance of objects. This loss of meaning for both verbal and nonverbal concepts (semantics) contrasts with the preservation of visuospatial skills and day-to-day memory. The predominant pathologic finding in SD is ubiquitinated inclusions.

The *logopenic* variant refers to the combination of features of both PPA and SD. This syndrome may be associated with Alzheimer's pathology. Logopenic progressive aphasia (LPA) is characterized by impaired repetition and naming difficulty. In contrast to semantic dementia, where naming is impaired and word meaning is lost, in LPA the naming deficit is due to a retrieval deficit. Patients may experience a loss of fluency and comprehension of single words, although comprehension of objects is preserved.

62. **What are the neurobehavioral characteristics of *vascular dementia* (VaD)?**
    VaD is the second most common type of dementia, either alone or in combination with AD. It is a highly heterogeneous entity commonly associated with executive dysfunction and relatively preserved verbal memory. Cognitive impairment depends on the vessels involved and may onset in a stepwise manner. Small vessel disease causing lacunar infarcts can cause a subcortical dementia, like *Binswanger's syndrome*. *CADASIL* is an autosomal dominant arteriopathy associated with mutations in the Notch 3 gene that can also cause dementia.

63. **What are the neurobehavioral characteristics of *Huntington's disease* (HD)?**
    Development of neuropsychiatric disturbances is a common feature of HD. Minor alterations in personality and behavior are the initial symptoms in a vast majority of cases. A wide range of neuropsychiatric symptoms have been reported, including depression, apathy, anxiety, irritability, poor self-control, perseveration, personality changes, and in many cases even frank psychosis.

    Progressive neurocognitive decline is also a hallmark of HD. Deficits in executive functioning, short-term memory, and long-term memory (including deficits in episodic, procedural, and working memory) gradually progress to development of an NCD.

64. **How are NCDs commonly treated? How are their associated neurobehavioral syndromes treated?**
    It is useful to consider the A-B-Cs of dementia: affect, behavior, and cognition.

    The cognitive deficits of dementia include memory loss, disorientation, apraxia, anomia, etc. Acetylcholinesterase inhibitors (donepezil, rivastigmine, galantamine) are the mainstays for treating the cognitive symptoms in mild to severe AD. Rivastigmine also has butyrylcholinesterase inhibiting properties, but the clinical significance of that is unclear. Memantine, an N-methyl-D-aspartate receptor antagonist, is also useful for AD, especially when there are behavioral problems, and it acts synergistically with the cholinesterase inhibitors. These medications may improve cognition and functioning in the first few months of treatment and delay or improve behavioral symptoms. They may then slow cognitive decline during the remainder of the disease. There is increasing evidence for clinical efficacy of these drugs in other dementias like VaD and DLB. Some investigators have found donepezil to be useful in MCI. Acetylcholinesterase inhibitors are generally not used in FTLD.

    Affect is frequently altered in the dementias, presenting as depression and anxiety. These symptoms are treated the same as in persons without dementia except that the doses required to be efficacious may be higher. On the other hand, since these dementias frequently occur in the elderly who are more sensitive to medications, it may be difficult to increase their doses. Selective serotonin reuptake inhibitors are most commonly used for mood and anxiety-related symptoms but are initiated at lower doses than in young patients.

    Behavior is commonly altered in dementia and includes the development of aggression, agitation, apathy, disinhibition, hallucinations, delusions, and illusions, etc. Behavioral issues worsen as the disease progresses, contribute significantly to caregiver burden, and can be a major factor in nursing home placement. It is important that they are identified and treated effectively to reduce suffering. Effective agents include antiepileptics, antidepressants, and atypical antipsychotics. There is a black box warning regarding increased rate of death associated with the use of atypical antipsychotics in dementia patients, so other agents should be used if possible, and the side effect profile should be discussed with the family. Impulsive and irritable behaviors respond well to mood stabilizers like lamotrigine or valproic acid.

    There are other treatments associated with the individual dementias where there is another underlying process. For example, controlling vascular risk factors is an important treatment strategy for preventing progression of VaD.

65. **What effects does *obstructive sleep apnea* (OSA) have on cognition?**
    OSA is associated with significant cognitive and behavioral dysfunction. It causes impaired executive functioning that is due, at least in part, to sleepiness. Visual ability, verbal ability, and long-term memory are relatively preserved localizing the deficit to prefrontal cortex. Symptoms usually improve with use of continuous positive airway pressure. OSA can also produce cognitive dysfunction through increasing hypertension and vascular disease.

66. **What effects does *alcohol* have on cognition?**
    Alcoholism can be associated with acute nutritional syndromes producing encephalopathy, such as Wernicke's encephalopathy and Marchiafava–Bignami. The acute syndromes can lead to chronic amnestic syndromes, such as Korsakoff's.

    Alcoholism can cause slowly progressive, chronic cognitive impairment, which is referred to as *alcoholic dementia*. It is characterized by executive dysfunction, such as attention deficits, frontal release signs, and problems with sequencing. It is also associated with visuospatial dysfunction, such as poor clock drawing. There may also be associated balance and gait dysfunction due to cerebellar involvement.

TRAUMATIC BRAIN INJURY

67. **What is *traumatic brain injury* (TBI)?**
    TBI refers to an alteration in brain function or other evidence of brain pathology resulting from an impact and/or acceleration/initialization of the brain. Both closed head injury and penetrating head injuries are classified as TBI. Additionally, a milder form of TBI is clinically termed a *concussion*.

    TBI causes both an acute injury due to direct damage and disruption of brain tissue and neural circuitry, plus secondary or delayed injury from other sources. These include ongoing hemorrhage, hypoxia, ischemia, elevated intracranial pressure, changes in metabolic function, coagulopathy and/or pyrexia, and dementia.

68. **What are the prognostic indicators after TBI?**
    Initial Glasgow Coma Scale, length of loss of consciousness, and duration of posttraumatic amnesia are good predictors of long-term prognosis and outcome.

69. **What are the criteria for mild TBI?**
    The diagnostic criteria for mild TBI/concussion set out by the American Congress of Rehabilitation Medicine are that a patient has had head trauma with loss of consciousness (LOC) up to 30 minutes, loss of memory for the events before or after the accident up to 24 hours, dazed/disoriented/confused feelings, or focal neurologic deficits. It would not be mild TBI if the LOC exceeds 30 minutes, the amnesia persists after 24 hours, or the Glasgow Coma Scale score after 30 minutes falls between 13 and 15.

70. **What are the neurobehavioral symptoms associated with TBI?**
    The TBI severity spectrum ranges from mild impact with no behavioral syndromes, resulting in no lasting structural injury and producing only transient and temporary changes in neurologic function, to patients in prolonged coma/vegetative state from catastrophic brain injury.

    Cognitive impairments after a concussion can include difficulty concentrating, difficulty remembering, feeling in a "fog," feeling slowed down, forgetting recent events, confusion, repeating questions, answering slowly, and amnesia.

    The duration of posttraumatic amnesia (PTA) can also provide an indication of injury severity ranging from very mild (<5 minutes) to extremely severe (>4 weeks). Retrograde amnesia involving minutes, or more rarely days, immediately preceding the accident frequently accompanies PTA.

71. **How are the neurocognitive symptoms of a *penetrating head injury* (PHI) different from those of a *closed head injury*?**
    Diffuse damage after a closed head injury may manifest usually as slowed mental speed, poor attention, and cognitive inefficiency but can also lead to impairment in high-level concept formation, complex reasoning, and executive actions. The inability to concentrate or perform complex mental operations, confusion, irritability, fatigue, and the inability to do things as before the accident are commonly reported.

    PHI can cause similar problems with attention and concentration, memory functions (most commonly short-term memory), mental slowing, and changes in capacity to deal with everyday intellectual demands.

In addition, PHI can cause specific cognitive deficits related to the site of the lesion. Hence, it can also include lateral and posterior functions, such as language impairment and constructional changes. These may show improvement over time after PHI, but the general effects of brain damage (distractibility or slowing) might never return to premorbid levels of functioning.

72. **What is *chronic traumatic encephalopathy* and who is at risk for it?**
Repetitive mild TBI (mTBI), such as can occur in professional sports, has been linked to a progressive disorder called *chronic traumatic encephalopathy* (CTE).
    It can be associated with the progressive development of cognitive decline, behavioral changes (aggression, impulsivity), changes in mood (depression, fatigue, apathy, suicidality), and motor/parkinsonian symptoms. The combination of a mood disorder and impulsivity has led to several suicides.
    The definitive diagnosis of CTE can only be established after death upon postmortem examination of the brain, which demonstrates hyperphosphorylated tau protein deposits in the depths of sulci.

73. **What are some possible long-term sequelae of TBI?**
TBI is a risk factor for later life dementia, including AD and FTD. Another late consequence of TBI can be a seizure disorder, which can be a significant cause of mortality and morbidity. mTBI has also been linked to parkinsonism (dementia pugilistica) and ALS, or Lou Gehrig's disease.

NEUROPSYCHIATRIC DISORDERS

74. **What are the new diagnostic criteria for *posttraumatic stress disorder* (PTSD)?**
DSM-5 has placed PTSD in a separate trauma- and stressor-related disorders category.
    The diagnostic criteria of PTSD require exposure to actual or threatened death, serious injury, or sexual violence leading to development of symptoms lasting >1 month, which cause significant distress or impairment in functioning. These symptoms include intrusive thoughts, reexperiencing symptoms, avoiding situations, negative alterations in cognition and mood, and marked alterations in arousal and reactivity.

75. **What are the associations between *TBI* and *PTSD*?**
TBI, in particular co-occurring mild TBI, may dramatically increase the risk of developing PTSD.
    Surprisingly, TBI and PTSD result in similar neurochemical abnormalities. Damage to the prefrontal cortex, ventral portions of the frontal lobe, and the anterior temporal lobe may be evident in cases of TBI as well as in PTSD. Disruption of attention, impaired short-term memory, persisting deficits in motor speed, and reduced learning capacity are also hallmarks of both TBI and PTSD.

76. **What is the evidence regarding a biological basis for the development of PTSD?**
The neural circuitry implicated in PTSD has been hypothesized to involve interactions between the thalamus, the hippocampus, the amygdala, the posterior cingulate, parietal and motor cortex, and the medial prefrontal cortex. Structural neuroimaging studies have revealed diminished hippocampal volume, reduced left amygdala volumes, and significantly smaller anterior cingulate cortex in persons with PTSD.
    Functional neuroimaging has further shown hyperresponsive amygdala and dorsal anterior cingulate cortex in PTSD. However, the most replicated functional neuroimaging finding in PTSD has been the hyporesponsivity of the ventromedial prefrontal cortex (vmPFC). Increased activity in the amygdala secondary to reduced inhibition by the vmPFC has therefore been suggested as a key component in the development of some PTSD symptoms.
    Patients with PTSD also demonstrate heightened autonomic response and electromyographic reactivity (especially in the facial musculature) to external trauma-related stimuli and to startling stimuli.

77. **What are some long-term sequelae of PTSD?**
Multiple organ systems change in PTSD, leading to an increased risk of vascular comorbidities, dementia, and many other disorders later in life.

78. **What are the new diagnostic criteria for *major depressive disorder*?**
The diagnostic criteria for major depressive disorder in DSM-5 include the presence of five or more of the following symptoms during the same 2-week period: depressed mood, anhedonia, significant weight loss or weight gain, insomnia or hypersomnia, psychomotor agitation or retardation, fatigue or loss of energy, feelings of worthlessness or excessive guilt, diminished concentration, and recurrent

thoughts of death and suicide. Additionally, the episode must include either depressed mood or anhe-donia, should cause significant distress and significant impairment in daily functioning, should not be due to substance use or another medical condition, is not better explained by the occurrence of any psychotic disorder, and is not in a patient who has had a manic or hypomanic episode.

79. What lesions are more commonly associated with *depression*?
   Structural or functional lesions in the left anterior frontal lobe are more often associated with depres-sion than other focal brain lesions.

80. What cognitive deficits are associated with depression, and what are they called?
   Depression is associated with deficits in episodic memory, learning and executive function, especially in set-shifting tasks. Most studies have implicated disruption of the prefrontal cortex in these impair-ments. Many have found that these deficits are independent of age and depression severity. The syndrome of dementia due to depression is called *pseudodementia*.

81. What are the new diagnostic criteria for *bipolar disorder*?
   The diagnostic criteria for a manic episode in DSM-5 include the presence of abnormally and persistently elevated/expansive/irritable mood and abnormally and persistently increased activity or energy lasting ≥1 week and present for most of the day. Additionally, during this period, three or more of the following symptoms should be present: inflated self-esteem or grandiosity, decreased need for sleep, rapid or increased speech, flight of ideas or racing thoughts, distractibility, an increase in goal-directed activity or psychomotor agitation, or involvement in activities that have a high potential for regretful consequences. This episode should cause significant impairment in daily functioning, necessitate hospitalization to prevent harm, or be associated with psychotic features but should not be due to substance use or another medical condition.

   A hypomanic episode, on the other hand, lasts ≥4 days, is associated with a change in mood and functioning observable by others. However, it is not severe enough to cause marked impairment of social or occupational functioning or necessitate hospitalization and is not associated with any psychotic features.

   For the diagnosis of bipolar disorder type 1, criteria should be met for at least one manic episode in the lifetime. For the diagnosis of bipolar disorder type 2, it is necessary to meet criteria for a current or past hypomanic episode and one must also meet criteria for a current or past major depressive episode.

82. What are the new diagnostic criteria for *schizophrenia*?
   The diagnostic criteria for schizophrenia in DSM-5 include the presence of two or more of the fol-lowing symptoms for a significant portion of time during a 1-month period: delusions, hallucinations, disorganized speech, grossly disorganized or catatonic behavior, or negative symptoms (flat affect, avolition, social withdrawal, decreased talking, neglect of personal hygiene, decreased emotional expression, etc.). Additionally, level of functioning should be markedly below baseline for a significant portion of time since the onset of the disturbance, and continuous signs and symptoms should persist for at least 6 months (may include prodromal or residual periods). Of note, the symptoms should not be due to substance use or another medical condition or be attributable to schizoaffective disorder or major mood disorders.

83. What are the new diagnostic criteria for *schizoaffective disorder*?
   The diagnostic criteria for schizoaffective disorder in DSM-5 include an uninterrupted period during which there is a major mood episode (depressive or manic) concurrent to meeting the diagnostic criteria for schizophrenia. Additionally, delusions and hallucinations should be present in the absence of a mood episode for ≥2 weeks. The symptoms of the major mood episode should be present for the majority of the duration of both active and residual illness. Of note, the symptoms should not be due to substance use or another medical condition.

84. What is *catatonia*?
   Catatonia has been described as a state of apparent unresponsiveness to external stimuli in a person who is apparently awake. DSM-5 characterizes catatonia as resistance to instructions (negativism); motoric immobility or excessive motor activity (catatonic excitement); a complete lack of verbal and motor responses (mutism and stupor); repeated stereotyped movements; peculiarities of voluntary movement (staring, grimacing); and echoing of speech (echolalia or echopraxia). Catatonic symptoms have been reported in the setting of multiple psychiatric as well as many general medical disorders.

85. **What lesions are associated with *obsessive-compulsive behavior*?**
    The majority of structural lesions associated with the development of obsessive-compulsive behavior have involved the frontal lobe and/or frontal-basal ganglia network connections.

KEY POINTS: MEMORY AND NEUROPSYCHIATRIC DISORDERS

Memory

1. There are several memory systems in the brain, and each has multiple phases utilizing different anatomic loci. Determining which memory phase is dysfunctional in a patient is essential for determining the underlying disorder since the loci are selectively vulnerable.
2. The hippocampal system is critical for encoding and consolidating declarative memory and is vulnerable to Alzheimer's and herpes simplex encephalitis.
3. Apraxia is the loss of ability to perform previously learned, purposeful motor tasks in the absence of a primary disturbance in attention, comprehension, motivation, coordination, or sensation that would preclude that act.
4. Amnestic mild cognitive impairment, or aMCI, is the isolated loss of anterograde episodic memory, i.e., learning new time-based facts such as what happened earlier today. It is important to recognize aMCI as it is often a harbinger of AD.

Neuropsychiatric Disorders

1. MCI is characterized by cognitive decline in single or multiple domains without functional impairment, i.e., lacking changes in ADLs.
2. Repetitive mild TBI in athletes can lead to CTE.
3. Even a single manic episode in a lifetime with a duration of ≥1 week is sufficient to establish a diagnosis of bipolar disorder type 1 in DSM-5.

 References available online at expertconsult.com.

Acknowledgments

The authors would like to acknowledge the contributions of Heike Schmolck, MD, PhD, and Salah Qureshi, MD, who contributed to this chapter in previous editions.

WEBSITES

http://www.nia.nih.gov/alzheimers
http://www.ptsd.va.gov/professional/index.asp
http://neuro.psychiatryonline.org/
http://dsm.psychiatryonline.org/
http://journals.lww.com/continuum/pages/default.aspx

BIBLIOGRAPHY

1. Arciniegas DB, Anderson CA, Filley CM: Behavioral Neurology and Neuropsychiatry, Cambridge, Cambridge University Press, 2013.
2. Brazis PW, Masdeu JC, Biller J: Localization in Clinical Neurology, 6th ed. Philadelphia, Lippincott Williams & Wilkins, 2011.
3. Heilman KM, Valenstein E (eds): Clinical Neuropsychology, 5th ed. New York, Oxford University Press, 2011.
4. Lezak MD, Howieson DB, Bigler ED, et al.: Neuropsychological Assessment, 5th ed. New York, Oxford University Press, 2012.
5. Love S, Louis DN, Ellison DW (eds): Greenfield's Neuropathology, 8th ed. Boca Raton, FL, CRC Press, 2008.
6. McKee AC, Cantu RC, Nowinski CJ, Hedley-Whyte ET, Gavett BE, Budson AE, et al.: Chronic traumatic encephalopathy in athletes: progressive tauopathy following repetitive head injury. J Neuropathol Exp Neurol 68(7):709-735, 2009.
7. Mesulam MM (ed): Principles of Behavioral and Cognitive Neurology, 2nd ed. New York, Oxford University Press, 2000.
8. Sadock BJ, Sadock V, Ruiz P: Kaplan and Sadock's Synopsis of Psychiatry: Behavioral Sciences/Clinical Psychiatry, Philadelphia, Lippincott Williams & Wilkins, 2014.

CHAPTER 18

CEREBROVASCULAR DISEASE

Sharyl R. Martini, Thomas A. Kent

STROKE BASICS

1. **What is a stroke?**

   Stroke is a *focal* disturbance of blood flow into or out of the brain, either primarily ischemic (87%) or hemorrhagic (13%). Stroke is not a single disease but the end result of many different pathophysiologies leading to cerebrovascular occlusion or rupture. The key clinical feature of a stroke is *very rapid symptom onset:* "it hit me like a ton of bricks" or "like someone flipped a light switch." While the initial onset is *sudden*, symptoms may fluctuate.

2. **What is a transient ischemic attack (TIA)?**

   TIA is an abrupt onset neurologic deficit due to interruption of blood flow to a portion of the brain, followed by complete symptom resolution. If the interruption continues long enough, an ischemic stroke will result. By classic definition TIA deficits resolve within 24 hours; however, contemporary definitions define it as lasting under 1 hour. In fact, most resolve within 5 to 15 minutes. Transient neurologic symptoms of unclear etiology are most appropriately referred to as *spells*; only those thought to be due to brain ischemia should be referred to as *TIAs*.

3. **Why is prompt recognition of TIAs important?**

   TIAs herald the possibility of a completed stroke: appropriate intervention may prevent strokes and thus permanent disability. Ninety-day stroke rates for patients with TIA are >10% in some series, with the greatest risk within 48 hours to 7 days. Longer symptom duration and presence of large cerebral artery (e.g., carotid) stenosis are associated with higher risk of stroke following TIA. All patients with a recent TIA (within 2 weeks) need an expedited workup to determine cause.

4. **How common are stroke and TIA?**

   According to the Centers for Disease Control, there are more than 795,000 strokes per year in the United States, and it is the leading cause of disability. There are at least 250,000 TIAs each year in the United States, but this number is likely an underestimate because many are not reported.

5. **What types of symptoms can strokes cause?**

   Focal weakness, numbness, facial asymmetry, or speech difficulties are classic presentations. Altered level of consciousness, vertigo, and cranial nerve deficits are often seen with posterior circulation (vertebrobasilar/brain stem) and cerebellar strokes. Table 18-1 lists common stroke syndromes. Diminished level of consciousness is unusual for ischemic strokes.

6. **How are stroke and TIA diagnosed?**

   Stroke and TIA are diagnosed clinically, and no imaging correlation is required for the acute diagnosis. Imaging studies are performed to rule out other causes such as tumor and to determine whether there is brain hemorrhage. Focal neurologic deficits with sudden onset should be considered vascular (e.g., stroke or TIA) until proven otherwise because of the possibility of recurrence or progression of the deficit.

7. **What are the most important risk factors for having a stroke?**

   The biggest predictor for ischemic stroke is prior stroke, and the second biggest risk factor is age. The most important modifiable risk factor for stroke is hypertension. Other risk factors for ischemic stroke include diabetes and smoking. A lipid profile with low high-density lipoprotein and high triglycerides is also associated with ischemic stroke, whereas high low-density lipoprotein is most closely associated with cardiac disease. Cardiac diseases such as atrial fibrillation and valvular disease are ischemic stroke risk factors. The most significant risk factor for the commonest type of hemorrhagic stroke is hypertension.

KEY POINTS: STROKE BASICS

1. The main clinical feature of stroke is sudden onset of a focal neurological deficit.
2. TIA serves as a warning for a completed stroke with the greatest risk for stroke in the first 72 hours to 2 weeks following the TIA.
3. The biggest predictor of ischemic stroke is a prior stroke.
4. The most important modifiable risk factor for stroke is hypertension.

Table 18-1. Stroke Syndromes

SYNDROME	SYMPTOMS
Anterior cerebral artery	Contralateral leg > arm numbness and weakness; akinetic mutism/abulia (especially bilateral infarcts)
Middle cerebral artery	Ipsilateral eye deviation; contralateral face and arm > leg weakness, sensory loss, contralateral hemianopsia; aphasia (left) or neglect (right)
Posterior cerebral artery	Contralateral hemianopsia, memory loss
Top of the basilar	Coma or somnolence/inattention, cortical blindness
Brain stem infarction	Ataxia, vertigo, diplopia, "crossed" findings: contralateral weakness with ipsilateral cranial nerve deficits
Cerebellar infarction	Ataxia (unilateral appendicular or truncal), vertigo, nausea/vomiting
Lateral medullary (Wallenberg's) syndrome	Loss of pain and temperature sensation from the contralateral body and ipsilateral face; dysarthria, dysphagia, ataxia, hiccups
Pure motor*	Contralateral face/arm/leg weakness
Pure sensory*	Contralateral face/arm/leg sensory loss
Sensorimotor*	Contralateral face/arm/leg weakness and sensory loss
Ataxic hemiparesis*	Contralateral ataxia out of proportion to mild weakness
Clumsy hand dysarthria*	Weak face and clumsy ipsilateral hand, dysarthria, dysphagia

*The five classic lacunar syndromes result from occlusion of a single penetrating artery, which may be caused by small vessel vasculopathy, cardioembolism, or large artery atherosclerosis.

ISCHEMIC STROKE—CAUSES

8. What stroke syndromes are associated with occlusion of the cerebral arteries?
   Stroke signs and symptoms depend on the part of the brain that is damaged. Although there is person-to-person variation in arterial supply, classic syndromes are frequently seen (see Table 18-1).

9. What are the major etiologies of ischemic stroke?
   The major etiologies of ischemic stroke are (1) cardioembolism; (2) small vessel vasculopathy (arteriosclerosis, lipohyalinosis) involving the penetrating arteries branching off the middle cerebral artery, anterior cerebral artery, posterior cerebral artery, or basilar arteries; and (3) large vessel atherosclerosis due to plaque rupture involving the intracranial or extracranial cerebral arteries. Table 18-2 lists characteristics of these etiologic stroke subtypes.

10. What cardiac conditions are considered sources of cardioembolic stroke?
    Cardiac conditions associated with stroke include atrial fibrillation or flutter, mechanical valves, septic emboli, and marantic endocarditis. Patent foramen ovale (PFO) is prevalent and is not considered a likely cardioembolic source unless left-to-right shunting and a venous clot can be demonstrated.

11. What are some less common causes of ischemic stroke?
    Dissection of the cervical vessels needs to be considered, especially if there is neck/face pain or a history of trauma. Horner's syndrome may be seen with carotid injury. Illicit drug use (cocaine, stimulant-induced spasm) can be a cause of ischemic stroke. Rarer causes of stroke include hypercoagulable states (e.g., active cancer, genetic clotting disorder, or autoimmune conditions such as lupus/antiphospholipid antibody

Table 18-2. Clues to the Most Common Ischemic Stroke Etiologies

ETIOLOGY	CLINICAL FEATURES
Large vessel atherosclerosis	Plaque rupture results in *in situ* large artery thrombosis or artery-to-artery thromboembolism Often occurs in early morning hours/on waking History of TIAs in same vascular distribution Symptoms may fluctuate
Cardioembolism	History or clinical features of heart disease Stroke symptoms are maximal at onset as clot is preformed TIA symptoms are usually different from one another, representing emboli to different vascular distributions Often occurs during waking hours Can be associated with Valsalva Caused by embolism, usually from left atrial appendage (in the setting of atrial fibrillation) or left ventricle (in the case of akinetic segment) May have strokes of different ages in different vascular territories
Small vessel vasculopathy	Strong association with hypertension and diabetes Diameter <1.5 cm Occurs in subcortical regions such as basal ganglia, thalamus, or brain stem Never see cortical findings (aphasia, neglect) Symptoms may fluctuate dramatically May have TIAs with similar symptoms Occlusion of small penetrating arteries is not always due to small vessel etiology—alternate etiologies must be evaluated

TIA, Transient ischemic attack.

syndrome) and genetic disorders such as cerebral autosomal dominant arteriopathy with subcortical infarcts and leukoencephalopathy (CADASIL) and fibromuscular dysplasia. PFO remains controversial as a cause of stroke. Cases in which no specific cause is identified are called *cryptogenic*.

12. How do ischemic strokes appear on imaging?
On computed tomography (CT), most ischemic strokes eventually become visible as hypodensities of the brain parenchyma (Fig. 18-1), but CT is largely normal for at least 6 hours. The earliest CT signs are loss of the cortical ribbon and gyral edema. On magnetic resonance imaging (MRI), strokes will appear hyperintense on T2-weighted sequences. Diffusion-weighted imaging (DWI) detects cytotoxic edema that accompanies ischemic cell death and can appear very shortly after onset of ischemia. True diffusion positivity will appear dark on the apparent diffusion coefficient (ADC) map sequence. Onset of DWI positivity may be delayed up to 48 to 72 hours, particularly in the brain stem, and typically lasts 10 to 14 days. The ADC map normalizes more quickly, often 4 to 7 days after onset.

KEY POINTS: ISCHEMIC STROKE CAUSES

1. Determining stroke etiology is key to proper acute management and secondary prevention.
2. Major ischemic stroke subtypes include (1) large artery stroke due to atherosclerotic plaque rupture; (2) cardioembolism, usually due to atrial fibrillation; and (3) small vessel vasculopathy.
3. Other causes of stroke include arterial dissection, hypercoagulable state, substance abuse, and infectious/inflammatory conditions.

ISCHEMIC STROKE—ACUTE MANAGEMENT

13. What are the initial steps if ischemic stroke is suspected?
Head CT rules out hemorrhage, subdural hematoma, and tumor. It is the first and most important test when evaluating for thrombolysis. In cases of suspected stroke, page the service responsible

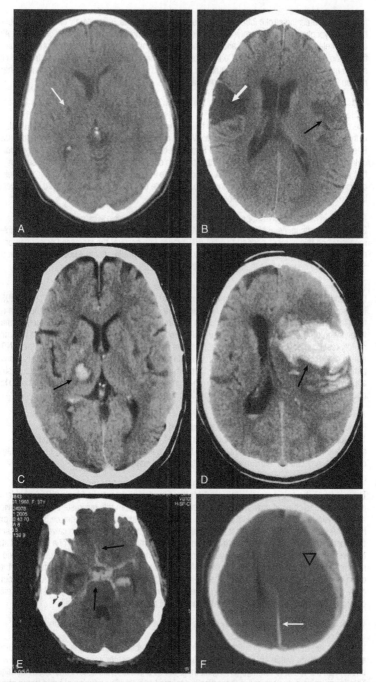

Figure 18-1. Computed tomography of strokes and stroke mimics. **A,** Lacunar ischemic stroke (*arrow*), typical of small vessel vasculopathy. **B,** Multiple ischemic strokes of different ages in different vascular territories (*arrows*), typical of cardioembolism. **C,** Subcortical intracerebral hemorrhage (*arrow*), typical of hypertensive hemorrhage. **D,** Cortical intracerebral hemorrhage (*arrow*), typical of cerebral amyloid angiopathy. **E,** Subarachnoid hemorrhage (*arrow*), typical of aneurysm rupture. **F,** Subdural hematoma (*arrowhead*) with a small amount of subarachnoid hemorrhage along the falx (*arrow*). (*From Levine G: Cardiology secrets, 4th edition, Philadelphia: Elsevier, 2014.*)

for rapidly addressing stroke (stroke team)—every minute counts. Immediately check blood glucose because hypoglycemia or hyperglycemia can cause focal neurologic deficits mimicking stroke. Also obtain an electrocardiogram (ECG) and a troponin test, as initial cardiac workup can reveal atrial fibrillation or myocardial infarction. Coagulation studies, basic chemistries, and complete blood count should be drawn, but thrombolysis should not be delayed while awaiting these results unless there is reason to suspect that they would be abnormal.

14. **What are the Food and Drug Administration (FDA)-approved treatments for acute ischemic stroke?**
The only medication currently approved by the FDA to improve outcome after acute ischemic stroke is intravenous tissue plasminogen activator (IV tPA), administered within 3 hours of symptom onset. Based on the European Cooperative Acute Stroke Study III (ECASS III), American Heart Association guidelines recommend treatment in selected patients out to 4.5 hours after symptom onset, but this extended time window was not FDA approved. The earlier IV tPA is given, the better the clinical outcome: an estimated 1 million neurons die each minute that thrombolysis is delayed. Only alteplase is approved for acute stroke thrombolysis.

15. **How much do patients benefit from tissue plasminogen activator?**
Eight stroke patients need to be treated with IV tPA to give one patient a complete or near-complete recovery, and this number-needed-to-treat (NNT) takes into account the increased risk of hemorrhage after tPA administration. Patients of any age benefit from tPA: recent studies suggest that those >80 years may benefit more than younger patients.

16. **What are contraindications to intravenous tissue plasminogen activator?**
Contraindications are based on the National Institute of Neurological Disorders and Stroke (NINDS) tPA trial: some, such as hemorrhage on CT head scan, are considered absolute, whereas others are relative (Table 18-3). The most frequent exclusion is time from when the patient was last seen normal (not when symptoms were discovered)—a particular problem for "wake-up strokes." Patients with minor/rapidly resolving deficits (possible TIAs) and seizure at stroke onset were excluded from the NINDS trial in order to avoid treating conditions that would return to baseline without thrombolysis. However, patients may be left disabled by "mild" or "improving" strokes, and seizures complicate acute strokes approximately 15% of the time. Wording on the package insert for IV tPA changed slightly in 2015. It is not yet clear whether this change will affect clinical guidelines.

17. **How are patients monitored after administration of IV tPA?**
Frequent clinical examinations are crucial, and blood pressure must be controlled to less than 180/105 mm Hg to prevent bleeding into the infarcted brain tissue. Subcutaneous heparin and antiplatelet agents are held for 24 hours, until follow-up imaging confirms absence of hemorrhagic conversion. Any change in exam warrants a stat CT head scan.

18. **When should intra-arterial (IA) therapy be used for acute ischemic stroke?**
The role for IA therapy is rapidly evolving. After three randomized controlled trials (RCTs) of older IA devices failed to show improved clinical outcomes, four RCTs primarily using stent retriever devices all demonstrated improved clinical outcomes, although it is not clear that the device is the sole explanation for the better outcomes. Most but not all patients in these recent trials received IV tPA. Each trial used different selection criteria, mostly enrolling patients without evidence of a completed stroke on imaging and residual perfusion by vascular imaging. These trials are being carefully assessed, and recommendations for the appropriate use of IA are pending. Until then, IA therapy with stent retriever devices is reasonable in patients with device-accessible proximal large vessel occlusions without early ischemic changes on brain imaging. Given the dangers of reperfusion injury and device-related complications (11% to 16%), rapid therapy and careful patient selection are vital.

19. **What if the patient is not a candidate for intravenous tissue plasminogen activator?**
In patients not treated with thrombolysis, aspirin (orally or rectally) reduces the chances of recurrent stroke when given within 48 hours. Optimal blood pressure for nonthrombolysed patients is not known but is often permitted to run high as long as there are no signs of hypertensive end-organ damage. This "permissive hypertension" is theoretically designed to increase perfusion of brain tissue at continued risk for ischemia, but it is not clear that this strategy improves outcomes. Avoid sudden drops or rises in blood pressure: relative hypotension associated with neurologic worsening should be treated with IV fluids. Lowering the head of the bed and administering vasopressors may also be considered.

Table 18-3. Contraindications to Intravenous Tissue Plasminogen Activator

Absolute Contraindications

Greater than 4.5 hours from the time patient was last seen normal

Initial head CT suggests time of onset is inaccurate

Suggestion of intracranial hemorrhage on pretreatment imaging

Subarachnoid hemorrhage

Intracerebral hemorrhage

Intracranial neoplasm or arteriovenous malformation

Active internal bleeding

Uncontrolled hypertension greater than 185/110 mm Hg despite antihypertensive treatment

Current bacterial endocarditis

Head trauma, intracranial/intraspinal surgery, or myocardial infarction within 3 months

Known bleeding diathesis:
- INR > 1.7 or PT > 15 seconds
- Platelets <100,000 mm^3
- Heparin within 48 hours if PTT is elevated
- PTT outside of the normal range
- Dose of nonwarfarin oral anticoagulant within past 12 hours

Relative Contraindications

Minor or rapidly resolving deficits

Seizure

Major surgery in the previous 2 weeks

GI or urinary hemorrhage in the previous 3 weeks

Puncture at noncompressible site within 7 days (including lumbar puncture)

PTT, Partial thromboplastin time; PT, prothrombin time; INR, international normalized ratio; GI, gastrointestinal; CT, computed tomography.

20. **What are the major clinical concerns in the initial days following an ischemic stroke?**
Clots may propagate, particularly those due to large artery atherosclerosis. Expeditious identification of this subtype is recommended. The most life-threatening complication of stroke is herniation due to cerebral edema, which manifests 12 hours to 5 days after onset. Clinical signs include somnolence, pupillary dilation from third nerve compression, and signs of increased intracranial pressure (nausea, vomiting). Herniation may occur either upward or downward through the tentorium or under the falx cerebri. Large hemispheric and cerebellar strokes are most likely to cause herniation. Manipulation of serum osmolarity (mannitol, hypertonic saline) or hyperventilation may be used, though definitive treatment is surgical decompression.

21. **When is hemicraniectomy recommended?**
Patients with malignant middle cerebral artery occlusion are at risk of death from cerebral edema and herniation. Every 2 hemicraniectomy procedures for malignant MCA infarction saves 1 life. Although fewer people die, less than 10% achieve functional independence. Surgical decompression is often suggested for large strokes within the cerebellar hemispheres as patients tend to recover well from these strokes if they survive the acute period. Early consultation with neurosurgery is suggested.

22. **What is hemorrhagic transformation (hemorrhagic conversion)?**
Ischemic strokes can develop a hemorrhagic component, especially if they are large or if the degree of ischemia is severe. This hemorrhagic transformation occurs because all tissue downstream of an ischemic stroke becomes ischemic—brain and vasculature. In many cases, blood flow to the ischemic area is reestablished too late to benefit the brain and returns via weakened, damaged vessels. These vessels may leak, resulting in petechial hemorrhage, or burst, resulting in a hematoma. Hemorrhagic transformation is most likely in the first days to a week after stroke. This is why clinical worsening in an ischemic stroke patient should be immediately evaluated with noncontrast head CT.

KEY POINTS: ISCHEMIC STROKE ACUTE MANAGEMENT

1. Noncontrast CT is used acutely to rule out hemorrhage or tumor (not to diagnose stroke).
2. For IV tPA eligibility, stroke onset is defined as the time the patient was last seen normal, not when he or she was discovered to have symptoms.
3. Clinical deterioration in the acute period following stroke may be due to clot propagation (large vessel subtype), cerebral edema/herniation, or hemorrhagic transformation.

ISCHEMIC STROKE—WORKUP AND MANAGEMENT

23. **What are the goals of hospitalization for an ischemic stroke?**
The goals of stroke hospitalization are to (1) prevent complications such as stroke progression, aspiration pneumonia, and pulmonary embolism; (2) develop a plan for functional recovery with the help of physical, occupational, and speech therapy; and (3) determine the stroke mechanism in order design an optimal secondary stroke prevention strategy.

24. **How can systemic complications of stroke be prevented?**
In all cases of stroke, ensure adequate deep vein thrombosis (DVT) prophylaxis to prevent pulmonary emboli. Keep patients nil per os (NPO) until safe swallowing can be confirmed to prevent aspiration and subsequent pneumonia. Frequent turning prevents skin breakdown. Catheters should be removed as soon as possible. Patients should be mobilized as soon as safely possible, although many are at high risk of falls and may need constant supervision—those with neglect in particular as they are unaware of their deficits.

25. **What is considered a complete ischemic stroke workup?**
Patients with anterior circulation strokes need urgent carotid imaging. Intracranial as well as extracranial imaging is performed in most cases. MRI is useful for detecting strokes not apparent on head CT: small strokes in multiple vascular distributions point to a cardioembolic source. In patients with suspected cardioembolism, echocardiogram (ECG) is indicated. All patients should have telemetry for atrial fibrillation identification—ECGs are inadequate for detection of this important risk factor. Implantable event monitors reveal subclinical atrial fibrillation in a substantial proportion of patients with cryptogenic stroke and are warranted in cases where clinical suspicion is high.

26. **How would stroke workup differ for a young person or someone without the usual stroke risk factors?**
Stroke workup in the young patient begins with a detailed history including personal or family history of clotting, autoimmune disease, trauma, and cardiac disease. Careful examination of eyes and skin may provide clues to neurofibromatosis, Fabry's disease, connective tissue diseases, or endocarditis. As young stroke patients are more likely to have cardiac abnormalities, a detailed cardiac evaluation including transesophageal echo should be performed. MRI brain, vessel imaging, and hypercoagulable workup are standard, as are toxicology, autoimmune, and vasculitis labs (erythrocyte sedimentation rate, C-reactive protein, antinuclear antibody, antineutrophil cytoplasmic antibody, rheumatoid factor, complement). Rapid plasma reagin and human immunodeficiency virus testing are vital. Lumbar puncture may reveal additional infectious or inflammatory conditions.

27. **What is a hypercoagulable workup?**
Family history of clotting, miscarriages, or a paucity of vascular risk factors should raise suspicion for a hypercoagulable state. Hormone use (oral contraceptives, testosterone replacement, hormone replacement) is associated with an increased thrombotic risk and should be specifically sought from history. Laboratory tests include antithrombin III, protein C, protein S, activated protein C resistance/ factor V Leiden mutation, and prothrombin mutation. Lupus anticoagulant and anticardiolipin or beta2 glycoprotein antibodies point to antiphospholipid antibody syndrome. Cancer produces a hypercoagulable state, so malignancy evaluation should be considered.

28. **What is the best strategy to prevent additional strokes?**
The best strategy depends on the causative etiology: options for carotid stenosis, intracranial stenosis, and atrial fibrillation are presented below. Small vessel disease secondary stroke prevention relies solely on aggressive risk factor management. Goals for secondary stroke prevention include target blood pressure <140/90, antiplatelet or anticoagulant as appropriate, statin, hemoglobin A1C <7, smoking cessation, regular exercise, and BMI <25. Obstructive sleep is associated with increased stroke risk independent of its association with hypertension, so treatment seems prudent.

29. **What options exist for evaluating cerebral vessels?**
Carotid duplex ultrasound is cost-effective but inadequate for evaluation of intracranial vessels or the posterior circulation. Transcranial Doppler ultrasound evaluates intracranial vessels but is operator dependent and not widely available. CT angiogram is fast, readily available, and provides detailed information from the aortic arch to the intracranial vessels. Disadvantages include radiation exposure and the need for iodinated contrast. MR angiogram also evaluates the entire cerebrovascular tree, although motion artifacts can obscure the arch and great vessel origins. Its major disadvantage is the need to lie still for 30 to 45 minutes. Gadolinium-based contrast agents provide additional resolution but cannot be given in renal insufficiency due to the possibility of systemic sclerosis.

30. **How should carotid stenosis be managed?**
Patients with symptomatic carotid stenosis >70% should be treated with carotid endarterectomy (CEA) or stenting within 2 weeks of a TIA or nondisabling stroke: risk of recurrent stroke is 15% per year, and CEA cuts it in half. Patients with 50% to 70% symptomatic stenosis benefit less from carotid intervention but have the same upfront procedure risk. Asymptomatic patients with ≥60% stenosis have a 2% to 4% annual stroke rate that is cut in half after CEA; however, upfront risk of death or stroke from the procedure is 3% to 6%, so overall benefit is less than for symptomatic disease. The Carotid Revascularization Endarterectomy versus Stenting Trial (CREST) comparing CEA with stenting showed higher stroke and death rates in the stenting group, but higher myocardial infarction rates with CEA: overall rates of the combined endpoint were not different. Older patients fared better with CEA than carotid stenting, and quality of life was better in those with myocardial infarction than in those with stroke.

31. **How should intracranial stenosis be managed?**
In the Stenting and Aggressive Medical Management for Preventing Recurrent stroke in Intracranial Stenosis (SAMMPRIS) trial, patients with recent mild stroke or TIA due to 70% to 99% intracranial stenosis were randomized to stenting plus aggressive medical management, versus aggressive medical management alone. All subjects received aspirin plus clopidogrel for 90 days, followed by aspirin alone. In addition to blood pressure and lipid goals, lifestyle coaches developed goals for weight loss, regular exercise, and smoking cessation with each participant. The trial was stopped early because 14.7% in the stenting arm had a stroke within 30 days (most within 1 day of stenting) compared with 5.8% in the medical management group; 1-year stroke rates were 20% and 12.2%, respectively. As such, intracranial atherosclerosis is now managed medically.

32. **What if the patient has a PFO?**
PFOs are present in up to 25% of the population and in most cases confer little if any stroke risk. Large PFOs with a right-to-left shunt and those with atrial septal aneurysms are of greater concern. If a concerning PFO is found the next step is to identify a venous source. Pelvic vein MRI may identify DVTs not apparent by standard vascular ultrasound techniques. PFO closure has been hotly debated: CLOSURE I compared PFO closure to best medical management in subjects with cryptogenic stroke and did not find a benefit of PFO closure after 2 years of follow-up. Most subjects with recurrent stroke had evidence of a mechanism other than paradoxical embolism. At this point, PFO closure is best done in the setting of an RCT.

33. **How well do anticoagulants work to prevent stroke in the setting of atrial fibrillation?**
All patients with stroke and atrial fibrillation merit consideration for long-term anticoagulation because it reduces ischemic stroke by more than 60%. Other high-risk groups include those age >75 (especially women), and those with poorly controlled hypertension, diabetes, poor left ventricular function, or recent heart failure. The CHA_2DS_2-VASc risk stratification scheme integrates risk factors to assist in the decision for anticoagulation therapy: the greater the number of risk factors, the higher the risk of stroke. Stroke or TIA automatically places a patient in the high-risk category, so secondary prevention of stroke in patients with atrial fibrillation should involve oral anticoagulation unless there is a contraindication.

34. **Do patients who have ablation or surgery for atrial fibrillation still need anticoagulation?**
Restoring sinus rhythm, resecting the left atrial appendage, and transcatheter closure of the left atrial appendage opening have thus far not demonstrated a sufficient reduction of stroke risk to warrant discontinuing anticoagulation. Atrial Fibrillation Follow-up Investigation of Rhythm Management (AFFIRM) found that restoring sinus rhythm did not reduce stroke risk. The Watchman trial similarly

did not find a reduction in stroke risk; additional device trials are ongoing. The Left Atrial Appendage Occlusion Study III is an ongoing phase 3 trial comparing surgical excision of the left atrial appendage with best medical therapy. At this time, anticoagulation is the only intervention proven to reduce stroke in the setting of atrial fibrillation.

35. **What about anticoagulation in patients at high risk for bleeding?**
Although elderly patients are at high risk for bleeding they are also at high risk for stroke from atrial fibrillation; thus, age is not a contraindication to anticoagulation. Contraindications include history of severe gastrointestinal (GI) bleeding, history of falls, or an extremely high fall risk. The HAS-BLED score is a simple method for assessing bleeding risk. After stroke, many patients are at risk for falls: as they recover, reconsider anticoagulation. The decision for anticoagulation should be an ongoing collaborative discussion of the risks, benefits, and monitoring schedule so that the patient can make an informed decision.

36. **What is the role of the new anticoagulants (dabigatran, rivaroxaban, apixaban)?**
New oral anticoagulants include the direct thrombin inhibitor dabigatran and the factor Xa inhibitors apixaban and rivaroxaban. The benefit of these agents over warfarin is due to better stroke prevention as well as lower bleeding risk. Intracerebral hemorrhage, the most dreaded complication of anticoagulation, was substantially reduced. Dabigatran and rivaroxaban had higher rates of GI bleeding than warfarin; apixaban showed no such trend. Dabigatran showed a small but consistent increase in myocardial infarction, although it decreased overall vascular events and mortality. One disadvantage is a higher risk of thrombotic events when these agents are stopped, so patients must be extremely compliant. Significant renal impairment is a contraindication.

37. **How soon after a stroke should anticoagulation be started?**
Large strokes and those due to cardioembolism are most likely to bleed. As such, it is common practice to wait 1 month after a large stroke before initiating anticoagulation for atrial fibrillation. Patients with very small cardioembolic strokes may be started on anticoagulation within 1 to 2 days. In patients with large strokes at high risk for embolization (mechanical valves, cardiac thrombus), anticoagulation may be started cautiously after 5 to 15 days. Retrospective data suggest bridging with heparin or low-molecular-weight heparin causes more bleeding. In the absence of a hypercoagulable state, it is acceptable to start warfarin at low doses to achieve therapeutic anticoagulation slowly. Some clinicians suggest aspirin until an international normalized ratio (INR) of 2 is achieved.

38. **How are antiplatelet agents used after stroke?**
Patients who do not meet criteria for anticoagulation should receive antiplatelet therapy: aspirin, clopidogrel, or extended-release dipyridamole plus aspirin. All are similarly efficacious, decreasing stroke risk 14% to 18%. Ensuring adherence is probably more important than the agent used, so choice should be guided by comorbidities, tolerability, and cost. Clopidogrel may be preferred for patients with peripheral vascular disease, chronic nonsteroidal antiinflammatory drug use, or drug-eluting stents. Aspirin is a good choice when not contraindicated, particularly for patients on proton pump inhibitors or when the cost of alternatives would hinder compliance. Antiplatelet therapy should be initiated immediately in patients who are not tPA candidates and do not have any hemorrhagic component. Wait 24 hours after tPA to start antiplatelet medications.

39. **Should aspirin and clopidogrel be used together for stroke prevention?**
Aspirin should not be combined with clopidogrel for long-term secondary stroke prevention due to unacceptably high bleeding risk without additional protection from strokes (SPS3 [Secondary Prevention of Small Subcortical Strokes] and MATCH (Management of Atherothrombosis with Clopidogrel in High-risk patients) trials). The CHANCE (Clopidogrel in High-risk patients with Acute Nondisabling Cerebrovascular Events) trial found that aspirin plus clopidogrel for the 21 days after stroke reduced the odds of a second stroke within 90 days. Most participants were from China where blood pressure control is less frequently achieved. In the absence of definitive data, either short-term dual antiplatelets or a single antiplatelet agent may be used for secondary stroke prevention. Patients on dual antiplatelets for other indications may be continued on this combination after stroke with the understanding that bleeding risk may be elevated.

40. **Should aspirin be added to anticoagulation?**
In patients requiring anticoagulation, bleeding risk increases with the addition of antiplatelet agents. Except in cases of unstable coronary disease or mechanical valves, this increased bleeding risk is not offset by a decrease in thrombotic events. Because ischemic stroke and intracerebral hemorrhage

increase dramatically with age, patients presenting with stroke are quite different from those presenting with acute coronary syndromes. As such, it is not valid to extrapolate stroke secondary prevention from cardiac studies, as the MATCH trial exemplified. The decision to add aspirin to anticoagulation is a difficult one, best made collaboratively among patient, neurologist, and cardiologist.

41. **What if a patient has a stroke while taking an antiplatelet agent?**
The notion of treatment "failure" has been proposed if a patient has a stroke or TIA while on a specific agent. Genetic variation in antiplatelet response has been convincingly established for clopidogrel and suggested for aspirin, but genetic testing is not routinely used in the selection of antiplatelet agents. Currently, only limited retrospective data support changing to a different antiplatelet agent after stroke. In the absence of definitive data, it may be more fruitful to address risk factor reduction strategies and medication adherence. The role of laboratory platelet inhibition measures in choice of antiplatelet agent remains to be established.

42. **How well do patients recover following ischemic stroke?**
Younger patients and those with smaller strokes tend to recover better, but there is remarkable person-to-person variation. The best predictor of how a person will recover is the initial stroke severity and the trajectory of recovery within the first weeks following the stroke. Much of the recovery occurs within the first month, and the majority of recovery is complete by 3 months. Recovery occurs after 3 months, especially for higher cortical function such as language, but at a slower pace. In cases of motor weakness, recovery usually begins proximally and moves distally as recovery progresses. The FLAME (Family Lifestyle, Activity, Movement and Eating) study found that fluoxetine initiated within 5 to 10 days of ischemic stroke was associated with lower rates of depression and improved motor recovery.

43. **What are additional considerations when stroke patients return for follow-up?**
Stroke follow-up visits should address new neurologic symptoms, stroke risk factors, depression, and recovery. New neurologic symptoms may represent stroke, TIA, or seizure. Those with ongoing paralysis should be assessed for conditions that may adversely affect their recovery including depression, spasticity, shoulder subluxation or frozen shoulder, and post-stroke pain. Complex regional pain syndrome is characterized by intermittent symptoms (cold feeling, purplish mottled skin, swelling) in the areas affected by the stroke.

KEY POINTS: ISCHEMIC STROKE WORKUP AND MANAGEMENT

1. Diffusion-weighted MRI can identify cytotoxic edema from ischemic strokes but may be negative in small strokes or TIAs.
2. CT angiogram or MR angiogram can suggest stroke etiology by identifying arterial thrombus, dissection, or atherosclerotic stenosis.
3. Symptomatic carotid stenosis requires urgent intervention; asymptomatic carotid stenosis does not.
4. For strokes due to atrial fibrillation, anticoagulation decreases risk of a subsequent stroke by 60%.

HEMORRHAGIC STROKE SUBTYPES

44. **What are the major types of hemorrhagic strokes?**
Hemorrhagic strokes include subarachnoid hemorrhage (SAH, usually due to aneurysm rupture) and parenchymal intracerebral hemorrhage (ICH). Overall, approximately 6% of strokes are due to deep ICH, 3% are due to lobar ICH, and 3% are due to SAH. Although ischemic strokes are more frequent, hemorrhagic strokes have a higher morbidity and mortality. Because subdural and epidural hematomas are extra-axial, these bleeds are not considered strokes (see Fig. 18-1).

45. **How can you distinguish hemorrhagic from ischemic strokes?**
Clinical clues pointing to a hemorrhagic etiology include an early diminished level of consciousness and worsening of symptoms over minutes to hours. Headache is more common in hemorrhagic stroke and is the cardinal feature of SAH. Head CT is the most reliable way to distinguish ischemic and hemorrhagic strokes, with acute hemorrhage appearing hyperdense (see Fig. 18-1).

46. **Why is the location of an intraparenchymal hemorrhage important?**
Intraparenchymal ICHs are classified by their location: deep or subcortical ICHs are associated with uncontrolled hypertension in 60% of cases; lobar or cortical ICHs are more concerning for underlying mass, arteriovenous malformation, or cerebral amyloid angiopathy.

47. **What is the typical clinical profile of a hypertensive hemorrhage?**
Hypertensive hemorrhages occur most frequently in patients with a history of poorly controlled hypertension. They are associated with small vessel ischemic changes and microbleeds of the basal ganglia, deep white matter, brain stem, and cerebellum. These hemorrhages occur more frequently and at younger ages in black and Hispanic individuals.

48. **What is the typical clinical profile of cerebral amyloid angiopathy?**
Cerebral amyloid angiopathy (CAA) is most common in elderly Caucasian individuals. It is associated with Alzheimer's disease, particularly in those carrying the ApoE4 allele. CAA hemorrhages have a predilection for the occipital cortex but may occur in any cortical region.

49. **How is ICH managed?**
ICHs are managed by reversing coagulopathy. Clot evacuation for lobar ICHs and ventriculostomy in cases with hydrocephalus or intraventricular blood may be considered. Intraventricular clot lysis with tPA is being studied. High blood pressure is associated with hematoma expansion and rebleeding, so systolic blood pressure is maintained below 180 mm Hg. The INTERACT (intensive blood pressure Reduction in Acute Cerebral haemorrhage Trial) and ATACH (Antihypertensive Treatment of Acute Cerebral Hemorrhage) trial have found that further lowering systolic blood pressure to 140 mm Hg is safe and feasible, but clinical benefit has not been demonstrated. DVTs are common following ICH, and pneumatic compression devices are more effective than compression stockings alone. Some practitioners add subcutaneous heparin after 48 hours.

50. **What is considered a complete workup for ICH?**
The urgency and possibly extent of workup will depend on the clinical scenario: an octogenarian with Alzheimer's disease and an occipital ICH may require less etiologic workup than would a 65-year-old with a basal ganglia ICH and decades of poorly controlled hypertension. Cases that do not fit these profiles require vessel imaging to evaluate for arteriovenous malformations (AVMs) or aneurysms and MRI with contrast to evaluate for tumors. Aneurysm rupture can cause intraparenchymal hemorrhage, so it is important to consider SAH as well as cerebral venous sinus thrombosis (see below). If initial workup is unrevealing, repeat studies after the hematoma has resolved (2 to 3 months) may be useful.

51. **What causes SAH?**
SAH can be traumatic but is commonly caused by a ruptured berry aneurysm. Hypertension, larger size (especially >7 mm), and posterior circulation location are associated with aneurysm rupture. Hypertension and smoking contribute to aneurysm growth. Polycystic kidney disease and inherited connective tissue defects are also associated with intracranial aneurysms.

52. **How is SAH diagnosed?**
SAH due to aneurysm rupture classically presents with the worst headache of one's life; loss of consciousness, nausea/vomiting, nuchal rigidity, and focal neurologic signs are also common. Although large amounts of subarachnoid blood are readily apparent on CT, even small amounts of subarachnoid blood can provoke symptoms. Detection of these small "sentinel bleeds" are vital, as they herald aneurysm rupture. Sensitivity of CT declines with time from symptom onset, so spinal fluid should be examined for red blood cells or xanthochromia if head CT is negative and clinical suspicion high. Because of its ready availability, CT angiogram is often performed acutely in lieu of conventional angiogram for surgical planning.

53. **How is SAH managed?**
SAH is managed by securing the aneurysm as soon as possible and monitoring for vasospasm in an intensive care unit setting for up to 2 weeks. Vasospasm may be evaluated by transcranial Doppler or CT angiogram. Cardiac arrhythmias are common following SAH. Pneumatic compression devices and subcutaneous heparinoid (once the aneurysm is secure) are used for DVT prophylaxis.

CEREBRAL VENOUS SINUS THROMBOSIS

54. **What causes cerebral venous sinus thrombosis (CVST)?**
CVST is caused by clot formation in large draining veins or dural sinuses. Congenital or acquired hypercoagulable states, dehydration, and oral contraceptive use are associated with CVST.

55. How is CVST diagnosed?

CVSTs usually present with continuous headache, worse in the morning or after lying down. If intracranial pressure is elevated, patients may experience impaired consciousness or blurry vision due to cerebral edema and subsequent papilledema. Venous infarctions are frequently hemorrhagic and can result in focal neurologic signs and symptoms that do not respect typical arterial distributions. Seizures are common and may be a presenting symptom. A high index of suspicion is needed to diagnose and appropriately treat CVST, as cases may be easily missed during the course of a standard ischemic or hemorrhagic stroke workup. CVST is diagnosed with CT or MR venogram.

56. How is CVST managed?

Venous sinus thrombosis is most commonly managed by anticoagulation, which may be counterintuitive in cases of venous infarction with hemorrhage. Other options include mechanical thrombectomy and intrasinus thrombolysis, especially if the patient is worsening despite anticoagulation. This is a fairly uncommon condition, so no RCTs have been performed to compare treatment strategies.

KEY POINTS: HEMORRHAGIC STROKE AND CEREBRAL VENOUS SINUS THROMBOSIS

1. Hemorrhagic strokes are more likely to be fatal than ischemic strokes.
2. Hemorrhagic stroke location suggests etiology: deep = hypertensive; lobar = CAA, AVM, or tumor; SAH = aneurysm rupture or trauma.
3. Clinically hemorrhagic strokes present with headache, diminished level of consciousness, and (in the case of SAH) meningeal signs.
4. CVST may cause venous infarction—often hemorrhagic—which is treated with anticoagulation.

 References available online at expertconsult.com.

WEBSITES

http://www.merck.com/mmpe
http://emedicine.medscape.com

BIBLIOGRAPHY

1. Martini SR, Grossman AW, Kent TA: Stroke. In Levine GN (ed): Color Atlas of Cardiovascular Disease, Philadelphia, Jaypee Brothers Medical Publishers, 2015.

CHAPTER 19

NEUROCRITICAL CARE

Pramod Gupta, Jose I. Suarez

INTRODUCTION

1. **What is neurocritical care?**
   Neurocritical care is a branch of critical care medicine that deals with the intensive care management of patients with life-threatening disorders due to either neurologic and neurosurgical illnesses or other systemic diseases affecting the central nervous system (CNS), the peripheral nervous system, or both. Neurocritical care provides the interface between the brain and other organ systems in the setting of critical illness. One of the main goals of treatment is the prevention of secondary CNS insults to prevent further damage.

2. **What is a neurointensivist?**
   A neurointensivist is an intensivist who specializes in the care of the neurocritically ill patient. Care of the neurocritically ill patient also includes prognostication of neurologic outcome and brain death determination. Neurointensivists may come from a number of medical and surgical backgrounds including neurology, neurosurgery, internal medicine, anesthesiology, emergency medicine, and pediatrics.

3. **What are the most common diseases treated in a neurocritical care unit?**
   The most common clinical disorders in the neurocritical care unit are ischemic stroke, intracerebral hemorrhage, subarachnoid hemorrhage, brain tumors, brain trauma, status epilepticus (SE), neuromuscular emergencies (e.g., myasthenia gravis crisis, Guillain–Barré syndrome), spinal cord injury, infection of brain and spinal cord, and the cardiopulmonary complications of brain injury.

GENERAL MANAGEMENT IN THE NEUROCRITICAL CARE UNIT

AIRWAY MANAGEMENT

Airway management is the first step in the evaluation and resuscitation of the critically ill patient (Table 19-1).

4. **How do we evaluate airway?**
   The initial evaluation includes an assessment of airway patency, protective reflexes, respiratory drive, and oxygenation. A depressed level of consciousness (defined as a Glasgow Coma Scale [GCS] score <8) is the greatest risk factor for airway obstruction and aspiration.

5. **When should a patient be intubated?**
   Common general indications for endotracheal intubation include the following: either cardiac or respiratory arrest; failure to protect the airway; inadequate oxygenation or ventilation; and impending or existing airway obstruction.

6. **What are the goals of ventilator management?**
   The goals are to reverse apnea, respiratory distress, severe hypoxemia, and hypercapnia. These goals can be accomplished either invasively (i.e., tracheal intubation) or noninvasively (i.e., noninvasive positive pressure ventilation [NIVPPV] used for chronic obstructive pulmonary disease exacerbation with hypercapnia, pulmonary edema, myasthenia gravis crisis, and at home for amyotrophic lateral sclerosis).

7. **What are the modes of ventilation?**
   There are four basic modes of assisted ventilation: assist control, synchronized intermittent mandatory ventilation, pressure support (PSV), and continuous positive airway pressure (CPAP).

8. **What are the targets of ventilation modes?**
   There are two targets of ventilation modes:
   1. Volume targeted in which the ventilator delivers a set tidal volume (Vt); and
   2. Pressure targeted in which the ventilator delivers a fixed inspiratory pressure.

9. **How can ventilator settings be adjusted to improve oxygenation?**
   Increase either fraction of inspired oxygen (FiO_2) or positive end-expiratory pressure (PEEP).

Table 19-1. General Management of the Neurocritically Ill Patient

	GENERAL	ISCHEMIC STROKE	ICH	SAH	TBI
Blood pressure goal	BP >100/80 MAP >70	BP <220/120 with no thrombolytics BP <180/105 after thrombolytics for 24 hours	BP <160/100	BP <160/100 for unsecured aneurysm BP >160-220/100 for secured aneurysm	SBP >90
Target	Oxygen delivery	Save penumbra	Avoid hematoma expansion	Avoid rebleeding	Avoid ischemia
Volume status	Euvolemia	Euvolemia	Euvolemia	Euvolemia	Euvolemia
DVT prophylaxis*	On admission unless contraindicated	Within 24 hours if no thrombolytics >24 hours with thrombolytics	Low dose 1-4 days after onset	24 hours after aneurysm repair	Timing unknown
Seizure prophylaxis	Not needed	Not needed unless documented seizure	Not needed unless documented seizure	3-7 days (avoid phenytoin)	7 days
Fever	Normothermia	Normothermia	Normothermia	Normothermia	Normothermia
Glucose	<180 (NICE SUGAR trial)	Not known, recommend normoglycemia	140-180 mg/dL based on (NICE SUGAR trial)	Not known, 80-200 mg/dL	Avoid hypoglycemia

ICH, Intracranial hemorrhage; SAH, subarachnoid hemorrhage; TBI, traumatic brain injury; BP, blood pressure; MAP, mean arterial pressure; SBP, systolic blood pressure; DVT, deep vein thrombosis.
*Sequential compression device (SCD) on all patients and heparin 5000 U SQ bid if <60 kg or tid if >60 kg or enoxaparin 40 SQ mg daily adjusted for renal function.

10. **How can ventilator settings be adjusted to remove carbon dioxide in hypercapnia?**
    The most efficient way is to increase minute ventilation, which represents the total volume of gas passing into and out of the lungs per minute and is calculated by multiplying respiratory rate (RR) × Vt. Thus, you can increase RR, Vt, or both.

11. **What is the lung protective strategy to prevent ventilator-induced lung injury?**
    The goal of the lung protective strategy is to improve alveoli recruitment while limiting derecruitment and overdistention. Currently, there is wide consensus that Vt restriction to 6 mL/kg ideal body weight and/or plateau airway pressures (PPlat) limited below 30 cm H_2O may prevent lung injury. Vt could be decreased to a minimal value of 4 mL/kg of predicted body weight in both groups in case of PPlat higher than 32 cm H_2O, or it could be increased to a maximal value of 8 mL/kg of predicted body weight in case of severe acidosis defined as arterial pH lower than 7.15. Patients with intracranial processes pose a unique challenge since carbon dioxide elevations can lead to increased intracranial pressure (ICP). Therefore, these patients need to be monitored closely and their ICP measured.

12. **What are the criteria to wean from ventilators?**
    It is important to wean patients from mechanical ventilation as soon as possible to minimize the risk of ventilator-associated pneumonia. In general, the following criteria need to be met to ensure successful ventilator weaning and extubation:
    • The cause of respiratory failure has been reversed or is improving;
    • Patient is breathing spontaneously;

- Patient is awake and alert or is easily arousable and cooperative;
- Sedation has been discontinued;
- Patient has achieved hemodynamic stability;
- Patient has adequate cough and minimal secretions;
- Adequate oxygenation is present, defined as a partial pressure of O_2 in arterial blood (PaO_2)/FiO_2 ratio >150 to 200; requiring PEEP ≤5 to 8 cm H_2O; FiO_2 ≤0.4 to 0.5; and pH (e.g., ≥7.25); and
- Rapid shallow breathing index (RSBI) <105. RSBI is calculated as RR/Vt (L). A value of >105 breaths/min/L predicts weaning failure (negative predictive value 95%).

A successful spontaneous breathing trial (SBT) with PSV of ≤5 or T piece for 30 to 120 minutes is currently thought to be the best predictor of successful weaning. SBT must be performed once a day.

GASTROINTESTINAL MANAGEMENT

13. What agents are used for peptic ulcer prophylaxis?
Famotidine is the first line of treatment. Pantoprazole should be used if the patient is already on a proton pump inhibitor at home or has gastrointestinal bleeding.

14. What bowel regimen should be used?
Docusate, senna, polyethylene glycol, bisacodyl, and lactulose on an as needed basis are acceptable medications used either individually or in combination.

15. How are nutrition and electrolytes managed?
- Nutritional support is indicated for any critically ill patient who cannot take oral feeds and in whom oral intake is not expected to cover the full energy needs. There are two routes for nutrition administration in these patients, enteral and parenteral. Enteral nutrition is always the first choice and should be started 24 hours after intensive care unit (ICU) admission if no procedures are planned. Parenteral nutrition should be restricted to those situations in which there are contraindications to enteral nutrition.
- Electrolytes: Electrolyte imbalances need to be worked up and corrected aggressively. Refeeding syndrome must be recognized in severe protein–calorie malnutrition, bearing in mind that hypophosphatemia is the hallmark of biochemical abnormality. Correction of hypophosphatemia should precede feeding.

TEMPERATURE MANAGEMENT

16. What are the workup and management of fever in the ICU?
Fever is defined as a core temperature above 38.3° C. Fever has been associated with worse neurologic outcome in brain injury patients. Ventilator-associated pneumonia, catheter-related sepsis, and sinusitis are the three major causes of ICU fever of recent onset. Antipyretic agents (acetaminophen alone or in combination with ibuprofen for central fever) are the first line of therapy. Surface cooling devices are more effective and should be used if drug therapy fails. Antishivering medications may be used as needed (Fig. 19-1).

MULTIMODALITY NEUROMONITORING

17. What systemic hemodynamic monitoring is indicated in patients with acute brain injury?
See Table 19-2.

18. What are the different hemodynamic parameters in the etiology of shock?
See Table 19-3.

19. What are the ways to monitor the brain during acute brain injury?
Clinically: The serial neurologic examination is still the best option.
Physiologically: ICP and cerebral blood flow (CBF).
- **ICP:** Both intraparenchymal monitors and ventricular catheters measure ICP and indirectly measure cerebral perfusion pressure (CPP). ICP and CPP monitoring are recommended in patients who are at risk of elevated ICP based on clinical and/or imaging features. Refractory ICP elevation is a strong predictor of mortality.

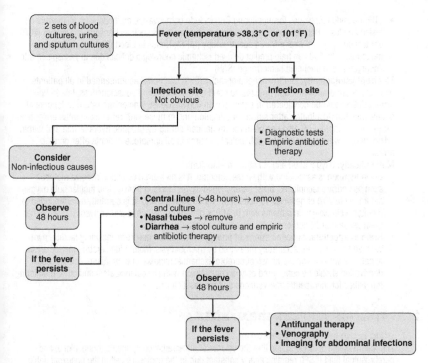

Figure 19-1. Approach to the febrile patient in the intensive care unit (ICU). *(From Dimopoulos G, Falagas ME: Approach to the febrile patient in the ICU.* Infect Dis Clin North Am *23(3):471-484, 2009.)*

Table 19-2. Systemic Hemodynamic Monitoring	
NONINVASIVE	**INVASIVE**
ECG	Invasive blood pressure monitoring
Arterial blood pressure	Central venous pressure monitoring
Pulse oximetry	Mixed venous oxygen (SvO$_2$) and serum lactate
Transthoracic echocardiogram (baseline when signs of cardiac dysfunction)	Arterial pressure waveform-derived (PiCCO, LiDCO) for cardiac output monitoring

Table 19-3. Hemodynamic Parameters in Different Shock			
ETIOLOGY OF SHOCK	**CARDIAC OUTPUT (CO)**	**EJECTION FRACTION (EF)**	**MIXED VENOUS OXYGEN (SVO$_2$)**
Hypovolemic	↓	Normal/↑	↓
Cardiogenic	↓	↓	↓
Sepsis	Normal/↓	↓	Normal/↑
Obstructive	↓	↓	↓

- **CBF:** Bedside techniques for monitoring CBF include both invasive methods such as thermal diffusion and laser Doppler flowmetry and noninvasive methods such as transcranial Doppler (TCD) ultrasonography and near infrared spectroscopy (NIRS). Trends in blood flow velocity changes measured with TCD can help predict delayed ischemic neurologic deficits due to vasospasm after aneurysmal subarachnoid hemorrhage (SAH).

Electrophysiologically: Electroencephalography (EEG) has been recommended in all patients with any acute brain insult and unexplained and persistent altered consciousness. In addition, urgent EEG should be considered in patients with convulsive SE who do not return to functional baseline within 60 minutes after seizure medication and in those with refractory status epilepticus (RSE). Furthermore, EEG also has been recommended during therapeutic hypothermia and within 24 hours of rewarming to exclude subclinical seizures in all comatose patients after cardiac arrest.

Metabolically: Oxygenation and substrate metabolism.

- **Brain hypoxia** is associated with worse outcome. It is measured by either invasive methods such as bedside techniques, brain parenchymal oxygen tension (PbtO$_2$), and jugular bulb oxygen saturation (SjvO$_2$) or noninvasive bedside methods such as NIRS. It is currently recommended to monitor brain oxygen in patients with or at risk of cerebral ischemia and/or hypoxia using either brain tissue (PbtO$_2$) and/or jugular venous bulb oximetry (SjvO$_2$).
- **Brain extracellular concentrations of energy metabolism markers**, including lactate, pyruvate, and glucose, are accurately measured by microdialysis. Monitoring cerebral microdialysis in patients with or who are at risk of cerebral ischemia, hypoxia, energy failure, and glucose deprivation should be considered only in combination with clinical indicators and other monitoring modalities for therapeutic interventions and prognostication.

ELEVATED ICP AND CEREBRAL EDEMA

20. What is the Monro–Kellie doctrine?

The Monro–Kellie doctrine states that the volume of intracranial components (brain, blood, and cerebrospinal fluid [CSF]) remains nearly constant due to the enclosure within the nonexpandable skull, after closure of the fontanelles. Additional volume will lead to the displacement of another of the contents and results in increased ICP.

21. What is elevated ICP?

The normal ICP ranges from 5 to 15 mm Hg (7.5 to 20 cm H$_2$O) in an adult and 3 to 7 mm Hg (4 to 9.5 cm H$_2$O) in children. The threshold that defines intracranial hypertension is uncertain but generally is considered to be >20 cm H$_2$O for >10 minutes.

22. What is the Cushing's triad?

The Cushing's response, the classic triad of severe hypertension, bradycardia, and irregular respiration, occurs during terminal brain herniation.

23. What are the different herniation syndromes?

See Table 19-4.

24. What is the threshold for intervention to reduce ICP?

When ICP is >20 cm H$_2$O for >10 minutes or when there are clinical signs of herniation.

25. What is CPP?

CPP is the driving arterial pressure gradient across the cerebral vasculature and is defined as the difference between the mean arterial pressure (MAP) and ICP.

$$[CPP = MAP - ICP]$$

The CPP goal is patient specific, and hence it is debatable. Based on studies, the recommended goal is 50 to 70 mm Hg, and values <50 mm Hg are associated with ischemia and poor outcome.

26. What is cerebral autoregulation?

Cerebrovascular resistance (CVR), which is determined by the diameter of small arteries and arterioles, modulates CBF.

$$[CBF = CPP/CVR]$$

Table 19-4. Herniation Syndromes

TYPES	ANATOMY	EXAM FINDINGS
Uncal (lateral transtentorial)	Inferior displacement of medial temporal lobe (uncus) past free edge of tentorium cerebelli	Ipsilateral oculomotor nerve palsy, posterior cerebral artery infarction Kernohan's notch phenomenon
Subfalcine	Cingulate gyrus forced under falx cerebri	Behavioral changes Contralateral leg weakness Anterior cerebral artery infarction
Central (transtentorial)	Progressive downward displacement of diencephalon and brain stem	Rostral to caudal progression of brain stem dysfunction
Tonsillar	Downward displacement of cerebellar tonsils through foramen magnum	Medullary dysfunction Cardiorespiratory arrest

A constant CBF over a wide range of systemic blood pressures, MAP 60 mm Hg–160 mm Hg, maintains CPP due to CVR. Outside this range of autoregulation, CBF varies directly with CPP. Below the lower limit of CPP, CBF decreases as vasodilation becomes insufficient to promote CBF, resulting in ischemia. Above the upper limit of CPP, increased intraluminal pressure results in a forceful dilation of arterioles ("luxury" perfusion), leading to disruption of the blood–brain barrier and brain edema. The upper and lower limits of cerebrovascular autoregulation vary from one person to another, so the targeted CPP must be individualized.

27. What is the etiology of elevated ICP and cerebral edema?
    See Table 19-5.

28. How is intracranial hypertension managed?
    Medical management: The initial steps in the medical management of elevated ICP are the universal mandates of assessing airway patency, breathing, and circulation. These goals should be followed sequentially and include the following:

Table 19-5. Mechanism and Etiology of Elevated Intracranial Pressure (ICP)

MECHANISM	ETIOLOGY
Increased intracellular brain water (cytotoxic edema)	Ischemic stroke, lead intoxication, anoxic brain injury, fulminant hepatic failure, Reye's syndrome
Increased extracellular brain water (vasogenic edema)	Hypertensive encephalopathy, eclampsia, posterior reversible encephalopathy syndrome, brain tumors, abscess, encephalitis, high-altitude cerebral edema
Transependymal edema (hydrocephalus)	Subarachnoid hemorrhage, idiopathic intracranial hypertension, meningitis
Osmotic edema	Hyponatremia, reverse urea syndrome, osmotherapy rebound effect, diabetic ketoacidosis, and hyperglycemic nonketotic coma (correction phase)
Ionic edema	Ischemic stroke
Venous obstruction	Sinus venous thrombosis, jugular vein thrombosis
Increased brain volume	Brain tumor, abscess, empyema, intracerebral hemorrhage
Increased blood volume	Hypercarbia, anoxia, severe anemia, hyperperfusion syndrome (i.e., postcarotid endarterectomy), vein of Galen malformation, arteriovenous malformation, arteriovenous fistula
Mass effect	Subdural hematoma, epidural hematoma, empyema, tension pneumocephalus

1. Maintenance of adequate oxygenation helps with both brain and systemic perfusion. Additionally, normothermia, normoglycemia, euvolemia, and normonatremia help optimize outcomes.
2. Elevation of the patient's head to 30° and positioning in midline facilitates cerebral venous drainage to decrease cerebral blood volume (CBV).
3. Controlled hyperventilation for a short period as a bridge to definitive therapy. Hyperventilation vasoconstricts cerebral arterioles and reduces CBV. Prolonged hyperventilation causes ischemia. The goal should be a minute ventilation to keep $PaCO_2$ ~ 30 to 35 mm Hg.
4. Sedation and analgesia help decrease cerebral metabolism. Agitation and pain increase cerebral metabolic rate of oxygen ($CMRO_2$) and CBF. Propofol and barbiturates reduce $CMRO_2$ and CBF. Patients should receive adequate sedation with propofol and adequate analgesia with fentanyl.
5. Neuromuscular blockade may lower ICP by both muscle relaxation and preventing Valsalva-induced spikes in ICP related to coughing and straining. Disadvantages are loss of the neurologic exam and an increase in the risk of critical illness neuromyopathy.
6. Osmotherapy with mannitol and/or hypertonic saline exerts osmotic and vasoconstrictive effects to reduce CBV. Doses of 0.5 to 1.5 g/kg intravenous (IV) bolus of 20% mannitol, followed by 0.25 to 1 g/kg every 6 hours via peripheral line are recommended. Electrolytes, renal function, and serum osmolarity must be monitored every 6 hours. Check osmolar gap = measured − calculated. Hold mannitol if the gap >20 serum osmoles. Hypertonic saline also is available for management of elevated ICP before or concomitantly with mannitol administration. Doses and concentrations include 23% saline 30 cc × 1 over 10 minutes via central line to avoid hypotension followed by 30 cc every 6 hours; 3% infusion 40 to 50 cc/h can also be used via central line. The serum sodium goal is 145 to 155 mEq/L.
7. Steroids should be used for vasogenic edema due to either brain tumors or encephalitis. Dexamethasone 10 mg IV × 1, then 4 mg q6h. Steroids must be avoided in traumatic brain injury (TBI) patients due to higher mortality.
8. Targeted temperature management has been advocated after the above measures have been utilized. The main goal is to prevent fever as fever has been associated with poor outcome. Active cooling to 32 to 34° C is used for refractory elevated ICP. It reduces $CMRO_2$ and CBV. However, induced hypothermia in TBI with elevated ICP should be used in conjunction with available management protocols.

Surgical management: CSF diversion via an intraventricular catheter reduces CSF volume and decreases ICP. It is indicated in obstructive hydrocephalus, diffuse cerebral edema, or mass effect due to space-occupying lesions.

Craniectomy reduces mass effect and CBV. The main indication for craniectomy is either a large hemispheric ischemic stroke or posterior fossa lesion with significant mass effect. Hemicraniectomy should be performed as early as possible, preferably before significant changes in the neurologic examination are observed. There is currently no evidence of benefit of craniectomy in TBI patients.

INFECTIONS

29. **What is systemic inflammatory response syndrome (SIRS)?**
    SIRS refers to the clinical manifestations of systemic inflammation. The presence of SIRS requires that two or more of the following criteria are met:
    1. Fever (>38° C) or hypothermia (<36° C)
    2. Tachycardia (>90 b/min)
    3. Either tachypnea (>20/min) or a fall in arterial $PaCO_2$ (<32 mm Hg)
    4. Either leukocytosis (>12.0×10^9/L) or leukopenia (<4.0×10^9/L) or >10% immature (band) forms

30. **What is sepsis, and what is severe sepsis?**
    Sepsis is defined as the presence (either probable or documented) of infection together with SIRS. Severe sepsis is sepsis-induced organ dysfunction or tissue hypoperfusion.

31. **What is septic shock?**
    Severe sepsis plus hypotension not reversed with fluid resuscitation.

32. **How should septic patients be evaluated?**
    The initial workup should focus on the identification of the infectious source including careful history and physical examination, two sets of blood cultures, urine culture, sputum culture, stool culture, and CSF studies.

33. How should septic patients be treated?
Early goal-directed therapy is a protocol for the first 6 hours of treatment of septic patients with shock refractory to fluids and vasopressors and requires administration of fluids, vasopressors, broad-spectrum antibiotics, and hydrocortisone.

KEY POINTS: GENERAL MANAGEMENT IN THE NEUROCRITICAL CARE UNIT

1. A depressed level of consciousness (GCS <8) is the greatest risk factor for airway obstruction and aspiration.
2. In assessing the airway, always recognize the potential for cervical spine injuries.
3. Hypocapnia constricts coronary and cerebral arteries and hampers oxygen unloading.
4. Always treat fever aggressively.
5. Avoid hypovolemia.

INTRACRANIAL HEMORRHAGE (ICH)

34. What percentage of strokes is due to intracerebral hemorrhage?
10% to 15%.

35. What is the overall 30-day mortality of ICH?
34%.

36. What are the typical locations for nontraumatic ICH?
Basal ganglia, thalamus, pons, cerebellum, and lobar.

37. What is the etiology of nontraumatic ICH?
See Table 19-6.

Table 19-6. Etiology of Spontaneous Hemorrhage

Hypertension: most common cause ~70%
Amyloid angiopathy: most common cause in the elderly
Arteriovenous malformations: most common cause in children
Intracranial aneurysm
Vascular malformations: cavernous angioma, venous angioma
Dural venous sinus thrombosis
Coagulopathy
Intracranial neoplasm
Cocaine, methamphetamine, or alcohol
Vasculitis
Hemorrhagic ischemic stroke

38. What neuroimaging modalities should be used in ICH evaluation and management?
Noncontrast computed tomography (CT) head scan is the imaging modality of choice to assess for ICH location, volume, ventricular extension, hydrocephalus, and mass effect. Hematoma volume can be calculated using the ABC/2 formula. A = longest diameter, B = largest diameter perpendicular to A, and C is the number of CT slices with hematoma × thickness of 10-mm slices in cm (if 5 mm divide C by 2). In most cases a noncontrast CT of the head is the only imaging modality that is required particularly in those patients with ICH located in the basal ganglia and thalamus.

Magnetic resonance imaging (MRI) of the brain may be needed to assess for ischemic stroke, underlying tumor, vascular lesion, and prior microbleeds or macrobleeds on gradient echo (GRE) sequence. Abnormalities in the latter would indicate the presence of cerebral amyloid angiopathy (CAA) (superficial lobar region) or hypertension-related changes (deep subcortical and infratentorial region).

CT angiography (CTA) spot sign is an indicator of active hemorrhage, which has been associated with increased risk of hematoma expansion, mortality, and poor outcome (Fig. 19-2). However, further studies are under way to determine the significance of the spot sign in daily clinical practice.

Vascular imaging: Noninvasive imaging such as CTA and MR angiogram (MRA) and/or an invasive modality such as digital subtraction angiography (DSA) should be considered in those patients where a vascular abnormality is suspected.

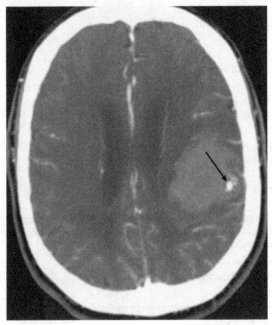

Figure 19-2. Computed tomography angiography (CTA) spot sign (*arrow*). *(From Law M, Som P, Naidich T:* Problem solving in neuroradiology. *Philadelphia, Elsevier, 2011.)*

39. **How rapidly does hematoma volume expand in acute ICH?**
    Twenty-six percent within 1 hour and another 12% within 20 hours after the initial CT scan.

40. **What are the imaging predictors for hematoma expansion (>33% growth from baseline CT)?**
    Irregular shape, heterogeneous density, and the spot sign.

41. **When should a head CT be repeated in an ICH patient?**
    Follow-up head CT scanning is usually performed 6 to 24 hours after presentation or earlier if there is a change in neurologic examination. Given the chance of hemorrhage expansion, repeat imaging is common, but it is expensive and may be dangerous. It is important to recognize that without a clinical change, the yield of repeat CT is low. It may be safely deferred in most circumstances. Some exceptions may include patients with increased ICP, a GCS score <12, or epidural hematoma, as the clinical examination may be less sensitive and the likelihood of intervention greater in these circumstances.

42. **When does swelling peak in ICH?**
    Days 3 to 7.

43. What are the predictors of poor outcome in ICH?
    - GCS on admission
    - High degree of systolic blood pressure variability or episodic hypertension
    - Hematoma location (extension to ventricles)
    - Hematoma volume
    - Hyperglycemia and fever

44. What are the best predictors of 30-day mortality in ICH?
    See Table 19-7.

Table 19-7. Intracranial Hemorrhage (ICH) Score

COMPONENT	FINDING	ICH SCORE POINT
GCS	3-4	2
	5-12	1
	13-15	0
ICH volume (cc)	>30	1
	<30	0
Intraventricular hemorrhage	Yes	1
	No	0
Infratentorial origin	Yes	1
	No	0
Age (years)	>80	1
	<80	0
Total score		0-6

30-day mortality based on ICH score (0, 1, 2, 3, 4, 5, and 6) →30-day mortality (0, 13, 26, 72, 97, and 100%).
GCS, Glasgow Coma Scale.

45. What are the risk factors for recurrence of ICH?
    Lobar location of the initial ICH, older age, ongoing anticoagulation, presence of the apolipoprotein
    E e2 or e4 alleles, and greater number of microbleeds on MRI are currently considered the main
    factors associated with ICH recurrence.

46. What are the diagnostic criteria for CAA?
    Definite CAA:
    - Full postmortem examination demonstrating:
      - Lobar, cortical, or corticosubcortical hemorrhage
      - Severe CAA with vasculopathy
      - Absence of other diagnostic lesion
    Probable CAA with supporting pathology:
    - Clinical data and pathologic tissue (evacuated hematoma or cortical biopsy) demonstrating:
      - Lobar, cortical, or corticosubcortical hemorrhage
      - Some degree of CAA in specimen
      - Absence of other diagnostic lesion
    Probable CAA:
    - Clinical data and MRI or CT demonstrating:
      - Multiple hemorrhages restricted to lobar, cortical, or corticosubcortical regions (cerebellar
        hemorrhage allowed)
      - Age >55 years
      - Absence of other cause of hemorrhage
    Possible CAA—clinical data and MRI or CT demonstrating:
    - Single lobar, cortical, or corticosubcortical hemorrhage
    - Age >55 years
    - Absence of other cause of hemorrhage

47. What are the predictors of symptomatic ICH recurrence in CAA?

The number of microbleeds and the presence of superficial siderosis on brain MRI predict recurrence risk of intracerebral hemorrhage in patients with CAA.

See Tables 19-8 and 19-9.

Table 19-8. Micro- or Macro-Bleeds on Gradient Echo (GRE)

NUMBER OF MICRO- OR MACRO-BLEEDS	3-YEAR CUMULATIVE RISK OF RECURRENT SYMPTOMATIC ICH (%)
1	14
2	17
3-5	38
>6	51

ICH, Intracranial hemorrhage.

Table 19-9. Cortical Superficial Siderosis on Gradient Echo (GRE)

Cortical superficial siderosis	No	Focal	Disseminated
4-year cumulative risk of recurrent symptomatic ICH	25%	28.9%	74%

ICH, Intracranial hemorrhage.

48. What is the blood pressure goal in the acute phase of ICH?

The 2010 AHA Stroke Council Guidelines recommended to keep blood pressure <160/90 mm Hg or MAP <110 mm Hg. However, data from the INTERACT trial suggested that intensive systolic blood pressure lowering to <140 mm Hg is safe and was associated with better functional outcome on ordinal analysis of modified Rankin scale scores. In practice, many neurointensivists recommend keeping systolic blood pressure <140 mm Hg pending the results of ongoing ATACH 2 phase 3 clinical trials comparing intensive blood pressure lowering (<140 mm Hg) versus standard blood pressure (<180 mm Hg).

49. How is recurrent ICH prevented?

Blood pressure control is still the best treatment to prevent ICH recurrence. After the acute ICH period, a goal target of a normal blood pressure of <140/90 mm Hg (<130/80 mm Hg is diabetes or chronic kidney disease) is reasonable and would be in accordance with current guidelines.

50. When should an ICH patient receive a platelet transfusion?

Studies of the effect of prior antiplatelet agent use or platelet dysfunction on ICH hematoma growth and outcome have found conflicting results.

The usefulness of platelet transfusions in ICH patients with a history of antiplatelet use and normal platelet count is unclear and is considered investigational. For patients with a coagulation factor deficiency and thrombocytopenia (platelet count <100,000), replacement of the appropriate factor or platelets is indicated.

51. When and how should coagulopathy be reversed?

Warfarin is both a risk factor for hematoma enlargement even after 24 hours and for worse outcomes after ICH. There are no randomized clinical trials available comparing the efficacy of different reversal agents and their impact on clinical outcome. Consequently there is considerable variability in clinical practice.

Patients with ICH whose international normalized ratio (INR) is elevated due to oral anticoagulants should have their warfarin withheld, receive therapy to replace vitamin K–dependent factors, correct the INR, and receive intravenous vitamin K with a goal INR of <1.4.

Prothrombin complex concentrates (PCC) have not shown improved outcome compared with fresh frozen plasma (FFP) but may have fewer complications compared with FFP and are reasonable to consider as an alternative to FFP.

FVIIa does not replace all clotting factors, and although the INR may be lowered, clotting may not be restored in vivo; therefore, rFVIIa is not routinely recommended as a sole agent for oral anticoagulant reversal in ICH.

There is currently no specific antidote available to antagonize the effects of novel oral anticoagulants.

52. **When is it safe to resume anticoagulation after spontaneous ICH?**
   Anticoagulation after nonlobar ICH and antiplatelet therapy after all ICH might be considered 2 to 4 weeks after symptom onset, particularly when there are definite indications for these agents.

53. **When is it safe to resume antiplatelet agents?**
   In practice many recommend restarting antiplatelet medications within ~1 week after ICH.

54. **What is the role of surgery in ICH?**
   For most ICH patients, the role of surgery remains uncertain. Patients with cerebellar hemorrhage who are either deteriorating neurologically or who have brain stem compression and/or hydrocephalus from ventricular obstruction should undergo surgical removal of the hemorrhage as soon as possible. Surgical evacuation also may be considered for those patients presenting with lobar clots >30 mL and within 1 cm of the brain surface.

55. **What are the indications for external ventricular drain (EVD) placement and ICP monitoring?**
   Patients with a GCS score of <8, those with clinical evidence of transtentorial herniation, or those with significant IVH or hydrocephalus might be considered for ICP monitoring and treatment.

56. **How should thrombolytic-related symptomatic ICH be managed?**
   The following recommendations have been proposed for patients experiencing thrombolytic-related ICH: keep systolic blood pressure <140 mm Hg; check platelet count, fibrinogen, thromboplastin time, and activated partial thromboplastin time; and infuse both platelets (6 to 8 U) and cryoprecipitate, which contains factor VIII to rapidly correct the systemic fibrinoytic state created by tissue plasminogen activator. If fibrinogen is <100 mg/dL administer cryoprecipitate 0.10 µ/kg IV. Repeat fibrinogen in 1 hour, and if it is <100 mg/dL, repeat cryoprecipitate dose IV and consult neurosurgery.

KEY POINTS: INTRACRANIAL HEMORRHAGE

1. Hematoma expansion usually occurs in the hyperacute setting.
2. Intensive blood pressure lowering to systolic blood pressure values <140 mm Hg is safe and results in better functional outcome on ordinal analysis of modified Rankin scale scores.
3. Rapid reversal with IV vitamin K and PCC in warfarin-induced ICH is indicated.
4. Consider surgery for lobar hematomas >30 mL and within 1 cm of the surface and cerebellar hemorrhage >3 cm.
5. Avoid corticosteroid administration in ICH.
6. Think of CAA in spontaneous lobar ICH age >55.

CRITICAL CARE MANAGEMENT OF ANEURYSMAL SUBARACHNOID HEMORRHAGE (aSAH)

57. **Why should we document a clinical severity scale?**
   The initial clinical severity of aSAH should be determined rapidly by use of simple validated scales (e.g., Hunt and Hess, World Federation of Neurological Surgeons) because it is the most useful indicator of outcome after aSAH.

58. **What are the complications of aSAH?**
   See Table 19-10.

59. **What is the initial management of aSAH?**
   - Ensure adequacy of airway patency, breathing, and circulation.
   - Avoid administration of hypotonic fluid administration.
   - Provide analgesia with narcotics and antiemetics if necessary.

Table 19-10. Complications in Aneurysmal Subarachnoid Hemorrhage (aSAH)

NEUROLOGIC COMPLICATIONS	SYSTEMIC COMPLICATIONS
Aneurysm rebleeding	Neurogenic pulmonary edema
High ICP/hydrocephalus (early and delayed)	Takotsubo cardiomyopathy
Vasospasm and delayed cerebral ischemia	Hyponatraemia (CSW/SIADH)
Seizures	Fever/SIRS/hyperglycemia/venous thromboembolism

CSW, Cerebral salt wasting; SIADH, syndrome of inappropriate antidiuretic hormone secretion; ICP, intracranial pressure; SIRS, systemic inflammatory response syndrome.

- Control blood pressure.
- Administer nimodipine for 21 days or until day of discharge.
- Place an external ventricular drain if hydrocephalus develops.
- Treat seizures (avoid phenytoin as literature suggests it worsens cognitive and functional outcome).
- Secure the ruptured aneurysm early.

60. What is the blood pressure goal prior to securing the ruptured aneurysm?
The magnitude of blood pressure control to reduce the risk of rebleeding has not been established, but a decrease in systolic blood pressure to <160 mm Hg has been recommended.

61. When should the aneurysm be treated?
Either surgical clipping or endovascular coiling of the ruptured aneurysm should be performed as early as feasible in the majority of patients to reduce the rate of rebleeding after aSAH. There is currently no clear absolute timeline, but treatment of the ruptured cerebral aneurysm should be undertaken within 24 to 48 hours of presentation.

62. What is the blood pressure goal after the ruptured aneurysm is secured?
Liberal blood pressure goals should be set for patients with aSAH after the aneurysm is secured. Although blood pressure goals should be individualized to account for patient-specific characteristics, most centers apply the AHA guidelines for acute ischemic stroke and do not use antihypertensive medications unless the systolic blood pressure exceeds 220 mm Hg or the diastolic blood pressure exceeds 120 mm Hg.

63. What are the causes of poor outcome in aSAH patients?
At admission: Poor grade SAH, high blood pressure, older age, thicker subarachnoid clot, preexisting medical conditions and posterior circulation aneurysm.
Later: Delayed cerebral ischemia (DCI), stroke, fever, and use of phenytoin.

64. How do we manage acute symptomatic hydrocephalus related to aSAH?
Acute symptomatic hydrocephalus related to aSAH should be managed by cerebrospinal fluid diversion (EVD or lumbar drainage, depending on the clinical scenario).

65. What is the incidence of convulsive seizure at onset of SAH?
Clinical seizures are uncommon after the initial aneurysm rupture (occurring in 1% to 7% of patients). When they do occur in patients with an unsecured aneurysm, they are often the manifestation of aneurysmal rerupture.

66. What is the incidence of nonconvulsive seizure at onset of SAH?
In comatose (poor-grade) aSAH patients, nonconvulsive seizures may be detected on continuous EEG (cEEG) in 10% to 20% of cases.

67. What cardiopulmonary complications occur after SAH?
Cardiac: Elevated troponin, electrocardiogram (ECG) changes, regional or global wall motion abnormality, stunned myocardium, and Takatsubo cardiomyopathy.
Pulmonary: Pulmonary edema (either cardiac or neurogenic), acute lung injury, or adult respiratory distress syndrome (ARDS).
Mechanism for both complications: Most likely a catecholamine surge at aSAH onset.

68. **How should cardiopulmonary complications be managed?**

    In cases of either pulmonary edema or lung injury, the goal of therapy should include avoiding excessive fluid intake and judicious use of diuretics targeting euvolemia.

    Standard management of heart failure is indicated with the exception that cerebral perfusion pressure should be maintained as appropriate for the neurologic condition.

69. **What is vasospasm?**

    Vasospasm is defined as either segmental or diffuse narrowing of large arteries that can be detected angiographically in up to 70% of patients beginning 4 to 12 days after aneurysm rupture and that resolves over 2 to 4 weeks.

70. **What is DCI?**

    DCI is defined as any neurologic deterioration (focal or global) presumed secondary to cerebral ischemia that persists >1 hour and cannot be explained by any other neurologic or systemic condition such as significant hydrocephalus, sedation, hypoxemia, seizures, electrolyte imbalances, renal injury, or hepatic impairment. Thus, DCI is a diagnosis of exclusion. DCI occurs in 30% of patients at any time within the first 21 days after symptom onset. However, the peak incidence of DCI is between 4 and 12 days after symptom onset.

71. **How should the aSAH patient be assessed for vasospasm?**

    Serial neurologic examination is the mainstay in the monitoring for cerebral vasospasm. Serial measurements, rather than a single transcranial Doppler (TCD) ultrasound measurement, are indicated to assess for trends in the mean CBF velocities and to help predict vasospasm. CTA, MRA, DSA, or CT perfusion may be considered in patients who do not have adequate temporal bone windows for TCD and in those high-risk patients with poor-grade aSAH and too poor an exam to document the presence of cerebral vasospasm.

72. **What are the TCD criteria for evidence of middle cerebral artery vasospasm?**

    The main criteria for vasospasm are as follows:
    - Mean middle cerebral artery (MCA) blood flow velocity >200 cm/s;
    - Rapid rise (>50 cm/s) between serial TCD measurements within 24 to 48 hours; and
    - Lindegaard index (MCA/ICA [intracranial artery] ratio) >6.

73. **How can DCI be prevented?**

    Oral nimodipine should be administered to all patients with an SAH. Oral nimodipine 60 mg q4h has a neuroprotective effect as it improves neurologic outcomes but does not reduce cerebral vasospasm. Avoidance of hypovolemia is the mainstay of preventive therapy for delayed cerebral ischemia. Patients with hyper- or hypovolemia have a significantly higher mortality. Maintenance of euvolemia and normal circulating blood volume is recommended to prevent DCI.

74. **Should central venous pressure (CVP) be used to guide fluid management in aSAH?**

    CVP appears to be an unreliable indicator of intravascular volume. Fluid management based solely on CVP measurements is not recommended.

75. **How is DCI treated?**

    The primary goal of treating DCI is prevention of ischemic strokes. Induced hypertension has become the major component of hemodynamic augmentation therapy. Patients clinically suspected of DCI should undergo a trial of induced hypertension, which should be maintained for at least 72 hours or until stability is achieved and is slowly weaned off after that. Blood pressure augmentation should progress in a stepwise fashion with assessment of neurologic function at each MAP level to determine if a higher blood pressure target is appropriate.

76. **What is the role of prophylactic hypervolemia and angioplasty in vasospasm?**

    Neither prophylactic hypervolemia nor balloon angioplasty before the development of symptomatic angiographic spasm is recommended.

77. **When should endovascular treatment to treat symptomatic vasospasm be considered?**

    Cerebral angioplasty and/or selective intra-arterial vasodilator therapy is reasonable in patients with symptomatic cerebral vasospasm, particularly those who are not rapidly responding to hypertensive therapy.

78. **What is the etiology of hyponatremia after aSAH?**

Hyponatremia is common after aSAH and has been associated with development of DCI and poor clinical outcome. It can be secondary to either cerebral salt wasting or inappropriate secretion of antidiuretic hormone.

79. **How do we treat hyponatremia in aSAH?**

Hyponatremia should not be treated with volume restriction, as hypovolemia is associated with poor outcome. In patients with a persistently negative fluid balance, use of fludrocortisone or hydrocortisone may be considered. These agents help correct the negative sodium balance and reduce the need for fluids. The administration of 1.5% to 3% saline also has been recommended.

80. **What is nonaneurysmal perimesencephalic SAH (NAPSAH)?**

In 15% of SAH patients imaging studies fail to demonstrate the source of bleeding. Approximately 38% of these patients have NAPSAH. NAPSAH is confirmed in the presence of a negative CTA or DSA in patients with the following head CT scan pattern:

- Center of hemorrhage is located immediately anterior to the midbrain, with or without extension of blood to the anterior part of the ambient cistern or to the basal part of the Sylvian fissures;
- No complete filling of the anterior interhemispheric fissure and no extension to the lateral Sylvian fissures, except for minute amounts of blood; and
- Absence of frank intraventricular blood.

81. **When should family members of patients with aSAH be screened for the presence of an aneurysm?**

It may be reasonable to offer noninvasive screening to patients with familial (at least one first-degree relative) aSAH and/or a history of aSAH to evaluate for de novo aneurysms or late regrowth of a treated aneurysm. The risks and benefits of this screening require further study.

KEY POINTS: ANEURYSMAL SUBARACHNOID HEMORRHAGE

1. Angiographic vasospasm and DCI contribute to poor outcome after aSAH.
2. Nimodipine is neuroprotective as it improves outcome but has not been shown to reduce vasospasm.
3. Hypovolemia is common in patients with aSAH and is associated with DCI.
4. Refrain from using prophylactic hypervolemia, induced hypertension, or hemodilution and cerebral angioplasty.
5. Induced hypertension is the mainstay treatment for DCI, whereas hypervolemia and hemodilution are not beneficial.

CRITICAL CARE MANAGEMENT OF LARGE HEMISPHERIC AND CEREBELLAR ISCHEMIC STROKES

82. **What is the clinical presentation of malignant edema after MCA stroke?**

The most common findings are hemiplegia, global or expressive aphasia, severe dysarthria, neglect, gaze preference, and a visual field defect. Pupillary abnormalities are a reflection of significant brain stem shift, typically not expected on initial presentation, and develop within the first 3 to 5 days. The initial National Institutes of Health Stroke Scale score is often >20 with dominant hemispheric infarction and >15 with nondominant hemispheric infarction, which is a reflection of stroke severity and infarct volume, not a marker of tissue swelling.

83. **What are the clinical signs of deterioration following hemispheric stroke?**

The most commonly described signs in deterioration from hemispheric supratentorial infarction are decreased level of consciousness, ipsilateral pupillary dysfunction, varying degrees of mydriasis, and adduction paralysis.

84. **What are the risk factors for the development of cerebral edema after ischemia?**

The main risk factors include the following: occlusions of the internal carotid artery, MCA, or both; involvement of additional vascular territories; incomplete circle of Willis; and marginal leptomeningeal collateral supply.

85. What are the predictors for the development of cerebral edema after MCA stroke?
    See Table 19-11.

Table 19-11. Predictors of Developing Edema after Middle Cerebral Artery (MCA) Stroke

CLINICAL	IMAGING
Early reduced GCS—most specific	Frank hypodensity within first 6 hours
Early nausea vomiting <24 hours	Involvement of >1/3 MCA territory
Younger patients <50 year	Dense MCA sign
Female sex	T occlusion of distal ICA/proximal MCA occlusion
CHF	Septum pellucidum midline shift ≥5 mm within the first 2 days
Leukocytosis	MRI DWI volume >80 cm^3 within 6 hours predicts rapid fulminant course

GCS, Glasgow Coma Scale; *ICA*, internal carotid artery; *MRI*, magnetic resonance imaging; *DWI*, diffusion-weighted imaging; *CHF*, congestive heart failure.

86. When does the neurologic deterioration occur?
    Neurologic deterioration usually occurs within 72 to 96 hours in most patients. Some patients may experience deterioration at 4 to 10 days.

87. What should be the blood pressure goal?
    There are insufficient data to recommend a specific systolic or mean arterial blood pressure target. Blood pressure–lowering drugs may be considered for the treatment of extreme hypertension. Specific blood pressure targets have not been established.

88. What fluids should be used?
    Use of adequate fluid administration with isotonic fluids should be considered, while avoiding hypotonic or hypo-osmolar fluids.

89. What is the role of hyperosmolar therapy?
    Osmotic therapy for patients with clinical deterioration from cerebral swelling associated with cerebral infarction is reasonable. Use of prophylactic osmotic diuretics before apparent swelling is not recommended.

90. Should ICP be monitored in patients with large hemispheric strokes?
    Clinical deterioration is more often the result of displacement of midline structures such as the thalamus and the brain stem rather than of a mechanism of globally increased ICP. Therefore routine ICP monitoring is not indicated in hemispheric ischemic strokes.

91. What is the role of surgery in the management of malignant MCA stroke?
    Decompressive hemicraniectomy reduces mortality by reducing progression to brain death and reduces the probability of permanent coma that eventually may lead to de-escalation of care and death.
    Decompressive craniectomy with dural expansion is effective in patients <60 years of age with unilateral MCA infarctions who deteriorate neurologically within 48 hours despite medical therapy. The effect of later decompression is not known, but it should be strongly considered. Although the optimal trigger for decompressive hemicraniectomy is unknown, it is reasonable to use a decrease in level of consciousness and its attribution to brain swelling as selection criteria.
    The efficacy of decompressive hemicraniectomy in patients >60 years of age and the optimal timing of surgery are uncertain. Recently the Destiny 2 trial showed improved survival but more moderate to severe disability in patients older than 60 years.
    Timing of decompressive hemicraniectomy remains unresolved, but it is generally agreed that the surgery is best undertaken before clinical signs of brainstem compression usually between 24 and 48 hours.

CEREBELLAR INFARCTION

92. When does peak swelling occur?
Peak swelling occurs several days after the onset of ischemia.

93. What are the clinical and radiologic markers of deterioration following cerebellar infarction?
Similar to hemispheric infarction, the most reliable clinical symptom of tissue swelling is decreased level of consciousness and thus arousal secondary to brain stem compression and/or obstructive hydrocephalus. Effacement of the fourth ventricle is a key radiologic marker, followed by basal cistern compression, followed by brain stem deformity, hydrocephalus, downward tonsillar herniation, and upward transtentorial herniation.

94. What is the role of surgery in the management of cerebellar infarction?
Suboccipital craniectomy with dural expansion should be performed in patients with cerebellar infarctions who deteriorate neurologically despite maximal medical therapy.
EVD insertion is recommended in obstructive hydrocephalus after a cerebellar infarct but should be followed or accompanied by decompressive craniectomy to avoid deterioration from upward cerebellar displacement.

KEY POINTS: LARGE HEMISPHERIC AND CEREBELLAR ISCHEMIC STROKES

1. Peak swelling occurs 72 to 96 hours after large hemispheric infarcts.
2. There is no role for prophylactic hyperosmolar therapy in large hemispheric infarction.
3. ICP monitoring is not useful in large hemispheric infarcts.
4. Early decompressive hemicraniectomy after large hemispheric stroke within 48 hours for age <60 improves survival and functional outcome.
5. Suboccipital craniectomy with dural expansion and ventriculostomy is recommended in obstructive hydrocephalus after a cerebellar infarct if the patient is deteriorating despite maximal medical therapy.

NEUROMUSCULAR WEAKNESSES IN THE ICU

95. What is the definition of myasthenia gravis crisis (MC)?
MC is defined as myasthenia gravis (MG) exacerbation leading to respiratory failure requiring assisted ventilation.

96. What is the incidence of MC?
Overall, 15% to 20% of patients with MG will experience an MC crisis, occurring within the first 2 years after diagnosis of MG in most patients (74%).

97. What are the predisposing factors for MC?
The most common identifiable precipitant of MC is an infection (40%), usually respiratory, such as pneumonia (Table 19-12).

98. What are the arterial blood gas findings in MC?
Arterial blood gas results can be misleading because patients with MC usually become hypoxemic only at a late stage. Earlier findings may include initial respiratory alkalosis with mild tachypnea,

Table 19-12. Triggers of Myasthenia Gravis Crisis

Infections (40%)—pneumonia, upper airway infection
Aspiration (10%)
Medications—botulinum toxins, prednisone
Stress—surgery, trauma
Idiopathic (30%)

progressing later to respiratory acidosis as the diaphragm weakens further. Normal $PaCO_2$ in a tachypneic patient means impending respiratory failure.

99. **When should an MC patient be intubated?**
The most common reasons for intubation include the following:
- A wet, gurgling voice, dysarthric/staccato speech, and stridor indicating poor airway protection;
- Abdominal paradoxical breathing indicating diaphragmatic weakness;
- Failure to manage secretions;
- Arterial blood gases showing a PaO_2 <60 mm Hg or $PaCO_2$ >60 mm Hg; and
- Increased work of breathing.
    The 20/30/40 rule (forced vital capacity <20 mL/kg; negative inspiratory pressure <30 cm H_2O; and positive expiratory pressure <40 cm H_2O) is probably the most helpful guide to decide when to intubate.

100. **When should an MC patient be weaned off the ventilator?**
General criteria have already been mentioned in the general management section of this chapter. For patients with MC the following criteria should additionally be considered:
- Improving strength (caution: degree of limb weakness does not correlate with diaphragm weakness);
- Improving bedside pulmonary function test (vital capacity >15 mL/kg, negative inspiratory pressure >30, and positive expiratory pressure >40);
- Absence of either severe atelectasis or pleural effusion; and
- Ability to manage secretions.

101. **What is the ventilatory test in MC?**
See Table 19-13.

Table 19-13. Ventilatory Test in Myasthenia Gravis Crisis (MC)

PARAMETERS	NORMAL VALUES	THRESHOLD FOR INTUBATION	INITIATION OF WEANING OFF VENTILATOR	CONSIDERATION FOR EXTUBATION
FVC (mL/kg)	>60	<20	>15	>25
NIP (cm H_2O)	>−70	<−30	>20	>40
PEP (cm H_2O)	>100	<40	>40	>50

FVC, Forced vital capacity; *NIP*, negative inspiratory pressure; *PEP*, positive expiratory pressure.
Modified from Godoy DA, Mello LJ, Masotti L, et al.: The myasthenic patient in crisis: an update of management in neurointensive care unit. *Arq Neuropsiquiatr* 71(9A):627-639, 2013.

102. **What is the role of NIVPPV?**
NIVPPV may be useful in either preventing intubation or reintubation except when $PaCO_2$ ≥45 mm Hg as the failure rate is higher.

103. **What should be done with home anticholinesterase inhibitors when the patient is intubated?**
Stopping pyridostigmine upon intubation is recommended as it causes increased secretions. Pyridostigmine should be started as soon as the patient improves and weaning is initiated.

104. **What is the role of steroids in MC?**
Patients who are taking steroids should not stop them. Initiation of high-dose steroids in patients with MG may lead to a paradoxical worsening of muscle weakness.

105. **What is the first line of treatment for MC?**
Either plasma exchange (PLEX) 1.5 L of plasma (20 to 25 mL/kg) per session for approximately five sessions or until the patient experiences clinical improvement or intravenous immunoglobulin (IVIG) 0.4 g/kg for 5 days are the first-line options for treatment of patients with MC. They are equally

effective in crisis. Although never compared in a controlled study, PLEX seems to work faster after two to three session days compared to 5 days after IVIG initiation and might be preferable for managing MC. Check IgA level prior to IVIG administration as anaphylaxis may be a serious adverse event in IgA-deficient individuals.

106. **What are the indications for ICU admission of Guillain–Barré (GBS) patients?**
The most common reasons for ICU admission in GBS are rapidly progressive weakness, worsening respiratory function, and autonomic dysfunction (cardiac arrhythmia, urinary retention, ileus). The two most common causes of death in GBS are airway failure and dysautonomia.

107. **What is the role of immunotherapy in the critical care management of GBS?**
Treatment with either PLEX or IVIG hastens recovery from GBS. The effects of IVIG and PLEX are equivalent. PLEX is recommended for nonambulant patients within 4 weeks of onset and for ambulant patients within 2 weeks of onset. IVIG is recommended for patients with GBS who require aid to walk within 2 or 4 weeks from the onset of neuropathic symptoms. Sequential treatment with PLEX followed by IVIG is not recommended.

108. **What is the role of steroids in the critical care management of GBS?**
Corticosteroids are not recommended for the treatment of patients with GBS.

109. **What is ICU-acquired weakness?**
It is weakness acquired in the ICU, which is due to several underlying pathophysiologic processes that may be present concomitantly. The two most common pathologic entities associated with ICU-acquired weakness are critical illness polyneuropathy (CIP) and critical illness myopathy (CIM).

110. **What is CIP?**
CIP is an acute length-dependent sensorimotor axonal polyneuropathy most often associated with sepsis and multiorgan system failure occurring after days to weeks of illness onset.

111. **What is CIM?**
CIM is an acute rapidly progressive myopathy most often seen in patients with sepsis and multiorgan system failure who are exposed to high-dose steroids and neuromuscular blocking agents (NMBAs) and occurs after days to weeks of illness onset.

112. **What are the differences between CIP and CIM?**
CIP is often difficult to clinically distinguish from CIM (Table 19-14).

KEY POINTS: NEUROMUSCULAR WEAKNESSES IN THE ICU

1. MC typically occurs within the first 2 years of MG diagnosis.
2. Pneumonia is the most commonly identified trigger for MC.
3. Patients with MC typically become hypercarbic before becoming hypoxemic.
4. The 20/30/40 rule for intubation is forced vital capacity<20 mL/kg; negative inspiratory pressure <30 cm H_2O; and positive expiratory pressure <40 cm H_2O.
5. The initiation of high-dose steroids in patients with MG leads to a paradoxical worsening of muscle weakness.
6. PLEX and IVIG are equally effective in crisis. However, PLEX is preferred as it works faster in MG crisis.
7. Bedside pulmonary function tests are more reliable in monitoring and weaning GBS and MC patients from assisted ventilation.
8. Combining or sequential treatments of PLEX followed by IVIG in GBS is not beneficial.
9. Steroids and neuromuscular blocking agent administration are the most important risk factors for CIM.

MANAGEMENT OF STATUS EPILEPTICUS

113. **What is the current definition of SE?**
SE is defined as 5 minutes or more of the following:
1. Continuous clinical and/or electrographic seizure activity; or
2. Recurrent seizure activity without recovery of consciousness (returning to baseline) between seizures.

Table 19-14. Difference between Critical Illness Polyneuropathy (CIP) and Critical Illness Myopathy (CIM)

CONDITION	INCIDENCE	CLINICAL FEATURES	ENMG FINDINGS	SERUM CK	MUSCLE BIOPSY	TREATMENT	PROGNOSIS
CIP	Common	Flaccid limbs; respiratory weakness	Axonal degeneration of motor and sensory fibers	Nearly normal	Denervation atrophy	Supportive, treat sepsis and avoid hyperglycemia	Variable
CIM	Common with steroids (NMBAs), and sepsis	Flaccid limbs; respiratory weakness	Abnormal spontaneous activity	Mildly elevated	Loss of thick (myosin) filaments	Supportive Judicious with high-dose steroids and NMBAs	Good

NMBAs, Neuromuscular blocking agents; CK, creatinine kinase.
From Bolton CF: Neuromuscular manifestations of critical illness. *Muscle Nerve* 32(2):140-163, 2005.

114. What is the definition of convulsive SE?

Convulsive SE is defined as convulsions that are associated with rhythmic jerking of the extremities. Characteristic findings of generalized convulsive SE are generalized tonic–clonic movements of the extremities and mental status impairment (coma, lethargy, confusion). Focal neurologic deficits may be associated with the postictal period.

115. What are the underlying etiologies of SE?

See Table 19-15.

Table 19-15. Underlying Etiologies of Status Epilepticus (SE)

ACUTE PROCESSES	CHRONIC PROCESSES
Toxic–metabolic disturbances: electrolyte abnormalities, hypoglycemia, renal failure Drugs: toxicity, withdrawal, AED noncompliance	Chronic ethanol abuse in setting of ethanol intoxication or withdrawal
CNS inflammation: meningitis, encephalitis, abscess, autoimmune encephalitis, paraneoplastic syndromes	CNS tumors
Vascular: ischemic stroke, intracerebral hemorrhage, subarachnoid hemorrhage, cerebral sinus thrombosis, hypertensive encephalopathy, PRES	Remote CNS pathology (e.g., stroke, abscess, TBI, cortical dysplasia)
Head trauma with or without epidural or subdural hematoma, hypoxia, cardiac arrest, sepsis	Preexisting epilepsy: breakthrough seizures or discontinuation of AEDs

CNS, Central nervous system; *AED*, antiepileptic drugs; *TBI*, traumatic brain injury; *PRES*, posterior reversible encephalopathy syndrome.

116. What is the initial workup for convulsive SE?

See Table 19-16.

Table 19-16. Workup for Status Epilepticus (SE)

ALL PATIENTS	BASED ON CLINICAL PRESENTATION
Finger stick glucose	LP
CBC, BMP, calcium (total and ionized), magnesium	Liver function tests, serial troponins, type and hold, coagulation studies, arterial blood gas
Head CT scan (appropriate for most cases), rule out stroke, ICH, cerebral venous sinus thrombosis	Brain MRI
AED levels	Comprehensive toxicology panel
Continuous EEG monitoring	Autoimmune disease screening

CBC, Complete blood count; *BMP*, basic metabolic panel; *LP*, lumbar puncture; *CT*, computed tomography; *ICH*, Intracranial hemorrhage; *MRI*, magnetic resonance imaging; *AED*, antiepileptic drug; *EEG*, electroencephalograph.

117. How should SE be managed?

The principal goal of treatment is to stop both clinical and electrographic seizure activity immediately. The following timeline should be followed:

- 0 to 2 minutes: Evaluate airway patency, breathing, and circulation, and obtain finger stick glucose.
- 0 to 5 minutes: Obtain peripheral IV access, reverse thiamine deficiency, treat hypoglycemia (thiamine given before dextrose), administer benzodiazepines, resuscitate hemodynamics, and then send basic laboratory studies.

- Administer first-line treatment benzodiazepines (Table 19-17).
- 6 to 10 minutes: Administer second-line treatment, screen for the underlying cause of SE, and immediately begin treatment of life-threatening causes of SE (e.g., meningitis, intracranial mass lesion).

If the patient stops seizing, the next goal is rapid attainment of therapeutic levels of an antiepileptic drug (AED) and continued dosing for maintenance therapy. If first-line drugs fail, then second-line agents must be given to stop SE.

In patients with known epilepsy who have been on an AED before admission, it is reasonable to provide an IV bolus of this AED, if available, prior to initiating an additional agent. This may include additional boluses that will result in higher than normal target concentrations of the AED to achieve the desired therapeutic response (i.e., cessation of seizure activity).

Table 19-17. First-Line Benzodiazepines

MEDICATIONS	LORAZEPAM (IV)	MIDAZOLAM (IM, INTRANASALLY, BUCCALLY)	DIAZEPAM (IV, RECTALLY)
Dose	0.1 mg/kg IV up to 4 mg per dose, may repeat in 5-10 minutes	0.2 mg/kg IM up to maximum of 10 mg	0.15 mg/kg IV up to 10 mg per dose, may repeat in 5 minutes. 20 mg rectally
Adverse events	Hypotension, respiratory depression	Hypotension, respiratory depression	Hypotension, respiratory depression
Half-life	12-14 hours	1-7 hours	18-20 hours IV, about 46 hours rectally

IM, Intramuscularly; *IV*, intravenously.

118. **What are the preferred second-line agents for SE?**
   See Table 19-18.

119. **What is refractory SE?**
   RSE is diagnosed when patients continue to experience either clinical or electrographic seizures after receiving adequate doses of an initial benzodiazepine followed by a second acceptable AED.

120. **What is the treatment of RSE?**
   Treatment recommendations are to use continuous infusion AEDs to suppress seizures. Patients with RSE require assisted ventilation and cardiovascular monitoring (Table 19-19).

121. **What is the goal target in RSE?**
   Dosing of continuous infusion AEDs for RSE should be titrated to cessation of electrographic seizures or burst suppression.

122. **How long should the infusions be maintained?**
   A period of 24 to 48 hours of electrographic control is recommended prior to slow withdrawal of continuous infusion AEDs for RSE. During the transition from continuous infusion AEDs in RSE, it is recommended to use maintenance AEDs and monitor for recurrent seizures by continuous EEG during the titration period.

123. **What are the indications for continuous EEG monitoring?**
   Continuous EEG monitoring should be initiated within 1 hour of SE onset if ongoing seizures are suspected. The duration of continuous EEG monitoring should be at least 48 hours in comatose patients to evaluate for nonconvulsive seizures (Table 19-20).

124. **When after the cessation of convulsive seizures should nonconvulsive SE be suspected?**
   If the patient's level of consciousness does not improve after 20 to 30 minutes following cessation of convulsive movements or mental status remains abnormal 30 to 60 minutes after convulsive activity ceases, ongoing nonconvulsive SE must be considered.

Table 19-18. Second-Line Treatment Agents

MEDICATION	FOSPHENYTOIN	VALPROIC ACID	PHENOBARBITAL	LEVETIRACETAM	MIDAZOLAM CI
Dose	20 mg PE/kg IV, may give an additional 5 mg/kg	20-40 mg/kg IV, may give an additional 20 mg/kg	20 mg/kg IV, may give an additional 5-10 mg/kg	1000-3000 mg IV	Initial dosing 0.2 mg/kg; rate of 2 mg/min CI: 0.05-2 mg/kg/h
Adverse events	Hypotension, arrhythmias	Pancreatitis, thrombocytopenia, hepatotoxicity, hyperammonemia,	Hypotension, respiratory depression	None	Respiratory depression, hypotension
Half-life	12-29 hours	10-12 hours	24-110 hours	6-8 hours	1-7 hours
Total level	15-20 µg/mL	80-140 µg/mL	20-50 mg/mL	12-46 mg/mL	NA

CI, Continuous infusion; PE, phenytoin equivalent; NA, not available.

Table 19-19. Infusions Used in Refractory Status Epilepticus (RSE)

MEDICATIONS	MIDAZOLAM	PROPOFOL	PENTOBARBITAL	THIOPENTAL
Dose	Initial: 0.2 mg/kg; administer at an infusion rate of 2 mg/min CI: 0.05-2 mg/kg/h Breakthrough SE: 0.1-0.2-mg/kg bolus, increase CI rate by 0.05-0.1 mg/kg/h every 3-4 hours	Loading dose: 1-2 mg/kg, start at 20 mcg/kg/min CI: 30-200 mcg/kg/min Breakthrough SE: increase CI rate by 5-10 mcg/kg/min every 5 minutes or 1-mg/kg bolus plus CI titration	Initial: 5-15 mg/kg, at an infusion rate ≤50 mg/min CI: 0.5-5 mg/kg/h Breakthrough SE: 5-mg/kg bolus, increase CI rate by 0.5-1 mg/kg/h every 12 hours	2-7 mg/kg, administer at an infusion rate ≤50 mg/min CI: 0.5-5 mg/kg/h Breakthrough SE: 1-2-mg/kg bolus, increase CI rate by 0.5-1 mg/kg/h every 12 hours
Adverse events	Respiratory depression, hypotension (less compared to other three agents, hence preferred)	Hypotension (especially with loading dose in critically ill patients), respiratory depression, cardiac failure, rhabdomyolysis metabolic acidosis renal failure (PRIS)	Hypotension, respiratory depression, cardiac depression, paralytic ileus At high doses, complete loss of neurologic function	Hypotension, respiratory depression, cardiac depression
Half-life	1-7 hours	3-12 hours	15-50 hours	

CI, Continuous infusion; *PRIS,* propofol-related infusion syndrome.

Table 19-20. Indication for Continuous Electroencephalogram (cEEG) Monitoring

Recent clinical seizure or SE without return to baseline >10 minutes
Coma, including postcardiac arrest
Epileptiform activity or periodic discharges on initial 30 minutes EEG
Intracranial hemorrhage including TBI, SAH, ICH
Suspected nonconvulsive seizures in patients with altered mental status

SE, Status epilepticus; *TBI,* traumatic brain injury; *SAH,* subarachnoid hemorrhage; *ICH,* intracranial hemorrhage.

125. What is the semiological spectrum of nonconvulsive seizures?

Positive symptoms include agitation/aggression, automatisms, blinking, crying, delirium, delusions, echolalia, facial twitching, laughter, nausea/vomiting, nystagmus/eye deviation, perseveration, psychosis, and tremulousness.

Negative symptoms include anorexia, aphasia/mutism, amnesia, catatonia, coma, confusion, lethargy, and staring.

126. What is the benzodiazepine trial for the diagnosis of nonconvulsive SE?

A patient experiencing rhythmic or periodic focal or generalized epileptiform discharges on EEG with neurologic impairment should have EEG, pulse oximetry, blood pressure, ECG, and respiratory rate monitored, and sequential small doses of rapidly acting short-duration benzodiazepine such as

midazolam at 1 mg/dose should be administered. Between doses, repeated clinical and EEG assessment must be performed. The trial is stopped after any of the following:
- Persistent resolution of the EEG pattern (and exam repeated);
- Definite clinical improvement;
- Respiratory depression, hypotension, or other adverse effect; or
- A maximum dose is reached (such as 0.2 mg/kg midazolam, though higher may be needed if on chronic benzodiazepines).

127. How should nonconvulsive SE be treated?

Management is less well defined for nonconvulsive SE as compared to convulsive SE due to the lack of randomized studies. Expert opinion recommends using noncoma-inducing agents initially such as IV fosphenytoin, valproate, and levetiracetam in addition to intermittent benzodiazepines to avoid intubation and drug-induced coma. For refractory nonconvulsive SE treatment should be individualized but can include either midazolam or propofol infusions.

KEY POINTS: STATUS EPILEPTICUS

1. Remember maintenance of airway patency, breathing, and circulation when treating convulsive SE.
2. Treat early and aggressively with benzodiazepines in convulsive SE while simultaneously screening and treating underlying etiologies.
3. Suspect nonconvulsive SE if the patient's level of consciousness is not improving by 20 to 30 minutes after cessation of movements, or mental status remains abnormal 30 to 60 minutes after convulsive activity ceases.

MENINGITIS AND ENCEPHALITIS

128. When do we need to obtain a CT head prior to lumbar puncture (LP)?

A head CT scan is generally recommended prior to a lumbar puncture in all patients suspected of having meningitis or encephalitis. Patients who are particularly at risk of experiencing cerebral tissue shifts and/or herniation are those with the following features: abnormal level of consciousness, new-onset seizures, immunocompromised state, focal neurologic deficit, history of CNS disease, and papilledema.

129. What specific empirical antimicrobial agent(s) should be used in patients with suspected encephalitis?

Although a wide range of viruses have been reported to cause encephalitis, specific antiviral therapy for viral encephalitis is generally limited to disease caused by the herpes viruses, especially herpes simplex virus (HSV). Because the earlier the treatment is started for herpes simplex encephalitis, the less likely death or serious sequelae will result, acyclovir (10 mg/kg intravenously every 8 hours in children and adults with normal renal function) should be initiated in all patients with suspected encephalitis as soon as possible, pending results of diagnostic studies.

130. What are the available therapies for specific viruses?

See Table 19-21.

Table 19-21. Therapy for Specific Viruses

VIRUSES	HSV	VZV	CMV
Antiviral	Acyclovir	Acyclovir, ganciclovir, adjunctive corticosteroids	Ganciclovir plus foscarnet is recommended

HSV, Herpes simplex virus; VZV, varicella zoster virus; CMV, cytomegalovirus.

131. When should we consider repeating herpes simplex polymer chain reaction (PCR) in suspected encephalitis?

In patients with encephalitis who have a negative initial herpes simplex PCR result, consider repeating the test 3 to 7 days later in those with either a compatible clinical syndrome or temporal lobe localization on neuroimaging.

132. What is the role of adjunctive dexamethasone therapy in patients with bacterial meningitis?

Dexamethasone has been shown to improve functional outcome and reduce mortality in patients with acute community-acquired bacterial meningitis. Administration of dexamethasone (0.15 mg/kg q6h for 2 to 4 days with the first dose administered 30 minutes before, or at least concomitantly with, the first dose of antimicrobial therapy) in adults with suspected or proven pneumococcal meningitis has been recommended. Dexamethasone should only be continued if either the CSF Gram stain reveals gram-positive diplococci or if blood or CSF cultures are positive for *Streptococcus pneumoniae*. Adjunctive dexamethasone should not be given to adult patients who have already received antimicrobial therapy because administration of dexamethasone in this circumstance is unlikely to improve patient outcome.

133. What specific empirical antimicrobial agent(s) should be used in patients with suspected meningitis?

See Table 19-22.

Table 19-22. Empiric Antimicrobial Coverage for Meningitis/Encephalitis

PREDISPOSING FACTOR	COMMON BACTERIAL PATHOGENS	ANTIMICROBIAL THERAPY
2-50 years of age	*Neisseria meningitidis, Streptococcus pneumoniae*	Vancomycin plus a third-generation cephalosporin*,†
>50 years	*S. pneumoniae, N. meningitidis, Listeria monocytogenes*, aerobic gram-negative bacilli	Vancomycin plus ampicillin plus a third-generation cephalosporin*,†
Basilar skull fracture	*S. pneumoniae, Haemophilus influenzae*, group A β-hemolytic streptococci	Vancomycin plus a third-generation cephalosporin*
Penetrating trauma	*Staphylococcus aureus*, coagulase-negative staphylococci (especially *Staphylococcus epidermidis*), aerobic gram-negative bacilli (including *Pseudomonas aeruginosa*)	Vancomycin plus cefepime, vancomycin plus ceftazidime, or vancomycin plus meropenem
Post neurosurgery	Aerobic gram-negative bacilli (including *P. aeruginosa*), *S. aureus*, coagulase-negative staphylococci (especially *S. epidermidis*)	Vancomycin plus cefepime, vancomycin plus ceftazidime, or vancomycin plus meropenem
CSF shunt	Coagulase-negative staphylococci (especially *S. epidermidis*), *S. aureus*, aerobic gram-negative bacilli (including *P. aeruginosa*), *Propionibacterium acnes*	Vancomycin plus cefepime,‡ vancomycin plus ceftazidime,‡ or vancomycin plus meropenem‡

CSF, Cerebral spinal fluid.
*Ceftriaxone or cefotaxime.
†Some experts would add rifampin if dexamethasone is also given.
‡In infants and children, vancomycin alone is reasonable unless Gram stains reveal the presence of gram-negative bacilli.
From Tunkel AR, Hartman BJ, Kaplan SL, et al.: Practice guidelines for the management of bacterial meningitis. *Clin Inf Dis* 39(9):1267-1284, 2004.

134. How is bacterial meningitis managed in adults in the neuro ICU?

In patients with a high risk of brain herniation, consider monitoring ICP and administering intermittent doses of osmotic diuretics (mannitol [25%] or hypertonic [3%] saline) to maintain an ICP of <15 mm Hg and a cerebral perfusion pressure of ≥60 mm Hg. Initiate repeated lumbar puncture, lumbar drain, or ventriculostomy in patients with acute hydrocephalus. EEG monitoring is recommended in patients with a history of seizures and fluctuating scores on the GCS. Either intubate or provide noninvasive ventilation in patients with worsening consciousness (clinical and laboratory indicators for intubation include poor cough and pooling secretions, a respiratory rate of >35 per minute, arterial oxygen saturation of <90% or arterial partial pressure of oxygen of <60 mm Hg, and arterial partial pressure of carbon dioxide of >60 mm Hg) as indicated under general care above. All general principles of ICU care as mentioned above should be followed.

KEY POINTS: MENINGITIS AND ENCEPHALITIS

1. Consider dexamethasone before or with first dose of antibiotic in suspected bacterial meningitis.
2. Consider repeating HSV PCR in 3 to 7 days if clinical suspicion is high and the initial HSV PCR was negative.
3. Identify patients at risk of hydrocephalus and herniation and treat aggressively.

COMATOSE SURVIVORS OF CARDIAC ARREST

135. What is the status of targeted temperature management (TTM)?

The 2010 American Heart Association Guidelines for Cardiopulmonary Resuscitation and Emergency Cardiovascular Care recommend that comatose (i.e., lack of meaningful response to verbal commands) adult patients with return of spontaneous circulation (ROSC) after out-of-hospital ventricular fibrillation cardiac arrest be cooled to 32 to 34° C (89.6 to 93.2° F) for 12 to 24 hours. Induced hypothermia also may be considered for comatose adult patients with ROSC after in-hospital cardiac arrest of any initial rhythm or after out-of-hospital cardiac arrest with an initial rhythm of pulseless electric activity or asystole.

Active rewarming should be avoided in comatose patients who spontaneously develop a mild degree of hypothermia (>32° C [89.6° F]) after resuscitation from cardiac arrest during the first 48 hours after ROSC.

The TTM after a cardiac arrest clinical trial published in 2013 included patients with both shockable and nonshockable rhythms experiencing out-of-hospital cardiac arrest. The TTM trial showed that hypothermia at a targeted temperature of 33° C did not confer a benefit as compared with a targeted temperature of 36° C in the first 24 hours and both groups did not differ in complication rates. It is left at the discretion of the hospital policy to use either 36 or 33° C pending further guidance. It is important to highlight that 36° C in this trial was not intended to represent the normothermia arm but rather the TTM arm. Maintaining this temperature target still requires similar active interventions as the induced hypothermia protocol.

136. How do we prognosticate after cardiac arrest?

The neurologic examination is the best way to prognosticate outcome in comatose survivors of cardiac arrest. The prognosis is invariably poor in comatose patients with absent pupillary or corneal reflexes or absent or extensor motor responses 3 days after cardiac arrest. The best possible outcome for these patients after hospital discharge would be vegetative state or only fragmentary response to external stimuli. These recommendations were based on data prior to the availability of induced hypothermia or TTM protocols. Even though there are no new data to guide prognostication with the advent of these protocols, the general consensus is to determine prognosis 72 hours after rewarming has been achieved.

BRAIN DEATH

137. What are the criteria to determine brain death?

The determination of brain death can be considered to consist of four steps:

1. The clinical evaluation (prerequisites).
   a. Establish irreversible and proximate cause of coma.
      i. Establish by history, examination, neuroimaging, and laboratory tests.
      ii. Exclude the presence of a CNS-depressant drug effect by history, drug screen, calculation of clearance using five times the drug's half-life (assuming normal hepatic and renal function), or, if available, drug plasma levels below the therapeutic range.
      iii. Prior use of hypothermia (e.g., after cardiopulmonary resuscitation for cardiac arrest) may delay drug metabolism.
      iv. Blood alcohol content (<0.08%) is a practical threshold below which an examination to determine brain death could reasonably proceed.

 v. No recent administration or continued presence of neuromuscular blocking agents (assessed by the presence of a train of four twitches with maximal ulnar nerve stimulation).
 vi. No severe electrolyte, acid–base, or endocrine disturbance (defined by severe acidosis or laboratory values markedly deviated from the norm).
 vii. Achieve normal core temperature >36° C.
 viii. Systolic blood pressure ≥100 mm Hg.
 2. The clinical evaluation (neurologic assessment).
 a. Presence of coma.
 b. Absence of brain stem reflexes.
 c. Apnea as demonstrated by an apnea test.
 3. Ancillary tests: EEG, cerebral angiography, nuclear scan, TCD, CTA, and MRI/MRA.
 Brain death is a clinical diagnosis. Ancillary testing can be used when uncertainty exists about the reliability of parts of the neurologic examination or when the apnea test cannot be performed.
 4. Documentation.
The time of brain death is documented in the medical records.

138. **How is the apnea test performed?**
Adjust vasopressors to a systolic blood pressure ≥100 mm Hg. Preoxygenate for at least 10 minutes with 100% oxygen to a PaO_2 ≥200 mm Hg. Reduce ventilation frequency to 10 breaths per minute to eucapnia. Reduce PEEP to 5 cm H_2O (oxygen desaturation with decreasing PEEP may suggest difficulty with apnea testing). If pulse oximetry oxygen saturation remains >95%, obtain a baseline blood gas (PaO_2, $PaCO_2$, pH, bicarbonate, base excess). Disconnect the patient from the ventilator. Preserve oxygenation (e.g., place an insufflation catheter through the endotracheal tube and close to the level of the carina and deliver 100% O_2 at 6 L/min).
 Look closely for respiratory movements for 8 to 10 minutes. Respiration is defined as abdominal or chest excursions and may include a brief gasp.
 Abort if systolic blood pressure decreases to <90 mm Hg. Abort if oxygen saturation measured by pulse oximetry is <85% for >30 seconds. Retry procedure with T-piece, CPAP 10 cm H_2O, and 100% O_2 12 L/min.
 If no respiratory drive is observed, repeat blood gas (PaO_2, $PaCO_2$, pH, bicarbonate, base excess) after approximately 8 minutes.
 If respiratory movements are absent and arterial PCO_2 is ≥60 mm Hg (or 20-mm Hg increase in arterial PCO_2 over a baseline normal arterial PCO_2), the apnea test result is positive (i.e., supports the clinical diagnosis of brain death).
 If the test is inconclusive but the patient is hemodynamically stable during the procedure, it may be repeated for a longer period of time (10 to 15 minutes) after the patient is again adequately preoxygenated.

KEY POINTS: COMATOSE SURVIVORS OF CARDIAC ARREST

1. Hyperthermia after cardiac arrest is associated with bad outcome.
2. Hypothermia at a targeted temperature of 33° C did not confer a benefit as compared with a targeted temperature of 36° C in the first 24 hours.
3. Absent pupillary or corneal reflexes or absent or extensor motor response, bilateral absence of cortical somatosensory evoked potentials (N_2O response), serum neuron-specific enolase levels >33 μg/L within 1 to 3 days, and myoclonus SE within the first day post cardiac arrest predict poor outcome.
4. Brain death is a clinical diagnosis.

MODERATE TO SEVERE TRAUMATIC BRAIN INJURY

139. **How is TBI classified?**
TBI is classified based on GCS after initial resuscitation.

Mild	Moderate	Severe
13-15 GCS	9-12 GCS	3-8 GCS

140. **What are the types of injuries we see in TBI?**

TBI is a heterogeneous condition with multiple mechanisms for injury. Primary injury occurs at time of impact, and secondary injury develops over hours to days. Injury can be either diffuse or perilesional. The mechanism of secondary injury is multifactorial; hypoxia–ischemia and CBF dysautoregulation are two of many secondary factors that influence outcome after TBI.

141. **What are the predictors of poor outcome in TBI?**

Hypoxia (oxygen saturation <90%) and hypotension (systolic blood pressure <90 mm Hg) are independent predictors of poor outcome. A sustained ICP >20 mm Hg or CPP <50 mm Hg are also associated with poor outcome.

142. **What are the blood pressure and oxygenation goals in TBI?**

Blood pressure should be monitored and hypotension (systolic blood pressure <90 mm Hg) avoided. Oxygenation should be monitored and hypoxia (PaO_2 <60 mm Hg or O_2 saturation <90%) avoided.

143. **What are the indications for ICP monitoring following TBI?**

Intracranial hypertension correlates with worse outcome. ICP >20 mm Hg is the threshold for treatment. The main indications for ICP monitoring are the following: (1) GCS 3 to 8 after resuscitation and an abnormal CT scan. An abnormal CT scan of the head is one that reveals hematomas, contusions, swelling, herniation, or compressed basal cisterns; and (2) GCS 3 to 8 after resuscitation with a normal CT scan if two or more of the following features are noted at admission: age over 40 years, unilateral or bilateral motor posturing, or systolic blood pressure <90 mm Hg.

144. **Should hyperventilation be used prophylactically?**

Prophylactic hyperventilation ($PaCO_2$ of 25 mm Hg or less) is not recommended. Hyperventilation is recommended as a temporizing measure for the reduction of elevated ICP. Hyperventilation should be avoided during the first 24 hours after injury when CBF is often critically reduced.

145. **What is the role of hyperosmolar therapy?**

Mannitol is effective for control of raised ICP at doses of 0.25 gm/kg to 1 g/kg body weight. Restrict mannitol use prior to ICP monitoring to patients with signs of transtentorial herniation or progressive neurologic deterioration not attributable to extracranial causes.

146. **Is there any role for prophylactic hypothermia?**

Pooled data indicate that prophylactic hypothermia is not significantly associated with decreased mortality when compared with normothermic controls. However, preliminary findings suggest that a greater decrease in mortality risk is observed when target temperatures are maintained for more than 48 hours. Prophylactic hypothermia is associated with significantly higher Glasgow Outcome Scale scores when compared to scores for normothermic controls.

147. **What is the goal CPP?**

Aggressive attempts to maintain CPP above 70 mm Hg with fluids and pressors should be avoided because of the risk of ARDS. CPP of <50 mm Hg should be avoided. The CPP value to target lies within the range of 50 to 70 mm Hg.

148. **What is the role of steroids?**

The use of steroids is not recommended for improving outcome or reducing ICP. In patients with moderate or severe TBI, high-dose methylprednisolone is associated with increased mortality and is contraindicated.

149. **What is the role of surgery?**

The Decompressive Craniectomy in Patients with Severe Traumatic Brain Injury (DECRA) clinical trial studied whether early decompressive craniectomy in patients with diffuse TBI and refractory ICP improved outcome. DECRA showed that intervention decreased ICP and length of stay but was associated with more unfavorable outcomes.

150. **What are the indications for surgery in epidural hematoma, acute subdural hematoma, and traumatic parenchymal lesions?**

Epidural hematoma: Volume >30 cm^3 regardless of the patient's GCS score; coma (GCS score <9) with anisocoria; and signs of herniation and elevated ICP.

Subdural hematoma (SDH): Acute, thickness >10 mm *or* a midline shift >5 mm regardless of the patient's GCS score; all patients in coma (GCS score <9) with an SDH <10 mm thick and a midline shift <5 mm should undergo surgical evacuation of the lesion if the GCS score decreased between the time of injury and hospital admission by 2 or more points on the GCS and/or the patient presents with asymmetric or fixed and dilated pupils and/or the ICP exceeds 20 mm Hg.

Traumatic parenchymal lesions: GCS scores of 6 to 8 with frontal or temporal contusions >20 cm^3 in volume with midline shift of at least 5 mm and/or cisternal compression on CT scan, and patients with any lesion >50 cm^3 in volume.

KEY POINTS: TRAUMATIC BRAIN INJURY

1. Hypoxia (oxygen saturation <90%) and hypotension (systolic blood pressure <90 mm Hg) are independent predictors of poor outcome.
2. Prophylactic hyperventilation in TBI is not recommended.
3. No role for steroids and surgery in diffuse TBI.

 References available online at expertconsult.com.

BIBLIOGRAPHY

General Management

1. Mercat A, Richard JC, Vielle B, et al.: Expiratory Pressure (Express) Study Group. Positive end-expiratory pressure setting in adults with acute lung injury and acute respiratory distress syndrome: a randomized controlled trial. JAMA 299(6):646-665, 2008.
2. MacIntyre NR, Cook DJ, Ely Jr EW, et al.: Evidence-based guidelines for weaning and discontinuing ventilatory support: a collective task force facilitated by the American College of Chest Physicians, the American Association for Respiratory Care, and the American College of Critical Care Medicine. Chest 120(Suppl.):375S-395S, 2001.
3. Bershad EM, Humphreis 3rd WE, Suarez JI: Intracranial hypertension. Semin Neurol 28: 690-702, 2008.
4. Dellinger RP, Levy MM, Rhodes A, et al.: Surviving sepsis campaign: international guidelines for management of severe sepsis and septic shock. Crit Care Med 41:580-637, 2013.

ICH

5. Qureshi AI, Mendelow AD, Hanley DF: Intracerebral haemorrhage. Lancet 373(9675): 1632-1644, 2009.
6. Demchuk AM, Dowlatshahi D, Rodriguez-Luna D, et al.: Prediction of haematoma growth and outcome in patients with intracerebral haemorrhage using the CT-angiography spot sign (PREDICT): a prospective observational study. Lancet Neurol 11(4):307-314, 2012.
7. Charidimou A, Peeters AP, Jager R, et al.: Cortical superficial siderosis and intracerebral hemorrhage risk in cerebral amyloid angiopathy. Neurology 81(19):1666-1673, 2013.
8. Morgenstern LB, Hemphill 3rd JC, Anderson C, et al.: Guidelines for the management of spontaneous intracerebral hemorrhage: a guideline for healthcare professionals from the American Heart Association/American Stroke Association. Stroke 41(9):2108-2129, 2010.

SAH

9. Macdonald RL: Delayed neurological deterioration after subarachnoid haemorrhage. Nat Rev Neurol 10:44-58, 2014.
10. Connolly Jr ES, Rabinstein AA, Carhuapoma JR, et al.: Guidelines for the management of aneurysmal subarachnoid hemorrhage: a guideline for healthcare professionals from the American Heart Association/American Stroke Association. Stroke 43:1711-1737, 2012.
11. Diringer MN, Bleck TP, Claude Hemphill 3rd J, et al.: Critical care management of patients following aneurysmal subarachnoid hemorrhage: recommendations from the Neurocritical Care Society's Multidisciplinary Consensus Conference. Neurocrit Care 15:211-240, 2011.

Large Hemispheric and Cerebellar Ischemic Stroke

12. Wijdicks EF, Sheth KN, Carter BS, et al.: Recommendations for the management of cerebral and cerebellar infarction with swelling: a statement for healthcare professionals from the American Heart Association/American Stroke Association. Stroke 45:1222-1238, 2014.

Neuromuscular Weaknesses in the ICU

13. Bershad EM, Feen ES, Suarez JI: Myasthenia gravis crisis. South Med J 101:63-69, 2008.
14. Rabinstein A, Wijdicks EF: BiPAP in acute respiratory failure due to myasthenic crisis may prevent intubation. Neurology 10:1647-1649, 2002.
15. Hughes RA, Wijdicks EF, Barohn R, et al.: Practice parameter: immunotherapy for Guillain-Barré syndrome: report of the Quality Standards Subcommittee of the American Academy of Neurology. Neurology 61(6):736-740, 2003.

Status Epilepticus

16. Brophy GM, Bell R, Claassen J, et al.: Guidelines for the evaluation and management of status epilepticus. Neurocrit Care 17:3-23, 2012.
17. Jirsch J, Hirsch LJ: Nonconvulsive seizures: developing a rational approach to the diagnosis and management in the critically ill population. Clin Neurophysiol 118:1660-1670, 2007.
18. Hirsch LJ, Gaspard N: Status epilepticus. Continuum (Minneapolis, Minn.) 19:767-794, 2013.

Meningitis and Encephalitis

19. de Gans J, van de Beek D: European Dexamethasone in Adulthood Bacterial Meningitis Study Investigators: Dexamethasone in adults with bacterial meningitis. N Engl J Med 347(20):1549-1556, 2002.
20. Tunkel AR, Hartman BJ, Kaplan SL, et al.: Practice guidelines for the management of bacterial meningitis. Clin Inf Dis 39(9):1267-1284, 2004.
21. Tunkel AR, Glaser CA, Bloch KC, et al.: The management of encephalitis: clinical practice guidelines by the Infectious Diseases Society of America. Clin Infect Dis 47(3):303-327, 2008.
22. Van de Beek D, de Gans J, Tunkel A, Wijdicks EFM: Community-acquired bacterial meningitis in adults. N Engl J Med 354:44-53, 2006.

Comatose Survivors of Cardiac Arrest

23. Bernard SA, Gray TW, Buist MD, et al.: Treatment of comatose survivors of out-of-hospital cardiac arrest with induced hypothermia. N Engl J Med 346(8):557-563, 2002.
24. Hypothermia after Cardiac Arrest Study Group: Mild therapeutic hypothermia to improve the neurologic outcome after cardiac arrest. N Engl J Med 346(8):549-556, 2002.
25. Nielsen N, Wetterslev J, Cronberg T, et al.: Targeted temperature management at 33° C versus 36° C after cardiac arrest. N Engl J Med 369:2197-2206, 2013.
26. Wijdicks EF, Hijdra A, Young GB, et al.: Practice parameter: prediction of outcome in comatose survivors after cardio-pulmonary resuscitation (an evidence-based review): report of the Quality Standards Subcommittee of the American Academy of Neurology. Neurology 67:203-210, 2006.
27. Wijdicks EF, Varelas PN, Gronseth GS, et al.: Evidence-based guideline update: determining brain death in adults: report of the Quality Standards Subcommittee of the American Academy of Neurology. Neurology 74(23):1911-1918, 2010.

TBI

28. Brain Trauma Foundation American Association of Neurological Surgeons Congress of Neurological Surgeons: Guidelines for the management of severe traumatic brain injury. [erratum published in J Neurotrauma 2008; 25(3):276-278] J Neurotrauma 24(Suppl. 1):S1-S106, 2007.

NEURO-ONCOLOGY

Jacob Mandel

CHAPTER 20

PRIMARY BRAIN TUMORS

1. **How are brain tumors classified?**
   Unlike most other malignant cancers, which are classified by the TNM (tumor size, lymph nodes, and metastasis) system, tumors arising from the central nervous system (CNS) are classified into four grades according to the World Health Organization (WHO) grading system.

2. **Describe the four grades of the WHO grading system for CNS tumors.**
   Grade I tumors are typically *well circumscribed*, slow growing, nonmalignant, and associated with long-term survival. Grade II tumors are relatively slow growing but sometimes recur as higher grade tumors and are defined histopathologically by *nuclear atypia* (abnormal appearance of cell nuclei). Grade III tumors are malignant and often recur as higher grade tumors and are defined histopathologically by *mitosis* (a process in cell division by which the nucleus divides). Grade IV tumors are fast growing and defined histopathologically by *microvascular proliferation* (blood vessels that have multiple layers of enlarged endothelial cells) and/or *necrosis* (cell death).

3. **What causes brain tumors?**
   For most patients the cause is unknown. The only definitive environmental risk factor for brain tumors is ionizing radiation. An elevated risk of several brain tumors such as meningiomas, gliomas, and nerve sheath tumors has been seen in cohort studies of atomic bomb survivors and childhood cancer survivors who received cranial radiation. Additionally, a small percentage of brain tumors are related to specific genetic syndromes such as neurofibromatosis type 1, neurofibromatosis type 2, Turcot syndrome, Gorlin syndrome, von Hippel–Lindau syndrome, and Li–Fraumeni syndrome.

4. **What are the most common brain tumors?**
   The most common brain tumors in adults are gliomas and meningiomas. Pilocytic astrocytomas, malignant gliomas, and medulloblastomas are the most common in children.

5. **Name the three glial cell types that make up gliomas.**
   Astrocytes, oligodendrocytes, and ependymocytes. Astrocytes fix neurons to their blood supply and serve a number of important support and structural roles, oligodendrocytes coat axons in the CNS creating a myelin sheath allowing electrical signals in the nervous system to travel faster, and ependymocytes line the ventricular system of the brain and spinal cord, helping create and secrete cerebrospinal fluid (CSF).

6. **Are gliomas found in different brain regions depending on age?**
   Yes, gliomas are mostly supratentorial in adults but infratentorial in children.

7. **Which is the most frequent glioma?**
   Glioblastoma (grade IV astrocytoma) is the most common and most malignant brain tumor in adults. It typically occurs in patients in the fourth and fifth decades of life.

8. **What are the characteristic radiographic findings for a glioblastoma?**
   Glioblastomas often appear as ring-enhancing lesions with a necrotic center on contrast magnetic resonance imaging (MRI). They are usually in the cerebrum but can infrequently display the classic infiltration across the corpus callosum ("butterfly glioma") (Fig. 20-1). Even in cases of classical imaging findings, tumor resection and pathologic confirmation are necessary.

9. **Can a glioblastoma be treated with surgery alone?**
   No, unfortunately, even when a glioblastoma has been completely resected there are microscopic cells that are infiltrative and intermixed with the normal brain that remain requiring treatment. However, studies have shown that prognosis improves with a gross total resection of the imaged enhancement.

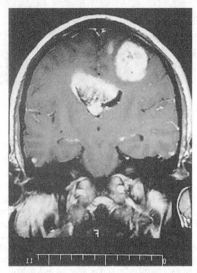

Figure 20-1. Gadolinium-enhanced T1-weighted magnetic resonance imaging (MRI) of the brain showing a malignant glioblastoma multiforme, with characteristic extension across the corpus callosum.

10. Describe the recommended treatment for a newly diagnosed glioblastoma.
Maximal surgical resection followed by concurrent chemoradiation with 75 mg/m^2 daily temozolomide for 6 weeks. After chemoradiation, patients have a month off of treatment and then undergo adjuvant temozolomide 150-200 mg/mg^2 for 5 days out of a 28-day cycle for 6 to 12 cycles.

11. What is "pseudoprogression"?
MRI may reveal an increase in contrast enhancement during the first few months after chemoradiation treatment. However, this imaging change may be due to treatment-related inflammation, postsurgical changes, ischemia, subacute radiation effects, or radiation necrosis and may not be because of tumor progression. Caution must be taken following chemoradiation treatment not to conclude that the tumor has progressed and treatment has failed, unless the new enhancement is outside of the previously radiated area.

12. How common is "pseudoprogression" in glioblastoma?
Twenty to thirty percent of patients undergoing their first postchemoradiation MRI show increased contrast enhancement that ultimately resolves without any change in therapy.

13. Are there any radiographic criteria to determine tumor progression?
The Response Assessment in Neuro-Oncology (RANO) criteria are used, which incorporates an increase in fluid attenuated inversion recovery hyperintensity as a way to measure nonenhancing tumor progression.

14. Have any second-line therapies been found for glioblastoma?
In 2009, the Food and Drug Administration approved the use of bevacizumab, a monoclonal antibody that binds vascular endothelial growth factor, for monotherapy in recurrent glioblastoma.

15. What is the prognosis for glioblastoma?
Glioblastoma has a poor prognosis with a median survival of 4 to 5 months without treatment and 16 to 18 months with standard of care treatment (concurrent chemoradiation with temozolomide followed by adjuvant temozolomide).

16. Have any clinical factors been shown to be useful in predicting prognosis in malignant (grade III and IV) gliomas?
Younger age, Karnofsky performance score (a scale used to quantify cancer patients' general well-being and activities of daily life), and larger extent of initial surgical resection have been shown to improve prognosis.

17. Are there any molecular alterations that are useful in the prognosis of malignant gliomas?

   Tumors with methyl guanine methyl transferase (MGMT) promoter methylation and mutations in the enzymes isocitrate dehydrogenase-1 (IDH1) and IDH2 have improved prognosis in malignant gliomas. Additionally, glioblastoma studies show MGMT may be predictive of response to temozolomide therapy as MGMT methylation silences an enzyme responsible for DNA repair following alkylating agent chemotherapy. Combined loss of genetic materials from chromosomes 1p and 19q is a major prognostic and predictive factor for improved survival and response to therapy in oligodendroglioma.

18. Which chemotherapy regimen has been shown to be the most beneficial in 1p/19q codeleted anaplastic oligodendrogliomas?

   For newly diagnosed 1p/19q codeleted anaplastic oligodendrogliomas, treatment with procarbazine, CCNU, and vincristine (PCV) either before or after radiation has been shown to nearly double the median overall survival.

19. Is there any standard of care treatment for patients with low-grade glioma?

   Currently, there is a lack of consensus regarding treatment because of a lack of randomized clinical trials. Recent data have suggested that high-risk (defined as biopsy/subtotal resection or age greater than 40) patients with low-grade glioma benefit more from treatment consisting of radiation followed by PCV compared to radiation alone. However, further studies and validation are needed.

20. Describe the classical histopathologic finding in ependymomas.

   Ependymoma is the most common primary tumor of the spinal cord in adults. Perivascular pseudo-rosettes (anuclear zones formed by radially arranged tumor cell processes surrounding central blood vessels) are the key histologic feature of ependymomas. Myxopapillary ependymoma is commonly located in the region of the conus medullaris/cauda equina/filum terminale (Fig. 20-2). These tumors are often encapsulated. Patients who undergo a complete resection without a breach of the capsule are unlikely to experience tumor spread and have been found to have an improved prognosis.

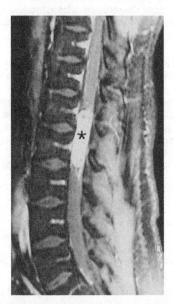

Figure 20-2. Gadolinium-enhanced T1-weighted magnetic resonance imaging (MRI) of the spine showing a myxopapillary ependymoma located in the region of the conus medullaris/cauda equina/filum terminale (*asterisk*). *(From Smith JK, Lury K, Castillo M: Imaging of spinal and spinal cord tumors.* Semin Roentgenol *41(4):274-293, 2006.)*

21. Describe the radiographic finding typically seen in meningioma.

Homogeneous contrast enhancement is seen on imaging often with a "dural tail" sign as a result of thickening of the dura (Fig. 20-3).

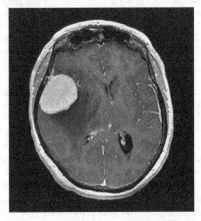

Figure 20-3. Gadolinium-enhanced T1-weighted magnetic resonance imaging (MRI) of the brain showing homogeneous contrast enhancement with thickening of the dura ("dural tail" sign). *(From Colnat-Coulbois S, Kremer S, Weinbreck N et al: Lipomatous meningioma: report of 2 cases and review of the literature.* Surg Neurol *69(4):398-402, 2008.)*

22. How are meningiomas treated?

Asymptomatic patients with incidentally discovered tumors may just be monitored with periodic MRI. Patients typically undergo a surgical resection if either they are symptomatic or the tumor is growing. Radiation may be performed if residual tumor is left after resection. Unlike benign (Grade I) meningioma, atypical and anaplastic meningioma (grades II and III) can be very aggressive and may require several surgeries and/or radiation. Chemotherapy including hydroxyurea, interferon-alfa, imatinib, and somatostatin has been tried with little evidence of either efficacy or increase in survival.

23. What medication should be avoided in patients where primary CNS lymphoma is on the differential?

Corticosteroids may alter the histopathology of the tumor and delay the diagnosis. It is essential that they not be given unless absolutely necessary before pathologic confirmation of biopsy results.

KEY POINTS: PRIMARY BRAIN TUMORS

1. CNS tumors are classified into four grades according to the WHO grading system.
2. Glioblastoma (grade IV astrocytoma) is the most common and malignant primary brain tumor in adults.
3. IDH-mutated malignant gliomas have an improved prognosis.
4. Corticosteroids may alter the histopathology of the tumor and delay the diagnosis in patients with primary CNS lymphoma.
5. Medulloblastomas have a high propensity to disseminate through the CNS; therefore a spinal MRI and lumbar puncture for CSF cytology should be performed.

24. Which chemotherapeutic agent should be used when treating newly diagnosed primary CNS lymphoma?

High-dose systemic methotrexate either alone or in combination with other agents such as cytarabine, rituximab, temozolomide, procarbazine, or vincristine.

25. Why is the use of radiation therapy in initial treatment of primary CNS lymphoma controversial?

Despite primary CNS lymphoma being extremely sensitive to radiation therapy, it is often withheld due to high rates of cognitive problems especially in elderly patients. For patients who are not candidates for high-dose systemic methotrexate (i.e., renal failure), it has continued to be an option for palliative treatment. Additionally for younger patients with a good cognitive performance status, radiation therapy after initial methotrexate therapy may be beneficial and continues to be further studied.

26. In addition to a brain MRI what other testing should be performed in patients following a diagnosis of medulloblastoma?

    Spine MRI and lumbar puncture for CSF cytology should be performed, as one-third of medulloblastomas metastasize throughout the CNS. Patients with spread of disease into the CSF have been shown to have a worse prognosis.

27. Are there any molecular markers that have shown to be useful in predicting prognosis in medulloblastoma?

    Integrative genomic studies propose that medulloblastoma can be divided into four molecular subgroups (WNT, SHH, Group 3, and Group 4). WNT tumors have the best prognosis, whereas Group 3 tumors with amplification of the *MYC* proto-oncogene have the worst prognosis.

28. Which syndrome is associated with surgical resection of medulloblastomas in children?

    Posterior fossa syndrome (cerebellar mutism) is a unique postoperative complication that is produced by damage to the cerebellar vermis or dentate nuclei. Impaired language production as well as emotional lability is seen a few days following surgery. Symptoms often resolve over the course of weeks to months but some patients may not completely recover language skills.

29. How is risk of tumor recurrence (average risk versus high risk) defined in medulloblastoma?

    Average-risk disease is defined as total or near-total resection and no evidence of disseminated disease by brain and spine MRI and CSF analysis. High-risk disease is defined as the presence of residual tumor ≥1.5 cm^2 following resection and/or evidence of disseminated or metastatic disease.

30. What is the initial treatment for medulloblastomas following surgical resection in children?

    For children older than 3 years, average-risk patients receive craniospinal irradiation with weekly vincristine and then adjuvant chemotherapy (vincristine, cisplatin, and CCNU or vincristine, cisplatin, and cyclophosphamide) whereas high-risk patients receive craniospinal irradiation with concurrent carboplatin and vincristine, followed by six cycles of cyclophosphamide and vincristine with or without cisplatin. Children younger than 3 years who receive craniospinal radiation are at high risk for serious damage to their developing nervous systems. Therefore, treatment is limited to multichemotherapeutic drug regimens without radiation.

31. If available, which type of craniospinal radiation should be performed in children?

    Proton beam irradiation can reduce the amount of radiation to normal tissue without compromising the radiation dose delivered to the tumor, thus decreasing long-term morbidity. However, this therapy is not widely available and needs expensive, specialized equipment.

32. Pituitary tumors can present with which neurologic finding on exam?

    Pituitary adenoma classically presents with bitemporal hemianopsia (peripheral vision loss affecting both eyes).

33. What is pituitary apoplexy?

    Pituitary apoplexy is sudden hemorrhage into the pituitary gland. Patients usually present with a severe headache and visual changes. Neurosurgery should be consulted as surgical decompression of the pituitary may be necessary. Additionally, stress doses of hydrocortisone should be given intravenously emergently because of the risk of adrenal failure (disruption in adrenocorticotropic hormone production) and subsequent shock.

34. What are prolactinomas and which medications are used to treat them?

    Prolactin-producing pituitary adenomas (prolactinomas) are benign tumors of the pituitary gland that produce prolactin. Prolactinomas are most common in women under the age of 50. Dopamine agonists such as bromocriptine and cabergoline are used to treat them.

35. Pineal gland tumors may present with which syndrome?

    Parinaud's syndrome which is characterized by paralysis of vertical gaze, pseudo-Argyll Robertson pupils, convergence–retraction nystagmus, upper eyelid retraction, and conjugate downward gaze.

36. What brain tumor is part of the diagnostic criteria of neurofibromatosis type 1?

    Optic nerve glioma.

BRAIN AND SPINE METASTATIC DISEASE

37. Are primary brain tumors more common than brain metastases?

No, brain metastases are the most common intracranial tumors in adults, occurring nearly 10 times more often than primary brain tumors.

38. Where are brain metastases usually located in the brain?

Eighty percent are located in the cerebral hemispheres, 15% in the cerebellum, and 5% in the brainstem (Fig. 20-4). This distribution correlates with the blood flow to each area of the brain as the most common mechanism of metastasis to the brain is by hematogenous spread. Brain metastases tend to develop in "watershed" areas where the vasculature is narrow as well as at the gray–white matter junctions.

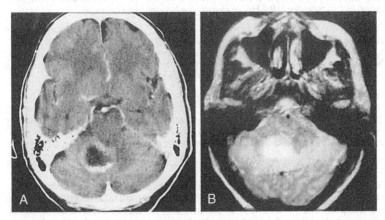

Figure 20-4. Small-cell carcinoma of the lung metastatic to the cerebellum shown on contrast-enhanced computed tomography (CT) scan (**A**) and proton-density magnetic resonance imaging (MRI) (**B**).

39. Brain metastases typically arise from which primary cancers?

Lung cancer, breast cancer, and melanoma are the most common. Melanoma has the highest tendency to spread to the brain, with up to 50% of advanced melanoma patients ultimately developing brain metastases.

40. What is the prognosis for patients with brain metastases?

Most studies show a median overall survival of less than 6 months. Patients with a good performance score, age less than 65 years, and a controlled primary tumor with no known extracranial metastases have the best prognosis.

41. Should patients with brain metastases undergo surgical resection of the lesion?

Surgery can be useful for symptomatic relief and local tumor control and provide a histologic diagnosis in patients with single brain metastases, controlled primary cancer, and no extracranial disease. Patients with a few small brain metastases (diameter of 3 cm or less) are treated with stereotactic radiosurgery. Treatment with whole brain radiation following surgery or stereotactic radiosurgery is controversial as it improves local control but not overall survival. It also increases the risk of cognitive decline following radiation. Patients with either large or multiple metastases should be treated with whole brain radiation.

42. Do any primary cancer types benefit from prophylactic cranial irradiation?

Prophylactic cranial irradiation has been shown to decrease the incidence of brain metastases and lengthen overall survival in patients with small-cell lung cancer who have responded to initial treatment and have limited stage disease (confined to one hemithorax).

43. Which primary cancers are the most common underlying cancer diagnoses in neoplastic epidural spinal cord compression?

Lung cancer, breast cancer, and multiple myeloma are the most common primary cancers. Patients with multiple myeloma have the highest incidence, with rates around 15%.

KEY POINTS: BRAIN AND SPINE METASTATIC DISEASE

1. Brain metastases are the most common intracranial tumors in adults, occurring nearly 10 times more often than primary brain tumors.
2. Melanoma has the highest tendency to spread to the brain, with up to 50% of advanced melanoma patients ultimately developing brain metastases.
3. Pain is usually the first and most common (80% to 90%) symptom of neoplastic epidural spinal cord compression.
4. Pretreatment neurologic status is the single most important prognostic factor for being ambulatory after neoplastic epidural spinal cord compression.

44. **What symptom is usually the first reported in neoplastic epidural spinal cord compression?**
Pain is usually the first and most common (80% to 90%) symptom of neoplastic epidural spinal cord compression. Other possible symptoms include weakness, sensory findings, bladder/bowel dysfunction, and ataxia. Neoplastic epidural spinal cord compression most frequently is located in the thoracic spine. Approximately 60% of cases occur in the thoracic spine, 30% in the lumbosacral spine, and 10% in the cervical spine.

45. **How is neoplastic epidural spinal cord compression treated?**
Patients should receive high-dose corticosteroids initially. Radiation therapy has shown to be beneficial in improving pain and preserving neurologic function. If patients have an unstable spine and limited primary disease burden, a decompressive resection and stabilization followed by radiation therapy should be performed. Early diagnosis and urgent treatment are critically important to maintain neurologic function. Pretreatment neurologic status is the single most important prognostic factor for being ambulatory after neoplastic epidural spinal cord compression.

LEPTOMENINGEAL DISEASE

46. **How common is leptomeningeal disease (LMD)?**
LMD is diagnosed in 5% of patients with metastatic cancer. The most common primary tumors associated with the development of LMD are breast, lung, and melanoma.

47. **Which sites are typically affected in LMD?**
The cerebellar folia, cortical surface and basal cisterns of the brain, as well as the dorsal aspect of the spinal cord (especially the cauda equina).

48. **What tests should be ordered in a person suspected of having LMD?**
MRI of the entire neuroaxis with contrast and a lumbar puncture to send CSF for cytology. MRI should be performed prior to the lumbar puncture as pachymeningeal enhancement may be seen on imaging following a lumbar puncture.

49. **Are CSF cytology results sensitive for LMD?**
An initial cytology sample has a sensitivity of only around 70%. The sensitivity increases to 86% after two samples and 90% after three samples. At least 10 mL of CSF should be collected with each sample for cytologic analysis alone. Flow cytometry should also be ordered in hematologic malignancies.

50. **Is there a difference in survival in LMD patients with primary solid versus primary hematologic malignancies?**
Prognosis for patients with LMD is extremely poor. Patients with solid tumors have a median survival around 2 to 3 months whereas those with hematologic malignancies have a slightly better median survival of around 4 to 5 months.

51. **How are poor-risk versus good-risk patients defined in LMD?**
Poor-risk patients have a low Karnofsky performance status (KPS) <60, severe neurologic deficits, or extensive systemic cancer with limited therapeutic options. These patients have a poor prognosis, and treatment should be focused on alleviating symptoms with steroids, analgesics, and/or radiation therapy. Good-risk patients have a KPS of 60 or greater, no major neurologic impairments, little systemic disease, and/or a cancer for which there are treatment options. Good-risk patients receive treatment with radiation to bulky/symptomatic areas of LMD followed by intrathecal chemotherapy.

52. What is an Ommaya reservoir?

An Ommaya reservoir is an intraventricular catheter system used for the aspiration of CSF and/or for the delivery of chemotherapy into the CSF. It is made up of a reservoir implanted under the scalp attached to a catheter in a lateral ventricle (Fig. 20-5). Prior to starting intrathecal chemotherapy via an Ommaya reservoir a CSF flow study via a radionuclide cisternogram should be performed to detect any areas of obstruction that may stop the chemotherapy from being circulated throughout the CSF. Radiation to areas of blockage can reverse the flow abnormality, thus improving the efficacy of intrathecal chemotherapy.

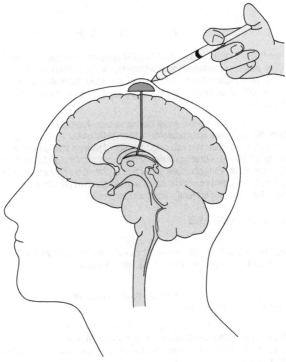

Figure 20-5. An Ommaya reservoir is made up of a reservoir implanted under the scalp attached to a catheter in a lateral ventricle used for the aspiration of cerebrospinal fluid and/or for the delivery of chemotherapy into the cerebrospinal fluid.

53. Name the three most commonly used intrathecal chemotherapies in patients with LMD.

Methotrexate, liposomal cytarabine, and thiotepa.

KEY POINTS: LEPTOMENINGEAL DISEASE

1. LMD is diagnosed in 5% of patients with metastatic cancer.
2. Methotrexate, liposomal cytarabine, and thiotepa are the three most commonly used intrathecal chemotherapies in patients with LMD.
3. A CSF flow study via a radionuclide cisternogram should be obtained prior to starting intrathecal chemotherapy.

NEUROLOGIC COMPLICATIONS FROM CANCER AND THERAPY

54. What complication should be suspected in cancer patients with lower extremity erythema swelling and pain?
Venous thromboembolism including deep vein thrombosis (blood clot) is increased in cancer patients. It is especially common in patients with malignant gliomas, affecting 20% to 30% of patients.

55. Intrathecal methotrexate use has been associated with which neurologic complications?
Aseptic meningitis, transverse myelopathy, encephalopathy, and leukoencephalopathy.

56. Systemic therapy of high-dose methotrexate is associated with failure of which organ?
Renal failure can be seen during treatment with high-dose methotrexate. Patients should be given aggressive hydration, urinary alkalinization, and leucovorin rescue when treated with high-dose metho-trexate. Additionally, glucarpidase was recently approved as a rescue treatment of toxic methotrexate plasma concentrations in patients with delayed methotrexate clearance due to impaired renal function.

57. Posterior reversible encephalopathy syndrome can be seen after treatment with which chemotherapies?
Cisplatin, cyclophosphamide, gemcitabine, sorafenib, and bevacizumab.

58. Which medication should be given to prevent aseptic meningitis from intrathecal liposomal cytarabine?
Dexamethasone should be given orally (4 mg twice daily) for a total of 5 days starting therapy 1 day before treatment with liposomal cytarabine.

59. Describe the type of ototoxicity reported with cisplatin use.
Ototoxicity from cisplatin use is characterized by a dose-dependent, high-frequency sensorineural hearing loss with tinnitus.

60. Pharyngolaryngeal dysesthesias can occur 24 to 72 hours after administration of which chemotherapeutic agent?
Oxaliplatin.

61. Peripheral neuropathies are associated with which chemotherapeutic agents?
Bortezomib, cisplatin, oxaliplatin, vincristine, paclitaxel, and thalidomide.

KEY POINTS: NEUROLOGIC COMPLICATIONS FROM CANCER AND THERAPY

1. Deep vein thrombosis risk is increased in cancer patients.
2. Intrathecal methotrexate use has been associated with aseptic meningitis, transverse myelopathy, encephalopathy, and leukoencephalopathy.
3. Peripheral neuropathies can be seen after treatment with bortezomib, cisplatin, oxaliplatin, vincristine, paclitaxel, or thalidomide.

62. Which medications are used for treatment of painful chemotherapy-induced peripheral neuropathies?
Duloxetine is recommended according to the American Society of Clinical Oncology clinical practice guidelines. Nortriptyline, gabapentin, and a compounded topical gel containing baclofen, amitriptyline hydrochloride, and ketamine can also be used.

63. Which features are useful in distinguishing radiation-induced brachial plexopathy from malignancy?
Characteristics favoring the diagnosis of recurrent tumor instead of radiation-induced brachial plexopathy include severe pain, Horner's syndrome, lower brachial plexus involvement, and a radia-tion dose less than 60 Gy. Additionally, myokymic discharges on electromyography are often seen in patients with radiation-induced plexopathy.

PARANEOPLASTIC SYNDROMES

64. Describe the proposed mechanism of neurologic paraneoplastic syndromes.
    Paraneoplastic syndromes are thought to occur when an immunologic response is focused against common antigens present on the tumor but also expressed in the nervous system. Patients suspected of having a paraneoplastic syndrome should be evaluated for paraneoplastic antibodies in their serum and CSF (Table 20-1).

Table 20-1. Antibody Testing for Paraneoplastic Syndrome

ANTIBODY	TUMOR	PARANEOPLASTIC SYMPTOMS
Anti-Hu (ANNA-1)	Small-cell lung cancer, neuroblastoma, prostate cancer	Paraneoplastic encephalomyelitis, paraneoplastic sensory neuronopathy, paraneoplastic cerebellar degeneration, autonomic dysfunction
Anti-Yo (PCA-1)	Ovarian, breast, and lung cancers	Paraneoplastic cerebellar degeneration
Anti-Ri	Breast, gynecologic, lung, and bladder cancers	Ataxia with or without opsoclonus–myoclonus
Anti-Tr	Hodgkin's lymphoma	Paraneoplastic cerebellar degeneration
Anti-VGCC	Small-cell lung cancer	Lambert–Eaton myasthenic syndrome
Antiretinal (antirecoverin protein)	Small-cell lung cancer, melanoma, gynecologic cancers	Cancer-associated retinopathy, melanoma-associated retinopathy
Antiamphiphysin	Breast and small-cell lung cancers	Stiff person syndrome, paraneoplastic encephalomyelitis
Anti-CRMP5 (anti-CV2)	Small-cell lung cancer, thymoma	Paraneoplastic encephalomyelitis, cerebellar degeneration, chorea, sensory neuropathy
Anti-PCA-2	Small-cell lung cancer	Paraneoplastic encephalomyelitis, cerebellar degeneration; Lambert–Eaton myasthenic syndrome
Anti-Ma1	Lung and other cancers	Brainstem encephalitis, cerebellar degeneration
Anti-Ma2 (-Ta)	Testicular cancer	Limbic brain stem encephalitis
ANNA-3	Lung cancer	Sensory neuronopathy, encephalomyelitis
Anti-mGluR1	Hodgkin's lymphoma	Paraneoplastic cerebellar degeneration
Anti-VGKC	Thymoma, small-cell lung cancer	Neuromyotonia
Anti-MAG	Waldenström macroglobulinemia	Peripheral neuropathy

From Darnell RB, Posner JB: Paraneoplastic syndromes involving the nervous system. *N Engl J Med* 349:1543-1554, 2003.

65. How common are paraneoplastic syndromes?
    Myasthenia gravis is seen in 15% of thymoma patients and Lambert–Eaton myasthenic syndrome in 3% of patients with small-cell lung cancer. However, for other solid tumors the incidence of paraneoplastic syndromes is far less than 1%.

66. Opsoclonus–myoclonus syndrome in children is associated with which neoplasm?
    Neuroblastoma.

67. An ovarian teratoma may be detected with which paraneoplastic syndromes?
    Anti-*N*-methyl-D-aspartate receptor (NMDAR) encephalitis can present with psychiatric changes, seizures, orofacial dyskinesias, and autonomic instability. Half of female patients older than 18 years with NMDAR have uni- or bilateral ovarian teratomas.

68. Name the two antibodies primarily associated with paraneoplastic cerebellar degeneration.
    Anti-Yo and anti-Tr.

69. Which antibody is most frequently found in paraneoplastic limbic encephalitis?
    Anti-Hu.

70. What is the treatment for paraneoplastic disorders?
    Elimination of the antigen source by treatment of the underlying tumor and suppression of the immune response with steroids, intravenous immunoglobulin, and/or plasma exchange are the two main approaches attempted. Rituximab and cyclophosphamide also have been reported to have some benefit in patients who failed first-line treatment.

KEY POINTS: PARANEOPLASTIC SYNDROMES

1. Paraneoplastic syndromes are thought to occur when an immunologic response is focused against common antigens present on the tumor but also expressed in the nervous system.
2. Patients suspected of having a paraneoplastic syndrome should have their serum and CSF checked for paraneoplastic antibodies.

Acknowledgment

The author would like to acknowledge the contributions of Yvonne Kew, MD, who was the author of this chapter in the previous edition.

 References available online at expertconsult.com.

WEBSITES

http://www.braintumor.org
http://cern-foundation.org
http://www.abta.org/

BIBLIOGRAPHY

1. Bernstein M, Berger M: Neuro-Oncology: The Essentials, New York, Thieme, 2008.
2. DeAngelis L, Posner J: Neurologic Complications of Cancer, New York, Oxford, 2008.
3. Mehta M: Principles & Practice of Neuro-Oncology: A Multidisciplinary Approach, New York, Demos Medical, 2010.
4. Newton H: Neurological Complications of Systemic Cancer and Antineoplastic Therapy, New York, Informa Healthcare, 2010.
5. Schiff D: Principles and Practice of Neuro-Oncology, New York, McGraw-Hill, 2005.

CHAPTER 21

HEADACHES

Randolph W. Evans

GENERAL PRINCIPLES

1. **What is the prevalence of headaches?**

   Having had any type of headache is a near universal experience, with a lifetime prevalence of 90% and a 1-year prevalence of over 50% (migraine 12% and tension type 38%). Migraine is the third most prevalent disorder and seventh highest specific cause of disability worldwide. Approximately 90% of headaches in patients with a normal neurologic examination are primary (such as migraine, tension type, and cluster). The remaining 10% are due to numerous secondary causes. There are over 300 different types and causes of headaches. Since there are only so many ways your head can hurt, there is overlap between the symptoms of primary and secondary headaches, although different headache types may have signature features.

   This chapter will often use definitions and present headaches in the order found in the *International Classification of Headache Disorders*, 3rd edition, beta version (ICHD-3), which is the international standard for classification and diagnosis of headache disorders.

2. **Which cranial structures are sensitive to pain?**

   Although all pain is registered in the brain, the brain itself is not pain sensitive. The arachnoid, ependyma, and dura (except portions near blood vessels) are also insensitive to pain. The following are sensitive to pain: cranial nerves V, VII, IX, and X; the circle of Willis and proximal continuations; meningeal arteries; large veins in the brain and dura; and structures external to the skull (including scalp and neck muscles, cutaneous nerves and skin, the mucosa of paranasal sinuses, external auditory canal and tympanic membrane, orbital structures and eyeballs, salivary glands, teeth, temporomandibular joints, cervical nerves and roots, and the external carotid arteries and branches).

3. **What are the key questions to ask for a headache history?**

   A detailed headache history is essential for establishing the diagnosis (Table 21-1).

4. **What are the reasons to consider neuroimaging for headaches?**

   Most patients do not need neuroimaging. Again, 90% of patients have primary headaches with a diagnosis made by a detailed history and normal neurologic examination.

   Neuroimaging should be considered for those patients whose temporal and headaches features include the following: (1) the "first or worst" headache; (2) subacute headaches with increasing frequency or severity; (3) a progressive or new daily persistent headache; (4) chronic daily headache; (5) headaches always on the same side; (6) headaches not responding to treatment; and (7) headaches triggered by cough, exertion, or Valsalva manuever. Patient demographics and comorbidities that should prompt consideration of neuroimaging include headaches cooccurring with seizures, a history of cancer or immunosuppression (human immunodeficiency virus [HIV]-infected or iatrogenically immunosuppressed), pregnancy or the postpartum period, and new-onset headache in those over 50 years of age. Worrisome associated symptoms and signs prompting neuroimaging include headaches associated with fever, stiff neck, nausea, and vomiting, headaches other than migraine with aura associated with focal neurologic symptoms or signs, and headaches associated with papilledema, cognitive impairment, or personality change. The likelihood that either computed tomography (CT) or magnetic resonance imaging (MRI) will reveal an abnormality responsible for the headache in patients with any headache and a normal neurologic examination is approximately 2%. Table 21-2 provides a mnemonic to help remember to "SNOOP for the red flags."

5. **Which imaging modality—CT or MRI—is the preferred neuroimaging for the evaluation of headaches?**

   When available, MRI is the preferred study for the evaluation for headaches. CT is preferable in acute situations such as head trauma, acute headache to rule out subarachnoid hemorrhage, as well as in patients with contraindications to MRI.

Table 21-1. Key Questions to Ask for the Headache History

- Do you have different types of headaches or just one?
- Where does the headache hurt?
- When did you first start having these headaches?
- What were you doing when the headache started?
- How long before the headache reaches maximal intensity?
- How long does the headache last?
- Does the headache recur? If so, how often?
- What is the pain like? Is it a pressure, throbbing, pounding, aching, or stabbing?
- On a scale of 1 to 10, with 10 the worst and 1 the least, how would you rate the headache?
- Do you have trouble with your vision before or during the headache?
- Do you have other symptoms (e.g., nausea, vomiting, light sensitivity, noise sensitivity, cranial autonomic symptoms) with the headache?
- During a headache, would you prefer to be in bright sunlight or in a dark room?
- During a headache, would you prefer to be in a room with loud music or in a quiet room?
- Are signs present (e.g., fever, ptosis, miosis)?
- Do you have triggers of your headaches (e.g., menses, stress, foods, beverages, lack of sleep, oversleeping, strong odors, trigger zones)?
- What makes the headache worse (e.g., coughing, Valsalva, physical activity)?
- What makes the headache better (e.g., sleep, lying down in a quiet room)?
- Do your headaches have any impact on your life (missed work, school, family or social activities)?
- Do you take over-the-counter medications, vitamins, or herbs for your headaches? If so, how much and how often?
- Do you drink caffeinated beverages? If so, what types and how many?
- What prescription drugs have you tried, what doses, for what duration, and with what effect? Any side effects?
- What doctors have you seen in the past for your headaches?
- What other treatments have you tried and with what success (e.g., acupuncture, chiropractic, biofeedback, stress management, massage)?
- Have you been under much stress lately?
- Have you been depressed?
- Do you have any parents or siblings with a history of migraines or bad headaches?

From Evans RW: Diagnosis of headaches. In: Evans RW, Mathew NT, editors: Handbook of headache. 2nd ed. Philadelphia: Lippincott Williams & Wilkins, 2005, p. 1.

Table 21-2. SNOOP: Red Flags to Consider Neuroimaging for Headaches

- Systemic symptoms (fever, weight loss) or
  Secondary headache risk factors (HIV, systemic cancer, pregnancy and postpartum)
- Neurologic symptoms or abnormal signs (confusion, impaired alertness, or consciousness)
- Onset: sudden, abrupt, or split-second-thunderclap
- Older: new onset and progressive headache, especially in age >50 years (e.g., giant cell arteritis)
- Previous headache history or headache progression: first headache or different (change in attack frequency, severity, or clinical features)

Data from Dodick DW. Diagnosing headache: clinical clues and clinical rules. Advanced Studies in Medicine 3:87-92, 2003. (Galen Publishing)

The following causes of headache can be missed on a routine CT scan of the head: vascular disease (saccular aneurysms, arteriovenous malformations—especially posterior fossa), subarachnoid hemorrhage, carotid or vertebral artery dissections, infarcts, cerebral venous thrombosis, vasculitis (white matter abnormalities), cerebral vasospasm, and subdural and epidural hematomas; neoplastic disease (neoplasms especially in the posterior fossa, meningeal metastases, and pituitary tumor and hemorrhage), cervicomedullary lesions (Chiari malformations and foramen magnum meningioma); infections (paranasal sinusitis, meningoencephalitis, cerebritis, and brain abscess); and low cerebrospinal fluid (CSF) pressure syndrome.

CT of the head also exposes the patient to ionizing radiation (2 mSv without contrast) where there may be a delayed increased risk for various cancers with a greater potential for younger people (see www.xrayrisk.com).

PRIMARY HEADACHES

6. How do you distinguish between episodic migraine, tension type, and cluster headaches (CHs)?

Table 21-3 compares and contrasts these headaches.

Table 21-3. Features of Some Primary Headaches

FEATURE	EPISODIC MIGRAINE	EPISODIC TENSION TYPE	EPISODIC CLUSTER
Epidemiology	• 18% of women • 6% of men • 4% of children before puberty	• 90% of adults • 35% of children aged 3-11 years	• 0.4% for men • 0.08% for women
Female/male	• 3/1 after puberty • 1/1 before puberty	5/4	1/5
Family history	80% of first-degree relatives	Frequent	Rare
Typical age at onset	• 92% before age 40 • 2% after age 50	20-40	20-40
Visual aura	In 30%	No	Occasional
Location	• Unilateral, 60% • Bilateral, 40%	Bilateral > unilateral	Unilateral maximal orbital, supraorbital, and/or temporal
Quality	Pulsatile or throbbing in 85%	Pressure, aching, tight, squeezing	Boring, burning, or stabbing
Severity	Mild to severe	Mild to moderate	Severe
Onset to peak pain	Minutes to hours	Hours	Minutes
Duration	• 4-72 hours • 2-72 hours in children	Hours to days	15-180 minutes
Frequency	Rare to frequent	Rare to frequent	1-8 per day during clusters
Periodicity	Menstrual migraine	No	Yes. Average bouts 4-8 weeks Average 1 or 2 bouts yearly
Associated features	• Nausea in 90% • Vomiting in 30% • Light and noise sensitivity in 80%	Occasional nausea	• Ipsilateral conjunctival injection and/or lacrimation in 95% • Nasal congestion and/or rhinorrhea in 77% • Ptosis and miosis in 30% • Eyelid edema in 21%
Triggers	Present in 85%	Stress, lack of sleep	Alcohol, nitrates
Behavior during headache	Still, quiet, tries to sleep	No change	Often paces
Awakens from sleep	Can occur	Rare	Frequently

Data from Evans RW: Diagnosis of headaches. In: Evans RW, Mathew NT, eds: Handbook of Headache. *2nd ed. Philadelphia: Lippincott, Williams & Wilkins, 2005, pp. 14-15.*

7. Can primary headaches awaken people from sleep or be present upon awakening in the morning?

Yes, often with migraine, CHs, tension type, paroxysmal hemicranias, and hypnic headache (see Question 55). Exploding head syndrome is a rare disorder where the person is awoken from sleep by a sensation of a momentary loud noise in the head lasting a few seconds without headaches (several reports of associated migraines), and 10% of these patients describe an associated flash of light. This disorder may occur at any age but is more common in those over the age of 50 years.

8. What are chronic daily headaches of long duration?

Chronic daily headaches are the primary headache disorders in which patients experience headaches lasting 4 or more hours per day (without treatment), 15 or more days a month for 3 or more months. This disorder affects 3% to 5% of the worldwide population. These headaches include chronic migraine, chronic tension-type headache, new daily persistent headache, and hemicrania continua. In contrast, chronic daily headaches of short duration (headaches lasting less than 4 hours per day untreated) are rare and include chronic CH, chronic paroxysmal hemicrania, and short-lasting unilateral neuralgiform headache attacks.

MIGRAINE

9. How common is migraine?

In a given year, migraine has a prevalence of 12% (17.1% in women and 5.6% in men). Annually, some 35 million people suffer migraine in the United States. The cumulative incidence of this disorder by age 85 years is 18.5% in men and 44.3% in women, with onset before the age of 25 years in 50% of cases, before the age of 35 years in 75%, and over the age of 50 years in only 2%. The median age of onset is 25 years. In children, approximately 8% of boys and 11% of girls have migraine. However, only about 56% of migraineurs know that they have migraine. They or their doctors have made a misdiagnosis of "sinus" or allergy headache, stress headache, or eye strain. Ninety percent of patients presenting to primary care physicians with recurrent headache meet the criteria for migraine.

9A. Is migraine more common in neurologists and family medicine physicians than in the general population?

Yes. The lifetime prevalence is 47% among male neurologists and 63% among females. The lifetime prevalence is even higher among male and female headache specialists, respectively, 72% and 82%. Another study found an increased lifetime prevalence of migraine among male and female family physicians, respectively, 37% and 61%. The reason for the higher prevalence is not certain, but possible explanations include the following: migraine is more common in the general population than studies suggest (physicians are better at self-diagnosis or recall of migraines); migraine is associated with a choice to become a physician; and occupational stress leads to migraine in susceptible individuals.

9B. Which US Presidents or First Ladies had migraines?

Jefferson had episodic severe headaches that may have been a migraine variant, episodic daily migraine. Lincoln, Grant, and Wilson were migraineurs. John Adams, Truman, Eisenhower, and Kennedy may have been migraineurs. First Ladies Abigail Adams, Lincoln, Eisenhower, and Kennedy all suffered from migraines. Grant, who treated some migraines with chloroform, had a severe migraine that immediately went away when he received a letter from Lee offering terms of surrender. To treat migraines and stomach cramps, Wilson's physician prescribed golf 6 days a week. He played at least 1200 rounds as president, perhaps as many as 1600, with an average score of 115. Nixon is cited as stating, "He also told the physician [White House physician Dr. Tkach] that he had never had a headache. He seemed to think headaches were imaginary—excuses for weak men...."

10. What are the phases of migraine?

The *prodrome* or *premonitory phase* occurs in about 80% of migraineurs and may precede the attack by hours or up to 1 or 2 days. Symptoms include changes in mental state (such as depression, hyperactivity, irritability, or drowsiness), neurologic symptoms (such as photophobia, phonophobia, and yawning), and general symptoms (such as stiff neck, food cravings, diarrhea, or constipation).

- *Aura* in about 30%
- *Headache* in most but not everyone
- *Resolution phase* or *postdrome* symptoms include changes in mood, weakness, tiredness, anorexia, irritability, and poor concentration ("mashed potato brain")

11. **What are the clinical features of migraine without aura?**
The location is easy to remember. Any part of the head or face may be affected, including the parietal region, the upper or lower jaw or teeth, the malar eminence, and the upper anterior neck. Pain is unilateral in 60% of cases and bilateral in 40%. Approximately 15% of migraineurs report so-called side-locked headaches in which migraine always occurs on the same side. The pain is often more intense in the frontotemporal and ocular regions before it spreads to the parietal and occipital areas. Throbbing pain is present in 85% of episodes of migraine, although up to 50% of patients describe steady pain during some attacks. As many as 75% of migraineurs report unilateral or bilateral tightness, stiffness, or throbbing pain in the posterior neck along with head pain. The neck pain can occur during the migraine prodrome, the attack itself, or the postdrome.
    Migraines last 4 to 72 hours if left untreated or if unsuccessfully treated. One that persists for more than 72 hours is termed *status migrainosus.* In children and adolescents (aged under 18 years), attacks may last 2 to 72 hours and the pain is more often bilateral (usually frontotemporal) than in adults.
    Without treatment, 80% of patients experience moderate to severe pain, and 20% have mild pain. Usually increased by physical activity or movement, the pain is associated with nausea in about 80% of episodes, vomiting in about 30%, photophobia in about 90%, and phonophobia in about 80%.
    Table 21-4 provides the International Headache Society criteria for the diagnosis of migraine.

Table 21-4. Diagnostic Criteria for Migraine without Aura

A. At least five attacks fulfilling criteria B-D
B. Headache attacks lasting 4-72 hours (untreated or unsuccessfully treated)
C. Headache has at least two of the following four characteristics:
   1. Unilateral location
   2. Pulsating quality
   3. Moderate or severe pain intensity
   4. Aggravation by or causing avoidance of routine physical activity (e.g., walking or climbing stairs)
D. During headache at least one of the following:
   1. Nausea and/or vomiting
   2. Photophobia and phonophobia
E. Not better accounted for by another ICHD-3 diagnosis

From Headache Classification Committee of the International Headache Society (IHS): The International Classification of Headache Disorders, 3rd edition (beta version), Cephalalgia 33(9):629-808, 2013.

12. **How often do migraines occur, is there associated impairment, and what are the genetics?**
A quarter of all migraineurs suffer four or more severe attacks a month, 35% have one to four severe attacks per month, 38% experience one or fewer severe attacks per month, and 37% have five or more headache days per month. In one study, during migraine attacks, most migraineurs (53.7%) reported severe impairment or the need for bed rest, whereas only 7.2% reported no attack-related impairment. Over a 3-month period, 35.1% of the migraineurs had at least 1 day of restricted activity related to headache.
    About 70% of migraineurs have an affected first-degree relative. Genetic heterogeneity is present.

13. **What are the common migraine triggers?**
Migraine triggers are present in 76% of migraineurs. One study reported the following triggers from affected patients: stress, 89%; female hormones, 65%; not eating, 57%; weather, 53%; physical exhaustion or travel, 53%; sleep disturbance, 50%; perfume or odor, 44%; bright lights, 38%; neck pain; 38%; alcohol, 38%; smoke, 36%; sleeping late, 32%; heat, 30%; food, 27%; and exercise, 22%.

14. **Why are migraines misdiagnosed as "sinus" headaches?**
Migraineurs and some physicians misdiagnose headaches as "sinus" because the pain occurs in the face or forehead, a change in weather is a common trigger, and the presence of cranial autonomic symptoms seems like sinus symptoms.

Cranial autonomic symptoms in migraine are caused by parasympathetic activation of the sphenopalatine ganglion, which innervates the tear ducts and sinuses. At least one symptom is present in 56% of migraineurs, usually bilaterally, but is not usually present during each attack. The most common cranial autonomic symptoms are forehead/facial sweating, conjunctival injection and/or lacrimation, and nasal congestion and/or rhinorrhea.

15. **Why are migraines misdiagnosed as stress or tension-type headaches?**
Migraines are confused with stress or tension-type headaches, because migraine pain is commonly experienced in the neck at some point during the attack (75%) and is often triggered by psychological stress (80%).

16. **What is the epidemiology of migraine with aura?**
In a given year in the United States, the prevalence of migraine with aura is 5.3% in women (30.8% of female migraineurs) and 1.9% in men (32% of male migraineurs). As many as 81% of those having migraine with aura also have attacks of migraine without aura.
   The reported age of onset is between a mean of 11.9 years (range, 4 to 17) and a mean of 21 years (range, 5 to 77). In one study, 54.9% of patients suffered less than one attack per month, and 9.7% reported more than three attacks per month.

17. **What are the clinical features of migraine aura?**
The visual aura is the most common, occurring in 99% of attacks, sensory (typically unilateral numbness, tingling, or pins and needles in the hand, which may spread to the face or either alone, can have unilateral tongue paresthesias) in 30%, and dysphasia (if the dominant hemisphere or can have slurred speech) in 20%. When more than one aura type occurs during an attack, symptoms typically follow one another in succession, beginning with visual, then sensory, and then dysphasia.
   Migraine aura meets International Headache Society criteria when the duration is 5 to 60 minutes. A duration of longer than 1 hour but less than a week defines probable migraine with aura. Visual aura lasts more than 1 hour in 6% to 10% of migraineurs with aura.
   Table 21-5 provides the International Headache Society criteria.

Table 21-5. Criteria for Migraine with Aura

Description
Recurrent attacks, lasting minutes, of unilateral fully reversible visual, sensory, or other central nervous system symptoms that usually develop gradually and are usually followed by headache and associated migraine symptoms.

Diagnostic Criteria
A. At least two attacks fulfilling criteria B and C
B. One or more of the following fully reversible aura
   Symptoms:
   1. Visual
   2. Sensory
   3. Speech and/or language
   4. Motor
   5. Brain stem
   6. Retinal
C. At least two of the following four characteristics:
   1. At least one aura symptom spreads gradually over ≥5 minutes, and/or two or more symptoms occur in succession
   2. Each individual aura symptom lasts 5-60 minutes
   3. At least one aura symptom is unilateral
   4. The aura is accompanied, or followed within 60 minutes, by headache
D. Not better accounted for by another ICHD-3 diagnosis, and transient ischemic attack has been excluded

Headache Classification Committee of the International Headache Society (IHS). The International Classification of Headache Disorders. 3rd ed (beta version). Cephalalgia 33(9):629-808, 2013.

18. Does the aura only occur before the onset of the headache?

Although many consider the migraine aura to be a distinct phase of the migraine attack preceding the headache, one prospective study found the aura phase occurring during the headache in 73% of patients. The aura may follow the headache in 3% to 8% of cases.

19. Can aura occur without headache?

Yes. This is termed *typical aura without headache* (acephalgic migraine), which may be more common with older age. Although usually just a visual aura, other aura symptoms may also occur. With the first or very short or prolonged episodes or when symptoms are just negative such as hemianopsia, other causes may need to be excluded.

20. What are the symptoms of the visual aura?

Fortification (looks like a fortified town as viewed from above) spectra or teichopsia ("seeing fortifications"), which is a jagged figure with fortification lines arranged at right angles to one another beginning from a paracentral area, may be experienced, which start in or adjacent to the center of the visual field in 50% or in the peripheral in 50% and then spread, leaving visual loss behind. There are often scintillations, which may be white or gray or have colors similar to a kaleidoscope in a semicircle or C shape surrounding the scotoma or area of visual loss. Scintillating scotomata are typically in one hemifield, with visual field defects beginning around fixation and spreading outward. Some patients may describe other phenomena including zigzag lines, flashes of bright light, or heat waves.

21. What distinguishes a migraine aura from cerebral ischemia and seizures?

Visual or sensory auras from migraine typically spread slowly across the visual field or body part followed by a gradual return to normal function in the areas first affected after 20 to 60 minutes. The onset of cerebral ischemic events is usually sudden with an equal distribution in the relevant vascular territory, although the affected area can expand stepwise if blood flow drops in additional vessels. The return of function in areas first affected while symptoms begin in newly affected areas occurs in migraine aura but not in ischemia or seizures.

Migraine aura often begins with positive phenomena such as shimmering lights, zigzags in vision, or tingling. It is then frequently followed minutes later by negative symptoms such as scotoma, numbness, or a loss of sensation. This symptom progression can also occur during seizures but usually with a faster progression of symptoms. This cycle from positive to negative symptoms is not typical of cerebral ischemia.

22. What is vestibular migraine (migrainous vertigo)?

Vestibular migraine has a lifetime prevalence of 1% in the general population. The vertigo can occur with (in 50%) or without a headache and can have a variable duration ranging from seconds (approximately 10%) to minutes (30%) to hours (30%) to several days (30%). Patients may describe lightheadedness, spinning, or a sensation of the environment spinning. For some patients, it may take weeks to recover fully from an attack. The attacks may occur days, months, or even years apart in an irregular fashion.

23. What is migraine with brain stem aura (formerly called basilar-type migraine)?

Migraine with brain stem aura is a rare disorder that usually affects patients aged 7 to 20 years and rarely presents in individuals older than 50 years. One study reported the following aura symptoms: vertigo, 61%; dysarthria, 53%; tinnitus, 45%; diplopia, 45%; bilateral visual symptoms, 40%; bilateral paresthesias, 24%; decreased level of consciousness, 24%; and hypoacusis, 21%. Visual symptoms—usually blurred vision, shimmering colored lights accompanied by blank spots in the visual field, scintillating scotoma, and graying of vision—may start in one visual field and then spread to become bilateral. The median duration of aura was 60 minutes (range, 2 minutes to 72 hours), with two or more aura symptoms always occurring.

24. How are episodic, intermittent, and chronic migraine defined?

Episodic migraine is 14 or fewer headache days per month, while chronic migraine is defined as 15 or more headache days (tension type-like and/or migraine-like) per month for 3 months or more having the features of migraine headache on at least 8 days per month.

Chronic migraine, or transformed migraine, is a complication of intermittent migraine, with 2.5% progressing yearly from episodic to chronic migraine. In the United States, 3.2 million people have chronic migraine and 80% are women. It may occur with or without medication overuse. The pain is often mild to moderate and not always associated with photophobia, phonophobia, nausea, or vomiting and may resemble a mixture of migraine and tension-type headaches with intermittent severe migraine-type headaches. Depression is present in 40% and anxiety in 30%.

24A. Who described the first case of chronic migraine?

In 1672, Thomas Willis (1621-1675) provided the first description of chronic migraine when he reported the case of the philosopher Anne, Viscountess Conway, who was also treated by William Harvey and Robert Boyle without benefit. (Lady Conway's disabling migraines inspired her concept that pain and suffering were purgative with the ultimate aim of restoring creatures to moral and metaphysical perfection.)

Willis gave our field its name in 1664 by coining the Greek term *neurologie* and also coining the terms *lobe, hemisphere, pyramid, peduncle, corpus striatum,* and *reflexion* (later reflex). He demonstrated the functional significance and provided the best illustrations of the circle of Willis in 1664.

Willis also described the differentiation between diabetes insipidus and mellitus and described meningococcal meningitis, general paralysis, Jacksonian epilepsy, myasthenia gravis, transient ischemic attacks, carotid occlusion with headache (Willis headache), narcolepsy, and bipolar disorder. He introduced the doctrine of the gray cortex as the source of cerebral activities and the white matter as a mass of connections. Next time you are at Westminster Abbey, visit his burial site.

25. What are the risk factors for transformation from episodic to chronic migraine?

Risk factors for transformation include medication overuse (especially opiates and barbiturate combinations), high caffeine consumption, female gender, stressful life events, anxiety, depression, baseline high-attack frequency, individuals with lower educational and socioeconomic levels, white patients, lifetime injuries to the head or neck, obesity, snoring, arthritis, and presence of cutaneous allodynia.

26. What is a common abnormality on MRI scans of the brain in migraineurs?

White matter abnormalities are present on MRI scans more often in migraineurs (variably reported in 12% to 46%) than in controls (2% to 14%). White matter abnormalities are foci of hyperintensity on both proton density and T2-weighted images in the deep and periventricular white matter due to either interstitial edema or periventricular demyelination of uncertain etiology.

27. What is medication overuse headache (MOH) or medication rebound?

MOH or medication rebound is defined as headache occurring on 15 or more days per month and developing as a consequence of regular overuse of acute or symptomatic headache medication for more than 3 months. It is present in about 1% to 2% of the population who have preexisting migraine or tension-type headache. MOH can result from the following: combination over-the-counter medications, triptans, or opiates 10 or more days per month. Some evidence suggests nonsteroidal antiinflammatory drug (NSAID) use 15 or more days per month may cause MOH; however, other evidence suggests NSAIDs may be used for migraine prevention. Caffeine-withdrawal headache may develop within 24 hours after regular consumption of caffeine in excess of 200 mg/day for more than 2 weeks. Some migraineurs benefit from avoiding caffeine completely.

28. How is MOH treated?

Overused medications can be tapered off. For those taking high-frequency butalbital combinations, phenobarbital 30 mg twice a day (bid) can be substituted for 2 weeks followed by 15 mg bid for 2 weeks (abrupt withdrawal can result in seizures). For those taking high doses of opioids, clonidine 0.1 to 0.2 mg three times a day titrated up or down based on symptoms or clonidine patch 0.1 to 0.2 mg/24 hours for 1 to 2 weeks.

Naproxen 500 mg bid may be used alone or can be combined with tizanidine starting at 2 mg at bedtime and titrating up to 16 mg at bedtime (for 6 weeks in one study) as tolerated. Steroids are probably not effective.

29. How effective are triptans (serotonin 1b/1d agonists) for acute migraine treatment?

Oral sumatriptan, almotriptan, eletriptan, rizatriptan, and zolmitriptan relieve the pain in about 65% to 70% with better efficacy than frovatriptan and naratriptan (Table 21-6). Sumatriptan subcutaneous (SC) 6 mg provides headache relief in 70% by 2 hours and 80% by 4 hours. Sumatriptan 20 mg nasal spray (NS) and zolmitriptan 5 mg NS are second fastest. Sumatriptan SC, NS, and iontophoretic transdermal patch are preferred for those with prominent nausea/vomiting or who do not respond to oral triptans. All acute medications are more effective when taken when the pain is mild.

Table 21-6. Available Triptan Preparations

DRUG (BRAND NAME)	FORMULATION	STRENGTHS (mg)
Almotriptan (Axert)	Tablets	12.5
Eletriptan (Relpax)	Tablets	40
Frovatriptan (Frova)	Tablets	2.5
Naratriptan (Amerge)	Tablets	1, 2.5
Rizatriptan (Maxalt)	Tablets	5, 10
	Orally disintegrating preparation* (Maxalt MLT)	5, 10
Sumatriptan (Imitrex)	Subcutaneous injection	6
	Tablets	25, 50, 100
	Nasal spray	5, 20
Sumatriptan patch (Zecuity)	Iontophoretic transdermal patch worn for 4 hours	6.5
Sumatriptan/naproxen (Treximet)	Tablet	85/500
Zolmitriptan (Zomig)	Tablets	2.5, 5
	Orally disintegrating preparation* (Zomig ZMT)	2.5, 5
	Nasal spray	5

*Dissolves on the tongue; can be taken without water (efficacy similar to that of tablet form).
Modified with permission from Evans RW: Headaches. In: ACP Medicine, BC Decker, 2009.

30. **What are contraindications to triptans? What about the risk of serotonin syndrome (SS)?**
   According to the package insert (PI), contraindications to use include those with ischemic heart disease, Prinzmetal's angina, Wolff–Parkinson–White syndrome or arrhythmias associated with other cardiac accessory conduction pathway disorders, cerebrovascular syndromes (including strokes and transient ischemic attacks), peripheral vascular disease (including ischemic bowel disease), uncontrolled hypertension, hemiplegic or basilar migraine, and use within 24 hours of ergotamine derivatives.
   The PI also warns that SS may occur with 5-HT$_1$ agonists, particularly when used concomitantly with other serotonergic drugs. The American Headache Society's position paper concludes, "The currently available evidence does not support limiting the use of triptans with selective serotonin reuptake inhibitors or selective serotonin/norepinephrine reuptake inhibitors, or the use of triptan monotherapy, due to concerns for serotonin syndrome."

31. **What is recurrence?**
   Recurrence refers to an initial reduction in pain intensity or resolution of pain of the acute migraine in response to analgesic treatment with subsequent pain recurrence within 24 hours. Its occurs depending on the initial analgesia used with a low of 14% of the time with a combination of sumatriptan and naproxen, 20% of the time with frovatriptan, and a high of 40% with sumatriptan SC.

32. **What are emergency department (ED) options for treatment of severe migraine?**
   Five million visits to US EDs annually are due to patients with migraine. Intravenous hydration is important for those who have been vomiting.
   The Canadian Headache Society systemic review strongly recommends use of the following: intravenous (IV) prochlorperazine 10 mg (which may be given with diphenhydramine 25 mg IV to prevent extrapyramidal side effects; diphenhydramine can also be given with metoclopramide); metoclopramide 10 mg IV; sumatriptan 4 to 6 mg SC (not used first line if another triptan has been taken in the past 24 hours); and ketorolac intramuscularly (IM) and IV 60 mg. Dihydroergotamine 0.5 mg IV with an antiemetic is a reasonable first-line option in the appropriate patient who has not had a triptan within

24 hours. Meperidine 75 to 100 mg IM is weakly recommended. The Society strongly recommends against the use of dexamethasone for the acute treatment of migraine pain.

33. **How is menstrual migraine (MM) treated?**
About 50% of female migraineurs report migraines with their menses, and 14% have MM only. Many women respond to the usual acute medications. For nonresponders, perimenstrual prevention with triptans may be effective beginning 2 to 3 days prior to the expected onset of the menses and continuing for a total of 5 days (frovatriptan 2.5 mg bid or zolmitriptan 2.5 mg three times a day [tid] or bid). Transcutaneous estradiol gel 1.5 mg or a 0.1 mg/24 h patch applied 2 days prior to the onset of menses and continued for 7 days may also be effective. For those with refractory MM or with irregular menses, daily migraine prevention can be tried. For those already using estrogen–progestin oral contraceptives, continuous contraception for 3 months or more can be effective.

34. **What are indications for starting preventive medications in migraine?**
The following factors may indicate the need for preventive medication treatment: recurring migraines that in the patient's opinion significantly interfere with daily routine, despite acute treatment; contraindication to or failure or overuse of acute therapies; adverse events with acute therapies; and patient preference. In addition to medication, triggers are avoided as much as possible, and adequate and regular sleep, avoiding missed meals, and regular exercise may be beneficial.

35. **How are preventive medications used and which are effective for episodic migraine?**
A preventive medication is slowly titrated to the target dose and taken for a minimum of 8 weeks to see if effective. Contraception should be discussed with women of childbearing potential and the potential risk of medication with pregnancy. A paper or electronic headache diary should be kept to monitor progress.
   Table 21-7 provides the American Headache Society/American Academy of Neurology Migraine Prevention Guidelines. Choose a medication based upon efficacy, the patient's preferences, the medication side effects, and the presence or absence of coexisting or comorbid conditions. One medication may be used for migraine and another disorder, a "two for" (such as depression, epilepsy, or hypertension). The most effective medications reduce the frequency of headaches by about 50% in about 50% of migraineurs.

36. **How well are preventive medications tolerated?**
Perhaps 20% of patients discontinue each of the preventive medications due to side effects. The physician should discuss the side effect profile with the patient before starting. For example, divalproex can cause nausea, somnolence, tremor, dizziness, weight gain, and hair loss. Caution should be used in prescribing divalproex or any valproic acid derivative to women of childbearing potential because of the risk for teratogenicity including major malformations and adverse cognitive and developmental outcomes. Topiramate can cause paresthesias, changes in taste (soft drinks may taste flat), depression, kidney stones in about 1%, reversible cognitive impairment in about 10%, weight loss, and rarely glaucoma.

37. **Are alternative or nonmedication treatments effective for episodic migraine prevention?**
Relaxation training, thermal biofeedback combined with relaxation training, electromyographic biofeedback, and cognitive behavioral therapy have grade A evidence for prevention of migraine. Acupuncture may be helpful. The evidence is inconclusive for spinal manipulation.
   Regular aerobic exercise may be helpful. Weight loss may help to reduce the frequency of migraines in overweight patients. Treatment of insomnia and obstructive sleep apnea may also be helpful.

38. **What medications are effective for chronic migraine prevention?**
The evidence for efficacy of preventive medication is different for chronic migraine than for episodic migraine (Table 21-8).

39. **What is dihydroergotamine (DHE) IV transitional therapy and what is its efficacy?**
For those with refractory chronic migraine, 67% have headache attack freedom during treatment and 75% have headache freedom within 1 month of completion, with duration of effect of an average of 28 days. DHE has the same contraindications as triptans.

Table 21-7. AHS/AAN Migraine Prevention Guidelines 2012

Drugs Recommended for Use

DRUG	EXAMPLES OF STUDIED DOSES
Level A: Established as Effective	
Should be offered to patients requiring migraine prophylaxis	
Divalproex/sodium valproate	400-1000 mg/day
Metoprolol	47.5-200 mg/day
Petasites (butterbur)*	50-75 mg bid
Propranolol	120-240 mg/day
Timolol	10-15 mg bid
Topiramate	25-200 mg/day
Level B: Probably Effective	
Should be considered for patients requiring migraine prophylaxis	
Amitriptyline	25-150 mg/day
Fenoprofen	200-600 mg tid
Feverfew	50-300 mg bid; 2.08-18.75 mg tid for MIG-99 preparation
Histamine	1-10 ng subcutaneously twice a week
Ibuprofen	200 mg bid
Ketoprofen	50 mg tid
Magnesium	600 mg trigmagnesium dicitrate qd
Naproxen/naproxen sodium	500-1100 mg/day for naproxen
	550 mg bid for naproxen sodium
Riboflavin	400 mg/day
Venlafaxine	150 mg extended release/day
Atenolol	100 mg/day
Level C: Possibly Effective	
May be considered for patients requiring migraine prophylaxis	
Candesartan	16 mg/day
Carbamazepine	600 mg/day
Clonidine	0.75-0.15 mg/day; patch formulations also studied
Guanfacine	0.5-1 mg/day
Lisinopril	10-20 mg/day
Nebivolol	5 mg/day
Pindolol	10 mg/day
Flurbiprofen	200 mg/day
Mefenamic acid	500 mg tid
Coenzyme Q10	100 mg tid
Cyproheptadine	4 mg/day

Data from Silberstein SD, Holland S, Freitag F, et al.; Quality Standards Subcommittee of the American Academy of Neurology and the American Headache Society. Evidence-based guideline update: pharmacologic treatment for episodic migraine prevention in adults: report of the Quality Standards Subcommittee of the American Academy of Neurology and the American Headache Society. Neurology 78(17):1337, 2012.

*Advise patients of rare risk of hepatotoxicity and monitor liver function tests if they wish to assume risk of use. Don't use in children and pregnancy. (Tepper SJ. Nutraceutical and Other Modalities for the Treatment of Headache. Continuum. 2015;21(4):1018-31).

Table 21-8. Preventive Medications for Chronic Migraine with Target Doses or Dose Ranges

Randomized Controlled Trials
OnabotulinumtoxinA 155 units (FDA approved)
Topiramate 100-200 mg daily
Divalproex sodium 500 mg bid
Gabapentin 800 mg tid
Tizanidine 8 mg tid
Amitriptyline 100 mg daily
Fluoxetine 40 mg daily
Candesartan 16 mg daily
Propranolol 160 mg long acting daily

Open Label
Pregabalin 150 mg bid
Zonisamide 100-400 mg daily
Atenolol 50 mg daily
Olanzapine 2.5-35 mg daily
Methylergonovine maleate 0.2-0.4 mg tid
Memantine 10-20 mg daily in divided doses
Combined?
Anecdotal
Venlafaxine 150 mg extended release daily

From Evans RW: An update on the management of chronic migraine. Pract Neurol November/December, 27-32, 2013. Available at http://practicalneurology.com/pdfs/PN1113_SF_ChronicMigraine.pdf.

Pretreatment is given with 4 mg of ondansetron (obtain baseline electrocardiogram risk of QT prolongation, pregnancy test as appropriate—some clinicians prefer metoclopramide 10 mg IV instead) before each dose of DHE (no triptan for 24 hours before). Day 1: DHE 0.5 mg in 100 mL of normal saline IV over 1 hour. If well tolerated (if not tolerated, dose is not titrated up or can be decreased to a lower dose), second dose 8 hours later of 0.75 mg in 250 mL of normal saline IV over 1 hour. Days 2 to 5: third and subsequent doses 1 mg in 250 mL of normal saline over 1 hour IV every 8 hours with the goal of a cumulative total dose of 11.25 mg ($\pm$1 mg) over 5 days.

For moderate or severe nausea, options are an additional dose of ondansetron 4 mg IV every 8 hours as necessary or promethazine 12.5 to 25 mg IV every 12 hours. DHE can also be given over 2 to 3 hours or the dose decreased or not escalated. Ketorolac 30 mg IV every 12 hours prn headache can be used for 3 days.

Some clinicians use IV valproate when DHE is contraindicated or in addition to DHE (loading dose of 15 mg/kg infused over 30 minutes followed by 5 mg/kg infused over 15 minutes every 8 hours).

TENSION-TYPE HEADACHES

40. How common are tension-type headaches and what are the clinical features?
    The 1-year prevalence of the episodic type is 38% and chronic (15 or more days per month for 3 or more months) is 2%. Most have headaches less than 1 day per month.
    The typical headache is a bilateral mild to moderate intensity, nonthrobbing headache described as dull, pressure, a tight cap, band, or a heavy pressure without associated symptoms. The headache is unilateral in 10% and occasionally pulsating. Stress is a common trigger.

41. How are tension-type headaches treated?
    For acute treatment, most patients respond to over-the-counter medications such as NSAIDs and simple analgesics that may be combined with caffeine. Opioids and butalbital combinations should be avoided.
    Preventive treatment is indicated for those with frequent or chronic tension-type headaches. Amitriptyline (nortriptyline and protriptyline are alternatives) is started at 10 to 25 mg at bedtime and titrated to a target dose of 100 mg as tolerated. Studies also suggest benefit from the use of mirtazapine, venlafaxine, topiramate, and gabapentin. Biofeedback and relaxation techniques may also be beneficial.

TRIGEMINAL AUTONOMIC CEPHALALGIAS

42. What are the trigeminal autonomic cephalalgias (TACs)?

TACs are a group of primary headache disorders characterized by unilateral trigeminal distribution pain that occurs in association with prominent ipsilateral cranial autonomic features. TACs include CH, paroxysmal hemicrania, short-lasting unilateral neuralgiform headache attacks with conjunctival injection and tearing (SUNCT), short-lasting unilateral neuralgiform headache attacks with cranial autonomic symptoms (SUNA), and hemicrania continua. Table 21-9 provides a comparison of the clinical features of the shorter duration TACs. These are typically diagnoses of exclusion with neuroimaging (preferably MRI scans including the pituitary) to exclude secondary causes.

Table 21-9. Clinical Features of the Trigeminal Autonomic Cephalalgias

	CLUSTER HEADACHE	PAROXYSMAL HEMICRANIA	SUNCT SYNDROME	HEMICRANIA CONTINUA
Sex F:M	1:3.5–7	2.13–2.36:1	1:2.1	2.4:1
Pain				
Type	Stabbing, boring	Throbbing, boring, stabbing	Burning, stabbing, sharp	Background dull ache, throbbing/stabbing exacerbations
Severity	Excruciating	Excruciating	Severe	Moderate background pain; severe exacerbations
Site	Orbit, temple	Orbit, temple	Periorbital	Orbit, temple
Attack frequency	1 every other day–8 daily	1–40/day	1/day–30/hr	Continuous
Duration of attack	15–180 min	2–45 min	5–250 seconds	Continuous background pain; exacerbations quite variable and lasting minutes to days
Autonomic features	Yes	Yes	Yes (prominent conjunctival injection and lacrimation)	Yes—mainly with exacerbations; less prominent than with other TACs
Migrainous features*	Yes	Yes	Yes†	Yes—during exacerbations
Alcohol trigger	Yes	Occasional	No	Rare
Indomethacin effect	–	++	–	++
Abortive treatment	Sumatriptan injection or nasal spray Oxygen	Nil	Nil	Nil
Prophylactic treatment	Verapamil Methysergide Lithium Prednisolone	Indomethacin	Lamotrigine Topiramate Gabapentin	Indomethacin

TACs, Trigeminal autonomic cephalalgias.
*Nausea, photophobia, or phonophobia.
†Photophobia homolateral to pain.
From Goadsby PJ. Migraine and the trigeminal autonomic cephalalgias. In: McMahon SB, Koltzenburg M, Tracey I, et al., editors. Wall & Melzack's Textbook of Pain, 6th ed. Philadelphia: Elsevier; 2013. p. 815–831.

HEMICRANIA CONTINUA

43. **What is hemicrania continua (HC)?**
HC is a rare disorder that may have a prevalence of up to 1% of the population. HC is more common in females than males, 1.6:1. The onset is often during the third decade of life with a range from the first to seventh decades.

    The pain is strictly unilateral most commonly in the orbital, frontal, and temporal areas but can be occipital or other areas of the head or neck. The pain can be mild to severe throbbing or sharp. The pain is typically constant, but 20% have pain-free periods for 1 day to several months. Exacerbations occur in 75% of patients and typically last 20 minutes to several days. The pain can be associated with nausea, vomiting, light and noise sensitivity, and rarely a visual aura. Cranial autonomic symptoms, most commonly tearing and conjunctival injection, occur in 75% of patients. HC is a mimic of chronic migraine.

44. **What is the treatment for HC?**
HC is defined by the fact that is resolves completely with indomethacin. One regimen is the following: 25 mg three times a day for 3 days, subsequently increasing, if ineffective, to 50 mg three times a day for a further 3 days and then, if ineffective, to 75 mg three times per day for 3 days. The lowest effective dose is continued. Because of the risk of gastroduodenal mucosal injury, indomethacin is typically taken with a proton pump inhibitor.

    For those who cannot tolerate indomethacin, other treatments, although much less effective, include topiramate, melatonin 6 to 12 mg at bedtime, verapamil, and gabapentin.

CLUSTER HEADACHES

45. **What is the epidemiology of CH?**
The lifetime prevalence is about 0.1% and the 1-year prevalence is 53 per 100,000, with a male to female ratio of 4:1. Onset is typically from ages 20 to 40 years although the range is from 4 to 96 years, with onset occurring after the age of 50 years in 10% of cases.

    Five to 20% have a family history. The risk of CH for first-degree relatives is increased by 14- to 39-fold. Up to 85% of patients are chronic cigarette smokers, but quitting smoking has no effect on the disease. During cluster periods, trigger factors include alcohol ingestion and nitric oxide donors or promoters such as nitroglycerin or sildenafil.

46. **What are the clinical features of CH (Table 21-10)?**
The strictly unilateral pain is behind the eye in about 90%, over the temple in 70%, and over the maxilla in 50% although the pain may be in the occipital neck region. The pain is usually severe in intensity and is sharp, stabbing, piercing, burning, or pulsating in quality. Most have one to three attacks per day. About 15% report that the pain shifts sides between bouts of attacks and, less often,

---

Table 21-10. Diagnostic Criteria for Cluster Headache

A. At least five attacks fulfilling criteria B-D

B. Severe or very severe unilateral orbital, supraorbital, and/or temporal pain lasting 15-180 minutes (when untreated)*

C. Either or both of the following:
   1. At least one of the following symptoms or signs, ipsilateral to the headache:
      a. Conjunctival injection and/or lacrimation
      b. Nasal congestion and/or rhinorrhea
      c. Eyelid edema
      d. Forehead and facial sweating
      e. Forehead and facial flushing
      f. Sensation of fullness in the ear
      g. Miosis and/or ptosis
   2. A sense of restlessness or agitation

D. Attacks have a frequency between one every other day and eight per day for more than half of the time when the disorder is active

E. Not better accounted for by another ICHD-3 diagnosis

*During part (but less than half) of the time course of cluster headache, attacks may be less severe and/or of shorter or longer duration.

during a bout, but never during a single attack. Untreated, each headache lasts 15 to 180 minutes, during which patients usually are either restless or agitated and prefer to pace, rock back and forth, or bang their heads. Nocturnal attacks occur in 70%.

Migrainous symptoms of light and noise sensitivity are reported by 70%, vomiting or nausea in more than 20%, and perhaps 14% report an aura (including visual and paresthesia). About 97% have ipsilateral cranial autonomic symptoms such as conjunctival injection, lacrimation, nasal congestion and/or rhinorrhea, eyelid edema, ptosis, and miosis.

47. **How often do attacks of CHs occur and what is the difference between episodic and chronic CHs?**

An "attack" is a single attack of pain, and a bout is a series or "cluster" of attacks. In the absence of preventive medications, episodic CH is characterized by bouts lasting 7 days to 1 year separated by remission periods lasting 1 month or longer. Chronic CH is the absence of remission for 1 year or remissions of less than 1 month. Ten percent of CH is the chronic type. Chronic CH may either be chronic from onset or may evolve from the episodic type.

Most people have one bout per year, with a mean bout duration of 8.6 weeks. Some patients can go years without a bout, and others have frequent bouts each year.

48. **What is the acute and transitional treatment for CH?**

Triptans, especially subcutaneous sumatriptan 4 to 6 mg, are the mainstay of treatment. Subcutaneous sumatriptan can result in pain freedom within 20 minutes in 75% of CH suffers. Intranasal zolmitriptan 5 mg and sumatriptan 20 mg may be effective but less so than subcutaneous sumatriptan. Anecdotally, some patients report benefit from oral triptans. Dihydroergotamine 1 mg IM or 2 mg intranasally may also be effective. Inhalation of 100% oxygen administered through a nonrebreather face mask at a rate of 8 to 15 L/min for 15 to 20 minutes with the patient sitting upright is effective in about 80% of cases.

Some patients with episodic and chronic CH benefit from transitional or bridging therapy resulting in a temporary remission while waiting for either a preventive medication to work or for the bout to end. One regimen anecdotally suggested is prednisone 60 mg daily for 5 days and then tapered by 10 mg daily. Ipsilateral greater occipital nerve block with steroid and local anesthetic has also been reported as effective.

49. **What preventive treatment is effective for CH?**

Verapamil is the drug of choice for both episodic and chronic types. It is started at 120 to 240 mg a day and slowly increased (80-mg increase every 3 to 7 days as tolerated) to 480 mg if necessary. High doses may be required (maximum dose 960 mg/day) depending upon tolerability and response. The drug can be given in both a regular formulation three times daily and an extended-release formulation once a day although, anecdotally, the three-times-daily dosing may be more effective. With daily doses of 240 mg or higher, baseline and serial electrocardiograms, repeating the electrocardiograms 1 to 2 weeks after a dose change, usually in 80-mg increments, are indicated to monitor for the development of heart block, which becomes more frequent at higher doses.

Topiramate may be effective (starting at 25 mg/day and titrating up to 100 mg/day). Valproic acid is questionably effective. Melatonin is questionably helpful as a CH preventive. Lithium may be effective for chronic and episodic CHs typically starting at 300 mg bid or tid and increasing every 4 to 5 days based upon levels, with a typical maintenance dose of 900 to 1200 mg daily in three to four divided doses. The lithium plasma level should be monitored and kept between 0.6 and 1.2 mmol/L. Lithium has a narrow therapeutic window and numerous significant side effects.

OTHER PRIMARY HEADACHES

50. **What is primary cough headache?**

Primary cough headache, which has a lifetime prevalence of 1%, is a sudden-onset bilateral or unilateral headache lasting seconds to 2 hours without associated symptoms provoked by coughing, sudden postural movements, weightlifting, laughing, and defecating and usually occurring in people over the age of 40 years. Secondary pathology should be excluded including Chiari type 1 malformation, posterior fossa lesions, unruptured cerebral aneurysms, spontaneous intracranial hypotension, and subdural hematoma by obtaining an MRI of the brain with and without contrast, and MRA (magnetic resonance angiogram) of the brain.

The cough should be treated. Indomethacin 50 to 200 mg daily in divided doses can be very effective (combined with a proton pump inhibitor for prolonged use). Acetazolamide, topiramate, propranolol, and naproxen may also be effective.

51. What is primary exercise headache?

Primary exercise headache may occur in 10% of the population and is a typically bilateral throbbing headache lasting from minutes up to 48 hours brought on by or occurring only during or after sustained physical exercise not usually associated with nausea and vomiting although migraineurs may have exercise as a trigger. The average age of onset is 24 (±11) years. Secondary pathology such as space occupying lesions and vascular pathology should be excluded with an MRI of the brain and MRA of the brain and neck.

Indomethacin 25 to 150 mg in divided doses can be taken daily for dosing 30 to 60 minutes before exercise for prevention. Propranolol and naproxen may also be effective.

52. What is primary headache associated with sexual activity?

With a lifetime prevalence of 1%, this is a bilateral (33% unilateral) occipital or diffuse headache lasting from 1 minute to 24 hours with severe intensity and/or up to 72 hours with mild intensity. The preorgasmic headache is a dull, usually biocciptal pressure or aching occurring during sexual activity and increasing in intensity with increasing sexual excitement. Orgasmic headache has a sudden explosive onset followed by a severe throbbing generalized headache.

Secondary causes of headache such as subarachnoid hemorrhage, arterial dissection, reversible cerebral vasoconstriction syndrome, hemorrhage into a cerebral tumor, and pheochromocytoma should be excluded with testing such as an MRI of the brain and MRA of the brain and neck or other appropriate studies. Approximately 5% of aneurysmal subarachnoid hemorrhages occur during sex.

Triptans may be effective for acute treatment. For prevention, triptans can be taken 30 minutes to 4 hours before sexual activity (depending upon the half-life of the triptan, e.g., sumitriptan 20 mg NS 30 minutes before, sumatriptan 100 po 2 hours before, and frovatriptan 2.5 mg 4 hours before). Indomethacin (25 to 225 mg per day), propranolol (40 to 240 mg per day), and topiramate (titrated to 100 mg daily) may be effective for prevention.

53. What is primary thunderclap headache?

A thunderclap headache is a severe headache of sudden onset reaching maximum intensity in less than 1 minute and lasting 5 minutes. A secondary headache must be excluded with appropriate testing, especially subarachnoid hemorrhage, which is the cause of up to 25% of thunderclap and sentinel headaches. Headache after subarachnoid hemorrhage typically lasts at least an hour or two.

These disorders present with thunderclap headaches the following percentages of the time: reversible cerebral vasoconstriction syndrome, 85%; cervical artery dissection, 20%; spontaneous intracranial hypotension, 15%; and cerebral venous thrombosis, 2% to 10%. There are numerous other causes including pituitary apoplexy, retroclival hematoma, ischemic stroke, acute hypertensive crisis, colloid cyst of the third ventricle, meningitis, complicated sinusitis, and subdural hematoma.

54. What is primary stabbing ("ice pick") headache?

An idiopathic disorder with transient and localized stabs of pain lasting 3 seconds or less 80% of the time (rarely 10 to 120 seconds) anywhere on the head, unilateral > bilateral of mild to severe intensity occurring in children and adults. One study found 38% with single stabs, 30% with a series of stabs, and 32% with both. This disorder is comorbid with migraine as well as tension-type headache, hemicrania continua, and primary cough headache.

Secondary causes of short stabbing headaches include herpetic meningoencephalitis, intracranial meningioma, pituitary tumors, acute thalamic hemorrhage, temporal arteritis (age >50 years), multiple sclerosis, systemic lupus erythematosus, Sjogren's, Behçet's, vasculitis, Lyme, and antiphospholipid antibody syndrome.

Possible treatments include indomethacin 75 to 150 mg daily, celecoxib 100 mg bid, melatonin 3 to 12 mg daily, gabapentin, and botulinum toxin A injections as well as amitriptyline in children.

55. What is hypnic headache?

Hypnic headache is a rare disorder that occurs in patients over the age of 50 years in 92% (rarely in children). Females are affected 65% of the time. The headache occurs only during sleep and awakens the sufferer at a consistent time (often 2 to 4 am). Nausea is infrequent and autonomic symptoms are uncommon. The headache can be unilateral or bilateral, throbbing or nonthrobbing, and mild to severe in intensity. The headache's duration can range from 15 minutes to 10 hours, with most lasting less than 3 hours, and can occur frequently, as often as nightly, for many years.

The best treatments are caffeine (one cup of strong caffeinated coffee or a 40- to 60-mg caffeine tablet before bedtime—insomnia is usually not reported in these patients), lithium carbonate (150 to 600 mg at bedtime), and indomethacin 25 to 50 mg tid and then tapering off after several weeks. A number of other medications have been reported as effective in case reports.

56. What is new daily persistent headache (NDPH)?

NDPH is a rare, idiopathic, persistent headache with pain becoming continuous and unremitting within 24 hours of onset, present for more than 3 months. Most patients have a constant headache ranging from mild to severe and bilateral in 89%, and present in any head region. Migraine features are present in over 50%. The age of onset ranges from 6 to greater than 70 years. Preceding stressful life events are reported in 10%, a flu-like, upper respiratory infection in 14% to 30%, and extracranial surgery in 7% to 12%.

NDPH is a diagnosis of exclusion including neoplasms, chronic subdural hematoma, post-traumatic, spontaneous intracranial hypotension, idiopathic intracranial hypertension, cervical artery dissection, reversible cerebral vasoconstriction syndrome, cerebral venous thrombosis, arteriovenous malformation, dural arteriovenous fistula, sphenoid sinusitis, chronic meningitis, postmeningitis, Chiari malformation, temporal arteritis, cervicogenic, and greater occipital neuralgia. The headache is treated like the primary headache (migraine or tension type) it most resembles.

SECONDARY HEADACHES

57. What are the features of secondary headaches?

Table 21-11 compares and contrasts the features of selected secondary headaches.

58. What are the features of posttraumatic headaches (PTH)?

Headaches occur in 30% to 90% of those symptomatic after mild traumatic brain injury. The prevalence and lifetime duration are greater in those who have mild head injury compared with those who have more severe injury. According to ICHD-3, the onset should be within 7 days of trauma or injury or within 7 days of regaining consciousness and/or the ability to sense and report pain when these abilities have been lost.

In most civilian studies, migraine-type headaches occur in about 25% while in US military series after blast trauma, migraine type is reported by about 75%. In one study of PTH in athletes, migraine type was reported by 18%. The other headaches are predominantly tension type. PTH can also be due to occipital neuralgia, supra- and infraorbital neuralgia, scalp lacerations, and temporomandibular disorder. Rare causes include TACs, CSF leaks through a cribriform plate fracture, cervical arterial dissections, cerebral venous thrombosis, and carotid-cavernous fistula. Of course, subdural and epidural hematomas should be excluded.

59. What are the prognosis and treatment of PTH?

Persistent headaches are reported at 3 months in 47% to 78%, 1 year in 8.4% to 35%, and 4 years in 24%.

There are few randomized, placebo-controlled trials of medications. The headaches are treated like the primary headache it most resembles.

60. What is footballer's migraine?

Minor head trauma can sometimes trigger migraine attacks in migraineurs. Matthews reported migraine with aura sometimes repeatedly triggered by heading the ball in soccer in four young males (including a 12-year-old) and a 20-year-old boxer after being hit in the head.

The most famous example occurred in American football in the first quarter of Super Bowl XXXII viewed by 800 million when migraineur Terrell Davis of the Broncos was kicked in the helmet and developed a migraine with visual aura. He was taken out of the game and treated with his usual medication, DHE nasal spray. He returned headache free for the second half and had 20 carries for 90 yards, a Super Bowl record; three rushing touchdowns; and won the game's MVP award.

Early treatment of migraine can get your patients back to school or work or even enable them to be a Super Bowl MVP.

61. Do headaches occur with cerebral ischemia?

Headache is present with acute ischemic stroke or transient ischemic attack about 25% of the time and is more common with hemispheric rather than lacunar. The pain can be dull or throbbing and is more often unilateral to the side of the lesion, but it can be generalized. The mean duration of headache is 3.8 ± 2.1 days.

62. What is a sentinel headache?

A sentinel headache is a sudden, severe headache occurring preceding major aneurysmal subarachnoid hemorrhage by days or weeks in 10% to 43% of cases. The sentinel headache may be due to minor aneurysmal bleeding or expansion of the aneurysmal wall. Sentinel headache is not associated with neck stiffness, altered levels of consciousness, or focal neurologic signs.

Table 21-11. Features of Selected Secondary Headaches

HEADACHE TYPE	EPIDEMIOLOGY	AGE OF ONSET	LOCATION	QUALITY AND SEVERITY	FREQUENCY	ASSOCIATED FEATURES	COMMENTS
Trigeminal neuralgia	4.3/100,000/year; 60% females	Usually >40 years; if <40 years, consider multiple sclerosis	Unilateral, 97%; second or third trigeminal division greater than first	Stabbing; electrical bursts; burning; lasts few seconds to <2 min	Few to many a day	Trigger zone present in 91% of cases	Usually due to vascular compression of CN V; scan needed to exclude occasional tumor
Brain tumor	Persons/year; 41,000 primary (1/3 malignant), 150,000 metastatic	Any age	Often bifrontal, unilateral or bilateral; any location	Can be pressure or throbbing, mild to severe	Occasional to daily; usually progressive	Papilledema in 40%; at time of diagnosis, headache present in 30-70%	Primaries in adults; lung, 64%; breast, 14%; unknown, 8%; melanoma, 10%; colorectal, 3%; hypernephroma, 2%
Idiopathic Intracranial Hypertension (pseudotumor cerebri)	1-2/100,000/year; 90% are female; 90% obese	Mean of 30 years	Often bifrontotemporal but can occur in other locations and unilaterally	Pulsatile; moderate to severe	Daily	Papilledema in 95%; transient visual obscurations in 70%; intracranial noises in 60%; VI nerve palsy in 20%	MRI scan preferred to better exclude cortical venous thrombosis and posterior fossa lesions
Subarachnoid hemorrhage	30,000/year caused by saccular aneurysm	Mean of 50 years	Usually bilateral; any location	Usually severe but can be mild and gradually increasing in 19%	Paroxysmal	Often with nausea, vomiting, stiff neck, focal findings, syncope; stiff neck absent in 36%	CT scan abnormal on first day in 95%; third day, 74%; 1 week, 50%; lumbar puncture may be essential for diagnosis
Temporal arteriti	In age >50 years, annual incidence of 18/100,000; female-to-male ratio, 3:1	Rare before 50 years; mean age of 70 years	Variable, unilateral, or bilateral; often temporofrontal	Often throbbing; may be sharp, dull, burning, or lancinating; mild to severe	Intermittent to continuous	50% have PMR; jaw claudication in 38%; 50% have absent pulse or tender STA	ESR WNL in up to 36%; CRP usually elevated; STA biopsy false negative in up to 44%

Continued

Table 21-11. Features of Selected Secondary Headaches—cont'd

HEADACHE TYPE	EPIDEMIOLOGY	AGE OF ONSET	LOCATION	QUALITY AND SEVERITY	FREQUENCY	ASSOCIATED FEATURES	COMMENTS
Acute paranasal sinusitis	More common in children (in whom frontal and sphenoid sinusitis is rare) than in adults	Any age	Frontal (forehead), maxillary (cheek), ethmoid (between eyes), sphenoid (variable)	Dull, aching; can be severe	Acute lasts from 1 day to 3 weeks	Fever in about 50%; nasal congestion and purulent nasal drainage usually present (less often in sphenoid)	Well visualized on routine MRI but not on routine head CT scan; sinus CT is the best study
Subdural hematoma	Occurs in 1% after mild head injury; in chronic cases, up to 50% without history of head injury	Any age	Unilateral or bilateral	Mild to severe; may be aching, dull, or throbbing	Paroxysmal to constant	Normal neurologic exam in 50%; alteration in consciousness and focal findings may be present	MRI may detect the occasional isodense subdural hematoma, which can be missed on CT scan

CN V, Cranial nerve V; CRP, C-reactive protein; CT, computed tomography; ESR, erythrocyte sedimentation rate; MRI, magnetic resonance imaging; PMR, polymyalgia rheumatica; STA, superficial temporal artery; WNL, within normal limits.

Modified with permission from Evans RW: Diagnosis of headaches. In: Evans RW, Mathew NT, editors: Handbook of headache. 2nd ed. Philadelphia: Lippincott Williams & Wilkins, p. 1, 2005.

63. What are the features of headaches occurring with cervical artery dissection?

The incidence of dissections is 2.6/100,000/year. Headache or neck pain is the only symptom of spontaneous cervical artery dissection in 8%. The headache has a thunderclap onset in about 20% of cases. Headache occurs in 60% to 95% of those with internal carotid artery dissection (ICAD) preceding other neurologic symptoms and/or signs by a mean time of 4 days. The pain of ICAD, which is ipsilateral in 91% of cases, is typically localized to the frontal or temporal area, jaw, ear, and/or orbit and is more often aching than throbbing. A partial Horner's syndrome occurs in about 25% of cases with ptosis and miosis.

Headache occurs in 70% of those with vertebral artery dissection (VAD) with head or neck pain preceding other neurologic symptoms and/or signs by a mean time of 14.5 hours. VAD is typically an ipsilateral occipitonuchal throbbing or pressure but can be bilateral.

64. What types of headaches occur with reversible cerebral artery vasoconstriction (RCVS)?

About 60% of patients develop the syndrome either postpartum or after exposure to vasoactive drugs (cannabis, ecstasy, selective serotonin reuptake inhibitors, triptans, cocaine, amphetamine, intravenous immunoglobulin). This type of headache occurs more commonly in women (3:1) and typically presents between the ages of 20 and 50 years (range 10 to 76 years). Multiple thunderclap can be associated with nausea and/or vomiting. Photophobia is a presenting feature in 94% of cases. Multiple thunderclap headaches may occur over a mean period of 1 week and may occur spontaneously or be triggered by cough, exertion, or Valsalva. One of the defining features of RCVS is transient cerebral vasoconstriction, which resolves within 1 to 3 months. Rare patients may develop NDPH.

Complications of RCVS include cervical artery dissection (12%), ischemic or hemorrhagic stroke (6% to 30%), cortical subarachnoid hemorrhage (22% to 34%), posterior reversible encephalopathy syndrome (9%), and seizures (3% to 9%). Nimodipine, nifedipine, and verapamil have been used. However, there are no placebo-controlled trials.

65. What are the symptoms of postdural puncture headaches (PDPH) and how can they be prevented?

PDPH are typically bilateral frontal, occipital, or generalized pressure-like or throbbing headaches, worse when upright, which can be associated with nausea, vomiting, dizziness, tinnitus, neck stiffness, and visual symptoms. They occur up to 40% of the time following diagnostic lumbar punctures, usually within 6 to 72 hours of the procedure. In 80% of patients the headache lasts less than 5 days but rarely can last for up to 1 year.

Risk factors include female gender, ages 18 to 30, smaller body mass index, prior chronic or recurrent headaches, prior PDPH, use of a Quincke needle, a larger diameter needle, perpendicular orientation of the bevel, and not reinserting the stylet. Atraumatic needles (such as the 22-gauge Sprotte or Whitache) greatly reduce the frequency of PDPH. Bed rest following lumbar puncture does not reduce the frequency of PDPH.

Bed rest is the initial treatment. Oral caffeine 300 mg every 6 to 8 hours might help temporarily. Caffeine sodium benzoate 500 mg in 1000 mL normal saline over 1 hour followed by 1000 mL of normal saline over 1 hour may relieve the headache in perhaps 50%. Persistent headaches can be treated with a lumbar epidural blood patch.

66. What are the features of headache due to spontaneous intracranial hypotension (SIH) or low CSF volume syndromes?

SIH almost always results from spontaneous CSF leaks, typically at the spinal level (most commonly thoracic) and rarely at the skull base. The annual incidence may be 5/100,000 cases, with a peak age of onset of 40 years and a female-to-male ratio of 1.5:1. It can occur in patients of all ages.

Orthostatic headache (a headache while upright, relieved while lying down) is the most common clinical manifestation. The headache may either appear or be relieved after a change in posture. The headache may be dull, throbbing, or pressure-like, mild to severe in intensity, and is usually but not always bilateral. The headache can be frontal, fronto-occipital, generalized, or occipital. It can gradually evolve into a nonorthostatic chronic daily headache or be a nonorthostatic chronic daily headache from onset. Other, less common types include exertional headaches, cough headaches, acute thunderclap onset, second-half-of-the-day headaches, paradoxical orthostatic headaches (present in recumbency, relieved when upright), intermittent headaches, and the acephalgic form (no headaches).

67. **What are other common symptoms and test findings in SIH?**
The headache can be associated with neck stiffness or pain, nausea ± vomiting, light and noise sensitivity, muffled hearing, tinnitus, interscapular pain, upper extremity radicular symptoms, sense of imbalance, and subtle cognitive dysfunction. Less commonly, patients report visual changes (blurring, visual field defects, diplopia), facial pain or numbness, facial weakness, and dysgeusia.

    The MRI of the brain is abnormal in 80% of cases. The most common abnormality is diffuse pachymeningeal (dura and outer layer of the arachnoid mater) enhancement. The opening pressure on lumbar puncture will often be low, less than 60 mm of H_2O, but normal pressures are common. CSF may be clear or xanthochromic, with either normal or elevated protein (as high as 1000 mg/dL), normal glucose, and either a normal leukocyte count or a lymphocytic pleocytosis (as high as 222 cells/mm^2). The patient may also have an elevated erythrocyte count.

68. **Other than low CSF volume syndrome such as PDPH or SIH, what are some other causes of orthostatic headaches?**
Postural orthostatic tachycardia syndrome, after surgery for Chiari malformation, the syndrome of the trephined, increased compliance of the dural sac, and occasional cases of colloid cyst of the third ventricle.

69. **What is the association between headaches and epilepsy?**
Headaches and epilepsy are comorbid. The prevalence of migraine in epilepsy has ranged from 8% to 24% and of epilepsy in migraine from 1% to 17%. Headaches can occur in association with seizures as seizure-related or peri-ictal headaches. Pre-ictal headaches precede the seizure and occur in 5% to 15% of patients with epilepsy. Ictal headache is reported by less than 5% of patients with epilepsy. Post-ictal headache can occur immediately after a seizure and is reported in 10% to 50% of patients with epilepsy. The headaches can be migraine-like, tension-like, or unclassifiable. Migralepsy, referring to a seizure developing during or within 1 hour of a migraine aura, is extremely rare.

70. **What is an ictal epileptic headache?**
Ictal epileptic headache is a rare controversial disorder where a migrainous or tension-type headache is the sole manifestation of a seizure. Ictal epileptic headache has been reported in patients with focal seizures arising predominantly from the occipital lobes as well as with nonconvulsive status epilepticus and generalized idiopathic epilepsy.

71. **What types of headaches are associated with Chiari I malformation?**
Headache is the dominant feature associated with Chiari I malformation and is typically occipital with radiation to the vertex and retro-orbital or to the neck and shoulders. It is frequently triggered by physical activity, Valsalva, coughing, laughing, or change of body position, with a duration ranging from a few minutes to chronic. Most patients become symptomatic during the second or third decade of life, with a mean age of symptom onset of 24.9 ± 15.8 years.

72. **What are the features of alcohol hangover headache (AHH)?**
Alcohol hangover or "veisalgia" (from the Norwegian *kveis* for uneasiness following debauchery and the Greek *algia* for pain) may include physical symptoms (headache, anorexia, diarrhea, tremulousness, dizziness, fatigue, and nausea), sympathetic symptoms (tachycardia and sweating), and cognitive and mood symptoms (decreased attention and concentration, decreased visuospatial skills and dexterity, depression, anxiety, and irritability). AHH is typically a throbbing headache with a lifetime prevalence of 72%. The headache usually occurs on the morning after alcohol consumption when the blood alcohol concentration (BAC) is falling. Peak symptoms occur at about the time when the BAC is 0 and may continue for up to 24 hours afterward. Symptoms may correlate with the amount of alcohol consumed. Hangover is much more common in light to moderate drinkers than in regular heavy drinkers. Alcohol consumption may also trigger migraine and CH.

73. **How can you decrease the risk of and treat AHH?**
AHH occurs more often with dark-colored drinks with congeners (which are natural byproducts of alcohol fermentation) such as whiskey, bourbon, and red wine than in noncongeners such as vodka, gin, and white wine.

    The effects of AHH may be decreased by the following: drinking in moderation; sipping beverages slowly; eating greasy foods before alcohol consumption to slow or delay alcohol absorption; ingestion of honey, tomato juice, and food rich in fructose, which may allow for more effective metabolism of alcohol; adequate sleep; not smoking; remaining hydrated with electrolyte-rich fluids to prevent dehydration; caffeine intake; and use of NSAIDs such as mefenamic acid for symptomatic treatment (but gastroduodenal risk).

74. **What are high-altitude headaches (HAH)?**
    Acute ascent to an altitude above 2500 m can produce acute mountain sickness with a bilateral headache of mild or moderate intensity in up to 87%. It can be associated with nausea, photophobia, vertigo, poor concentration, and, in severe cases, impaired judgment. It resolves within 24 hours after descent to below 2500 m. High altitude is also a common migraine trigger.

75. **How can HAH be treated and the risk reduced?**
    The risk of HAH can be reduced with the use of aspirin 320 mg taken three times at 4-hour intervals starting 1 hour before ascent or ibuprofen 600 mg three times a day starting 6 hours before ascent to an altitude between 3480 m and 4920 m, four doses total. Acetazolamide 125 mg every 12 hours starting 1 day prior to ascent and continued for 2 to 3 days at maximum altitude may also be effective. Slow ascent, copious fluid intake, avoidance of alcohol, and 2 days of acclimatization prior to strenuous exercise at high altitude may help to prevent HAH.

    HAH can be treated with acetaminophen, ibuprofen, and antiemetics. Acetazolamide 125 to 250 mg bid or, as an alternative, dexamethasone 2 to 4 mg every 6 hours can be continued for 24 hours after symptoms either resolve or descent is complete. However, dexamethasone should be used for no longer than 7 days total.

76. **What is sleep apnea headache?**
    Sleep apnea headache is a recurrent morning headache, which is usually a bilateral pressing pain without associated symptoms with a duration of less than 4 hours caused by sleep apnea (diagnosed by polysomnography) and which resolves with successful treatment of the sleep apnea.

77. **What levels of hypertension are associated with headaches?**
    An often bilateral and pulsating headache may be associated with an acute rise in a systolic blood pressure to ≥180 mm Hg and/or diastolic to ≥120 mm Hg. It remits after normalization of blood pressure. Mild or moderate chronic hypertension does not appear to cause headache.

    Hypertensive encephalopathy presents with persistent elevation of blood pressure to ≥180/120 mm Hg (typically in those with a history of chronic hypertension) and at least two of the following: confusion, reduced level of consciousness, visual disturbance including blindness, and seizures. Headache is reported at presentation in 22%. In those previously normotensive, encephalopathy may develop with blood pressure as low as 160/100 mm Hg. At increasing levels of blood pressures beyond the upper range of cerebral autoregulation, endothelial permeability increases and cerebral edema occurs, most prominently in the parieto-occipital white matter on MRI.

78. **What other disorders can present with headaches and hypertension?**
    Severe frontal or occipital pulsating or constant paroxysmal headaches may occur in 51% to 80% of those with pheochromocytoma, variably accompanied by sweating, palpitations, pallor, anxiety, tremor, visual disturbances, abdominal or chest pain, nausea, vomiting, facial flushing, and occasionally paresthesias. The headaches typically last less than 1 hour in 70% of patients.

    Preeclampsia and eclampsia occur during pregnancy or up to 4 weeks postpartum with a blood pressure of >140/90 mm Hg on two readings at least 4 hours apart or a rise in diastolic pressure of ≥15 mm Hg or of systolic pressure of ≥30 mm Hg along with urinary protein excretion greater than 0.3 g/24 hours. The usually bilateral and pulsating headache occurs in 63% of those with preeclampsia.

    A severe throbbing headache can occur in 56% to 85% of those with a spinal cord injury (SCI) and autonomic dysreflexia. The headache of SCI and autonomic dysreflexia is associated with a paroxysmal rise above baseline in systolic pressure of ≥30 mm Hg and/or diastolic pressure ≥20 mm Hg and can be triggered by either noxious or nonnoxious stimuli such as bladder distention, urinary tract infection, bowel distention or impaction, gastric ulcer, decubiti, trauma, or procedures. The latency from onset after the SCI can range from 4 days to 15 years and is more common in those with a complete SCI.

79. **Can hypothyroidism cause headaches?**
    About 30% of patients with hypothyroidism experience a typically bilateral nonpulsatile headache that resolves with treatment. Migraineurs with subclinical hypothyroidism may also improve with treatment. Hypothyroidism can also be a manifestation of a pituitary adenoma.

80. **Can fasting cause headaches?**
    A generalized mild to moderate nonpulsating headache can occur during a fast of at least 8 hours and is relieved after eating (occurs in 47% after a 15-hour fast in one study). Fasting is a common trigger for migraineurs as reported by 57%.

81. **What is cardiac cephalalgia?**

    Cardiac ischemia rarely may cause a unilateral or bilateral headache in any part of the head brought on by exercise and relieved by rest. This type of headache is called *cardiac cephalalgia* or *anginal headache*. Headaches may occur alone or be accompanied by chest pain. In cases of unstable angina, headaches may occur at rest. A thunderclap headache may accompany the chest pain.

82. **What headaches are associated with temporomandibular disorders (TMDs)?**

    TMDs include musculoskeletal and neuromuscular conditions that involve the temporomandibular joints (TMJ), the masticatory muscles, and all associated tissues. A painful TMD may occur in 10% of the population. Other signs or symptoms of TMD such as clicking, limited range of motion, and pain on joint function have been reported in 46% of the US population.

    The pain associated with TMD is frequently of muscular origin and the symptoms are often self-limiting. The pain is typically ipsilateral when arising from the TMJ or may be bilateral when muscular. The headache may be exacerbated by either jaw movement or pressure applied to the TMJ or surrounding musculature.

    Sleep bruxism, which occurs in up to 31% of the population, may exacerbate TMD and/or headache symptoms, but a causal relationship is not evident.

    Those with asymptomatic clicking often do not require treatment. Therapy is indicated if pain, signification limitation in mandibular range of motion, or both are present.

83. **What are the features of classical trigeminal neuralgia (TN) due to neurovascular compression?**

    The annual incidence of TN is 4-13/100,000, with most cases starting after age 50 and a gradually increasing incidence with older age (although teens and young adults and rarely children may be affected). The male:female ratio is 1:1.7.

    According to ICHD-3, the facial pain is unilateral with at least three of the following four characteristics: recurring in paroxysmal attacks lasting from a fraction of a second to 2 minutes; severe intensity; electric shock-like, shooting, stabbing, or sharp in quality; precipitated by innocuous stimuli to the affected side of the face. There is no clinically evident neurologic deficit.

    TN is most commonly caused by compression of the nerve by the superior cerebellar artery. Imaging, preferably MRI, should be done, to exclude secondary causes such as multiple sclerosis (especially in patients under the age of 40 years), neoplasm, and basilar artery aneurysm.

84. **What are the features of classical TN in a prospective series and what is pretrigeminal neuralgia?**

    In a prospective series of 158 patients, the average age of onset was 52.9 years, with 60% being females. TN affects the right side of the face in 56%, left side in 41%, and both sides in 3%. Pain was reported in the following distributions: V1, 4%; V2, 17%; V3, 19%; V1 + V2, 10%; V2 + V3, 33%; and V1 + V2 + V3, 13%. Thirteen percent had a more dull persistent pain at the onset of the disorder ("pretrigeminal neuralgia") while 87% had stabbing paroxysmal pain. The paroxysmal pain was rated on average 10/10 by 58% of the patients. Forty-nine percent of the cohort reported concomitant persistent pain along with the paroxysmal pain.

    Forty percent suffered from more than 10 paroxysms of pain per day. Painful awakening at night because of pain attacks at least occasionally was reported by 49%. Trigger factors were reported by 91% included the following: chewing, 73%; touch, 69%; brushing teeth, 66%; eating, 59%; talking, 58%; and cold wind, 50%. During attacks of pain, 31% experienced ipsilateral autonomic symptoms, most commonly conjunctival tearing or injection. Of the surgery-naïve patients, 29% had sensory abnormalities on exam, most commonly hypesthesia confined to the painful area of the face. Most patients (63%) had periods of remission, with the average number per year of disease of 0.44 and 37% having months of remission and 63% experiencing years of remission.

85. **What is the treatment of classical TN?**

    The most effective medication for TN is carbamazepine (200 to 2400 mg daily depending upon efficacy and tolerability), with efficacy in 58% to 100% of patients depending upon the study while oxcarbazepine (titrated up to 1800 mg daily depending upon effect and tolerability) is probably as effective as carbamazepine and may be effective in patients not responsive to carbamazepine. Baclofen (40 to 80 mg daily in three doses slowly titrated up) and lamotrigine (up to 400 mg daily slowly titrated up) are possibly effective while there are limited data on the benefit of other medications including clonazepam, phenytoin, tizanidine, topiramate, pregabalin, misoprostol, and valproate. Those who fail carbamazepine monotherapy may benefit from combination therapy with baclofen, gabapentin, tizanidine, lamotrigine, or topiramate. One trial found benefit from onabotulinumtoxinA. Acupuncture may be helpful.

Perhaps 40% of patients with TN do not respond to medication treatment. A joint society position paper of the American Academy of Neurology and the European Federation of Neurological Societies concluded that microvascular decompression, percutaneous procedures on the gasserian ganglion (rhizotomy), and gamma knife are possibly effective.

86. **What is glossopharyngeal neuralgia?**
Typically severe stabbing pain along one side of the throat near the tonsillar area with occasional radiation to the ear lasting fractions of a second up to 2 minutes is present, which can be precipitated by swallowing, coughing, talking, or yawning. Most patients are believed to have an artery compressing the nerve as it exits the medulla and travels through the subarachnoid space to the jugular foramen although secondary causes should be excluded by MRI and other testing (including tumors, multiple sclerosis, Paget's disease, Sjögren's syndrome, and other causes).

The incidence is about 0.2 to 0.7 per 100,000 patients, with most presenting older than 50 years of age and with a female:male ratio of 1:1. Medical treatment is the same as for TN. If intractable, surgical options include microvascular decompression and rhizotomy.

87. **What are the features of persistent idiopathic facial pain (PIFP), formerly called atypical facial pain?**
According to ICHD-3, the diagnostic criteria are the following: "A) Pain in the face, present daily and persisting for all or most of the day, fulfilling criteria B and C; B) Pain is confined at onset to a limited area on one side of the face, and is deep and poorly localized; C) Pain is not associated with sensory loss or other physical signs; D) Investigations including X-ray of face and jaws do not demonstrate any relevant abnormality."

"Note: Pain at onset is commonly in the nasolabial fold or side of the chin, and may spread to the upper or lower jaw or a wider area of the face and neck."

PIFP has a lifetime prevalence of perhaps 0.03% with a female:male ratio of 2:1.

88. **What are secondary causes of PIFP and the treatment?**
Secondary causes such as TMD, dental pathology, nasopharyngeal tumors, and rarely lung carcinoma should be excluded by evaluation by a dentist and appropriate testing including an MRI of the brain and radiologic examination of the chest.

Treatment is difficult. Amitriptyline, fluoxetine, venlafaxine, and topiramate may be effective.

89. **What is occipital neuralgia?**
Greater occipital neuralgia (GON) can be caused by trauma or be unrelated to trauma. It may be due to compression or irritation of the nerve by the muscles as the nerve passes through the semispinal capitis and trapezius. Although "true" GON is described as paroxysms of electrical pain in the distribution of the nerve, other patients can have longer duration pain. The pain can be referred in a suboccipital, hemicranial, temporal, frontal, orbital, periorbital, or retro-orbital distribution. Similarly, lesser occipital neuralgia can occur with pain referred in the distribution of the nerve over the lateral scalp superior and posterior to the ear and sometimes in the ear. On examination, there is tenderness over the involved nerve with reproduction of symptoms. There may be hyperesthesia, dysesthesia, or paresthesia in the involved scalp.

Primary and secondary headaches including temporal arteritis can mimic occipital neuralgia so diagnostic testing may be indicated. Occipital nerve block with local anesthetic can be quite effective (but can also be effective for migraine). Other treatments may include physical therapy, NSAIDs, baclofen, carbamazepine, gabapentin, pregabalin, and tricyclic antidepressants.

KEY POINTS: HEADACHES

1. Ninety percent of headaches are primary, and 90% of headaches seen by primary care physicians are migraine.
2. Most headaches are diagnosed by the history and physical examination where diagnostic testing is not indicated.
3. Consider the risk of medication overuse when treating migraineurs with frequent headaches.
4. Consider subarachnoid hemorrhage as the cause of thunderclap headaches or worse headaches. Temporal arteritis should be considered as the cause of new-onset headaches in those over the age of 50 years.

References available online at expertconsult.com.

WEBSITES

http://www.americanheadachesociety.org/
http://www.ihs-headache.org/

BIBLIOGRAPHY

1. Evans RW (ed): Secondary headache. Neurol Clin 32(2):283-568, 2014.
2. Evans RW (ed): Migraine and other primary headaches. Neurol Clin 27(2):321-582, 2009.
3. Headache Classification Committee of the International Headache Society (IHS): The International Classification of Headache Disorders, 3rd ed (beta version). Cephalalgia 33(9):629-808, 2013.
4. Loder E, Weizenbaum E, Frishberg B, et al.: Choosing wisely in headache medicine: the American Headache Society's list of five things physicians and patients should question. Headache 53:1651-1659, 2013.

CHAPTER 22

SEIZURES AND EPILEPSY

Atul Maheshwari, Zulfi Haneef

DESCRIPTION AND CLASSIFICATION

1. What is the etymology of *epilepsy*?
   Epilepsy comes from the Greek "epi" meaning "upon," and *lambanein* meaning to "take hold of."

2. What is a seizure and what is *epilepsy*?
   A seizure is a single event characterized by the abnormal excessive synchronized firing of cortical neurons that usually results in altered sensation, perception, or motor activity. Between 2% and 4% of the population will have a seizure at some point in their lives. Epilepsy is defined as one or more of the following: (1) at least two unprovoked (or reflex) seizures occurring >24 hours apart; (2) one unprovoked (or reflex) seizure and a probability of further seizures; or (3) diagnosis of an epilepsy syndrome. Between 0.5% and 1% of the population currently has epilepsy, and the lifetime risk of epilepsy is about 1% to 2%.

3. How are seizures classified?
   Seizures are classified according to their clinical and electroencephalographic (EEG) characteristics. Classification schemes have been proposed in 1981, 1989, and most recently 2010. Terms from each scheme are still commonly in use (Table 22-1).

Table 22-1. Classification of Seizures and Epilepsy

YEAR	SEIZURES (DEFINED BY ONSET)	EPILEPSY (DEFINED BY ETIOLOGY)
1981	Partial (simple vs complex) vs generalized	N/A
1989	Localization related vs generalized	Symptomatic vs idiopathic vs cryptogenic
2010	Focal (retained consciousness vs dyscognitive) vs generalized	Structural/metabolic vs genetic vs unknown

4. What features distinguish focal- from generalized-onset seizures?
   Focal seizures start in a specific area of the brain and have clinical and electrographic features that indicate onset from a single unilateral brain region. Generalized seizures appear to arise from both cerebral hemispheres at once. The manifestations of focal seizures depend on the area of the brain involved. Consciousness is likely to be impaired if the focal seizure involves the limbic system or a sufficiently large region of the brain. Focal seizures may then spread to adjacent areas or to contralateral or other more distant regions through thalamocortical and interhemispheric pathways, eventually resulting in secondarily generalized seizures.

5. What are the clinical features (semiology), EEG patterns, and common causes of seizures from different areas of the brain?
   See Table 22-2.

6. What causes generalized-onset seizures? At what age do they usually start?
   Generalized-onset seizures (i.e., seizures that cannot be localized to one cerebral hemisphere at onset) usually have a genetic predisposition. The seizures typically begin before the age of 20 and are not associated with well-defined auras (an aura is the first subjective symptom of the seizure and represents a focal seizure).

Table 22-2. Localization Features and Common Causes of Seizures

REGION	TYPICAL SEMIOLOGY	EEG	ETIOLOGY
Frontal	Often nocturnal, occur in clusters, often brief <30 seconds. Other symptoms relate to subregion of frontal lobes (versive turning). Complex motor automatisms such as bicycling, pelvic thrusting, or other sexual gestures. Vocalizations common, minimal postictal symptoms.	Frontal or anterior vertex epileptiform discharges. Occasionally frontal bisynchronous discharges. Often no obvious change or obscured by muscle artifact.	Trauma, malformations such as cortical dysplasia or cavernous angiomas, strokes, tumors, infections, anoxia. Some genetic syndromes.
Mesial temporal	Auras common: olfactory, gustatory, rising epigastric sensation, déjà vu, "indescribable" feeling. Behavioral arrest, lip-smacking/swallowing (oroalimentary) and ipsilateral hand (manual). Semipurposeful or repetitive stereotypical movements. Contralateral dystonic posturing. Significant postictal confusion. Often ipsilateral postictal nose wipe.	Temporal epileptiform discharges localized to anterior temporal region or sphenoidal electrodes, if used. Rhythmic theta activity within 30 seconds of seizure onset.	Mesial temporal sclerosis, postinfectious, trauma.
Lateral temporal	Auras more likely to be auditory, vertiginous, visual distortions, early aphasia symptoms. Frequent secondary generalization.	Lateral temporal epileptiform discharges and rhythmic theta activity.	Lateral cortical lesions and dysplasias. Cavernous angiomas. Genetic.
Parietal	Rare. May reflect activity of association cortex activity and include elementary or unusual formed sensory phenomena, nausea/abdominal, dysphasia, or speech arrest.	Parietal epileptiform discharges.	Usually due to cortical lesions such as infarcts, cortical dysplasia, malignancies.
Occipital	Usually consist of unformed visual phenomena. May be negative visual symptoms.	Occipital epileptiform discharges, unilateral or bisynchronous.	Cortical lesions such as infarcts, dysplasia, or malignancies, but also as an idiopathic epilepsy syndrome (benign epilepsy with occipital paroxysms).

7. Construct a chart describing the major types of generalized-onset seizures.
   See Table 22-3.

8. How can focal seizures with behavioral arrest (focal dyscognitive or complex partial seizures) and absence seizures be differentiated clinically?
   Three main features may help to differentiate complex partial from absence seizures:
   1. Complex partial seizures, unlike absence seizures, may be preceded by a well-defined aura.
   2. On average, complex partial seizures last 60 to 90 seconds, whereas absence seizures usually last no more than 30 seconds.

Table 22-3. Features of Primary Generalized Seizures

SEIZURE TYPE	SEMIOLOGY	EEG
Absence	Sudden behavioral arrest, staring, may have some automatisms. No aura, no postictal confusion.	Generalized 3-Hz spike-and-wave discharges, exacerbated by hyperventilation. Background usually normal.
Atypical absence	Sudden behavioral arrest and staring, but more prolonged with more prominent automatisms than absence.	Generalized 1.5-2.5-Hz spike-and-wave discharges. Often less regular and less symmetric than absence. Background usually abnormal.
Atonic	Sudden loss of tone in postural muscles, resulting in drop attacks. Usually with brief impairment of consciousness. Minimal postictal state.	Low-voltage fast activity, polyspike and wave, or electrodecrement.
Tonic	Generalized or occasionally asymmetric hypertonia. May have sudden or gradual onset. Seldom lasts more than 1 minute. Respiratory muscle contraction—"ictal cry."	Often associated with generalized 10-Hz or faster activity.
Tonic–clonic	Loss of consciousness with initially generalized tonic contractions, followed by rhythmic generalized jerking of all four extremities.	Initially generalized 10-Hz activity in the tonic phase, followed by rhythmic spike-wave, slow-wave, or sharp-slow-wave activity.

3. After a complex partial seizure, the patient is usually confused or has some postictal cognitive problem. Absence seizures are not associated with a postictal state, and patients return to their baseline cognitive state at the end of the seizure.

4. Absence seizures are generally induced by hyperventilation while complex partial seizures are not. **Note**: Automatisms can occur with both absence and complex partial seizures.

9. **Define the term** *epileptic syndrome*.
An epileptic syndrome is a constellation of signs and symptoms that may be associated with certain acquired pathologies or etiologies (symptomatic or structural/metabolic), lack an identifiable pathology or etiology (cryptogenic or unknown), or are likely genetic and follow a well-defined and accepted characteristic pattern (idiopathic or genetic). Syndromes may be associated with focal seizures that begin in one area of the cortex (such as mesial temporal sclerosis) or generalized seizures that appear throughout the cortex at onset (such as childhood absence epilepsy). Syndromic classification is useful because it can often predict prognosis and guide antiepileptic drug therapy. The most recent list of epilepsy syndromes is found at the International League Against Epilepsy website (http://www.ilae-epilepsy.org).

10. **List the four most common presumed genetic epileptic syndromes.**
1. Febrile convulsions
2. Benign childhood epilepsy with centrotemporal spikes
3. Childhood absence epilepsy
4. Juvenile myoclonic epilepsy

The first three syndromes usually are associated with spontaneous remission with age. Juvenile myoclonic epilepsy persists and usually responds to treatment with antiepileptic drugs.

11. **Describe the Lennox–Gastaut syndrome.**
This epileptic syndrome usually begins before age 5 years and is characterized by generalized tonic–axial, atonic, and atypical absence seizures. Many patients also have myoclonic, partial, and tonic–clonic seizures. The EEG is characterized by a slow (2 to 2.5 Hz) frontocentral dominant spike and wave pattern, and patients have developmental delay. The seizures are usually refractory to medication, and status epilepticus is common. About 60% of patients have a clear underlying cause of encephalopathy (symptomatic or structural/metabolic).

12. What are "benign" febrile seizures?

Benign febrile seizures (convulsions) are an inherited predisposition to developing a tonic–clonic seizure with a high fever. The description is limited to convulsions associated with high fever in children younger than the age of 5 years (usually between 6 and 36 months of age), with no cause for the seizure other than the fever. Benign febrile seizures are common, occurring in 3% to 5% of children younger than the age of 5 years. Most patients have only one or two seizures. Recent genetic analysis of families with febrile convulsions has defined specific associated gene defects (see Question 21, Table 22-4).

13. Are febrile seizures a risk factor for the development of epilepsy?

A single, isolated febrile seizure of short duration probably does not greatly influence the later development of epilepsy. The overall risk of developing epilepsy in the general population is approximately 1%, and in those with febrile seizures, the risk increases to approximately 3%. In general, if there are no other reasons to suspect recurrent seizures, such children are not treated. The following features, however, have been identified as risk factors for the development of epilepsy:
1. Underlying neurologic or developmental abnormality
2. Family history of nonfebrile seizures
3. Prolonged febrile convulsions
4. Multiple febrile convulsions
5. Atypical or focal features (complex febrile seizures)

14. Describe the syndrome of benign childhood epilepsy with centrotemporal spikes.

This syndrome accounts for about 15 to 20% of epilepsy cases younger than the age of 15 years. The seizures, which are mostly nocturnal, are associated with focal motor activity of the face with salivation. The seizures may generalize secondarily. Sensory symptoms may occur around the mouth in addition to motor components. Speech may not be possible. The EEG is characterized by a prominent interictal centrotemporal sharp wave with otherwise normal background. The sharp waves occur more frequently during sleep. This epilepsy typically remits spontaneously by the age of 16, regardless of treatment. Treatment for this focal epilepsy may be instituted, depending on how disruptive the seizures are. Therapy is individualized and ranges from no therapy with counseling and observation to chronic antiepileptic drug (AED) therapy.

15. Characterize juvenile myoclonic epilepsy.

This syndrome is characterized by multiple seizure types including (1) myoclonic seizures that often occur shortly after wakening, (2) generalized tonic–clonic seizures that tend to be precipitated by sleep deprivation, and (3) absence seizures. Interictally, the EEG typically shows a 4- to 6-Hz generalized spike-wave pattern. The generalized myoclonic jerks are associated with a generalized spike-wave discharge, and usually consciousness is not lost. Unlike the other common idiopathic epilepsies, juvenile myoclonic epilepsy does not usually remit with age. Valproate, topiramate, lamotrigine, levetiracetam, and primidone have been successful in treating seizures. Some of the other newer AEDs also may prove to be beneficial.

PHYSIOLOGY

16. What systemic physiologic changes occur during a seizure?

For both absence and complex partial seizures, the patient may have a variety of autonomic alterations, including changes in pulse rate, perspiration, salivation, pupillary dilatation, and urinary incontinence. The most dramatic systemic changes occur during generalized tonic–clonic seizures, with increased blood pressure and pulse rate, increased autonomic nervous system activation, metabolic acidosis, and a drop in PO_2 and increase in PCO_2 during the apneic tonic phase. Prolonged generalized tonic–clonic seizures may have serious consequences including hyperkalemia or rhabdomyolysis.

17. What central nervous system physiologic changes occur during a seizure?

During a seizure, cerebral blood flow and glucose utilization in the brain are increased. There may be an accompanying increase in lactate and a decrease in pH, alterations in the concentration of neurotransmitters, an increase in extracellular potassium, and a decrease in extracellular calcium. Generalized tonic–clonic seizures and most complex partial seizures activate the hypothalamus and increase serum prolactin, a finding that may help to differentiate epileptic from nonepileptic (psychogenic) seizures with prolactin level assays postictally. Prolactin also may be elevated after syncope and hence cannot differentiate epileptic seizures from syncope.

Table 22-4. Genetic Epilepsies with Generalized Seizures

	EPILEPSY SYNDROME	GENE	GENE PRODUCT	INH*	TESTING
Neonates—Infants	Benign familial neonatal epilepsy	KCNQ2/KCNQ3	K+ channel subunits Kv7.2-Kv7.3	AD	Sequencing, deletion/duplication analysis
	Benign familial neonatal/infantile epilepsy	SCN2A	Na+ channel subunit Nav1.2		Sequencing
	Benign familial infantile epilepsy	PRRT2	Proline-rich transmembrane protein 2		Sequencing
		ATP1A2	Na+/K+ transporting ATPase		
	Early infantile epileptic encephalopathy with suppression-burst (Ohtahara syndrome)	ARX	Aristaless-related homeobox	XLD	Sequencing, deletion/duplication analysis
		CDKL5	Cyclin-dependent kinase-like 5		
		STXBP1	Syntaxin binding protein 1	AD	
		KCNQ2	Potassium channel subunit Kv7.2		
		PLB1	Phospholipase B1	AR	
	Familial infantile myoclonic epilepsy	TBC1D24	TBC1 domain family, member 24	AR	Sequencing (commercially unavailable in United States)
	Generalized epilepsy with febrile seizures plus (GEFS+)	SCN1B	Voltage-gated Na+ channel, type 1β	AD	Sequencing
		SCN1A	Voltage-gated Na+ channel, Nav1.1		Sequencing, deletion/duplication analysis
		GABRG2	GABAA receptor, γ2 subunit	?	Sequencing
		SCN2A	Na+ channel subunit Nav1.2	AD	
		GABRD	GABAA receptor, δ subunit	?	
	Severe myoclonic epilepsy of infancy (Dravet syndrome)	SCN1A	Voltage-gated Na+ channel, Nav1.1	AD	Sequencing, deletion/duplication analysis
		SCN2A	Na+ channel subunit Nav1.2		Sequencing
		GABRG2	GABAA receptor, γ2 subunit	?	

Continued on following page

Table 22-4. Genetic Epilepsies with Generalized Seizures (Continued)

	EPILEPSY SYNDROME	GENE	GENE PRODUCT	INH*	TESTING
Generalized	Childhood absence epilepsy	GABRG2	GABA$_A$ receptor, γ2 subunit	?	Sequencing
		GABRA1	GABA$_A$ receptor, α1 subunit	AD	
		SLC2A1	Solute carrier family 2, member 1	AD/AR	
		GABRB3	GABA$_A$ receptor, β3 subunit	?	
		CACNA1H	T-type Ca^{++} channel, α1H subunit		
		CACNG3	Ca^{++} channel subunit γ3		
	Juvenile absence epilepsy	LGI4	Leucine-rich repeat LGI family, member 4	AR	Commercially unavailable
		ME2	Mitochondrial malic enzyme 2	AR	
		INHA	Inhibin α	?	
	Juvenile myoclonic epilepsy	GABRA1	GABA$_A$ receptor, α1 subunit	AD	Sequencing
		EFHC1	EF-hand domain (C-terminal) containing 1	?	
		BRD2	Bromodomain containing 2		
		CACNB4	Ca^{++} channel subunit β4		
	Myoclonic-atonic epilepsy (myoclonic epilepsy of Doose)	SCN1A	Voltage-gated Na$^+$ channel, Nav1.1	AD	Sequencing, CNV† analysis
		SCN2A	Na$^+$ channel subunit Nav1.2	?	Sequencing
		GABRG2	GABA$_A$ receptor, γ2 subunit	?	Sequencing
		SLC2A1	Solute carrier family 2, member 1	AD/AR	Sequencing, CNV analysis
Focal	Autosomal dominant nocturnal frontal lobe epilepsy (ADNFLE)	CHRNA4	Nicotinic Ach receptor, α4 subunit	AD	Sequence analysis
		CHRNB2	Nicotinic Ach receptor, β2 subunit		
		CHRNA2	Nicotinic Ach receptor, α2 subunit		
	Autosomal dominant epilepsy with auditory features (ADEAF)	LGI1	Leucine-rich repeat LGI family, member 1		
	Benign epilepsy with centrotemporal spikes (BECTS)	ELP4	Elongator acetyltransferase complex, subunit 4	?	Commercially unavailable
		Other described genes include (gene products unknown): (4q13.2-q21.3), (7p21.3), (1q25 and 18q, digenic), (12q22-23.3)		?	Genes unknown

*Inheritance: AD, Autosomal dominant; XLD, X-linked dominant; AR, autosomal recessive; CNV, Copy Number Variant.

Courtesy of Zulfi Haneef.

ETIOLOGY

18. **What are the identifiable causes of seizures as a function of age?**
    The common causes of seizures vary by age. See Figure 22-1 for the common causes of seizure by age.

Cause of seizure

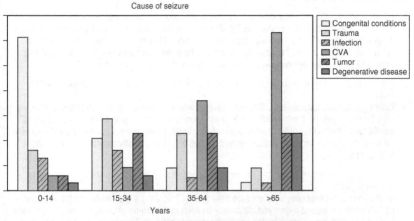

Figure 22-1. Common causes of seizure by age.

19. **Which electrolyte imbalances commonly lead to seizures?**
    Low electrolyte levels are common causes for seizures. Hypocalcemia is a common and reversible electrolyte imbalance leading to seizures. Others include hyponatremia and hypomagnesemia. Although not an electrolyte imbalance, hypoglycemia, and less commonly hyperglycemia (i.e., nonketotic hyperglycemic state) can also lead to seizures.

20. **What drugs are common causes of seizures?**
    Prescription medications leading to seizures include bupropion and clozapine, which both lower seizure threshold. Drugs causing seizures at toxic levels include penicillin, lidocaine, aminophylline, and isoniazid. Drug withdrawal may cause seizures, particularly with barbiturates and benzodiazepines. Drugs of abuse causing seizures include cocaine and amphetamines. Marijuana has not been shown to cause seizures. Alcohol may also cause seizures, both in excess and with withdrawal.

21. **What are genetic epilepsies? What are the genes described for epilepsy?**
    According to the 2010 ILAE Classification of Seizures and Epilepsy, epilepsy can be divided by etiology into genetic, structural/metabolic, or unknown. Genetic epilepsies, previously known as *idiopathic*, like other types of epilepsies, may have seizures that are focal in onset, appear to be "generalized" in onset, or both. The list of genes associated with epilepsy is rapidly expanding; a recent list is shown in Table 22-4. Newer gene associations are frequently being described as our knowledge of genetic epilepsies advances with new research.

22. **Which factors predict the development of epilepsy after head trauma?**
    Among all patients with head trauma who seek medical attention, about 2% develop posttraumatic seizures. The risk is 12% for those with severe traumatic brain injury (TBI) and up to 50% with penetrating injuries. Factors that predispose to the development of epilepsy after head trauma include a seizure within 2 weeks of injury, depressed skull fracture, loss of consciousness for longer than 24 hours, cerebral contusion, cortical subdural or subarachnoid hemorrhage, and age of injury older than 65 years.

23. **Should antiepileptic drugs be used after head trauma to prevent the development of epilepsy?**
    Seizure prophylaxis after moderate or severe TBI is often standard practice, but there is no definitive answer to this question. The most recent study assessing posttraumatic prophylactic treatment with phenytoin concluded that therapy was useful only during the first week after head trauma. At later

dates, the side effects produced by phenytoin appeared to be detrimental to patients with severe neurologic damage after head trauma. Valproate also has been found to be ineffective as a prophylactic agent after head trauma. At present, no drug clearly has been shown to be an effective prophylaxis against posttraumatic epilepsy.

DIAGNOSTIC TESTING

24. **How many EEGs are needed to establish the diagnosis of epilepsy?**
Between 29% and 69% of patients with the clinical diagnosis of epilepsy have interictal epileptiform activity on a single EEG. A greater number of EEGs increase the yield of diagnosis, with four EEGs enhancing the yield up to 92%. More EEGs than that have minimal additional yield. The diagnostic yield of EEG also may be increased by recording sleep and prolonging monitoring.

25. **Which patients with seizures should have magnetic resonance imaging (MRI) scans?**
Patients with focal features on EEG should have an MRI scan to look for a brain lesion associated with their seizures, particularly when epilepsy surgery is a consideration. Contrast-enhanced MRI should be performed for patients with new-onset epilepsy to diagnose acute lesions. Patients with clear-cut primary generalized epilepsy based on EEG and clinical features usually do not require MRI scanning.

26. **What is the value of positron emission tomography (PET) scanning in patients with epilepsy?**
Most patients with epilepsy who are evaluated with PET scans are studied during the interictal period, when an area of hypometabolism may be seen in the region of seizure onset. This reflects a decrease in glucose uptake by the involved abnormal brain. PET scanning can help to localize seizure onset in patients with intractable, complex partial seizures who are being evaluated for surgical therapy. Between 60% and 90% of patients with temporal lobe epilepsy, and 67% with extratemporal lobe epilepsy, show hypometabolism in PET imaging, while about 44% of "nonlesional" epilepsy may show hypometabolism in PET. When performed during or shortly following an epileptic seizure, PET imaging often reveals complex patterns of both hypometabolism and hypermetabolism. A common tracer used in PET to evaluate epilepsy patients is [18F] fluoro-2-deoxy-glucose.

27. **What is a single-photon emission computed tomography (SPECT) scan? What role does it have in evaluating patients?**
SPECT is a functional neuroimaging modality that compares differences in regional cerebral blood flow. It is performed in both the ictal and the interictal periods during the epilepsy surgery workup. Focal seizures are typically found to cause local hyperperfusion on SPECT. Subtraction of the interictal scan from the ictal scan and superimposition on an MRI scan can provide an anatomic and physiologic picture of the epileptogenic zone. This subtraction SPECT coregistered to magnetic resonance images is referred to as *SISCOM*. It has been claimed that ictal SPECT correctly identifies the seizure focus in more than 90% of patients with temporal lobe epilepsy, while extratemporal epilepsy has a lower sensitivity (66%). Common tracers used in SPECT to evaluate epilepsy patients are Tc-99m hexamethylpropyleneamine oxime and Tc-99m ethyl cysteinate dimer.

THERAPY

28. **When should antiepileptic treatment be initiated?**
In general, patients who have epilepsy as defined in Question 1 should be treated with antiepileptic medication. The seizure type or syndrome may help with this decision. For example, absence seizures are rarely isolated and so require therapy (the first line is ethosuximide), whereas simple febrile seizures are often isolated and therapy is not indicated. Between 20% and 70% of people with an isolated, unprovoked generalized tonic–clonic seizure will never have another seizure.

29. **Which patients are at highest risk for recurrent seizures?**
Seizure recurrence is more likely if the patient has focal neurologic deficits, developmental delay, a structural brain lesion, or an EEG that demonstrates epileptiform abnormalities. In these

patients, it is reasonable to begin antiepileptic therapy. In patients with a well-defined provocative etiology, it is best to treat the underlying process rather than or in concert with the seizures themselves, for example, in clear-cut cases of alcohol withdrawal seizures and drug-induced seizures.

30. **When should antiepileptic treatment be stopped?**
When considering stopping an antiepileptic, the risk of seizure recurrence should be weighed against the risk of side effects of continued AED therapy. Certain seizure types and benign epileptic syndromes may remit. Patients with absence epilepsy often cease having seizures after puberty, and therapy is no longer needed. Benign childhood epilepsy with centrotemporal spikes also remits. In general, after 2 years of seizure freedom, it is reasonable to consider withdrawing medications. However, approximately one-third of adult patients and one-fourth of children who are seizure free for 2 years will relapse after termination of antiepileptic medication. Evaluation at this stage typically includes an EEG.

31. **Which patients are most likely to have further seizures after their medications have been stopped?**
Risk factors for recurrence include:
    1. Prolonged period before seizures were controlled
    2. Previously high seizure frequency
    3. Neurologic abnormalities
    4. Developmental delay
    5. Complex partial seizures
    6. Consistently abnormal EEGs (both epileptiform and nonepileptiform abnormalities)

32. **Which antiepileptic drugs are most appropriate for focal- versus generalized-onset seizures?**
The choice of AED is dictated by the types of seizures that the patient has experienced. Generalized-onset seizures are typically treated with broad-spectrum medications, and focal-onset seizures may be treated with either narrow- or broad-spectrum medications (Table 22-5). One exception is absence epilepsy, which has generalized-onset seizures, but it is best treated with a narrow-spectrum medication (typically ethosuximide). If possible, monotherapy should be used.

Table 22-5. Broad- versus Narrow-Spectrum Antiepileptic Drugs (AEDs)

BROAD-SPECTRUM AEDS	NARROW-SPECTRUM AEDS
Treats focal- or generalized-onset seizures:	*Treats focal-onset seizures:*
Benzodiazepines	Carbamazepine
Felbamate	Eslicarbazepine
Lamotrigine	Ezogabine
Levetiracetam	Gabapentin
Phenobarbital*	Lacosamide
Tiagabine*	Oxcarbazepine
Topiramate	Perampanel
Valproic acid	Phenytoin
Vigabatrin*	Pregabalin
Zonisamide	Rufinamide
	Treats absence seizures:
	Ethosuximide

*May aggravate absence seizures.

33. **What guides the choice of an AED aside from spectrum of action?**
If an epilepsy syndrome is diagnosed, there are certain AEDs that are first line (Table 22-6). Otherwise, within the classes of broad- and narrow-spectrum medications, one medication is not clearly more efficacious than another; therefore, side effects and comorbidities are key reasons in choosing an AED.

Table 22-6. Preferred Antiepileptic Drugs (AEDs) for Specific Epileptic Syndromes

EPILEPTIC SYNDROME	AED OF CHOICE
Childhood absence epilepsy	Ethosuximide > valproic acid/lamotrigine/levetiracetam
Juvenile myoclonic epilepsy	Valproic acid/levetiracetam/lamotrigine > topiramate/ zonisamide
Lennox–Gastaut syndrome (LGS)	Valproic acid/lamotrigine/felbamate/clobazam (carbamazepine/tiagabine can lead to status epilepticus)
LGS with drop seizures	Rufinamide
West syndrome	Adrenocorticotropic hormone (vigabatrin if tuberous sclerosis)

Courtesy of Zulfi Haneef.

34. Construct a table of all major antiepileptic medications to compare their mechanism of action, metabolic profile, common dosages, and significant side effects. See Table 22-7.

35. In general, how often should AEDs be given?

AEDs should be given at least every half-life. Some medications may need to be given more frequently because of peak-dose side effects. For example, patients tolerate two or three daily doses of ethosuximide better than a single daily dose. In some cases, pharmacokinetics (i.e., drug metabolism, half-life) may not match pharmacodynamics (i.e., drug effect), and medication is given at intervals longer than the half-life. For example, levetiracetam has a half-life of 6 to 8 hours but is given twice daily.

36. What are the advantages of monotherapy?
    1. In most situations, one drug controls seizures as well as two or more drugs.
    2. Monotherapy prevents interactions between antiepileptic medications and limits interaction with other non-AEDs.
    3. Monotherapy is less expensive.
    4. Monotherapy improves compliance.

37. What are the two main mechanisms for drug interactions among AEDs?
    1. Inhibition/induction of hepatic enzymes: For example, valproic acid inhibits lamotrigine metabolism, so with initiation of lamotrigine while the patient is taking valproic acid, a slower titration needs to be performed to avoid lamotrigine toxicity. Carbamazepine induces its own metabolism so levels may drop many months after being therapeutic.
    2. The other main mechanism of drug interaction is through protein binding. Phenytoin, valproate, and tiagabine are highly bound (>90%) to plasma proteins and can compete for binding sites. For example, valproic acid binding can displace phenytoin so that free phenytoin levels increase, resulting in the potential for phenytoin toxicity.

38. When and how often should blood levels of AEDs be checked?
    AED levels in general do not need to be regularly checked. Monitoring of AED levels can help when the patient is initially loaded with the medication and when the drug reaches a steady-state concentration, usually after approximately five half-lives. Monitoring of drug levels is most helpful in determining patient compliance, in documenting high levels when the patient has symptoms concerning for possible drug toxicity, and documenting low levels with breakthrough seizure occurrence.

39. Which screening blood tests should be performed for patients taking AEDs? How often should they be done?
    Many AEDs may affect the ability of the bone marrow to produce blood cells or may cause liver dysfunction. It is reasonable to use complete blood count and comprehensive metabolic profile tests as baseline studies to identify predisposing problems. After this initial screening, it is usually not necessary to perform these studies routinely unless the patient is symptomatic. Possible exceptions are young children and developmentally delayed patients who cannot communicate their toxic symptoms. Other special situations include the use of felbamate and valproate, which require hematologic and hepatic function monitoring, and carbamazepine, which requires hematologic monitoring.

Table 22-7. Major Antiepileptic Medications

ANTIEPILEPTIC DRUG (AED), TRADE NAME, MANUFACTURER, YEAR RELEASED	MECHANISM	METABOLISM	COMMON DOSAGES	THERAPEUTIC LEVEL, HALF-LIFE	COMMON OR SIGNIFICANT SIDE EFFECTS
Phenobarbital, generic by various manufacturers, 1912	Prolongs opening of GABA-ergic Cl⁻ channels, increases GABA inhibition.	Hepatic > renal. Enzyme inducing. 20%–45% protein bound.	For status epilepticus: 20-mg/kg loading dose. Neonates: 2–5 mg/kg/day divided bid. Adults: 100–300 mg divided bid. Children: 3–7 mg/kg/day divided bid.	Therapeutic range: 15–40 mg/L. Half-life: 24–168 hours. Takes 2–3 weeks to achieve steady state if no loading dose given.	Sedation, depression, cognitive slowing, respiratory depression, hepatic dysfunction, lupus-like syndrome, erythema multiforme, osteomalacia.
Phenytoin, Dilantin by Parke-Davis, 1938	Blocks voltage-dependent Na⁺ and Ca²⁺ channels, reduces high-frequency firing.	Hepatic > renal. Enzyme inducing. 90% protein bound. Nonlinear kinetics.	Loading dose 20 mg/kg. Maintenance 5 mg/kg/day, may divide bid. Adjust dose based on level (nonlinear kinetics). For level 7–10 mg/L, increase dose by 50 mg/day. Level <7 increase dose by 100 mg/day.	Therapeutic range: 10–20 mg/L. Check unbound level (0.5–3 mg/L) if creatinine clearance <10, albumin <3.2 mg/dL, on valproate, pregnant, or suspected toxicity. Half-life: average 22 hours (range 7–42 hours, nonlinear kinetics).	Cerebellar atrophy, ataxia, megaloblastic anemia, neuropathy, gingival hyperplasia, nystagmus, osteomalacia.
Primidone, Mysoline by Athena Neurosciences, 1954	Enhances GABA inhibition, essentially as phenobarbital, but may also have additional activity.	Renal > hepatic. Enzyme inducing. Protein bound.	Adults: start 100–125 mg qhs, increase by 100–125 mg/day every 3 days to initial target of 250 mg tid. Children: start 50–60 mg/day, increase by 50 mg/day every 3 days to initial target of 10–25 mg/kg/day divided tid.	Therapeutic range: Primidone: 5–12 mg/L. Phenobarbital: 15–40 mg/L. Half-life: Primidone: 8–22 hours. Phenobarbital: 56–140 hours. Phenylethylmalonamide: 10–25 hours.	Sedation, depression, cognitive slowing, respiratory depression, hepatic dysfunction, lupus-like syndrome, erythema multiforme, osteomalacia.

Continued on following page

Table 22-7. Major Antiepileptic Medications *(Continued)*

ANTIEPILEPTIC DRUG (AED), TRADE NAME, MANUFACTURER, YEAR RELEASED	MECHANISM	METABOLISM	COMMON DOSAGES	THERAPEUTIC LEVEL, HALF-LIFE	COMMON OR SIGNIFICANT SIDE EFFECTS
Ethosuximide, Zarontin by Parke-Davis, 1960	Blocks T-type calcium channels, reduces thalamocortical excitability.	Hepatic > renal.	Adults: 1000 mg/day in divided doses tid. Children: 20 mg/kg/day	Therapeutic range: 40-100 mg/L. Half-life: 30-60 hours.	Sedation, nausea/vomiting, headache, personality changes, psychosis.
Carbamazepine, Tegretol, Tegretol XR by Novartis, Carbatrol by Shire, 1974	Blocks voltage-dependent Na⁺ and Ca²⁺ channels, reduces high-frequency firing.	Hepatic > renal. Active metabolite: carbamazepine 10-11 epoxide. Enzyme inducing.	Adults: 200-400 mg tid. Children <12: start 10-20 mg/kg/day divided bid or tid, increase by 5-10 mg/kg/day weekly, target 20-35 mg/kg/day divided bid or tid. Take with food.	Therapeutic range: 4-12 mg/L. Half-life: initially 25-65 hours with induction, 12-17 hours.	Sedation, ataxia, nausea, diplopia/blurred vision, nausea, hyponatremia, SIADH, elevated LFTs, osteomalacia, photosensitivity.
Valproic acid, Depakote, Depakote ER, Depakene ER by Abbott, 1978	Blocks voltage-dependent Na⁺ and Ca²⁺ channels, reduces high-frequency firing. Potentiates GABA.	Hepatic *N*-glucuronidation and beta-oxidation *CYP450.* >90% protein bound.	Adults and children: start 10-15 mg/kg/day bid or tid. Increase by 5-10 mg/kg/day weekly. Max 60 mg/kg/day.	Therapeutic range: 50-125 mg/L. Half-life: 9-12 hours, children, 5-13 hours, 20 hours with extended-release preparation.	Tremor, weight gain, elevated LFTs, increased bleeding, thrombocytopenia, hyperammonemia, polycystic ovary syndrome, fragile hair, osteomalacia.
Felbamate, Felbatol by Wallace, 1993	*N*-methyl-D-aspartate blocker (glycine site), enhances GABA inhibition, blocks Na⁺ channels.	Renal > hepatic.	Adults: start 1200 mg/day divided tid or qid. Increase by 1200 mg/day weekly. Max 3600 mg/day. Children: start 15 mg/kg/day divided tid, increase by 15 mg/kg/day weekly. Max 3600 mg/day.	Therapeutic range: 30-80 mg/L. Half-life: 20-23 hours.	Requires informed consent regarding idiosyncratic reactions—aplastic anemia and hepatic failure. Headache, drowsiness, agitation, weight loss, nausea/vomiting, tachycardia.

Drug	Mechanism	Metabolism	Dosing	Pharmacokinetics	Side effects
Gabapentin, Neurontin by Parke-Davis, 1993	Increases brain GABA levels, may work at Ca^{2+} channels.	Renal >95% unchanged	Adults: start 300 mg qhs, increase by 300 mg/day every 1-3 days. Max 3600 mg/day divided tid. Children: start 10-20 mg/kg/day divided tid, increase by 10-20 mg/kg/day. Max 50 mg/kg/day divided tid.	Therapeutic range: 2-12 mg/L. Half-life: 4-6 hours.	Somnolence, fatigue, ataxia, weight gain, edema, TTP, leukopenia, tinnitus.
Lamotrigine, Lamictal by Glaxo Wellcome, 1994	Voltage-dependent Na^+ channel blocker. Decreases release of excitatory neurotransmitters.	Hepatic > renal.	Starting titration varies if on other drugs. Adults (with valproate): start 25 mg every day, increase by 25 mg bid every 1-2 weeks, initial target 100 mg bid. Monotherapy or enzyme-inducing AEDs: start 25 mg bid, increase by 50 mg every week, target 200 mg bid. Children (with valproate): 0.15 mg/kg/day for 2 weeks, then 0.3 mg/kg/day for weeks 3-4. Children on monotherapy or enzyme-inducing AEDs: 0.6 mg/kg/day for first 2 weeks, then 1.2 mg/kg/day for weeks 3-4, target 5-15 mg/kg/day.	Therapeutic range: 4-15 mg/L. Half-life: 11-60 hours (depending if on inducer or inhibitor).	Rash or Stevens–Johnson syndrome more likely if increased rapidly. Nausea, lethargy, dizziness, headache.

Continued on following page

Table 22-7. Major Antiepileptic Medications (Continued)

ANTIEPILEPTIC DRUG (AED), TRADE NAME, MANUFACTURER, YEAR RELEASED	MECHANISM	METABOLISM	COMMON DOSAGES	THERAPEUTIC LEVEL, HALF-LIFE	COMMON OR SIGNIFICANT SIDE EFFECTS
Topiramate, Topamax by Ortho Biotech, 1996	Blocks repetitive neuron firing. Blocks kainate and AMPA receptors. Improves GABA inhibition, carbonic anhydrase inhibitor.	Predominantly renal, but has enzyme-inducing effects.	Adults: start 25 mg daily, increase by 25-50 mg divided bid weekly, target 100-200 mg divided bid. Children: 1-3 mg/kg/day, increase by 1-3 mg/kg/day every 1-2 weeks divided bid, target 5-9 mg/kg/day	Therapeutic range: 4-10 mg/L. Half-life: 18-30 hours.	Nephrolithiasis, acute angle closure glaucoma, metabolic acidosis, hyperthermia, tingling, altered taste, anorexia/weight loss, lethargy, word finding problems, diarrhea, dizziness.
Tiagabine, Gabitril by Cephalon, 1997	Potentiates GABA by blocking glial uptake.	Hepatic >90%. Protein bound.	Adults: start 4 mg daily, increase to 4 mg bid in 2 weeks, then increase by 4 mg day, divided bid weekly, target 32-56 mg divided bid. Children (12-16 years): start same as adult, but target 20-32 mg.	Therapeutic range: 0.1-0.3 mg/L. Half-life: 4-9 hours.	Fatigue, weakness, poor attention, ataxia, nausea, tremor.
Levetiracetam, Keppra by UCB Pharma, 1999	Decreased high-voltage N+-type Ca²⁺ channel current, reduces effects of Zn and beta-carbolines at GABA A and glycine receptors.	Renal > hepatic. Not enzyme inducing. <10% protein bound.	Adults: start 250 mg bid for 1 week, then target 500 mg bid. May increase to 1500 bid.	Therapeutic range: 5-40 mg/L. Half-life: 6-8 hours.	Personality changes, irritability, sedation, hallucinations.

Drug	Mechanism	Metabolism	Dosing	Therapeutic range/Half-life	Side effects
Oxcarbazepine, Trileptal by Novartis, 2000	Blocks Na+ and Ca2+ channels, stops high-frequency firing.	Hepatic = renal. Metabolized to active monohydroxy metabolite by cytosolic liver enzymes, then further glucuronidation and oxidation to other less active metabolites, then renal excretion. 40% protein bound.	Adults: start 300 mg bid, increase by 300 mg every 3 days, to initial target 600 mg bid. Max 2400 mg/day. Children (4-16 years): start 8-10 mg/kg every 2 weeks to target (all divided bid). 20-29 kg: 900 mg/day, 29-39 kg: 1200 mg/day, >39 kg: 1800 mg/day.	Therapeutic range: 10-monohydroxymetabolite 12-30 mg/L. Half-life: 8-12 hours.	Hyponatremia, fatigue, somnolence, ataxia, nausea, vomiting, diplopia, nystagmus.
Zonisamide, Zonegran by Elan, 2000	Blocks Na+ and Ca2+ channels, stops high-frequency firing, interacts with GABA_A channels, carbonic anhydrase inhibitor.	Hepatic > renal.	Adults: start 100 mg/day, increase by 100 mg every 2 weeks, target of 400 mg once daily (may divide bid). Children: start 1.2 mg/kg/day, increase by 0.5-1 mg/kg/day every 2 weeks to target of 5-8 mg/kg/day.	Therapeutic range: 15-40 mg/L. Half-life: 63 hours.	Nephrolithiasis, tingling, altered taste, anorexia/weight loss, lethargy, word finding problems, visual field defects, dizziness.
Pregabalin, Lyrica by Pfizer, 2005	Increases GABA and decreases glutamate, decreases influx through voltage-dependent Ca2+ channels.	Renal.	Start 75 mg bid, increase to 300 mg bid.	Therapeutic range: variable. Half-life: 6 hours.	Dizziness, drowsiness.
Vigabatrin, Sabril by Ovaron Pharma, under FDA consideration in 2009	Inhibits GABA transaminase to increase brain levels of GABA.	Renal.	Adults: start 500 mg bid, increase by 500 mg/day every week up to 3 gm/day bid. Infantile spasms: 50 mg/kg/day bid, titrate by 25-50 mg/kg/day every 3 days to max of 150 mg/kg/day.	Therapeutic range: unknown. Half-life: 5-12 hours.	Peripheral visual field defects, behavioral changes. Requires informed consent because of the visual field effects.

Continued on following page

Table 22-7. Major Antiepileptic Medications *(Continued)*

ANTIEPILEPTIC DRUG (AED), TRADE NAME, MANUFACTURER, YEAR RELEASED	MECHANISM	METABOLISM	COMMON DOSAGES	THERAPEUTIC LEVEL, HALF-LIFE	COMMON OR SIGNIFICANT SIDE EFFECTS
Lacosamide, Vimpat by Eisai, 2009	Enhances slow inactivation of Na⁺ channel.	Renal and hepatic.	Begin 25-50 mg bid and titrate by 50-100 mg/week to dose of 200 mg bid.	13 hours, therapeutic levels not established.	Dizziness, headache, nausea, diplopia. May be increased with other AEDS that block sodium channels.
Rufinamide, Banzel by Eisai, 2009	Sodium channel.	Hepatic.	Begin with 200-400 mg bid and increase weekly by 400-800 mg/day to target of 1600 mg bid.	6-10 hours, therapeutic levels not established.	Somnolence, vomiting, headache, can shorten QT interval at higher doses and contraindicated in individuals with short QT interval.
Ezogabine, Potiga by GlaxoSmithKline, 2011	Potassium channel (KCNQ) enhancer.	Hepatic.	Begin with 100 tid and increase weekly by 100-200 mg/day to target dose of 400 tid.	13-20 hours, therapeutic levels not established.	Retinal/scleral pigment change, blue skin discoloration, urinary retention.
Clobazam, Onfi by Lundbeck, 2012	GABA agonist (1,5-benzodiazepine).	Hepatic.	Begin with 5 mg bid and increase weekly by 10-20 mg/day to target of 40 mg bid.	36-42 hours, therapeutic levels not established.	Sedation (less than other benzodiazepines), tolerance/withdrawal.
Eslicarbazepine, Aptiom by Sunovion, 2014	Sodium channel blocker.	Hepatic.	Begin at 400 mg qhs and increase weekly by 400 mg to target of 1200 qhs.	13-20 hours, therapeutic levels not established.	Diplopia, hyponatremia.
Perampanel, Fycompa by Eisai, 2014	AMPA receptor blocker.	Hepatic.	Begin at 2 mg qhs and increase weekly by 2-4 mg weekly to target of 12 mg qhs.	105 hours, therapeutic levels not established.	Irritability.

SIADH, Syndrome of inappropriate antidiuretic hormone; *LFT*, liver function tests; *AED*, antiepileptic drug; *TTP*, thrombotic thrombocytopenic purpura; *AMPA*,

WOMEN AND EPILEPSY

40. What are the differences between the effects of estrogen and progesterone on seizures?
    In adults, estrogen is neuroexcitable, while progesterone (specifically one of its metabolites called *allopregnanolone*) is neuroinhibitory. As such, estrogen can increase the occurrence of seizures, while progesterone may tend to reduce seizures. The balance between these hormones has corresponding effects on seizures throughout the menstrual cycle, pregnancy, and other hormonal changes.

41. In catamenial epilepsy, how do hormone changes predispose to seizures?
    Catamenial epilepsy is defined as a significant increase in seizures during specific menstrual phases. The main trigger for this is the estrogen to progesterone ratio, which results in increased seizures during the periovulatory/perimenstrual phases. Such a catamenial pattern is said to occur in about one-third of women with focal epilepsy.

42. What effect do AEDs have on oral contraceptives and teratogenicity?
    Enzyme-inducing AEDs can induce the metabolism of oral contraceptives, leading to failure of contraception (Table 22-8). An implant or intrauterine device might provide better protection in this instance.

Table 22-8. Antiepileptic Drugs in Contraception and Pregnancy

AED	ORAL CONTRACEPTIVE EFFICACY	PREGNANCY CATEGORY*	KNOWN TERATOGENICITY ISSUES
Phenobarbital	Decrease	D	Cleft lip and palate and heart defects
Phenytoin	Decrease	D	Hypoplasia of the nails plus stiff joints, cleft lip and palate
Primidone	Decrease	D	Cleft lip and palate
Carbamazepine	Decrease	D	Neural tube defects 0.5%-1%, other major malformations, microcephaly, and growth retardation
Valproic acid	None	D	Neural tube defects 1%-2%, also cardiac anomalies, hypospadias, polydactyly, bilateral inguinal hernia, dysplastic kidney, and equinovarus clubfoot
Felbamate	None	C	Uncertain
Gabapentin	None	C	Uncertain
Lamotrigine	None	C	Uncertain
Topiramate	Decrease	C	Uncertain
Tiagabine	None	C	Uncertain
Levetiracetam	None	C	Uncertain
Oxcarbazepine	Decrease	C	May be more favorable than carbamazepine (no epoxide metabolite)
Zonisamide	None	C	Uncertain
Lacosamide	None	C	Uncertain
Pregabalin	None	C	Uncertain
Rufinamide	Decrease	C	Uncertain
Vigabatrin	None	C	Uncertain

*Pregnancy categories.
C: Risk not ruled out.
D: Positive evidence of risk.

Some AEDs used during pregnancy, particularly valproate, have been associated with increased incidence of birth defects. Because some AEDs cause neural tube defects, all sexually active and fertile women with epilepsy should be taking folate on a daily basis (0.4 to 5 mg/day).

SEIZURES AND EPILEPSY IN OLDER PATIENTS

43. **Are seizures in the elderly easily identified?**
Seizures in the elderly are notoriously underdiagnosed and misdiagnosed. The average delay to diagnosis in patients age 59 to 96 years is about 1.7 years. These patients tend not to seek help initially, but even after medical evaluation, only 28% of elderly patients with complex partial seizures and about 50% of the patients with generalized seizures are correctly diagnosed initially.

44. **What are some of the age-related changes that can affect AED pharmacokinetics and pharmacodynamics?**
Elderly patients frequently have progressive decline in AED protein binding by albumin, increased volume of distribution, and slow drug elimination. These patients also appear to have increased sensitivity to the side effects of many AEDs. They are often on many other medications, which can lead to drug interactions. More frequent monitoring of drug levels may be appropriate in this age group.

ACUTE EPILEPSY TREATMENT

45. **What is status epilepticus?**
Status epilepticus refers to a seizure that fails to remit. While traditionally defined as 30 minutes of continuous seizure activity, a widely accepted current definition is at least 5 minutes of continuous seizures or two or more seizures with incomplete recovery of consciousness in between them.

46. **How is status epilepticus classified?**
Status epilepticus may be classified into convulsive or nonconvulsive status epilepticus (Fig. 22-2). Convulsive status epilepticus is a medical emergency. It can be characterized as either primary or secondary generalized seizures. Nonconvulsive status epilepticus refers to either absence or complex partial status epilepticus. In either case, the patient does not have major motor seizures but is abnormal cognitively and may appear to be in a fugue state. Absence status appears to have no morbidity (unless injuries occur during the status), but complex partial status may lead to permanent cognitive deficits.

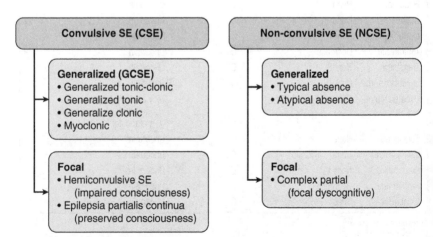

Figure 22-2. Classification of status epilepticus *(Courtesy of Zulfi Haneef.)*

47. What are the most common causes of status epilepticus?

The most common cause of status epilepticus is a low blood concentration of antiepileptic drugs in patients with chronic epilepsy (34%). Other frequent causes include remote symptomatic causes (24%), cerebrovascular accidents (22%), anoxia or hypoxia (10%), metabolic causes (10%), and alcohol and drug withdrawal (10%). The common causes of status epilepticus in a more or less descending order of frequency are given in Table 22-9.

Table 22-9. Most Common Causes of Status Epilepticus

Subtherapeutic antiepileptic drug (AED)
Remote brain injury
Stroke
Head trauma
Hypo- and hyperglycemia
Electrolyte imbalance (Mg, Ca, Na)
Hepatic/renal failure
Sepsis
Anoxic brain injury
Drug intoxications
Alcohol withdrawal
Hypertensive encephalopathy
Central nervous system infections
Neoplasms
Congenital malformations
Cryptogenic
Autoimmune encephalitis
Paraneoplastic syndromes

48. How is absence status epilepticus treated?

Absence status is treated with intravenous diazepam or derivatives, not with phenytoin or the barbiturates. Intravenous valproate also can be an effective therapy.

49. How is complex partial status epilepticus treated?

Complex partial status is usually not associated with life-threatening systemic complications but may result in impairment of memory function and should be treated aggressively, similar to generalized tonic–clonic status. However, one may decide to initiate therapy with nonsedating AEDs before using anesthetic agents.

50. How is convulsive status epilepticus treated?

Generalized tonic–clonic or convulsive status epilepticus is a medical emergency, and every effort should be made to stop the seizures as quickly as possible. Sequelae are more frequent if seizures are not stopped within 60 minutes of onset. The initial approach includes administration of thiamine followed by glucose when glucose levels are low or unknown and correction of electrolyte imbalances. Hyperthermia, which may accompany status epilepticus, should be aggressively controlled. Initial specific therapy should include a benzodiazepine (e.g., lorazepam, 0.1 mg/kg intravenously infused at 1 to 2 mg/min). If seizures continue, a second dose can be given. Regardless, second-line therapy in the form of a longer acting AED is initiated. Intravenous fosphenytoin should be given at a rate up to 150 mg/min with cardiac monitoring. If the patient still continues to have seizures, other options include intravenous valproate or phenobarbital. Intravenous levetiracetam and lacosamide have also been used in this situation. If the patient is resistant to phenytoin, phenobarbital, and lorazepam, anesthesia should be administered. Choices for this include midazolam, propofol, and pentobarbital. An outline for the treatment of status epilepticus is presented in Table 22-10.

Table 22-10. Protocol for Treatment of Generalized Tonic–Clonic Status Epilepticus

TIME	ACTION
0-5 minutes	Provide for maintenance of vital signs. Maintain airway. Give oxygen. Observe and examine patient.
6-10 minutes	Obtain 50 mL of blood for glucose, calcium, magnesium, electrolytes, blood urea nitrogen, liver functions, anticonvulsant levels, CBC, and toxicology screen. Begin normal saline IV and give 50 mL of 50% glucose and 100 mg of thiamine. Monitor ECG, blood pressure, and, if possible, EEG.
11-30 minutes	Use intravenous lorazepam to stop seizures, 0.1 mg/kg at 1-2 mg/min.
11-30 minutes	If seizures continue, load with phenytoin using fosphenytoin 20 mg phenytoin equivalents (PE)/kg at 150 mg PE/min. If cardiac arrhythmia or hypotension occurs, slow the infusion rate.
31-60 minutes	If seizures persist 10-20 minutes after administration of phenytoin, give an additional 10 PE/kg. If seizures continue, intubate patient. Consider phenobarbital at a rate of 50-100 mg/min until seizures stop or 20 mg/kg is given. Alternatively move to anesthetic agents.
After 60 minutes of status	Review laboratory results and correct abnormalities. Arrange for anesthesia, neuromuscular blockade, and EEG monitoring. Options include midazolam (0.15-0.2 mg/kg load, then 0.06-1.1 mg/kg/h) or propofol (1-2 mg/kg load, then 3-10 mg/kg/h), or barbiturate anesthesia (pentobarbital, 6-15 mg/kg loading dose, then 0.5-5 mg/kg/h). Pentobarbital often causes circulatory collapse, so be prepared to administer a pressor agent such as dopamine.

CBC, Complete blood count; ECG, electrocardiogram; EEG, electroencephalography.
Data from Lowenstein DH, Alldredge BK: Status epilepticus. *N Engl J Med* 338(14):970-976, 1998, and Treiman DM, Meyers PD, Walton NY, et al.: A comparison of four treatments for generalized convulsive status epilepticus. *N Engl J Med* 339(12):792-798, 1998.

51. What is epilepsia partialis continua? How is it treated?
   Epilepsia partialis continua is simple partial motor status epilepticus, which consists of rhythmic contractions of a restricted region of the body, usually the face and hand or fingers. The patient is usually fully conscious during these seizures. The most common causes include nonketotic hyperglycemic states, cerebral infarction, encephalitis (particularly Rasmussen's encephalitis), and cerebral neoplasms. Treatment is directed at correcting metabolic abnormalities when present. AEDs are used, but epilepsia partialis continua may be resistant to drug therapy short of anesthesia. In extreme cases, epilepsy surgery is considered.

52. Does continuous seizure activity cause nervous system damage?
   Certain seizure types, such as absence seizures, are not known to have any significant sequelae. In other settings, after a certain duration of epileptiform activity, there may be irreversible neuronal loss. A number of mechanisms probably mediate this neuronal death, including calcium loading of neurons and excitotoxicity produced by excessive glutamate release. Because continuous seizure activity can cause neuronal death, it is important to monitor the patient's EEG during the treatment of status epilepticus, particularly if the patient is paralyzed by neuromuscular blockade. It is also important to try to prevent any neuronal death by controlling the patient's status within the first 60 minutes after seizure onset.

EPILEPSY SURGERY

53. Which patients are good candidates for epilepsy surgery?
   Epilepsy surgery is effective in well-selected patients with pharmacoresistant focal epilepsy. Surgical resection can result in seizure freedom in approximately 80% of patients with seizures due to a structural lesion (e.g., cavernous angioma or low-grade neoplasm), 60% to 70% of patients with temporal lobe epilepsy, and 50% of patients with focal extratemporal epilepsy. Palliative epilepsy surgery may be performed when focal resection is not feasible and includes disconnections/neuroablation procedures (e.g., corpus callosotomy and hemispherotomy), and neuromodulation with implantable devices (e.g., vagus nerve stimulation and responsive neurostimulation).

54. At what point are epilepsy patients considered to be "refractory"?
   Pharmacoresistant (i.e., drug resistant, intractable, refractory) epilepsy is defined by the International League against Epilepsy as the failure of at least two tolerated, appropriately chosen AED trials in achieving seizure freedom. The definition has evolved over the years based on seminal trials showing that after two to three appropriate AED trials have failed to render a patient seizure free, the chances of that patient ever becoming seizure free on any AED is only about 5% to 10%. In general, approximately 47% of patients will become seizure free after the first AED and an additional 13% after the second AED. Further trials of AEDs result in seizure freedom in only 1% to 3%, which argues for the consideration of epilepsy surgery over further, likely futile, AED trials. Epilepsy surgery in appropriately chosen surgical candidates can still result in seizure freedom between 50% and 80% in pharmacoresistant epilepsy patients.

KEY POINTS: SEIZURES AND EPILEPSY, PART 1

1. Epilepsy is classified by etiology (structural/metabolic, genetic, or unknown), while seizures are classified by onset (focal or generalized).
2. Epilepsy with generalized-onset seizures is usually genetic in origin, but epilepsy with focal-onset seizures can be genetic or acquired.
3. The likely cause of epilepsy changes significantly with age at onset.
4. In patients with focal-onset seizures, an MRI scan should be considered.
5. Patients with epilepsy may have a normal EEG and MRI.

KEY POINTS: SEIZURES AND EPILEPSY, PART 2

1. Accurate seizure classification and if possible syndromic diagnosis guide therapeutic choices.
2. A significant change in antiepileptic drug levels should alert you to either noncompliance or a new drug interaction.
3. The most common cause of antiepileptic drug treatment failure is drug side effects.
4. Patients whose seizures are refractory to two appropriate and tolerated antiepileptic drug trials should be evaluated at an epilepsy center for definitive diagnosis and surgical evaluation.
5. Hippocampal sclerosis is a common cause of drug-resistant epilepsy, which is often remediated with anterior temporal lobe resection.

55. What is hippocampal sclerosis? How is it diagnosed?
   Hippocampal sclerosis is a disorder commonly associated with complex partial seizures of temporal origin. The term describes the pathology of the hippocampus that includes a loss of neurons and associated gliosis. MRI scans may demonstrate hippocampal sclerosis and volume loss of the hippocampal region. Unilateral hippocampal sclerosis associated with intractable complex partial seizures is important to identify because it is a potentially curable syndrome with surgery (Fig. 22-3).

56. What types of epilepsy surgeries are available?
   The most effective method to treat pharmacoresistant focal epilepsy is epilepsy surgery. Surgical treatment has been divided into (1) focal resections (e.g., anterior temporal lobe resection), (2) disconnections or neuroablation procedures (e.g., corpus callosotomy, hemispherotomy, and multiple subpial

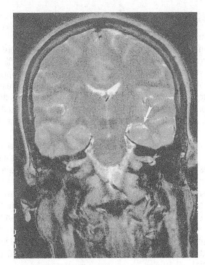

Figure 22-3. Magnetic resonance imaging (MRI) scan in a patient with partial complex seizures. The arrow shows sclerosis in the hippocampus of the left temporal lobe (mesial temporal sclerosis).

transections), and (3) neuromodulation (e.g., vagus nerve stimulation and responsive neurostimulation procedures). Focal resection results in the best seizure control among these procedures. However, it should be noted that only about half of the pharmacoresistant patients with epilepsy are candidates for epilepsy surgery. For the remaining patients, palliative procedures, such as disconnection or neuromodulation, may be considered, aiming at reduction in the seizure burden.

57. **What is vagus nerve stimulation (VNS)? How effective is it in reducing seizures?**
VNS is often advised when patients with pharmacoresistant seizures are not candidates for epilepsy surgery with resection/ablation or decline such surgery. An incision along the anterior left sterno-mastoid is used to implant wire electrodes to the left vagus nerve, which are stimulated with a pulse generator implanted in the left upper chest wall. The antiepileptic effect increases over months to years, and a greater than 50% seizure reduction is seen in 27% of patients. Seizure freedom may be attained in 5%. Adverse effects include hoarseness (from recurrent laryngeal stimulation), cough, dyspnea, and neck pain.

58. **What is responsive neurostimulation (RNS)? How effective is it in reducing seizures?**
RNS is a closed loop system where intracranially implanted electrodes (one to two depth or strip elec-trodes with a maximum of eight active contacts) are placed at the location of the presumed seizure onset. These electrodes continuously record cortical EEG and check for electrographic seizure activity using automated algorithms. When this activity is recognized, the system delivers current to decrease seizure frequency at preset thresholds (hence, it is called *responsive neurostimulation*). A seizure frequency reduction of >50% has been reported at 2 years with RNS use. In addition, improvement in the quality of life has also been reported with the use of RNS.

EPILEPSY AND DRIVING

59. **What recommendations about driving should a physician make to patients with epilepsy?**
It depends on the state where the patient is driving. While the American Academy of Neurology and American Epilepsy Society do not support mandatory reporting by physicians to driving authorities, some states do require it. In general, physicians should caution against driving if the seizures are not controlled and involve impairment of consciousness or motor function for the safety of both the patient and the public. It is usually appropriate to recommend that the patient volunteer to report this condition to the state's driver-licensing authorities.

Acknowledgments
The authors wish to thank Philip Kurle, MD, and Paul Rutecki, MD, for coauthoring the previous version of this chapter in Neurology Secrets.

 References available online at expertconsult.com.

WEBSITES

http://www.aesnet.org
http://www.efa.org
http://www.pslgroup.com/epilepsy.htm
http://epilepsy.org
http://ilae-epilepsy.org

BIBLIOGRAPHY

1. Engel J, Pedley TA, Aicardi J, Dichter M: Epilepsy: A Comprehensive Textbook, 2nd ed. Hagerstown, MD, Lippincott Williams & Wilkins, 2007.
2. Wilner AN: Epilepsy in Clinical Practice, New York, Demos, 2004.
3. Wyllie E (ed): The Treatment of Epilepsy, 4th ed. Baltimore, Lippincott Williams & Wilkins, 2005.

CHAPTER 23

SLEEP DISORDERS

Amee A. Patel, Daniel G. Glaze

GENERAL PRINCIPLES

1. **What is sleep?**
   Sleep is a dynamic physiologic process that affects physical, emotional, cognitive, and social development; however, the exact mechanisms that occur during sleep are not fully understood. The sleep cycle consists of an alternating pattern of nonrapid eye movement (NREM) sleep and rapid eye movement (REM) sleep at 50- to 60-minute intervals during the first year of age, which gradually increases to 75- to 90-minute intervals around 5 to 6 years of age, and remains relatively stable thereafter.

2. **What are the main features of NREM sleep?**
   The current American Academy of Sleep Medicine (AASM) scoring manual for polysomnography revised the Rechtschaffen and Kales (1968) sleep scoring manual, which subdivided NREM sleep into stages 1, 2, 3, and 4. The current AASM scoring manual designates the sleep stages as the following: N1, N2, N3, and REM. N1 (<5% of total sleep time) is the lightest stage of sleep. It is distinguished from wakefulness by the absence of alpha rhythm, which is seen in the occipital electroencephalogram (EEG) lead. N2 (40% to 60% of total sleep time) typically follows N1 and is characterized by K-complexes and spindles on EEG. N3 (10% to 20% of total sleep time in adults, 20% to 40% in children) represents the deeper stages of sleep and is also known as *slow-wave sleep* or *delta sleep* for its electroencephalographic characteristics. The amount of N3 sleep begins decreasing in puberty and continues decreasing into adulthood.

3. **What are the main features of REM sleep?**
   REM sleep is characterized by pronounced muscular atonia, phasic twitches, and bursts of rapid eye movements. During this state, the EEG is relatively low in amplitude and often is similar to that seen during drowsiness, although people in REM sleep appear deeply asleep by behavioral criteria. Most dreaming occurs during REM sleep. Newborns and infants have a higher proportion of REM sleep compared to NREM sleep. The proportion of REM sleep to NREM sleep gradually decreases as the pattern of sleep shifts with increasing age and remains stable (18% to 25% of total sleep time) through later childhood and adult life.

4. **Do the stages of sleep occur randomly during the night?**
   No. Normal individuals exhibit a fairly regular alternation of NREM sleep and REM sleep during the sleep period, with cycle times of approximately 60 to 90 minutes. There are usually a few awakenings (typically fewer than 10 per night), and the various stages of sleep are present in consistent amounts.

5. **Which areas of the brain control sleep?**
   Essentially every area of the brain is involved in sleep. Wakefulness is maintained by neurons in the brain stem reticular formation via the thalamocortical neurons, dorsal hypothalamus, basal forebrain, and locus ceruleus. NREM sleep is maintained by the neural systems of the forebrain (ventrolateral preoptic nucleus also known as *VLPO* and *basal forebrain*), solitary tract nuclei, midbrain raphe, amygdala, and thalamus. REM sleep is regulated in the pons (lateral tegmental nuclei, pedunculopontine nucleus), pontine reticular formation, and medullary and spinal neurons. The suprachiasmatic area of the hypothalamus is directly involved in the regulation of circadian cycles that determine when sleep occurs within a 24-hour day. A group of nuclei in the pontomesencephalic region (including locus ceruleus, dorsal raphe, and several cholinergic areas) are critical for the alternating sequence of REM sleep and non-REM sleep cycles.

6. **What processes control sleep?**
   There are two main intrinsic processes that influence the sleep cycle: homeostasis and circadian rhythm. Homeostasis, also known as *process S*, regulates the length and depth of sleep. The drive may be regulated by the accumulation of adenosine during prolonged periods of wakefulness.

After a prolonged period of wakefulness, there is an increased tendency to sleep. Circadian rhythm, also known as *process C*, is the internal process that directs the quality of sleep and duration of the sleep–wake cycle. The master circadian clock is located in the suprachiasmatic nucleus in the ventral hypothalamus. There are also different neurons and neural networks that maintain wake, NREM, and REM sleep.

7. **What are the major neurotransmitters involved during wakefulness, NREM sleep, and REM sleep?**
   The main neurotransmitters involved in promoting wakefulness include acetylcholine, dopamine, glutamate, histamine, hypocretin/orexin, norepinephrine, and serotonin. The main neurotransmitters involved in promoting sleep include acetylcholine, adenosine, gamma-aminobutyric acid (GABA), and glycine. Table 23-1 is a summary of the location and action of the major neurotransmitters that are known to participate in the sleep–wake cycle.

Table 23-1. Summary of Neurotransmitters Involved in the Sleep–Wake Cycle

NEUROTRANSMITTER	LOCATION	ACTIVITY LEVEL DURING SLEEP–WAKE CYCLE
Acetylcholine	Dorsal midbrain, pons, pendunculo-pontine, lateral–dorsal tegmental areas	High during wakefulness and REM sleep; low during NREM
Norepinephrine	Locus ceruleus	Active during wakefulness, less active during NREM, inactive during REM
Histamine	Tuberomammillary nucleus in posterior hypothalamus	High during wakefulness, lower in NREM, lowest in REM
Serotonin	Median and dorsal raphe	Active during wakefulness, less active during NREM, inactive during REM
Dopamine	Substantia nigra and ventral tegmental area	High during wakefulness, low in NREM/REM
Orexin/hypocretin	Lateral and posterior hypothalamus	Active during wakefulness, less active in NREM; controversial whether active during REM
GABA	Ventrolateral preoptic area, thalamus, hypothalamus, basal forebrain, cerebral cortex	Active during NREM, slightly less active in REM, inactive during wakefulness
Adenosine	Basal forebrain	High during wakefulness, low during NREM/REM sleep
Glycine	Forebrain and spinal cord	Promotes sleep; contributes to REM-sleep-related muscle atonia/hypotonia

REM, Rapid eye movement; *NREM,* nonrapid eye movement; *GABA,* gamma-hydroxybutyrate.

8. **How are sleep disorders classified?**
   1. Insomnia—includes chronic insomnia, short-term insomnia, and other insomnia disorders
   2. Sleep-related breathing disorders—include obstructive sleep apneas, central sleep apnea syndromes, and sleep-related hypoventilation/hypoxemic syndromes
   3. Central disorders of hypersomnolence—excessive daytime sleepiness not due to a circadian rhythm sleep disorder, sleep-related breathing disorder, or other cause of disturbed nocturnal sleep
   4. Circadian rhythm sleep–wake disorders—characterized by a persistent or recurrent pattern of sleep disturbance due to alterations of the circadian timing system or a misalignment between the

timing of the individual's endogenous circadian rhythm of sleep propensity and exogenous factors that affect the duration or timing of sleep

5. Parasomnias—include confusional arousals, sleepwalking, sleep terrors, REM sleep behavior disorder, nightmares, sleep enuresis, and sleep talking

6. Sleep-related movement disorders—include restless legs syndrome, periodic limb movement disorder, sleep-related leg cramps, sleep-related bruxism (teeth grinding), and rhythmic movement disorder

9. **How much sleep is required for optimal daytime function?**
Most adult individuals require about 6 to 8 hours of sleep per night, but there is a great deal of individual variability. As a general rule, if daytime performance is significantly impaired by excessive sleepiness, and this condition persists despite adherence to a regularly scheduled nocturnal sleep period of at least 8 hours, more definitive diagnostic tests are indicated. A significant change in sleep requirements may indicate an underlying sleep disorder.

10. **Do sleep needs in children differ from those in adults?**
Sleep needs in children differ from those in adults. During the newborn period, the amount of sleep newborns require is about 16 to 18 hours over a 24-hour period. By 6 months of age, sleep duration decreases to about 14 hours. Sleep during the day then begins to consolidate into one to two naps by 1 year of age. Most children stop taking naps by age 4 or 5 years in preparation for a full day of school. By childhood, sleep requirements gradually decrease to 10 to 11 hours. This decreases to 8 to 9 hours during adolescence into adulthood.

11. **What are the common medicolegal issues that arise in caring for patients with sleep disorders?**
Patients with sleep disorders, such as obstructive sleep apnea or narcolepsy, are at an increased risk for motor vehicle accidents. They should be counseled about avoidance of driving and participating in potentially dangerous activities, such as operating heavy machinery, during periods of drowsiness. Of particular importance, laws vary from state to state for commercial drivers.

KEY POINTS: GENERAL SLEEP PRINCIPLES

1. There are three major states that are unique for daily function: wakefulness, NREM sleep, and REM sleep. For example, REM sleep is important for learning.

2. Sleep problems are common in adults and children and should be screened routinely since treatment options are available to improve sleep quality.

3. Sleep architecture, sleep quality, and total sleep time are objective markers to evaluate overall growth and development.

DIAGNOSTIC EVALUATION

12. **What are some diagnostic tools that can objectively identify a sleep disorder?**
In addition to the history and physical examination, sleep testing is helpful for the evaluation of sleep disorders. This may include an overnight polysomnography (PSG), ambulatory home study (used in adults), actigraphy, mean sleep latency test (MSLT), sleep logs, and sleep questionnaires. The International Classification of Sleep Disorders-Third edition (ICSD-3) is a diagnostic and coding manual that provides a thorough review of sleep disorders that is available to all practitioners. The manual includes essential features, diagnostic criteria, predisposing factors, pathophysiology, clinical findings, and differential diagnoses.

13. **What is an overnight PSG?**
An overnight PSG is the most common diagnostic tool for most sleep medicine experts. During a PSG, multiple physiologic parameters are recorded simultaneously. The study includes EEG monitoring, electro-oculography to monitor eye movements, pulse oximetry, oronasal airflow, belts to determine abdominal and chest wall movements, chin electromyography (EMG) to determine chin movements, leg EMG to determine leg movements, transcutaneous carbon dioxide or end-tidal carbon dioxide monitoring ($ETCO_2$), electrocardiography, snore microphone, and video recording. PSG is the gold standard to diagnose many sleep disorders, such as sleep disordered breathing, periodic limb movement disorder, etc.

14. **What are the indications for PSG?**
PSG is routinely indicated for the diagnosis of sleep-related breathing disorders, such as obstructive sleep apnea syndrome, for titration of positive airway pressure (PAP) as therapy for sleep-disordered breathing, to evaluate for possible narcolepsy or idiopathic hypersomnia (combined with an MSLT), or to evaluate sleep-related behaviors such as periodic limb movement disorder or REM sleep behavior disorder. Follow-up PSG is indicated for the assessment of treatment results after surgical or dental treatment of patients with sleep-related breathing disorders or if there is a substantial amount of weight loss or gain (>10% of body weight). PSG is also indicated when evaluating for parasomnias that are either unusual or atypical, but it is not indicated for circadian rhythm disorders. Guidelines, specifically for adults and children, have been developed.

15. **What is an MSLT?**
An MSLT consists of a series of five 20-minute nap opportunities that measure the physiologic tendency to fall asleep in quiet situations, since it varies during the day. Mean sleep latencies should be considered a continuum of values in which below 5 minutes indicates sleepiness and those over 10 minutes indicates normal alertness. An MSLT may help identify the etiology of excessive daytime sleepiness. A PSG prior to MSLT testing is useful to exclude other major sleep disorders that could contribute to hypersomnia and to confirm that a sufficient amount of sleep is obtained (at least 6 hours) prior to the MSLT.

16. **Can medications alter the results of a PSG and MSLT?**
Many medications (e.g., hypnotics, sedatives, and stimulants) can significantly alter the results of these procedures. In particular, both periods of medication initiation and acute withdrawal are often associated with major alterations of sleep characteristics, and the resultant patterns may mimic other sleep disorders, including narcolepsy or sleep-disordered breathing. When it is not possible to discontinue medications that affect sleep, such medications should be continued at constant and stable levels for at least 2 weeks prior to testing. Patients should never be told simply to refrain from taking a medication on the night of a study or several nights before the examination as this approach may affect the outcome of study results.

SLEEP-RELATED BREATHING DISORDERS

17. **What sleep disorder is associated with excessive daytime sleepiness and snoring?**
Obstructive sleep apnea (OSA) syndrome. This condition affects 3% to 7% of the adult population and 1% to 4% of the pediatric population. Obstructive sleep apnea is characterized by repetitive episodes of apneas and partial upper airway obstruction (hypopnea) occurring during sleep, resulting in intermittent oxygen desaturation or fragmented sleep. Excessive daytime sleepiness is a common presenting symptom along with loud snoring. PSG may be helpful in diagnosing OSA as well as determining the severity of OSA.

18. **How is OSA defined on PSG in adults and in children?**
In adults, the polysomnographic recording will show at least five or more scorable respiratory events per hour of sleep, with evidence of increased respiratory effort during all or a portion of each respiratory event. In children, the polysomnographic recording will show at least one or more scorable respiratory events per hour of sleep. Table 23-2 compares the diagnostic criteria for OSA in adults and children per the ICSD-3.

19. **How is OSA treated?**
Therapy is directed toward correction of the upper airway obstruction (which can result from anatomic factors or abnormal relaxation of the musculature of the oropharynx). Administration of PAP by means of a nasal mask is currently the most frequently used therapeutic modality. Surgical procedures are often the first line of treatment in children with adenotonsillar hypertrophy. In rare cases, surgery may be helpful when a discrete structural abnormality producing airway obstruction can be identified. In mild cases, significant improvement is achieved by preventing sleep in the supine position or by elevation of the head and trunk (positional therapy). Tongue-retaining devices and other oral appliances may be beneficial in a small number of instances, particularly when the respiratory disturbance is mild. Weight loss is often beneficial in patients who are morbidly obese.

Table 23-2. Diagnostic Criteria of Obstructive Sleep Apnea in Adult and Pediatric Populations

ADULT (CRITERIA [A AND B] OR C MUST BE MET)	PEDIATRIC (CRITERIA A AND B MUST BE MET)
A. The presence of one or more of the following: 　1. The patient has excessive daytime sleepiness, fatigue, or insomnia symptoms 　2. The patient reports breath holding, gasping, or choking during sleep 　3. The bed partner reports habitual snoring, interruptions in breathing, or both during sleep 　4. The patient has hypertension, a mood disorder, cognitive dysfunction, coronary artery disease, stroke, congestive heart failure, atrial fibrillation, or type 2 diabetes B. Polysomnography demonstrates five or more obstructive respiratory events per hour of sleep 　OR C. Polysomnography demonstrates 15 or more obstructive respiratory events per hour of sleep	A. The presence of one or more of the following: 　1. Snoring 　2. Labored, paradoxical, or obstructed breathing during sleep 　3. Sleepiness, hyperactivity, behavioral problems, or learning problems B. PSG demonstrates one or both of the following: 　1. One or more obstructive respiratory events per hour of sleep 　OR 　2. A pattern of obstructive hypoventilation, defined as at least 25% or total sleep time with hypercapnia ($PaCO_2 > 50\,mm\,Hg$) in association with one or more of the following: 　　1. Snoring 　　2. Flattening of the inspiratory nasal pressure waveform 　　3. Paradoxical thoracoabdominal motion

20. **How does OSA syndrome differ between adults and children?**
    Most adults with OSA experience daytime sleepiness and snoring, whereas children tend to have behavioral issues such as inattentiveness, distractibility, irritability, hyperactivity, or impaired academic performance in addition to snoring. The most common anatomic finding in children is enlarged tonsils and adenoids. Children more frequently have obstructive hypopneas (partial upper airway obstruction), whereas adults are more likely to have obstructive apneas. The nocturnal sleep pattern is typically highly fragmented in adults whereas children may have fewer respiratory-related arousals than adults. Younger children may also demonstrate a pattern of obstructive hypoventilation. Obesity is common among adults and adolescents with OSA, while a significant number of young children have normal weight or even failure to thrive. Of note, cognitive and cardiovascular dysfunction can occur in both adults and children.

21. **What conditions predispose a child to OSA?**
    Tonsillar and adenoidal hypertrophy are strong risk factors for OSA in children. A number of neurogenetic disorders also predispose children to OSA including Down syndrome, Prader–Willi syndrome, cerebral palsy, mucopolysaccharidoses such as Hunter syndrome, muscular dystrophy and other neuromuscular disorders, Arnold–Chiari malformation and other structural abnormalities involving the brain stem, Pierre–Robin syndrome and other craniofacial malformations, and achondroplasia. In addition, obesity is also a risk factor. The recent obesity epidemic in children has been associated with an increased occurrence in OSA. Family history of OSA, race, and ethnicity are also risk factors for OSA in children. African-American children are at an increased risk for OSA.

22. **What is primary central sleep apnea (CSA)?**
    Primary CSA is characterized by recurrent central apneas of unknown etiology not caused by a medical or neurologic condition or medications. It is defined as a cessation of airflow during sleep associated with an absence of respiratory effort. Airflow and respiratory effort cease simultaneously in a repetitive pattern throughout the course of the night. As a result, there is fragmented sleep, yielding to excessive daytime sleepiness, frequent nocturnal awakenings, or both. $ETCO_2$ monitoring will show a low normal $PaCO_2$ during wakefulness (less than $40\,mm\,Hg$).

23. **What is congenital central alveolar hypoventilation syndrome (CCHS)?**
    CCHS is characterized by abnormal autonomic control of breathing during sleep. Age of onset is typically during the infancy period; however, there are cases of late-onset central hypoventilation with hypothalamic dysfunction. The majority of cases of CCHS have been linked to the mutation of the homeobox gene *PHOX2B*. During wakefulness, the control of breathing is normal. However, during NREM and REM sleep, respirations are shallow and irregular. CCHS is a diagnosis of exclusion. Neurologic, cardiac, and metabolic disorders must be ruled out. In addition, other forms of central hypoventilation secondary to Arnold–Chiari malformation, trauma, central nervous system tumors, and obesity hypoventilation syndrome should be distinguished from CCHS.

HYPERSOMNIAS

24. **What are the common patient-reported symptoms of excessive daytime sleepiness?**
    Patients with excessive daytime sleepiness will often report difficulty concentrating, focusing on daily tasks, irritable mood, and falling asleep at inappropriate times. Patients with certain conditions (such as sleep apnea or periodic limb movements) may awaken several times throughout the night, thus contributing to fragmented sleep.

25. **What are the clinical symptoms suggestive of narcolepsy?**
    Narcolepsy is a chronic disorder of hypersomnia in which there are sudden onsets of sleep episodes or "sleep attacks" that can be associated with cataplexy, sleep paralysis, hypnagogic/hypnopompic hallucinations, and disrupted nighttime sleep. The diagnosis of narcolepsy (type 1 and type 2) should be confirmed whenever possible by a PSG followed by an MSLT. In addition, the hypersomnia is not better explained by another sleep disorder, medical or neurologic disorder, psychiatric disorder, medication use, or substance abuse.

26. **What are the types of narcolepsies?**
    There are two types of narcolepsies. Narcolepsy type 1 is characterized by daily periods of an irrepressible need to sleep or daytime lapses into sleep occurring for at least 3 months. In addition, one or both of the following criteria must be met:
    1. cataplexy with a mean sleep latency of less than or equal to 8 minutes and two or more sleep onset REM periods (SOREMPs) on MLST
    2. cerebrospinal fluid (CSF) hypocretin 1 concentration is less than or equal to 110 pg/mL.
    Narcolepsy type 1 is caused by a deficiency of hypothalamic hypocretin (orexin) signaling. Narcolepsy type 2 is similar to type 1 except there is no cataplexy; CSF hypocretin is not measured or is greater than 110 pg/mL. For both types, the hypersomnolence and/or MSLT findings are not better explained by other causes such as insufficient sleep, sleep-disordered breathing, or effects of medications or substances.

27. **What is cataplexy?**
    Cataplexy is a condition characterized by sudden episodes of either muscular weakness or paralysis without loss of consciousness, precipitated by emotional changes such as laughter, excitement, or anger. Episodes typically last from a few seconds to several minutes and sometimes are terminated by a direct transition into sleep.

28. **What are the features of sleep paralysis?**
    Sleep paralysis is characterized by a recurrent inability to move the trunk and extremities either at sleep onset or upon awakening from sleep. Eye movements and respiratory effort are not impaired. Each episode lasts seconds to a few minutes and typically resolves spontaneously. The episodes cause clinically significant distress including either bedtime anxiety or fear of sleep. Sleep paralysis is seen in patients with narcolepsy but is not necessary for the diagnosis of either type of narcolepsy. Sleep paralysis can occur in normal individuals. Sleep deprivation and irregular sleep-wake schedules have been identified as predisposing factors to episodes of sleep paralysis. The disturbance is not better explained by another sleep disorder (especially narcolepsy), psychiatric disorder, medical condition, sleep deprivation, or medication or substance use.

29. **Do hypnagogic hallucinations occur during REM sleep?**
    No. Hypnagogic hallucinations occur during sleep–wake transitions (either when falling asleep or during arousals) and can involve various sensory modalities (most commonly visual). Although this entity is typically observed in association with narcolepsy, it occasionally occurs in normal individuals.

30. What are the diagnostic criteria for narcolepsy type 1?

    The current ICSD-3 (2014) diagnostic criteria for narcolepsy with cataplexy (type 1) include the following: (1) a complaint of excessive daytime sleepiness occurring almost daily for at least 3 months and (2) the presence of cataplexy with a mean sleep latency of ≤8 minutes and two or more SOREMPs on an MSLT. Alternatively, CSF hypocretin-1 concentration is ≤110 pg/mL or one-third of the mean normal control values.

31. What are the diagnostic criteria for narcolepsy type 2?

    The current ICSD-3 (2014) diagnostic criteria for narcolepsy without cataplexy (type 2) include all of the following: (1) excessive daytime sleepiness occurring almost daily for at least 3 months; (2) typical cataplexy is not present (but may include atypical or doubtful cataplexy); (3) mean sleep latency of ≤8 minutes and two or more SOREMPs on MSLT; and (4) CSF hypocretin-1 concentration is ≤110 pg/mL or one-third of the mean normal control values.

32. What is the etiology of narcolepsy?

    It is now firmly established that narcolepsy type 1 is caused by deficiencies in hypocretin (orexin) signaling, most likely due to a selective loss of hypothalamic hypocretin-producing neurons. The majority of patients (90% to 95%) with narcolepsy type 1 have undetectable or low levels in the CSF. There is a strong human leukocyte antigen (HLA) association in narcolepsy—HLA DQB1*0602—that has led to the hypothesis that there is an autoimmune mechanism that could potentially explain the selective destruction of the hypocretin-containing neurons in the hypothalamus. However, this is not diagnostic of narcolepsy.

33. How is narcolepsy treated?

    Treatment objectives for narcolepsy should include control of sleepiness and other sleep-related symptoms such as cataplexy. Nonpharmacological options include maintaining an appropriate sleep–wake schedule that promotes developmentally appropriate amounts of nighttime sleep and scheduled daytime naps. Scheduled 15- to 20-minute naps in conjunction with medical therapy can be beneficial in controlling the degree of daytime sleepiness. Modafinil is an effective pharmacologic treatment of daytime sleepiness in adults. Alternately, stimulant medications (e.g., methylphenidate, dextroamphetamine) are effective and are the standard therapy for children with narcolepsy. Sodium oxybate (a derivative of gamma-hydroxybutyrate) is effective for the treatment of daytime sleepiness, cataplexy, and disrupted sleep due to narcolepsy. It is administered at night at sleep onset and again midway through the sleep period. Alternately, cataplexy and sleep paralysis are often treated successfully with either tricyclic antidepressants (e.g., imipramine, protriptyline) or selective serotonin reuptake inhibitors (e.g., venlafaxine).

34. Are any other conditions, besides narcolepsy and sleep apnea, typically associated with excessive daytime somnolence?

    Yes. Table 23-3 lists a number of specific conditions that can be associated with excessive sleepiness and episodes of sleep at inappropriate times.

KEY POINTS: EXCESSIVE DAYTIME SLEEPINESS, OBSTRUCTIVE SLEEP APNEA AND NARCOLEPSY

1. Excessive daytime sleepiness is defined as the inability to stay awake and alert during the major waking episodes of the day, resulting in periods of irrepressible need for sleep or unintended lapses into drowsiness or sleep.
2. OSA is the result of decreased cross-sectional area of the upper airway lumen due to either excessive bulk of soft tissues (tongue, soft palate, lateral pharyngeal walls) or craniofacial abnormalities.
3. OSA is a risk factor for systemic hypertension and motor vehicle accidents. OSA in adults may also be associated with cardiac arrhythmias, stroke, pulmonary hypertension, and depression.
4. The occurrence of two or more SOREMPs during an MSLT is a more specific finding in narcolepsy than is a mean sleep latency of ≤8 minutes.
5. The maintenance of wakefulness test is a measure of the ability to remain awake during the daytime in a darkened, quiet environment and is usually administered to assess response to treatment. It should not be used for diagnostic purposes.

Table 23-3. Disorders Often Associated with Excessive Daytime Sleepiness

Sleep Disorders
- Insufficient sleep
- Obstructive sleep apnea
- Central sleep apnea
- Sleep-related hypoventilation/hypoxemia
- Circadian rhythm disorders
- Rhythmic movement disorders (restless legs syndrome, periodic limb movement disorder)

Central Disorders of Hypersomnolence
- Narcolepsy (type 1 or 2)
- Kleine–Levin syndrome
- Idiopathic hypersomnia
- Hypersomnia secondary to a medical condition
- Menstrual-related hypersomnia

Neurologic Disorders
- Neurodegenerative disease
- Myotonic dystrophy/neuromuscular disease
- Multiple sclerosis
- Amyotrophic lateral sclerosis
- Anatomic lesions affecting the thalamus, hypothalamus, or brain stem
- Posttraumatic
- Cerebral trypanosomiasis

Medical/Genetic Disorders
- Down syndrome
- Cerebral palsy
- Obesity
- Hypothyroidism
- End-stage renal disease
- Hepatic encephalopathy
- Niemann–Pick type C disease
- Prader–Willi syndrome
- Moebius syndrome
- Fragile X syndrome
- Postviral encephalitis (H1N1)

Psychiatric Disorders
- Depression
- Anxiety
- Substance abuse
- Psychogenic sleepiness

Medications
- Benzodiazepines
- Sedatives other than benzodiazepines
- Antipsychotics
- Opioid analgesics
- Antihistamines
- Anticonvulsants
- Sedative antidepressants

INSOMNIA

35. What is insomnia?

Insomnia is defined as a persistent difficulty with sleep initiation, duration, consolidation, or quality that occurs despite adequate opportunity and circumstances for sleep and results in some form of daytime impairment. The patient may report at least one of the following forms of daytime impairment related to difficulty in sleeping: fatigue, attention, impairment of concentration or memory, poor job or school performance, daytime sleepiness, irritable mood or disturbance, concerns or worries about sleep, increased tendency for errors or accidents at work or while driving, or nonspecific symptoms such as headaches, gastrointestinal symptoms in response to sleep loss. In past editions of the ICSD, insomnia has been classified under different subtypes (psychophysiologic insomnia, behavioral insomnia of childhood, paradoxical insomnia, inadequate sleep hygiene, insomnia due to a medical condition, etc.). However, the current ICSD-3 has classified these subtypes of insomnia into one of three categories: short-term insomnia, chronic insomnia, or other insomnia disorder.

36. How does insomnia in the pediatric population differ from that in adults?
In general, the causes of insomnia in children are numerous. It can be related to a medical condition, pain, medication side effects, lack of a routine schedule, attention seeking, or a combination of the aforementioned. In contrast to adult insomnia, the caregiver usually reports sleep issues, especially if they delay sleep onset or require prolonged intervention through the night, thereby contributing to insufficient sleep for the caregiver.

37. How is insomnia treated?
Treatment goals for insomnia involve improving sleep quality and quantity as well as improving insomnia-related daytime function. Psychological and behavioral interventions are effective and recommended in the treatment of chronic insomnia. Initial approaches to treatment should include at least one behavioral intervention such as stimulus control therapy or relaxation therapy or the combination of cognitive therapy, stimulus control therapy, and sleep restriction therapy with or without relaxation therapy (also known as *cognitive behavioral therapy for insomnia*). Short-term hypnotic treatment can be supplemented with behavioral and cognitive therapies when possible and should be directed by the following: symptom pattern, treatment goals, past treatment responses, patient preference, cost, availability of other treatments, comorbid conditions, contraindications, concurrent medication interactions, and side effects.

CIRCADIAN RHYTHM DISORDERS

38. What is jet lag syndrome?
Jet lag syndrome is characterized by a temporary mismatch between the timing of the sleep–wake cycle generated by the endogenous circadian rhythm and that of the sleep–wake pattern required by a change in time zone. Individuals typically report associated daytime impairment, general malaise, or somatic symptoms (gastrointestinal symptoms) within 1 or 2 days after travel. The severity and duration of symptoms are dependent on the number of time zones traveled, the ability to sleep while traveling, exposure to appropriate circadian time cues in the new location, and direction of the travel. Eastward travel (requiring advancing circadian rhythm and sleep–wake hours) is usually more difficult to adjust to than westward travel.

39. What is delayed sleep–wake phase disorder?
Delayed sleep–wake phase disorder is characterized by habitual sleep–wake timing that is delayed, usually by more than 2 hours, relative to the conventional or socially acceptable timing. Affected individuals will have difficulty falling asleep and waking up at a socially acceptable time, as required to obtain sufficient sleep duration on a school or work night. The condition is more common among adolescents and young adults. The symptoms last about 3 months. When allowed to follow the individual's preferred schedule, the individual's timing of sleep is delayed.

40. What is shift work disorder?
Shift work disorder is characterized by either insomnia or excessive daytime sleepiness that occurs in association with work hours that occur during the usual sleep time of that individual. The symptoms are usually present for at least 3 months or more. The disorder is closely linked to work schedules and typically resolves when the major sleep episode is scheduled at a conventional time.

PARASOMNIAS

41. What are parasomnias?
Parasomnias are undesirable behaviors or experiences that occur during the onset of sleep, during sleep itself, or during an arousal from sleep. They may occur during NREM sleep, REM sleep, or transitions to and from sleep. Table 23-4 lists the different types of parasomnias and the stage of sleep in which they occur.

Table 23-4. Examples of Parasomnias
Associated with NREM Sleep
• Confusional arousals
• Sleep walking
• Sleep/Night terrors
Associated with REM Sleep
• REM sleep behavior disorder
• Recurrent isolated sleep paralysis
• Nightmare disorder
Other
• Sleep-related enuresis
• Sleep-related groaning (catathrenia)
• Exploding head syndrome
• Sleep-related eating disorder
• Sleep-related dissociative disorders

NREM, Nonrapid eye movement; *REM*, rapid eye movement.

42. **Describe the major characteristics of sleep terrors.**
Sleep terrors, also known as *pavor nocturnus*, are episodes of apparent intense fear, often associated with crying or screaming, that occur during an arousal from NREM (typically N3) sleep. Elevated heart and respiratory rates characteristically accompany these events, and the patient may exhibit confusion and disorientation. They are common in children between 4 and 12 years of age but may persist into the adult years. Episodes typically end spontaneously after several minutes, but attempts to abruptly awaken the individual may prolong the duration of sleep terrors. Episodes are often more frequent in the setting of insufficient sleep. Treatment usually involves reassurance, but pharmacotherapy is sometimes indicated when episodes become frequent or if the risk of injury is high. Benzodiazepines are often effective for short-term use.

43. **What are the differences between night terrors and nightmares?**
Nightmares occur during REM sleep and are characterized by a frightening dream. The event typically results in a prolonged wake period. In comparison to night terrors, nightmares occur during the last third of the night and are intense during REM sleep. Most children are awake and are able to recall the events of the dream. In addition, nightmares have more of an emotional component as opposed to autonomic nervous system activation, which occurs in night terrors. Night terrors usually occur during the first third of the night or first half of the night, which consists of slow-wave sleep. Treatment involves education and reassurance.

44. **What is sleepwalking?**
Sleepwalking, or somnambulism, consists of a series of complex behaviors that are initiated during arousals from slow-wave sleep (N3) and finishes with the child walking with an altered state of consciousness. The episodes occur during the first third of the night, which consists of slow-wave sleep. The episodes often involve inappropriate behaviors such as urinating in the closet, moving furniture, climbing out of the window, etc. Most children cannot recall the episode in the morning. The predisposition to sleepwalking increases as the number of affected parents increases. Sleepwalking spontaneously resolves as the child transitions into adolescence. However, sleepwalking can occur during adulthood.

45. **What are confusional arousals?**
Confusional arousals consist of a state of confusion during or following an arousal from sleep. They occur during slow-wave sleep (N3) and occur during the first third of the night. The child may appear to be awake during some or most of a confusional arousal, despite the diminished response to external stimuli. Most episodes last about 5 to 15 minutes and occur in children age 3 to 13 years. Confusional arousals resolve as children age. Young children who have confusional arousals often go on to sleepwalk as an adolescent.

46. **What is REM sleep behavior disorder (RBD)?**
RBD is characterized by repeated episodes of sleep-related vocalization and/or complex motor behaviors, such as chewing, punching, singing, whistling, running, kicking, dancing, arm flaring, etc. These behaviors are either documented by PSG to occur during REM sleep or are presumed to occur during REM sleep based

on clinical history of dream enactment. PSG recording demonstrates REM sleep without atonia. The disturbance is not better explained by another sleep disorder, psychiatric disorder, medication, or substance use.

47. **What sleep disorders are associated with RBD?**
RBD can be strongly linked with narcolepsy type 1. The behavior associated with RBD may be precipitated or worsened by the pharmacologic therapy of the cataplexy. Per the ICSD-3, RBD associated with narcolepsy is now considered to be a distinct phenotype of RBD. The presence of RBD in the pediatric population may be an initial manifestation of narcolepsy type 1. RBD can be also associated with periodic limb movement disorder, and neurologic disorders such as ischemic or hemorrhagic cerebrovascular disease, multiple sclerosis, Lewy body dementia, Parkinson's disease, multisystem atrophy, Guillain–Barré syndrome, mitochondrial disorders, Tourette syndrome, autism, and normal pressure hydrocephalus. Medication use as well as medication withdrawal has been reported to be associated with RBD.

48. **How is RBD treated?**
Patients with RBD are at risk for sleep-related injury. Therefore, efforts in modifying the sleep environment to ensure patient safety are strongly recommended. This includes placing a mattress on the floor, padding corners of furniture, window protection, and removing potentially dangerous objects, such as guns or sharp objects, from the bedroom. When self-injury is present secondary to RBD, clonazepam is suggested for the treatment of RBD in adults but should be used with caution in patients with dementia, gait disorders, or concomitant OSA. Melatonin is suggested for the treatment of RBD because it has few side effects. Pramipexole, L-DOPA, zopiclone, benzodiazepines other than clonazepam, Yi-Gan San, desipramine, clozapine, carbamazepine, and sodium oxybate may also be considered to treat RBD; however, the clinical evidence available is limited.

49. **How are parasomnias generally treated?**
Generally, treatment involves ensuring the safety of the patient during the parasomnia as well as avoiding insufficient sleep. Sleep deprivation can cause the events to become more frequent. Caregivers should receive counseling to allow the parasomnia to occur without intervention. Abrupt interruptions of the parasomnia may prolong the episode. In addition, comorbid conditions such as sleep-disordered breathing, periodic limb movement disorder, and restless leg symptoms may contribute to developing chronic parasomnias.

50. **Which sleep disorders may be confused with epileptic seizures?**
    1. RBD
    2. Sleepwalking and other parasomnias
    3. Rhythmic movement disorder (head banging, body rocking)
    A detailed clinical history may be helpful in identifying the type of sleep behavior as this will help direct therapy. For example, night terrors tend to occur during the first third or half of the night during N3 sleep, while seizures may occur throughout the night and occur during the daytime. An overnight PSG with expanded EEG montage to record and precisely characterize the behavior may be indicated to make a correct diagnosis.

SLEEP-RELATED MOVEMENT DISORDERS

51. **What are the key features of periodic limb movement disorder (PLMD)?**
Periodic limb movements, formerly called *nocturnal myoclonus*, are characterized on PSG by frequent clusters of extremity movements (typically the legs, but occasionally the arms) that tend to recur periodically during sleep at intervals of 5 to 90 seconds. The frequency is >15/hr in adults and >5/hr in children. When these events produce arousals, as they often do, the sleep pattern may be severely disrupted, and the patient may experience significant daytime sleepiness. When there is clinical sleep disturbance or daytime impairment in conjunction with the PSG findings of periodic limb movements, then a diagnosis of PLMD can be made. PLMD is thought to be rare as periodic limb movements are typically associated with restless legs syndrome (RLS), RBD, or narcolepsy and represent a distinct diagnosis from PLMD.

52. **What are the diagnostic criteria for RLS?**
RLS is a clinical diagnosis that is characterized by an urge to move the legs that is usually accompanied by unpleasant or uncomfortable sensations in the lower (and occasionally the upper) extremities before sleep onset (and sometimes at other times as well). This sensation is typically described as a "crawling" or "creeping" feeling, and it resolves temporarily when the involved extremities are moved. The urge to move the legs begins or worsens during periods of rest or inactivity and occurs exclusively in the evening or night rather than during the day. The diagnosis is made clinically. PSG is not required to make the diagnosis.

53. How are PLMD and RLS treated?

There is insufficient evidence at present to evaluate the use of pharmacologic therapy in patients diagnosed with PLMD alone. However, there are several studies that have demonstrated a decrease in abnormal limb movements in the setting of RLS and PLMD. The standard medications for RLS include pramipexole and ropinirole. Medications reported to be beneficial include dopaminergics (e.g., L-DOPA, bromocriptine), opioids, gabapentin, pregabalin, carbamazepine, and clonidine. Supplemental iron may be used to treat RLS patients with low ferritin levels. It is important to identify medications or other factors that could aggravate RLS and PLMD. For instance, selective serotonin reuptake inhibitor, metoclopramide, diphenhydramine, sleep deprivation, nicotine, caffeine, and alcohol have all been shown to either promote or aggravate RLS and PLMD. There are no approved medications for the pediatric population. However, off-label use of certain medications such as gabapentin have been used to treat RLS in children.

54. What is sleep-related rhythmic movement disorder?

Sleep-related rhythmic movement disorder is characterized by repetitive, stereotyped, and rhythmic motor behaviors that occur near sleep onset. The movements are not tremors, involve large muscle groups, and include body rocking, head banging, head rolling, or a combination of the aforementioned. The behaviors result in sleep disturbance, significant impairment in daytime function, or self-inflicted bodily injury or likelihood of injury if preventive measures are not used. Typically, the disorder is seen in infants and children; however, it does occur in adolescents and adults. The rhythmic movements are not better explained by another movement disorder or epilepsy. Rhythmic movements have been reported to be associated with RLS, OSA, narcolepsy, RBD, and attention deficit-hyperactivity disorder.

 References available online at expertconsult.com.

WEBSITE

http://www.aasmnet.org

BIBLIOGRAPHY

1. Kryger M, Roth T, Dement W: Principles and Practice of Sleep Medicine, 5th ed. Philadelphia, Saunders, 2010.
2. Iber C, Ancoli-Israel S, Chesson A, Quan SF, for the American Academy of Sleep Medicine: The AASM Manual for the Scoring of Sleep and Associated Events. Rules, Terminology, and Technical Specifications, Westchester, IL, American Academy of Sleep Medicine, 2007.
3. International Classification of Sleep Disorders: Diagnostic and Coding Manual (ICSD-2), 3rd ed. Darien, IL, American Academy of Sleep Medicine, 2014.
4. Sheldon S, Kryger M, Ferber R: Principles and Practice of Pediatric Sleep Medicine, 2nd ed. Philadelphia, Elsevier, 2014.

CHAPTER 24

NEUROLOGIC COMPLICATIONS OF SYSTEMIC DISEASE

John D. Eatman, Ericka P. Simpson

CARDIAC DISEASE

1. **What is the major neurologic complication of cardiac disease?**
   Stroke is the most common neurologic sequela of cardiac disease. The risks for embolic, thrombotic, and hemorrhagic strokes are elevated in the presence of cardiac disease. Nonvalvular atrial fibrillation, followed by ischemic heart disease and valvular heart disease, is the most common type of cardiac abnormality causing embolic ischemic strokes. Infective endocarditis is frequently associated with embolic strokes with hemorrhagic conversion. A patent foramen ovale may be a risk factor for stroke in some, especially younger patients, but it may be merely an incidental finding unrelated to stroke in other patients with other vascular risk factors.

2. **What is the association between transient ischemic attack (TIA) and myocardial infarction (MI)?**
   Patients who suffer a TIA are more likely to suffer a fatal MI than a stroke, although the stroke incidence is three times higher in those who suffer from a TIA. Patients with a TIA are twice as likely to suffer an MI as the general population. Due to this increased risk, screening for cardiovascular disease and primary prevention of coronary artery disease are important in patients with a TIA.

3. **What is the association between sleep, MI, and stroke?**
   Profound changes in centrally mediated sympathetic activity occur during rapid eye movement (REM) sleep, with small increases in blood pressure, heart rate, skin conductance changes, as well as momentary restorations in muscle tone, mesenteric and renal vasodilation, and skeletal muscle vasoconstriction. In the elderly, it is hypothesized that large fluctuations in sympathetic activity associated with REM sleep also cause increased rates of arrhythmia and increased risk for cardiac vasospasm and subsequent stroke and MI. The presence of heart rate abnormalities during sleep in normotensive patients is also reported to be a predictor of future cardiovascular disease. Sleep-disordered breathing (SDB) also contributes to increased stroke risk in multiple ways. In patients with obstructive sleep apnea, apneic episodes can cause increased sympathetic activation and increases in blood pressure. Compared to control subjects, atrial fibrillation is more common in patients with SDB. Finally, hypoxia due to apnea may activate inflammatory pathways. These pathways increase oxidative stress in blood vessels, leading to accelerated atherosclerosis.

4. **What are the nonstroke-related neurologic complications of cardiac disease?**
   Cardiac arrhythmias (especially sick sinus syndrome) may produce decreased cardiac output, causing syncope, and, rarely, encephalopathy. Cerebral blood flow can be altered due to changes in cerebral autoregulation caused by abnormal autonomic vagal activity associated with cardiac disease. Persistent decreased brain perfusion, such as in the case of cardiac arrest or cardiogenic shock, may lead to laminar necrosis of the cerebral cortex or hippocampus.

GASTROINTESTINAL DISEASE

5. **What is the major cause of neurologic symptoms associated with gastrointestinal (GI) disease?**
   Most known neurologic complications of GI disease are the consequence of malabsorption of essential nutrients and vitamins. The consequences of some nutrient deficiencies have been well described, including those involving thiamine, folate, cyanocobalamin, niacin, vitamin D, vitamin E, and copper.

6. **What are the neurologic manifestations of celiac disease?**
   Celiac disease, or gluten enteropathy, is an autoimmune disease of the small intestine that produces chronic small bowel malabsorption of vitamins and other nutrients often with iron deficiency

anemia, osteoporosis and osteomalacia, and hypoalbuminemia. Individuals with the disease are intolerant to gluten proteins that are present in rye, wheat, barley, and in some adhesives, including that of stamps and envelopes. Ten percent of affected patients have neurologic complaints, the most notable being cerebellar dysfunction secondary to chronic fat malabsorption. Tremor, intra-nuclear ophthalmoplegia, encephalopathy, subacute combined degeneration, seizures, or myopathy are other features associated with the disease. The observed myopathy is often treatable by vitamin D replacement.

7. What is the triad of neurologic clinical features associated with Whipple's disease?
   Whipple's disease is a multisystem granulomatous infection caused by *Tropheryma whippelii*. Neurologic complaints develop in 10% of afflicted patients. The common triad of findings includes ocular disturbance (often ophthalmoparesis), gait ataxia, and dementia. Other associated abnormalities include seizures, myelopathy, meningoencephalitis, autonomic dysfunction, and steroid-unresponsive myopathy. Effective treatment involves antibiotic therapy directed against the organism. Untreated, most patients die within 1 year of the onset of neurologic symptoms.

8. What is the triad of neurologic complaints associated with Wernicke's encephalopathy?
   Wernicke's encephalopathy is associated with thiamine deficiency. Clinical symptoms include a triad of ophthalmoparesis, gait ataxia, and disturbances of mental function. An axonal sensorimotor neuropathy appears in half of patients with this deficiency state, and Korsakoff's psychosis (dementia associated with profound amnesia and confabulation) is also variably present. The mortality associated with Wernicke's encephalopathy is still greater than 10%, although this is more due to concomitant infections and malnutrition than to the neurologic disorders.

9. What is known about the etiology of nervous system impairment associated with vitamin B12 malabsorption?
   The deficiency of methionine synthetase activity secondary to absence of its cofactor (B12) leads to accumulation of homocysteine. The resulting impairment in DNA synthesis is responsible for the megaloblastic anemia associated with vitamin B12 deficiency, while neurologic abnormalities are the result of failure to maintain methionine biosynthesis.

10. What are the neurologic manifestations of vitamin B12 deficiency?
    Neurologic manifestations of vitamin B12 deficiency include cognitive, behavioral dysfunction, myelopathy, and peripheral neuropathy. Patients may manifest slowed cerebration, dementia, or delirium (with or without delusion), while others exhibit depression, amnesia, or acute psychotic states. Rare cases of reversible manic or schizophreniform states have also been reported. In addition to a sensorimotor neuropathy, vitamin B12 deficiency also can result in subacute combined degeneration of the spinal cord due to dorsal and lateral column involvement. Copper deficiency due to small bowel malabsorption or zinc overconsumption can produce a similar neurologic presentation.

11. Which vitamin deficiencies cause different neurologic syndromes in children from those in adults?
    Lack of absorption of vitamin D from the intestinal tract leads to rickets in children and osteomalacia in adults. In children with rickets, neurologic sequelae include head shaking, nystagmus, and increased irritability that may evolve into tetany with a sufficient fall in serum calcium concentrations. **Malabsorption of folate** in infants leads to mental retardation, seizures, and athetotic movements, whereas in adults, polyneuropathy and depression are the primary complications. **Pyridoxine deficiency** leads to seizures in infants but a sensory polyneuropathy in adults.

12. Malabsorption of which vitamins will lead to an increased risk for subdural hematoma?
    Malabsorption of vitamin C or vitamin K results in an increased tendency for hemorrhage, especially following trauma. Lack of thiamine, vitamin B12, or vitamin E all can result in ataxia, with an increased tendency for falls and head trauma.

13. Besides thiamine, malabsorption or dietary lack of which vitamin may produce a syndrome resembling Korsakoff's dementia?
    Nicotinic acid deficiency results in pellagra, whose major and often sole manifestation is psychiatric disturbance, sometimes mimicking Korsakoff's psychosis.

HEPATIC DISEASE

14. What are the five major neurologic syndromes associated with hepatic dysfunction?
    1. Encephalopathy
    2. Hepatocerebral degeneration
    3. Wilson's disease
    4. Reye's syndrome
    5. Intracranial hemorrhage (ICH)

15. What causes hepatic encephalopathy (HE)?
    This complication may occur with hepatic failure or with portal or hepatic circulatory dysfunction, as caused by acute or chronic hepatitis, hepatic necrosis, cirrhosis, or portocaval anastomosis. There are multiple theories about the pathogenesis of HE. Ammonia is thought to play an important role in the pathogenesis of HE. Patients with HE have been shown to have increased diffusion of ammonia through the blood–brain barrier. In the brain, cytoplasmic enzymes in the astrocyte medicate ammonia detoxification. Overloading of this system with excess ammonia generates free radicals in the mitochondria, causing cellular swelling and astrocytic dysfunction. Another important potential factor are nonpharmacologic ligands interacting with the gamma-aminobutyric acid (GABA) receptor. These ligands are normally occurring substances proposed to accumulate in brain tissue in HE. In addition, ammonia also plays a role in the affinity of GABA receptors to GABA itself. Reduction in the serum concentration of ammonia, or addition of centrally acting GABA antagonists, may temporarily improve hepatic encephalopathy, although correction of the precipitating causes of hepatic dysfunction is necessary for ultimate recovery.

16. How is HE treated?
    Acute therapy for HE requires either removal or blockade of neurologically acting toxins produced in the gut. Reduction of protein intake along with lactulose therapy to enhance ammonia excretion and reduce ammonia absorption is the mainstay of therapy. Oral antibiotics, such as either neomycin or rifaximin, and amino acids L-ornithine and L-aspartate, are used as second-line agents to reduce gut bacterial levels and ammonia formation. Long-term treatment of HE with medical therapies has only limited success and depends on whether the hepatic damage is reversible, static, or progressive. Ultimately, the most effective therapy involves treatments directed at reversing the hepatic failure, including surgical shunting procedures and liver transplantation for selected individuals.

17. What is Reye's syndrome?
    Reye's syndrome is a rare, acute noninflammatory encephalopathy that primarily affects children and adolescents. A correlation between the disease and a preceding viral infection (especially influenza and varicella) treated with salicylates has been reported, although other toxic, metabolic, or hypoxic insults may play roles in the pathogenesis. The clinical manifestations of Reye's syndrome include hyperammonemia, hypoglycemia, coagulopathy, and cerebral edema. Treatment is supportive and includes administration of intravenous glucose to prevent hypoglycemia, and in severe cases, hyper-ventilation and intravenous mannitol to reduce intracranial pressure.

    Defects in fatty acid oxidation, such as medium-chain acyl coenzyme A dehydrogenase deficiency, can also present as a Reye-like syndrome and may be more common than Reye's syndrome, warranting a workup for inborn errors of metabolism in affected children.

18. In addition to HE, what other diseases cause asterixis?
    Asterixis, or "flapping tremor," is best elicited by the extension of outstretched, opened hands. It results from the acute loss of muscle tone or contraction associated with passive or active hand/wrist extension ("negative" myoclonus), most likely induced by pathologic coupling of the thalamus and motor cortex. This sign is encountered in many metabolic encephalopathies, including uremia, malnutrition, severe pulmonary disease, and polycythemia rubra vera.

19. What electroencephalographic (EEG) abnormality is associated with hepatic encephalopathy?
    Slow triphasic waves are the abnormal EEG pattern reported with hepatic encephalopathy, and the pattern is commonly used to support the diagnosis. It can also be seen with encephalopathy associated with head trauma (especially with subdural hematoma), acute cerebral anoxia, uremia, electrolyte imbalance, and thyrotoxicosis.

20. **What are the neurologic manifestations of Wilson's disease?**
Wilson's disease is a rare disorder of copper metabolism resulting in accumulation of copper in the liver, kidneys, and central nervous system (CNS). In almost half of patients, neurologic manifestations are present, including tremors, dysarthria, clumsiness, drooling, and gait instability in order of decreasing frequency. Neuropsychiatric symptoms, including those of dementia, mania, depression, or psychosis, may dominate the presentation in up to 20% of patients. Kaiser–Fleischer rings, copper deposits in Descemet's membrane of the cornea, are present in 98% of patients with neurologic manifestations and are visualized by slit-lamp examination. Neurologic manifestations invariably follow liver involvement, even in silent, unrecognized liver disease.

21. **What is the treatment for Wilson's disease?**
Early diagnosis and copper chelation therapy are the mainstays of therapy. The chelation therapy of choice is oral D-penicillamine. D-Penicillamine should be administered concomitantly with pyridoxine to prevent vitamin B6 deficiency. Side effects include rash, fever, thrombocytopenia, relative eosinophilia with total leukopenia, and reversible lupus-like and myasthenia gravis-like syndromes. Trientene and zinc acetate are alternative agents with fewer side effects. Liver transplantation is recommended in patients with fulminant hepatic failure and end-stage liver cirrhosis but is not generally recommended for patients with neurologic disease without pronounced liver involvement.

22. **What are the neurologic complications of hemochromatosis?**
Hemochromatosis is a disorder of iron overload resulting in multiorgan fibrosis and dysfunction. Acquired causes result from excess total body iron due to multiple blood transfusions. Hereditary hemochromatosis is due to mutations in the *HFE* gene, which encodes for a protein involved in the regulation of GI iron absorption and uptake. Encephalopathy, truncal ataxia, and rigidity may all complicate hemochromatosis and invariably are due to liver disease (liver cirrhosis and failure) resulting from massive iron deposition in the liver. Neuritis is either a complication of the diabetes mellitus (DM) that accompanies most cases of hemochromatosis or is a result of local iron deposition.
    Treatment requires serial phlebotomies four to six times per year. Lifetime treatment with phlebotomies is currently the treatment of choice, although newer therapies using growth factor control over red blood cell production are being tested.

23. **Which porphyrias are associated with primarily neurologic manifestations?**
Hepatic porphyrias, acute intermittent porphyria (AIP), and variegate (South African) porphyria can be distinguished from the rare "erythropoietic" forms that produce dermatologic symptoms without neurologic disease. In AIP, clinical symptoms develop during crises, most often precipitated by ingestion or administration of drugs that adversely affect porphyrin metabolism. These clinical symptoms include the following: (1) abdominal pain with vomiting, constipation or diarrhea, and often a previous history of exploratory abdominal surgery; (2) psychiatric disorder, with symptoms suggesting conversion reactions, delirium, or psychosis; (3) peripheral neuropathy, primarily motor, often with autonomic abnormalities, that may be severe or fatal and mimic Guillain–Barré syndrome; and (4) central abnormalities, such as syndrome of inappropriate antidiuretic hormone or convulsions.

24. **Chronic ingestion of what substance may produce a condition similar to AIP?**
Lead poisoning produces a condition (termed *saturnism*) that closely resembles AIP clinically, and also appears to share heme synthetic dysfunction with accumulation of delta-aminolevulinic acid.

25. **What is the treatment for neurologic crises in AIP?**
Therapy is directed at modifying the biochemical abnormalities found in the disease, including overproduction of the neurotoxin delta-aminolevulinic acid and heme deficiency. Intravenous administration of hematin increases available heme and downregulates the patient's abnormal heme biosynthetic pathway, thus reducing delta-aminolevulinic acid levels. Prevention of crises is the primary goal in treating patients with AIP. Education of patients to the many precipitants of acute attacks is necessary for their survival.

RENAL DISEASE

26. **What are the most common neurologic complications of renal disease?**
Typical neurologic complications of renal disease are peripheral neuropathy and metabolic encephalopathy.

27. **What are the characteristics of uremic neuropathy?**
Uremic neuropathy appears as a symmetric distal sensorimotor axonal neuropathy and is almost invariably present in patients by the time they require dialysis. Other conditions that predispose to renal failure (e.g., diabetes and vasculitis) may also produce neuropathy, and thus symptoms can result from several different etiologies. Uremic neuropathy is at least partially reversible by repeated dialysis or by kidney transplantation.

28. **What are the characteristics of uremic encephalopathy?**
Patients with uremia often develop a metabolic encephalopathy. The mechanisms responsible for this encephalopathy remain unclear but presumably involve the retention of inorganic and organic acids, fluid alterations among cerebral cellular compartments, and abnormalities caused by hypertension, hypocalcemia, hyperkalemia, hypernatremia, hyperphosphatemia, and hypochloremia. Uremic encephalopathy is unusual because of the coexistence of signs of neuronal depression (lethargy, coma) with those of neuronal excitation (agitation, muscle cramps, myoclonus, tetany, asterixis, and seizures).

29. **Name three neurologic complications associated with dialysis.**
Dialysis disequilibrium syndrome, dialysis dementia, and ICH.

30. **What is dialysis disequilibrium syndrome?**
Dialysis disequilibrium syndrome is the name given to the cerebral edema produced by the rapid removal of urea and other osmoles and fluid and electrolyte shifts associated with dialysis. Dialysis disequilibrium is most likely to occur in patients either during or after their first treatment but can occur at any time in their treatment. The incidence appears to be decreasing, likely due to the earlier initiation of dialysis in the course of end-stage renal disease. The symptoms are nonspecific, but they are similar to those of ICH. They include persistent headache and fatigue. The syndrome may also be sufficiently severe to produce seizures, coma, and death. Due to the nonspecific nature of the symptoms, other causes of increased intracranial pressure must be ruled out. Recognition of this problem has led to newer protocols using more frequent, but less vigorous, dialysis.

KEY POINTS: COMMON ASSOCIATIONS WITH TRIPHASIC WAVES ON ELECTROENCEPHALOGRAPHY

1. Hepatic encephalopathy
2. Uremic encephalopathy
3. Acute cerebral anoxia
4. Thyrotoxicosis

---

31. **What is dialysis dementia?**
Dialysis dementia refers to reported cases in the 1980s of a rare but serious syndrome of irreversible progressive dementia with apraxias, dysarthria, hyperreflexia, myoclonus, and multifocal seizures. Clusters of patients with dementia presented from dialysis centers that used water contaminated with aluminum, and therefore the presence of aluminum in the dialysate was thought to be the primary agent causing CNS toxicity. Removal of aluminum with ion exchange resins prior to dialysis has significantly reduced the problem.

32. **What causes ICH in patients undergoing dialysis?**
Anticoagulation during dialysis and chronic hypertension associated with renal failure increases the incidence of ICH.

33. **What neurologic complications are associated with renal transplantation?**
Neurologic complications of renal transplantation can be due to either the renal disease necessitating transplantation or posttransplantation immunosuppression. Calcineurin inhibitors are the most common immunosuppressive medications in renal transplant patients and may cause tremors, paresthesia, a severe disabling pain syndrome, and posterior reversible encephalopathy syndrome. Reduction or discontinuation of the drug can either reverse or reduce the majority of the neurologic side effects. The monoclonal antibody OKT3 may induce severe neurologic syndromes such as

aseptic meningitis. Stroke occurs in about 8% of renal transplant patients. End-stage renal disease due to diabetes and/or peripheral vascular disease are the strongest risk factors. Guillain–Barré syndrome may also develop, triggered in some cases by either cytomegalovirus or *Campylobacter jejuni* infection. Infection represents the most frequent neurologic complication in transplant patients on immunosuppression. Acute meningitis, usually caused by *Listeria monocytogenes*, and subacute and chronic meningitis, caused by *Cryptococcus neoformans*, account for more than 90% of nonviral CNS infections. *Aspergillus fumigatus*, *Toxoplasma gondii*, and *Nocardia asteroides* result in focal brain infection and JC virus, a polyoma virus, and cause progressive multifocal leukoencephalopathy. Lymphomas are the most frequent brain tumors. They are usually associated with an Epstein–Barr virus infection and are more frequent in patients who receive aggressive immunosuppressive therapy. The overall risk of developing cancer following renal transplantation is approximately 6%, or about 100-fold greater than that expected for the general nonimmunosuppressed population.

PULMONARY DISEASE

34. **What are the neurologic signs and symptoms of respiratory insufficiency?**
    Neurologic features of this medical emergency result from hypoxemia and acute hypercapnia. Initial symptoms may be those of either a nocturnal or early morning headache associated with lethargy, drowsiness, inattentiveness, and irritability. Motor signs at this stage include tremor and twitching, caused by hypercapnia-induced stimulation of sympathetic nervous system output. More severe levels of hypoxia result in somnolence, confusion, and asterixis. Prolonged, severe hypoxia results in coma and generalized seizures. Ocular findings include papilledema in 10% of patients, probably from hypercapnia-induced increases in intracranial pressure. However, isolated chronic hypercapnia with PCO_2 measurements of up to 110 mm Hg may exist without apparent neurologic symptoms or signs.

KEY POINTS: NEUROLOGIC DISEASES ASSOCIATED WITH RESPIRATORY INSUFFICIENCY

1. Brain/brain stem
2. Spinal cord
3. Peripheral nerve
4. Neuromuscular junction
5. Muscle

---

35. **What neurologic diseases may result in respiratory insufficiency?**
    Brain and brain stem
    - Brain herniation
    - Muscular dystrophy (central apnea)

    Spinal cord
    - Upper cervical cord injury, transection ($\leq$ C6)
    - Lower motor neuron disease (amyotrophic lateral sclerosis, postpolio syndrome, spinal muscular atrophy)

    Peripheral nerve
    - Acute inflammatory polyradiculoneuropathy (Guillain–Barré syndrome)

    Neuromuscular junction
    - Myasthenia gravis
    - Botulism
    - Congenital myasthenic syndromes

    Muscle
    - Muscular dystrophy (peripheral/obstructive apnea)
    - Congenital myopathy
    - Inflammatory myopathies (polymyositis, inclusion body myositis)

36. Describe the clinical features of prolonged hyperventilation.
Anxious patients with acute psychogenic hyperventilation usually complain of lightheadedness, dyspnea, circumoral and acral paresthesias, and the presence of visual phosphenes. Visual blurring, tremor, muscle cramps, carpopedal spasm, and chest pain are found with prolonged hyperventilation. In addition to psychogenic etiologies, prolonged hyperventilation may be the result of drug effects, metabolic acidosis, CNS damage or edema, or response to heat stroke or overexercise.

37. What causes high-altitude sickness? How is it treated?
Cerebral hypoxia results from the lower partial pressure of oxygen at high altitudes. A shift of water and sodium into neurons may also occur as the result of the failure of glycolysis-dependent cellular enzymes and transporters, such as the Na^+/K^+ pump. Exercise in the cold temperatures encountered at high altitude worsens cerebral edema by further increasing cerebral blood flow. Treatment prophylactically with dexamethasone will prevent most cases of acute mountain sickness. The use of high-pressure oxygen, removal to lower altitudes, and acetazolamide therapy may reduce symptoms in patients with preexisting high-altitude sickness.

HEMATOLOGIC DISEASE

38. Name the most common symptoms associated with anemia.
Headache, lightheadedness, and fatigue are the most commonly reported neurologic complaints of the anemic patient.

KEY POINTS: SYSTEMIC DISEASES ASSOCIATED WITH AN INCREASED RISK OF STROKE

1. Hematologic disease (sickle cell anemia, hemophilia, platelet disorders)
2. Diabetes
3. Cardiac disease
4. Vitamin C and K deficiencies
5. Connective tissue disease and CNS vasculitides
6. Pregnancy

39. What is the most serious neurologic complication of sickle cell anemia?
Ischemic stroke, often affecting patients in childhood or adolescence, is the most frequent serious sequela of a vascular crisis in sickle cell disease. Intimal hyperplasia and stenosis of proximal cerebral vessels have been described in the pathogenesis for medium-vessel and large-vessel stroke in these patients. Hyperventilation (with associated vasoconstriction) is thus a common precipitating event for stroke in the young patient with sickle cell disease. Recurrence rates for stroke in patients with sickle cell disease exceed 67%. Intracranial hemorrhage may also be seen in patients with sickle cell disease. Rupture of intracranial aneurysms is the usual cause for ICH in affected individuals. Other neurologic complications of sickle cell anemia include silent cerebral infarcts, which occur in one-fourth of pediatric sickle cell patients before the age of 6 and one-third of pediatric sickle cell patients before the age of 14. These silent infarcts can be significantly detrimental to cognitive development and academic performance.

40. What are the primary neurologic manifestations of hyperviscosity states?
Hyperviscosity states are conditions in which red blood cells, white blood cells, or serum proteins are increased to a sufficient degree that impedance of blood flow and/or oxygen delivery results. Neurologic manifestations include symptoms of either chronic or acute vertebrobasilar insufficiency (tinnitus, lightheadedness, and headache); paresthesias; and problems with mentation, visual/auditory disturbances, seizures, stroke, stupor, or coma.

41. What red cell diseases can produce a hyperviscosity state?
Polycythemia rubra vera and "secondary" or "relative" polycythemia increase the hematocrit or the red cell volume/plasma volume ratio, respectively. These conditions thereby increase blood viscosity, producing symptoms. Either chronic reduction in hematocrit by phlebotomy or acute expansion of the plasma volume both reduce symptoms and may decrease the risk of serious sequelae.

42. **What diseases produce elevated serum proteins and cause hyperviscosity states?**

    Neurologic symptoms may be the presenting symptoms of hyperviscosity due to paraproteinemias. Multiple myeloma and Waldenström's macroglobulinemia are the most common causes of increased serum viscosity. In most cases, plasmapheresis is used in combination with corticosteroids and immunosuppressive drugs to prevent production of abnormal proteins and treat the underlying disease.

43. **What are the neurologic complications of hemophilia?**

    Intracranial hemorrhages of multiple types are the most serious consequence of factor VIII deficiency. A history of head trauma is often obtained, preceding symptoms of a subdural hemorrhage by days. Subarachnoid and intraparenchymal hemorrhages cause more rapid progression of symptoms and carry an increased risk for mortality. Intraspinal hemorrhage, while rare, rapidly produces cord compression and paralysis, while soft tissue hematomas may cause focal compressive neuropathies.

44. **Which platelet disorders produce neurologic disease?**

    Primary acute or chronic immune thrombocytopenia purpura (ITP), disseminated intravascular coagulation (DIC), thrombotic thrombocytopenic purpura (TTP), dysimmune thrombocytopenia (DIT) secondary to rheumatic disease (associated with anticardiolipin antibodies) or hyperviscosity states, and heparin-associated thrombocytopenia (HAT) all are associated with neurologic disease due to thrombocytopenic states. TTP produces a microangiopathic hemolytic anemia with prominent neurologic symptoms of headache, encephalopathy, or seizures, whereas DIC and (less commonly) ITP may produce larger intracerebral hemorrhages. HAT and DIT more commonly cause ischemic strokes. Thrombocytosis usually results from essential thrombocythemia, which produces symptoms of a hyperviscosity state when platelet counts exceed 600,000 to 1,000,000 per microliter. Cerebrovascular complications—TIAs and ischemic stroke—are the serious consequences of this disease.

45. **How are antiphospholipid antibodies related to neurologic disease?**

    Antibodies directed against phospholipids are associated with thrombotic states and are found with a high frequency in patients with retinal vascular thrombosis, amaurosis fugax, ischemic optic neuropathy, and stroke in young patients. The most common antibodies, lupus anticoagulant and anticardiolipin antibody, probably induce thrombosis via multiple mechanisms. The presence of these antibodies has also been associated with migraine, chorea, myelopathy, and orthostatic hypotension. Nonneurologic features may include miscarriage, livedo reticularis, and pulmonary hypertension. The pathophysiology of these symptoms is poorly understood.

46. **What is the treatment for antiphospholipid antibody syndrome?**

    Few controlled trials have been conducted, and there is no consensus about the optimal treatment for patients with antiphospholipid antibodies. Most authorities favor use of the antithrombotic agent warfarin, but plasmapheresis combined with immunosuppression and intravenous immunoglobulin (IVIG) increasingly is used in severe cases. Enoxaparin, rather than warfarin, and IVIG are the treatments of choice for pregnant women.

ENDOCRINE DISEASE

47. **Which endocrine diseases are commonly associated with neurologic complications?**
    1. Diabetes mellitus (DM)
    2. Hyperthyroidism
    3. Hypothyroidism
    4. Hyperparathyroidism
    5. Hypoparathyroidism
    6. Acromegaly
    7. Adrenal insufficiency
    8. Glucocorticoid excess
    9. Diabetes insipidus (DI)

48. **Which endocrine diseases are complicated by seizures?**

    Seizures most commonly occur after an acute change in endocrine function and usually result from electrolyte imbalance. They occur in 50% or more of patients with hypoparathyroidism because of the hypocalcemia. Although seizures are usually generalized, partial or absence seizures may also complicate hypoparathyroidism. Seizures do not occur in hyperparathyroidism.

Seizures may be the presenting sign in 20% of all hypothyroid patients and are nearly always generalized. In contrast, the incidence of seizures in thyrotoxicosis is only 5% to 10%.

In Addison's disease, seizures follow the rapid onset of serum hyponatremia (<115 mEq/L) and carry a subsequent mortality of greater than 50%. Seizures are seen in DI only with rapid elevation of serum sodium (usually to greater than 160 mEq/L). In DI, seizures are often partial and may occur as a result of either brain shrinkage with focal hemorrhage or during rehydration.

Seizures are observed with other endocrine causes of brain shrinkage, such as in nonketotic hyperosmolar states from DM. In this setting, up to 25% of patients develop partial or generalized motor seizures that may evolve into epilepsia partialis continua or generalized status epilepticus. Seizures may also be seen in DM as the result of hypoglycemia from insulin therapy but are distinctly uncommon in diabetic ketoacidosis. Seizures are not typically associated with Cushing's disease or acromegaly.

49. **Which endocrine diseases may cause coma?**
Coma is a rare and life-threatening complication of both hypothyroidism and hyperthyroidism. In the latter case, coma is almost always associated with thyroid storm. Decompensated hypothyroidism can cause myxedema coma, with mortality rates as high as 25% to 60%. Coma is also found in hyperparathyroidism when serum calcium is greater than 19 mg/dL, in adrenal hypofunction with severe hyponatremia, and in DM associated with severe hyperglycemia as well as with therapy-related hypoglycemia.

50. **What are the common neurologic features of hypothyroidism?**
Hypothyroidism causes headache, fatigue, slowness of speech and thought, apathy, and inattention in 90% of patients and is often mistaken for early dysthymia or depression. Reversible sensorineural hearing loss, with or without tinnitus, develops in 75% of hypothyroid patients, and reversible ptosis occurs in 60% of patients as a result of diminished sympathetic tone. Sleep apnea occurs in up to half of hypothyroid patients and usually results from obstructive problems due to associated obesity and myxedema. Seizures are reported in 20% of patients, often as the presenting neurologic sign. Prolonged relaxation time for deep tendon reflexes can be elicited in many hypothyroid patients but is not specific for the disease.

Rarely, hypothyroidism is associated with limb ataxia, nystagmus, carpal tunnel syndrome, demyelinating polyneuropathy, optic neuropathy, ophthalmoparesis, pseudotumor cerebri, trigeminal neuralgia, Bell's palsy, reversible dementia, or overt psychosis (myxedema madness).

Myopathy in hypothyroidism is common and ranges between 30% and 80% of cases. The major symptoms related are weakness, muscular cramps, and myalgia. The pseudohypertrophic form is called Hoffman's syndrome. Laboratory investigation shows increased levels of muscle enzymes, low serum thyroid hormones, and elevated thyrotropic-stimulating hormone.

51. **What are the most dangerous neurologic complications of hypothyroidism?**
Although myxedema coma develops in only 1% of hypothyroid patients, its often rapid onset with associated bradycardia, ventricular arrhythmias, hypotension, hypopnea, hypothermia, hypoglycemia, electrolyte disturbance, and seizures makes it life threatening. Treatment is supportive, with correction of metabolic abnormalities, rewarming, ventilatory and/or cardiovascular support, and adequate replacement of thyroxine and corticosteroids. In utero and in the newborn period, undiagnosed and untreated hypothyroidism leads to cretinism. Treatment requires early screening prior to the onset of symptoms and thyroid hormone replacement before permanent damage occurs.

52. **What are the neurologic features of hyperthyroidism?**
Thyrotoxicosis may manifest with reversible behavioral and cognitive changes, including emotional lability, euphoria, irritability, mania, and psychosis. Delirium may be observed as a manifestation of thyroid storm. Apathetic hyperthyroidism may appear as fatigue, with symptoms suggesting depression or dementia. Other features of thyrotoxicosis are tremor of the hands, eyelids, or tongue, as well as chorea, spasticity (sometimes with clonus and Babinski's signs), thyrotoxic periodic paralysis, and myopathy.

Neurologic problems usually resolve after treatment of the underlying thyrotoxicosis, but thyroid ophthalmopathy often requires surgical orbital decompression. Additionally, bulbar palsies and motor weakness may not recover following correction of hyperthyroidism secondary to coexistence of other dysimmune disease, such as acute myasthenia gravis.

53. **What are the neurologic features of parathyroid dysfunction?**
Up to 25% of patients with hyperparathyroidism have prominent psychiatric symptoms resembling mania, psychosis, or acute confusional state. An additional 50% of hyperparathyroid patients may have symptoms suggesting depression. Interestingly, 80% of patients with hypoparathyroidism also exhibit psychological manifestations of their disease, including symptoms resembling depression, pseudodementia, mania, psychosis, and delirium.

In hyperparathyroidism, hypercalcemia-induced coma and spinal cord or root compression caused by collapse of decalcified vertebrae are the major nonpsychiatric symptoms. Myopathy is also a common finding in hyperparathyroidism. In contrast, hypocalcemia resulting from hypoparathyroidism is more closely associated with seizures and tetany. Seizures are often difficult to control and require correction of the electrolyte imbalance. Latent tetany can present as laryngeal spasm and may also be evoked by mechanical stimulation of the facial nerve (Chvostek's sign), by hyperventilation, or by occlusion of venous return from an arm resulting in carpopedal spasm (Trousseau's sign).

54. **How may adrenal insufficiency lead to weakness?**
Up to 50% of patients with Addison's disease have a glucocorticoid-sensitive myopathy with associated cramping. Adrenal insufficiency results in decreased blood flow to the muscle, reduced muscle carbohydrate metabolism, and altered Na^+/K^+ pump function and potassium homeostasis with resulting reduced intracellular muscle potassium and altered muscle contractility. Decreased adrenergic sensitivity in patients with Addison's disease also results in reduced exercise tolerance and exercise-related hypotension. Abnormalities in potassium homeostasis may additionally result in the episodic appearance of extreme weakness, resembling hyperkalemic periodic paralysis.

55. **How does prolonged glucocorticoid excess lead to weakness?**
Most patients with Cushing's disease have frank weakness and demonstrable myopathic findings on electromyography and selective type IIb muscle fiber atrophy on muscle biopsy. Chronic treatment with glucocorticoids, especially with the fluorinated steroids, will reproduce these effects on ectopic adrenocorticotropic hormone production in 10% to 20% of patients. Glucocorticoids produce an insulin-resistant state in myotubes, in which both glycolytic (nonoxidative) carbohydrate metabolism and protein synthesis are adversely affected. Type IIb fibers, which are least able to compensate for this reduction of glycolytic metabolism, are most affected.

56. **What neurologic disorders are associated with excess growth hormone?**
Sustained excessive growth hormone (GH) appears to directly produce myopathy. GH-induced changes in the myotubule include impaired glycolytic carbohydrate metabolism, increased fatty acid oxidation, and increased protein synthesis with reduced protein degradation. The more highly oxidative type I and type IIa muscle fibers are typically most affected by GH. Myotubule hypertrophy from abnormal protein synthesis produces weakness in the face of increased muscle size. Although central sleep apnea may also be caused directly by excessive GH production, the obstructive sleep apnea, basilar impression, myelopathy, and compressive neuropathies reported in this disease are all indirect effects of bony, ligamentous, and soft-tissue hyperplasia with secondary compression of neural tissue.

57. **How does DM affect the peripheral nervous system?**
Damage to the peripheral nervous system accounts for the main neurologic manifestations of diabetes. Approximately 50% of diabetic patients will develop a neuropathy. Initially, a symmetric distal stocking-and-glove sensory neuropathy involving small, unmyelinated or thinly myelinated fibers appears and is often associated with painful, burning paresthesias. In more severe cases, larger proprioceptive fibers are also affected, leading to Charcot joints. The cumulative exposure to hyperglycemia is thought to be the most important risk factor. The typical diabetic neuropathy can be slowed or sometimes even improved with better glycemic control. Autonomic nerve damage causes atrophic skin changes, impotence, orthostatic hypotension, arrhythmias, gastroparesis, and sphincter incontinence. Motor fibers may also be damaged, leading to symmetric distal weakness, especially of the lower extremities. Focal destruction of nerves may cause cranial nerve palsies, diabetic amyotrophy, and thoracoabdominal neuropathy.

FLUID AND ELECTROLYTE DISORDERS

58. **What are the most common neurologic complications of hypokalemia and hyperkalemia?**
Myalgias and weakness can be found with serum potassium concentrations of 2.5 to 3.0 mEq/L. Prolonged hypokalemia of less than 2.5 mEq/L will lead to rhabdomyolysis, myoglobinuria, and cardiac arrhythmias.

Hyperkalemia (>6.0 mEq/L) likewise causes functional and structural muscle abnormalities, including weakness and cardiac arrhythmias. Ventricular asystole or fibrillation is life threatening and occurs long before neurologic symptoms are usually manifested. The few previous reports of drowsiness, lethargy, and coma in hypokalemia may actually be the result of acid–base disequilibrium.

59. **How do changes in serum sodium affect the nervous system?**
Because extracellular fluid volume changes as a direct function of total body sodium, patients who are hyponatremic are usually hyposmolar, whereas hypernatremic patients are hyperosmolar. Neurologic manifestations of sodium dysregulation mainly result from shrinkage or swelling of the brain, and the degree to which these changes occur depends both on the amount and the rapidity of the sodium changes.

60. **What are the most common neurologic complications of hyponatremia and hypernatremia?**
Alteration of mental status is the common neurologic alteration resulting from hyponatremia and may occur after acute reduction of serum sodium to below 130 mEq/L or with chronically depressed sodium concentrations of below 115 mEq/L. Seizures, seen in the presence of acute reduction of serum sodium to less than 125 mEq/L, are generalized in nature and signify a mortality risk of greater than 50%. Therapy includes fluid restriction or sodium replacement in severe hyponatremia. Rapid sodium replacement of sodium can result in myelinolysis (central pontine and/or extrapontine) throughout the brain due to rapid osmotic shifts. Other patients at particular risk for this complication, despite slow and carefully monitored sodium replacement, include alcoholics and those with renal disease.

Hypernatremia (serum sodium >160 mEq/L) may lead to an altered mental state, progressing to coma or seizures. Focal cerebral hemorrhage resulting from the tearing of parenchymal vessels or bridging veins (due to brain shrinkage) produces multiple neurologic symptoms, including hemiparesis, rigidity, tremor, myoclonus, cerebellar ataxia, and chorea, as well as signs of subarachnoid hemorrhage or subdural hematoma.

61. **What are the neurologic complications of hypercalcemia and hypocalcemia?**
Hypercalcemia (>12 mg/dL) leads commonly to symptoms of progressive encephalopathy and coma and more rarely to seizures or signs of corticobulbar, corticospinal, or cerebellospinal tract dysfunction. Elevated serum calcium may also produce weakness due to reduced membrane excitability at the level of the neuromuscular junction and may possibly cause a reversible myopathy.

Hypocalcemia often presents with circumoral numbness, tetany, paresthesias, seizures, and changes in mental status. Some patients develop parkinsonism after prolonged hypocalcemia. In chronic hypoglycemia, there can be calcification of the basal ganglia. Increased excitability at the neuromuscular junction with reduced serum calcium may manifest as tetany.

62. **What are the most common neurologic complications of hypomagnesemia and hypermagnesemia?**
Because, like potassium, magnesium is an intracellular ion whose intracellular concentrations are tightly controlled, the presence of neurologic complications may not directly correlate with extracellular magnesium concentrations. Hypomagnesemia, however, appears to present in patients with essentially the same findings as hypocalcemia. Because serum-ionized calcium concentrations are reduced in the presence of hypomagnesemia, some of these symptoms may, in fact, be the functional result of hypocalcemia.

Hypermagnesemia results in CNS depression and muscle paralysis. The first sign of hypermagnesemia is often a loss of deep tendon reflexes. The mechanism of CNS depression is not well understood; muscle paralysis occurs as a result of direct neuromuscular blockade.

RHEUMATOLOGIC DISEASE

63. **What are the neurologic manifestations of systemic lupus erythematosus (SLE)?**
Neurologic symptoms and signs appear as manifestations of SLE in 30% to 40% of patients, with 40% to 50% of these manifestations occurring within 1 to 2 years of diagnosis. Major risk factors for neurologic manifestations of SLE include generalized disease activity with treatment with cytotoxic agents or steroids, previous neurologic manifestations including stroke and seizure, and positive antiphospholipid antibodies. Central dysfunction includes neuropsychiatric and behavioral changes, such as dementia, psychosis, and confusional states (the most common central manifestation of SLE). While severe cognitive dysfunction occurs in only 2% to 5% of cases, mild to moderate cognitive

dysfunction is common. Localizing neurologic findings include hemiparesis, chorea, tremor, cerebellar ataxia, cranial neuropathies including optic neuritis, and transverse myelitis. Aseptic meningitis, seizures, and signs of increased intracranial pressure may also develop in SLE patients. The mean 5-year survival for patients with neurologic symptoms is 30% less than that of SLE patients without neurologic problems. Vasculitis with CNS hemorrhage accounts for a large portion of this difference.

SLE may result in a vasculitic peripheral neuropathy that may manifest as mononeuropathy, mononeuritis multiplex, a symmetric distal sensorimotor deficit. Myositis occurs in 25% of patients with SLE but is a serious complication only when the myocardium is involved.

64. **What are the major neurologic manifestations of rheumatoid arthritis (RA)?**
The major sequelae of RA are typically limited to the peripheral nervous system due to nerve entrapment near inflamed joints, perineural inflammation and demyelination of sensory nerves, and vasculitic destruction of large nerves giving rise to an asymmetric sensorimotor neuropathy. Diffuse nodular polymyositis may occur in 30% of patients with RA, although classic polymyositis is rare (5%). Focal ischemic myositis occurs as a result of a vasculitic attack on the muscle vasculature.

CNS manifestations are rare and include a polyarteritis nodosa (PAN)-like vasculitis affecting cerebral vasculature, hyperviscosity syndrome producing focal ischemic and hemorrhagic CNS lesions, and rheumatoid cervical spine disease with myelopathy most commonly occurring at C4-C5. Compression or laceration of the spinal cord may be the direct result of impaction or subluxation of one or more vertebral bodies or rings against the cord. Vascular compression syndromes may also be found in RA patients with cervical disease, especially involving the anterior spinal artery. These syndromes lead to ischemic central gray matter destruction and to necrosis of the dorsal columns and corticospinal tracts.

65. **Trigeminal neuropathy is found in which rheumatic diseases?**
Isolated trigeminal neuropathy may be the presenting sign in 10% of patients with neurologic manifestations of systemic sclerosis and occurs in 4% to 5% of all patients with systemic sclerosis. Fibrosis with nerve entrapment is the likely cause for this and other cranial neuropathies in progressive systemic sclerosis. Vasculitic damage to the trigeminal nerve is found in SLE and less commonly in mixed connective tissue disorder.

66. **What is the most common neurologic manifestation of Behçet's disease?**
CNS disease is found in 10% to 30% of Behçet's patients. An initially relapsing and remitting focal meningoencephalitis that predominantly affects the brain stem is the most common finding. Cranial nerve and long tract signs may eventually lead to spastic quadriplegia and pseudobulbar palsy. Subcortical dementia, pseudotumor cerebri, vasculitis with cerebral infarction, and peripheral neuropathy have also been reported in this disease.

VASCULITIDES

67. **Which vessels are affected by primary vasculitic disease?**
Although all vessels may be damaged in vasculitis, different vasculitides affect different vessel types. The aorta is selectively damaged in Takayasu's arteritis, whereas giant cell arteritis more commonly affects the temporal, vertebral, and carotid arteries. Medium-sized muscular intracerebral arteries are affected in polyarteritis nodosa (PAN), allergic granulomatosis, and granulomatous angiitis, whereas small muscular arteries are thrombosed in Wegener's granulomatosis. Hypersensitivity angiitis selectively involves capillaries and venules, sparing the arterial system.

68. **What are the neurologic manifestations of PAN?**
Half of patients diagnosed with PAN have evidence of peripheral neuropathy. The five following peripheral neuropathy syndromes have been identified: (1) mononeuritis multiplex of sensory and motor nerves; (2) extensive mononeuritis multiplex with severe, primarily distal weakness and sensory deficits; (3) isolated small cutaneous sensory nerve involvement; (4) distal symmetric sensorimotor neuropathy; and (5) radiculopathy. Myalgias have also been reported in 25% of patients with PAN, usually associated with weakness. Peripheral neuropathy is a common and early finding of PAN.

CNS manifestations of vasculitic disease can be found in 40% to 45% of patients with PAN, including encephalopathy, seizures (40%), and focal deficits related to infarction (50%). Cranial nerve palsies occur in 15% of patients, most commonly involving cranial nerves II, III, and VIII. Hypertensive CNS changes with papilledema and focal hemorrhages are observed in 10% of patients with an acute confusional state, and often signify a poorer prognosis. CNS sequelae are often late manifestations of this disease, occurring 2 to 3 years after the initial diagnosis.

69. **Does Churg–Strauss syndrome cause neurologic damage?**

Two-thirds of patients with allergic granulomatosis (Churg–Strauss syndrome) have CNS manifestations similar to those seen in PAN, including encephalopathy, seizures, and coma, and mononeuritis multiplex in the majority of patients. Hemorrhage is more common in this disorder than in PAN, but the clinical distinction between these two diseases rests on the almost invariable presence of pulmonary involvement with asthma in patients with Churg–Strauss syndrome, along with eosinophilia and elevated serum IgE levels.

70. **What are the neurologic effects of Wegener's granulomatosis?**

Wegener's granulomatosis presents as a triad of focal segmental glomerulonephritis, granulomas of the respiratory tract, and necrotizing vasculitis. Up to 67% of patients will have peripheral nervous system (PNS) involvement, with sensorimotor polyneuropathy and mononeuritis multiplex as the most common manifestations. Most PNS involvement develops within 2 years of disease onset. CNS manifestations are commonly the result of granulomatous invasion from the sinuses or nasal passages and may appear as exophthalmos, pituitary disease, or basilar meningitis with cranial neuropathies. The most common cranial neuropathy is of the optic nerve due to orbital granulomatous masses. Up to 5% of patients will have ICH secondary to either focal vasculitis or intragranulomatous hemorrhage.

71. **What is the clinical triad associated with temporal arteritis?**

Headache, jaw claudication, and constitutional symptoms compose the triad of clinical symptoms often found in temporal arteritis. The headache is typically boring, throbbing, or lancinating, radiating from one or both temples to the neck, jaw, tongue, or back of the head. Fever, malaise, night sweats, and anorexia with weight loss usually present early in the disease. Patients are usually older than 50 years of age, and 50% will have concomitant polymyalgia rheumatica. Mononeuritis multiplex may occur in 10% of afflicted patients. Untreated, one-third of patients will develop amaurosis fugax, monocular or binocular blindness, diplopia, or ophthalmoplegia. Cerebral infarctions or TIAs are common complications late in the disease.

72. **How is temporal arteritis diagnosed and treated?**

Evidence of an elevated sedimentation rate (>60 mm/hr by the Westergreen method) and characteristic findings of arteritis on biopsy of the temporal artery are helpful in making the diagnosis, but biopsy is frequently negative (70% diagnostic after bilateral biopsy). Treatment of temporal arteritis is with steroids and should not await biopsy (biopsy should be performed within the first few days of therapy). Treatment should continue at least 2 years with oral steroid therapy. Treatment effect is usually on the basis of sedimentation rates.

73. **What are five vasculitides whose effects are localized to the CNS?**

Cogan's syndrome produces vestibular and/or auditory dysfunction with episodic acute interstitial keratitis, scleritis, or episcleritis. **Eales' syndrome** is an isolated peripheral retinal vasculitis. Both of these rare syndromes tend to afflict young adults. **Spinal cord arteritis** is a diagnosis of exclusion, because many diseases may present with myelopathy. Among these diseases is **granulomatous angiitis of the nervous system**, the most severe isolated CNS vasculitic syndrome. **Susac syndrome** is characterized by encephalopathy, branch retinal artery occlusion, and hearing loss.

74. **What are the nervous system manifestations of granulomatous angiitis?**

Granulomatous angiitis of the nervous system is also called *isolated angiitis of the CNS.* Thirty percent of patients have elevated opening pressure on spinal tap with associated cerebrospinal fluid (CSF) pleocytosis in 65% of patients, and increased protein in 80% of patients. Cerebral angiography and brain biopsy may each be diagnostic in 50% of cases. The differential diagnosis includes other vasculitides, tuberculosis, multiple sclerosis, strokes due to emboli, sarcoidosis, syphilis, Lyme disease, drug abuse–associated CNS vasculopathy, neoplasm, and lymphomatoid granulomatosis.

PREGNANCY

75. **What is the most common neurologic symptom found during pregnancy?**

Headache is the most common neurologic symptom reported in pregnancy. While headaches occur no more frequently in pregnant women than nonpregnant reproductive age women, headaches beginning during pregnancy are a cause for concern for serious underlying illnesses that occur with higher frequency in pregnant women. These include subarachnoid hemorrhage, rapid expansion of a tumor, cortical venous thrombosis, posterior reversible encephalopathy syndrome, pseudotumor cerebri, *Listeria monocytogenes* meningitis, or preeclampsia and eclampsia. History and physical examination can usually exclude serious problems. Other headaches that may begin during pregnancy include migraines, even though the majority of female migraineurs improve during pregnancy. Onset of benign bifrontal nonmigrainous headaches is also seen in pregnancy and is most common during the first trimester. Postpartum headache is the most common self-limited headache of the puerperium and occurs in up to 40% of all women.

76. **What is eclampsia?**
Eclampsia, which means "to shine forth," is a state characterized by the neurologic complications of seizures and/or coma, presenting in a pregnant patient with preeclampsia (i.e., with signs of hypertension and proteinuria with or without edema). The risk factors for preeclampsia include nulliparity, high body mass index, family history of preeclampsia, chronic hypertension, and previous history of preeclampsia. Eclampsia occurs in 0.05% to 0.2% of all pregnancies extending beyond the 20th week of gestation. Seizures or coma develops in 50% of eclamptic patients prior to the onset of labor, with an additional 25% becoming symptomatic during labor. The remaining 25% of eclamptic patients have onset of symptoms after delivery, usually within the first 24 hours postpartum. The differential diagnosis for eclampsia includes posterior reversible encephalopathy syndrome, stroke, hypertensive encephalopathy, epilepsy, brain neoplasms and abscesses, meningitis/encephalitis, and metabolic diseases such as hypoglycemia or hypocalcemia.

77. **What is the cause of associated mortality in eclampsia?**
If present, eclampsia results in a maternal mortality of up to 14%, with associated fetal mortality of up to 28%. Maternal death from eclampsia is caused by complications of sustained intracranial and systemic hypertension. Death can be due to intracerebral hemorrhage, vasospasm, pulmonary edema, DIC, abruptio placentae, the HELLP syndrome (hemolysis, elevated liver enzymes, and low platelet count), or renal or hepatic failure from decreased organ perfusion. Systolic hypertension is the largest predictor of intracerebral hemorrhage and stroke with blood pressure reduction being associated with decreased maternal morbidity and mortality. Fetal mortality results from decreased uteroplacental perfusion.

78. **How is eclampsia treated?**
The primary objective of treatment is to reduce blood pressure without compromising either uteroplacental or maternal renal perfusion. Intracranial hypertension is usually present in patients with encephalopathy or coma, and thus intracranial pressure should be monitored in such persons and managed with intubation and hyperventilation. These patients should also be imaged by computed tomography to assess for ICH and cerebral edema.

Eclamptic seizures must be aggressively controlled due to increased fetal mortality and increased intracranial pressure in the mother. Magnesium sulfate is the treatment of choice for prevention of seizures from preeclampsia as well as treatment of seizures from eclampsia. Magnesium sulfate has been shown to be superior to both phenytoin and diazepam in reducing the risk of recurrence of seizures in the treatment of eclampsia.

The definitive treatment for eclampsia occurring before birth is termination of the pregnancy by delivery of the fetus. The risk of recurrent seizures decreases within 24 hours following delivery, and long-term prophylaxis of eclampsia-induced seizures is unnecessary. Although hypertension resolves more slowly, normalization of blood pressure occurs in the first postpartum week.

79. **Is the risk for stroke altered in pregnancy?**
Cerebrovascular ischemic events occur 13 times more frequently in pregnant patients than in age-matched nonpregnant women, with an overall stroke risk of 1 in 3000 pregnancies. Stroke accounts for 10% of all maternal deaths during pregnancy, and 35% of all strokes in female patients aged 15 to 45 years occur during pregnancy or in the puerperium. Atherosclerotic disease is less commonly a cause for stroke in this population than is arterial embolus or cerebral venous thrombosis (Fig. 24-1).

80. **How does the physician clinically distinguish puerperal cerebral venous thrombosis from arterial thrombosis?**
Cerebral venous thrombosis usually occurs in the first three postpartum weeks and commonly presents with headache, focal or generalized seizures, stupor or coma, transient focal deficits, and/or signs of increased intracranial pressure. Rare thromboses include superior sagittal sinus thrombosis, with paraplegia and sensory deficits of the leg and bladder dysfunction, and Rolandic vein thrombosis, with sensory and motor deficits of the leg, hip, and shoulder, sparing the face and arm. Mortality in sagittal sinus thrombosis approaches 40% but may be reduced to 20% with intensive care and anticoagulants. Recovery of survivors is usually complete.

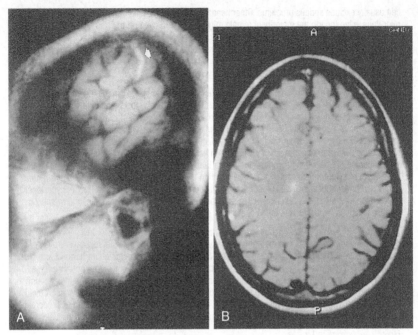

Figure 24-1. T1-weighted sagittal view of the superficial cerebral cortex of the parietal lobe, showing a cerebral vein thrombosis (**A,** *arrow*). The axial T1 view (**B**) shows the small hemorrhagic infarction caused by the venous thrombosis.

Arterial thrombosis is rarer than either arterial embolus or venous thrombosis, is more likely to occur in the second or third trimester than in the puerperium, and commonly presents with persistent focal deficit, such as hemiparesis, without alteration of consciousness, seizures, or signs of increased intracranial pressure.

An immune mechanism has been hypothesized for a significant percentage of pregnancy-related venous and arterial thromboses. The presence of antiphospholipid antibodies should be sought, especially when a history of previous miscarriages or preeclampsia is obtained.

81. What is the differential diagnosis for seizures during childbirth?

Eclampsia, **HELLP syndrome**, and **TTP** are the most commonly observed causes for seizures during the third trimester. **Amniotic fluid embolism**, **water intoxication**, **autonomic stress in patients with upper spinal cord injury**, and **toxicity from local anesthetics** are all intrapartum causes for seizures. **Cerebral venous thrombosis** usually occurs postpartum and may present with seizures.

Subarachnoid hemorrhage may occur at any time during pregnancy and may produce seizures, although aneurysms most commonly rupture during the third trimester, with greatest risk for rebleeding in the postpartum period. Arteriovenous malformations are more likely to rupture in the second trimester and rebleed during delivery or with subsequent pregnancies. **Epilepsy** may manifest at any time before, during, or after pregnancy and may require lifelong therapy. However, such patients must be distinguished from those with **gestational epilepsy**, which requires therapy only during pregnancy.

82. How should therapy of epilepsy change during pregnancy?

Because all anticonvulsants have some potential to be teratogenic or harmful to the fetus, treatment should be aimed toward monotherapy at the lowest functionally effective dose.

Due to physiologic changes that occur in pregnancy the pharmacokinetics of anticonvulsants are usually altered. Effective prepregnancy anticonvulsant levels should be used as the target levels during pregnancy. Drug levels should be measured as soon as pregnancy is diagnosed because blood concentrations of anticonvulsants may drop precipitously during the first trimester, as a result of alterations in drug absorption, metabolism, or protein binding. This is especially true for phenytoin, with its nonlinear kinetics, in which doses may need to be increased by 50% to 100% during pregnancy to maintain prepregnancy levels. Routine drug levels should be measured each trimester and more frequently if either seizure control worsens or if patients have a history of previous alterations in drug levels during pregnancy. Because drug clearance returns to prepregnancy norms within 3 to 6 weeks postpartum, prepregnancy anticonvulsant doses should be gradually introduced during this period.

All patients of childbearing age should take folic acid to lower risks of neural tube defects, which have a higher incidence in children born to women taking anticonvulsants. Women of childbearing potential on anticonvulsants should be on folic acid even prior to conception, and doses up to 4 mg should be prescribed as soon as pregnancy is suspected.

83. **What neuropathies are commonly associated with pregnancy and childbirth?**
Prior to birth, **carpal tunnel syndrome** is the most commonly associated neuropathy. Treatment is conservative with wrist splinting, and it commonly resolves within 3 months postpartum. **Meralgia paresthetica** (numbness or dysesthesia of the anterolateral thigh due to compression of the lateral femoral cutaneous nerve along the pelvic wall or obturator canal) occurs as the fetus enlarges, and also typically resolves within 3 months of delivery. Bell's palsy is seen with increased frequency in pregnant women. Treatment with corticosteroids during pregnancy for the treatment of Bell's palsy is still controversial.

Traumatic mononeuropathy usually occurs during childbirth. Trauma involving the obturator nerve may result from compression by the fetal head, from misplaced forceps, or from hyperflexion in the lithotomy position. Compression injuries during delivery have also been reported involving the femoral, saphenous, common peroneal, or sciatic nerves. Postpartum footdrop is an interesting example of traumatic mononeuropathy with generally excellent prognosis, most typically observed in short primigravid women with large infants.

IATROGENIC (DRUG INDUCED)

84. **What factors are important with regard to an increased risk for seizures due to drug therapy?**
High-dose intrathecal or intravenous administration, blood–brain barrier permeability, prior history or family history of epilepsy, preexisting cerebral or systemic disease (renal, liver disease), and abrupt withdrawal.

85. **What drugs are associated with increased seizure risk at therapeutic dose and serum levels?**
Tricyclic antidepressants (1%), aliphatic (chlorpromazine, promazine, prochlorperazine) phenothiazines (1% to 2%), and tetracyclic antidepressants.

86. **What drugs are associated with the development of pseudotumor cerebri?**
Pseudotumor cerebri is characterized by headache, papilledema, diplopia, and impaired vision due to raised intracranial pressure possibly due to CSF malabsorption. Drugs associated with its development include oral contraceptives, estrogens, tetracyclines, nalidixic acid, nitrofurantoin, ketamine, nitrous oxide, vitamin A, and retinoids such as isotretinoin and acitretin, minocycline, danazol, ampicillin, amiodarone, etretinate, and thyroxine. Abrupt withdrawal of corticosteroids has been associated with its development in children.

87. **What drugs induce movement disorders?**
Major classes of psychotropic drugs, antiparkinsonian agents, and tricyclic antidepressants may induce involuntary movements or changes in muscle tone and posture associated with action on dopaminergic neurotransmission.

88. **What extrapyramidal disorders can be induced by drugs?**
Acute dystonic–dyskinetic reactions, akathisia, tardive dyskinesia, chorea and choreoathetosis, drug-induced parkinsonism, neuroleptic malignant syndrome, tremor, tic, and myoclonus.

89. **What category of drugs affects or induces neuromuscular disorders?**
Peripheral neuropathy
- Antimicrobial (isoniazid, ethambutol, dapsone, fluoroquinolones, metronidazole, antiretrovirals)
- Antineoplastic (vinca alkaloids, platinum analogs, taxanes, sorafenib, thalidomide)

- Antirheumatic (chloroquine, gold treatment, D-penicillamine)
- Cardiovascular (amiodarone)
- Other: colchicine

Neuromuscular junction (* aggravation or unmasking of myasthenia gravis)
- Antimicrobial (aminoglycosides, fluoroquinolones, telithromycin)*
- Anticonvulsants (phenytoin)
- Antirheumatic (D-penicillamine, chloroquine)
- Cardiovascular (quinidine, propranolol)*
- Psychotropic (lithium, chlorpromazine)*
- Muscle relaxants*

Muscle (rhabdomyolysis,* neuroleptic malignant syndrome,** cramps/myalgias,[†] myopathy[‡])
- Amphotericin B*
- Antirheumatic (gold,[†] D-penicillamine,[†] steroid*)
- Psychotropic (lithium,* haloperidol,** fluphenazine**)
- Sedatives (barbiturates, diazepam)*
- Analgesics (heroin, morphine, salicylates, codeine)*
- Cardiovascular (statins,[‡] clofibrate,* labetalol,[†] captopril[†])
- Anesthetics (suxamethonium*)

 References available online at expertconsult.com.

WEBSITES

http://www.wilsonsdisease.org
http://www.sjogrens.com
http://www.neuropathy.org

BIBLIOGRAPHY

1. Aminoff MJ, Josephson SA: Aminoff's Neurology and General Medicine, 5th ed. Philadelphia, Elsevier, 2014.
2. Daroff RB, Jankovic J, Mazziotta JC, Pomeroy SL: Bradley's Neurology in Clinical Practice, 7th ed. Philadelphia, Elsevier, 2015.
3. Rosenbaum RB, Campbell SM, Rosenbaum JT: Clinical Neurology of Rheumatic Diseases, Boston, Butterworth-Heinemann, 1996.
4. Samuels MA, Feske S (eds): Office Practice of Neurology, 2nd ed. New York, Churchill-Livingstone, 2003.

CHAPTER 25

INFECTIOUS DISEASES OF THE NERVOUS SYSTEM

Rohini Samudralwar, Colin Van Hook, Joseph S. Kass

CEREBROSPINAL FLUID

1. What is the normal composition of cerebrospinal fluid (CSF)?
   See Table 25-1.

Table 25-1. Normal Composition of Cerebrospinal Fluid (CSF)

OPENING PRESSURE	WBC	RBC	PROTEIN	GLUCOSE
8-15 mm Hg or 100-180 mm H_2O	0-5/mm^3	0/mm^3	15-45 mg/dL	45-80 mg/dL

WBC, White blood cells; RBC, red blood cells.
From Irani DN: *Cerebrospinal Fluid in Clinical Practice*. Philadelphia, Elsevier, 2009.

2. List common contraindications to performing a lumbar puncture.
   - Infection: cellulitis, abscess
   - Space-occupying lesion
   - Uncal, central, transtentorial, or cerebellar herniation
   - Coagulopathy: thrombocytopenia, liver failure, anticoagulant use

3. List the major complications of a lumbar puncture.
   - Headache
   - CSF leak
   - Infection
   - Bleeding
   - Rarely herniation

4. Describe the basic technique involved in performing a lumbar puncture.
   - Obtain computed tomography/magnetic resonance imaging (CT/MRI) brain indicated for patients with papilledema, altered mental status, focal neurologic deficit, new-onset seizure, or immuno-compromised state.
   - Ensure that platelet count is >50,000, and international normalized ratio is <1.5.
   - Place patient in lateral decubitus position, with knees and neck flexed.
   - Ensure patient's back is as close to edge of bed as possible.
   - Palpate top of iliac crest and then place thumb of same hand in the interspace forming a vertical line with the top of the iliac crest.
   - The identified location indicates the L3-L4 space. The needle can be placed into the L3-L4, L4-L5, or L5-S1 interspaces.
   - Avoid L2-L3 interspace and higher since the conus medullaris terminates at L1-L2.
   - Insert needle, with the bevel parallel to longitudinal fibers of the supraspinous ligament.
   - Advance needle, and a "pop" should be felt, indicating the piercing of the needle through the supraspinous ligament. Advance needle into the subarachnoid space.

5. Describe the typical composition of CSF by type of infectious agent.
   See Table 25-2.

Table 25-2. Typical Findings in Cerebrospinal Fluid (CSF) by Type of Infection

	OPENING PRESSURE	WBC	PROTEIN	GLUCOSE
Bacterial	Elevated	>1000/mm^3 PMN predominance	>120 mg/dL	<30 mg/dL
Viral	Normal	<100/mm^3 Lymphocytic predominance	Normal-elevated	Normal
Fungal	Normal-slightly elevated	20-500/mm^3 Lymphocytic predominance	Elevated	Decreased
Tuberculosis	Elevated	10-500/mm^3 Lymphocytic predominance	100-500 mg/dL	35-40 mg/dL
Syphilis	Increased	Mononuclear predominance	Elevated	Normal
Lyme disease	Normal	Lymphocytic predominance	Increased	Normal

WBC, White blood cells; PMN, polymorphonuclear leukocyte.

BACTERIAL MENINGITIS

6. Name the common pathogens causing bacterial meningitis by population group, and indicate the typical empiric therapy for these bacterial pathogens.
   See Table 25-3.

Table 25-3. Bacterial Meningitis by Population Type and Appropriate Therapy

POPULATION GROUP	COMMON PATHOGENS	EMPIRIC THERAPY
Newborns	Gram negative: Escherichia coli, Klebsiella, Enterobacter, Proteus group B streptococci: Streptococcus agalactiae	Cefotaxime + Ampicillin
Infants and children	Neisseria meningitidis, Streptococcus pneumoniae, Hemophilus influenzae	Ceftriaxone or cefotaxime plus vancomycin
Healthy, immunocompetent	N. meningitidis, S. pneumoniae, Listeria monocytogenes	Third/fourth-generation cephalosporin plus ampicillin plus vancomycin
Nosocomial/postneurosurgical	Gram-negative Enterobacteriaceae, Pseudomonas aeruginosa, staphylococci	Meropenem plus vancomycin
Ventriculitis	Staphylococcus epidermidis, Staphylococcus aureus, gram-negative Enterobacteriaceae, P. aeruginosa	Meropenem plus vancomycin
Elderly	L. monocytogenes, gram-negative Enterobacteriaceae, P. aeruginosa, pneumococci	Third/fourth-generation cephalosporin plus ampicillin plus vancomycin

From Roos KL (Editor): *Principles of Neurologic Infectious Diseases: Principles and Practice.* New York, McGraw-Hill, 2004.

7. When is chemoprophylaxis for meningococcal meningitis appropriate, and what antimicrobials can be used?
   Every person sleeping in the same house and those contacts engaging in saliva exchanging oropharyngeal secretions should undergo chemoprophylaxis.
   • Rifampin: adults, infants

- Ciprofloxacin: adults
- Ceftriaxone: adults, children

8. What is the role of adjunctive corticosteroids in the treatment of bacterial meningitis?

    The benefits of intravenous corticosteroids in bacterial meningitis come from the reduction of the inflammatory process that leads to significant morbidity and mortality. Corticosteroids are thought to help decrease intracranial pressure (ICP) and reduce brain edema and meningeal inflammation. In children, corticosteroids have been shown to reduce the incidence of sensorineural hearing loss. Studies in adults showed protection in patients with *Streptococcus pneumoniae* meningitis. Treatment showed association with significant reduction in unfavorable outcome and mortality. The dosing regimen is dexamethasone 4 mg intravenously every 6 hours for 4 days with the first dose given 30 minutes prior to the first dose of antibiotics. If the CSF cultures indicate the pathogen is not *S. pneumoniae*, the dexamethasone may be discontinued.

9. Describe the pathogenesis, common clinical findings, diagnostic approach, neuroimaging findings, and complications of bacterial meningitis.

    See Table 25-4.

Table 25-4. Bacterial Meningitis

Pathogenesis	Bacteria enter subarachnoid space → replication and autolysis → release of bacterial components in CSF → release of proinflammatory host factors
Clinical findings	Stiff neck, headache, fever, photophobia, malaise, vomiting, lethargy → deterioration of level of consciousness
Diagnosis	Lumbar puncture: elevated opening pressure, polymorphonuclear leukocytic pleocytosis, elevated protein, low glucose, and elevated lactate in post-neurosurgical patients, gram-stained smear, CSF culture Blood cultures, CRP/ESR
CT/MRI findings	Cerebral edema, hydrocephalus, ventriculitis, vasculitis, septic embolism, sinus venous thrombus causing infarction, intracranial free air due to dural leak
Complications	Death with highest mortality in pneumococcal and *Listeria* meningitis Sensorineural hearing loss Hemiparesis, epileptic seizures, hemianopia, ataxia, cranial nerve palsies

CSF, Cerebrospinal fluid; *CRP*, C-reactive protein; *ESR*, sedimentation rate.
Data from Roos KL: Meningitis: 100 Maxims. London, Arnold, 1996

BRAIN AND EPIDURAL ABSCESSES AND SUBDURAL EMPYEMA

10. Compare the etiology, pathophysiology, clinical presentation, diagnostic approach, and treatment of a bacterial brain abscess, a cranial epidural abscess, and a subdural empyema.

    See Table 25-5.

11. Describe the epidemiology, pathogenesis, clinical features, diagnostic approach, and differential diagnosis of viral meningitis.

    See Table 25-6.

Table 25-5. Abscesses and Empyema

	ETIOLOGY	PATHOPHYSIOLOGY	CLINICAL PRESENTATION	DIAGNOSIS	TREATMENT
Bacterial brain abscess	MCC: streptococci and anaerobes Posttrauma/surgery: *Staphylococcus aureus*, Enterobacteriaceae, *Pseudomonas aeruginosa*	Direct spread from contiguous sites (e.g., sinusitis, mastoiditis, otitis media) Hematogenous spread from remote site of infection After cranial trauma/surgery	Fever, headache, focal neurologic deficit, seizures	CT with contrast: hypodense lesion with typically thin ring of contrast enhancement around edge MRI brain with contrast: ring-enhancing lesion	Antimicrobial therapy and, if amenable, aspiration, drainage, or excision
Cranial epidural abscess	Similar to brain abscess	Frontal sinus, middle ear, mastoid, orbit infection reaches epidural space through retrograde spread into emissary veins, direct spread of bone infection, or through craniotomy	Hemicranial headache with fever	MRI: crescent-shaped purulent fluid collection seen more prominently on T1 sequence	Immediate neurosurgical drainage, empiric antimicrobial therapy with third- or fourth-generation cephalosporin, metronidazole, and vancomycin for 4-6 weeks after drainage followed by 2-3 months of oral antibiotic
Subdural empyema	Aerobic, microaerophilic, and anaerobic streptococci; staphylococci from neurosurgical procedure	Collection of pus between dura and arachnoid, most common predisposing condition is paranasal sinusitis Less common: mastoiditis, neurosurgical procedure	Signs of infection, increased ICP from expanding lesion, stroke, headache, altered mental status, focal deficit	MRI with gadolinium: T1 and FLAIR sequences	Evacuation by drainage or craniotomy, empiric therapy with third- or fourth-generation cephalosporin, metronidazole, vancomycin for 2-3 weeks intravenously then oral antibiotic for 6 weeks

MCC, Most common cause; *CT*, computed tomography; *MRI*, magnetic resonance imaging; *ICP*, intracranial pressure; *FLAIR*, fluid attenuation inversion recovery.

Table 25-6. Viral Meningitis	
Epidemiology	**Enterovirus:** MCC, immunocompetent, hypogammaglobulinemia **Arbovirus:** immunocompetent, blood donors, organ transplant (WNV) **LCM:** mice/hamster owners/handlers **EBV:** oral secretions, allogeneic bone marrow transplant
Pathogenesis	**Enterovirus:** fecal–oral contamination → replication in intestinal lining → viremia and seeding of CNS. Clearance by antibody mechanism **Arbovirus:** mosquito/tick bite → local replication in tissues and lymph nodes → viremia and seeding of CNS **HSV:** inoculation during time of genital infection → latent infection in sacral DRG → reactivation of genital lesions, radiculitis, and meningitis
Clinical features	Fever, frontal/retro-orbital headache, pain on extraocular movements, photophobia, neck stiffness, maculopapular erythematous rash from face to trunk. Focal deficits and seizure not seen
Diagnosis, CSF studies	Lymphocytic pleocytosis, normal-mildly decreased (enterovirus, HSV-2, VZV) glucose, normal-mildly increased protein **Enterovirus:** RT-PCR, throat/stool culture (presumptive diagnosis) **Arbovirus:** antibody titer in serum, IgM antibody in CSF PCR: WNV, HSV, EBV, HIV
Differential diagnosis	Fungal (MCC: cryptococcal), *Mycobacterium tuberculosis*, and Lyme disease

DRG, Dorsal root ganglion; *WNV,* West Nile virus; *LCM,* lymphocytic choriomeningitis; *MCC,* most common cause; *EBV,* Epstein–Barr virus; *CNS,* central nervous system; *HSV,* herpes simplex virus; *VZV,* varicella zoster virus; *RT-PCR,* reverse transcription polymerase chain reaction; *CSF,* cerebrospinal fluid; *HIV,* human immunodeficiency virus.

12. **Describe the pathogenesis, clinical features, diagnostic approach, treatment, and common complications of viral encephalitis.**
    See Table 25-7.

13. **What are the epidemiology and pathogenesis of common forms of fungal meningitis?**
    Fungal meningitis typically results from lymphatic and hematogenous spread from the lungs. Typically, an immunocompetent host will eliminate the fungus by exhalation. At-risk patients include those with defective cell-mediated immunity due to human immunodeficiency virus (HIV), neutropenia, or immunosuppressive medications such as corticosteroids or cytotoxic chemotherapeutic agents. A notable exception to this pathogenesis are *Candida* species since they colonize human mucosa and may enter systemic circulation through both wounds and intravenous catheters. The epidemiology of central nervous system (CNS) fungal infections is rapidly changing with expanded use of antiretroviral therapy in HIV-infected patients. *Cryptococcus neoformans* remains by far the most common CNS fungal infection, with an annual global incidence of over 1 million cases, resulting in 600,000 deaths.

14. **What are the typical clinical features of fungal meningitis, and how is it diagnosed?**
    Fungal meningitis may follow an acute, subacute, or chronic course and commonly presents with fever, headache, and mental status changes. Focal neurologic symptoms and seizures may develop in the setting of space-occupying lesions.

15. **What is the differential diagnosis of fungal meningitis?**
    Fungal meningitis presents with a clinical course and CSF profile similar to that of partially treated bacterial or tuberculous meningitis. Noninfectious considerations include sarcoidosis, Beçhet's disease, and carcinomatous/lymphomatous meningitis.

16. **What are the expected CSF findings in common types of fungal meningitis?**
    The CSF will show a normal to slight elevation in opening pressure with 20 to 500 cells/cc, increased protein, decreased glucose, and a lymphocytic predominance (although *Coccidioides immitis* and other less common pathogens may show a neutrophil predominance early in the disease course).

	Other Diagnostic Testing
Cryptococcus species	CSF: India ink stain, cryptococcal antigen; stain and culture Serum: cryptococcal antigen Other: biopsy of skin lesions
Evacuation by drainage or craniotomy	CSF: +/– eosinophilia; serology; stain and culture Serum: eosinophilia
Histoplasma capsulatum	CSF: Histoplasma serology; stain and culture Blood and urine: histoplasma antigen
Candida species	CSF: stain and culture Other: biopsy of skin lesion, culture of catheters

Table 25-7. Viral Encephalitis

Pathogenesis: direct CNS invasion by virus or immune-mediated response	**Arthropod:** inoculation from mosquito → local replication → viremia → infection of cerebral capillary endothelial cells → neurons OR choroid plexus → intraventricular CSF → ventricular ependymal cells → periventricular cerebral tissue (prefer basal ganglia and thalami) **HSV:** retrograde axoplasmic flow of virus in the axons of a division of trigeminal nerve → latent infection in the ganglion and reactivation (prefer inferior and medial temporal lobes)
Clinical features	**Arthropod:** nonspecific, increased lethargy and behavioral changes, or brief single seizures, rashes in WNV, parkinsonian features, poliomyelitis-like syndrome **HSV:** subacute fever, headache, behavioral changes, focal seizure activity, and neurologic deficits **VZV:** subacute small and large vessel ischemic and hemorrhagic infarctions
Diagnosis, CSF studies	**Arthropod** **CSF:** antibody titer or immunoassay **MRI:** hyperintense lesions on FLAIR in subcortical areas, basal ganglia **HSV** **CSF:** +HSV PCR **MRI:** hyperintensity on T2 FLAIR sequence in medial and inferior temporal lobe up to insula with CSF correlation, at times hemorrhagic **EEG:** PLEDS over temporal lobes **VZV** **CSF:** antibody titer more sensitive than PCR **MRI:** large- and small-vessel ischemic and hemorrhagic infarctions and spherical subcortical white matter lesions
Treatment	**Arthropod:** supportive care and management of neurologic complications; ribavirin for La Crosse virus **HSV:** acyclovir 10 mg/kg q 8h × 3 weeks **VZV:** acyclovir 10 mg/kg q 8h × 3 weeks **CMV:** foscarnet and gancyclovir
Common complications	Seizures, increased ICP, multifocal neurologic deficits, cognitive impairment, myelitis, death

WNV, West Nile virus; *HSV*, herpes simplex virus-1; *VZV*, varicella zoster virus; *CNS*, central nervous system; *CSF*, cerebrospinal fluid; *VZV*, varicella zoster virus; *MRI*, magnetic resonance imaging; *EEG*, electroencephalogram; *PCR*, polymer chain reaction; *FLAIR*, fluid attenuation inversion recovery; *CMV*, cytomegalovirus; *ICP*, intracranial pressure.

17. What are the appropriate antimicrobial agents for cryptococcal meningitis?
The mainstay of treatment for fungal CNS infections remains intravenous amphotericin B, often in conjunction with flucytosine or azoles. Treatment of cryptococcal meningitis is often divided into induction, maintenance, and clearance phases.

18. What are some important complications of fungal meningitis?
Fungal CNS infections typically present as a basilar meningitis and may lead to cranial palsies and optic neuritis. Patients may also develop communicating hydrocephalus requiring neurosurgical shunt procedures. Patients with mass lesions >3 cm should be considered for surgical debridement. Such lesions may lead to the development of seizures or focal neurologic deficits. Cryptococcal meningitis is notorious for causing elevated ICP. Serial lumbar punctures may be needed to reduce ICP and prevent irreversible complications of increased ICP such as blindness.

CNS TUBERCULOSIS

19. What are the epidemiology and pathogenesis of CNS tuberculosis?
Incidence of tuberculosis (TB) remains highest in Southeast Asia, sub-Saharan Africa, and Eastern Europe. The Centers for Disease Control (CDC) estimated the incidence of TB to be 3.0 per 100,000 in 2013. Development of tuberculous meningitis is not limited to immunocompromised patients and may occur in up to 10% of untreated TB in the immunocompetent.
Mycobacterium tuberculosis has no natural reservoir other than infected hosts. It is spread by aerosolized droplets that allow bacilli to colonize the alveoli before spreading hematogenously to numerous sites throughout the body, including the CNS. Tubercles of mononuclear cells around a center of caseating necrosis form in secondary sites such as the brain, which then rupture, allowing spread throughout the CNS.

20. What are the typical clinical features of CNS tuberculosis, and how is it diagnosed?
CNS tuberculosis may present as an acute meningitic syndrome with headache, altered mental status, increased intracranial pressure, meningismus, seizures, and focal neurologic symptoms. Subacutely, it may present as cranial nerve deficits due to coating of the nerves by exudate as a result of a hyper-sensitivity reaction to basilar meningitis. Often, it may present chronically as a slowly progressive dementing illness with abulia and incontinence due to frontal lobe deficits.

21. What is the differential diagnosis of CNS tuberculosis?
Fungal or partially treated bacterial meningitis as well as viral encephalitis can present with a similar CSF profile. Noninfectious considerations include autoimmune encephalitis, carcinomatous o lymphomatous meningitis, neurosarcoidosis, CNS sarcoidosis, Behçet's syndrome, systemic lupus erythematosus, Mollaret's meningitis, and Wegener's granulomatosis.

22. What are the expected CSF findings in CNS tuberculosis?
Patients will have an elevated opening pressure, increased white blood cell count with 10 to 500 cells/cc with lymphocytic predominance, increased protein of 100 to 500 mg/dL, and decreased glucose. Cultures are positive in 75% of cases and require 3 to 6 weeks of growth.

23. What are the appropriate antimicrobial agents for CNS tuberculosis?
CNS tuberculosis is typically treated with 9 to 12 months of therapy consisting of 2 months of isoniazid, rifampin, pyrazinamide, and ethambutol followed by isoniazid and rifampin alone.

24. What are some common complications of CNS tuberculosis?
Patients may commonly develop communicating hydrocephalus, infarctions due to vasculitis or direct invasion of blood vessel walls, cranial nerve deficits, seizures, cognitive impairment, myelitis, and radiculitis.

25. What is the effect of coinfection with HIV on CNS tuberculosis?
The clinical presentation of tuberculous meningitis is very similar in HIV and non-HIV-infected individuals, although HIV-infected patients are more likely to have mass lesions and extrameningeal TB at time of presentation.

1. Patients suspected of having bacterial meningitis should be treated with antibiotics and dexamethasone emergently. Administration of antibiotics should not be delayed for lumbar puncture or CT scan, although these studies should be performed as rapidly after presentation as possible. The choice of empiric antibiotics depends on the patient's age and other clinical factors (recent neurosurgery, immunocompromised state, etc.) to cover the most likely organisms.
2. Clinicians should maintain a high index of suspicion for the presence of herpes simplex virus-1 (HSV-1) encephalitis as it is the most common cause of nonepidemic viral encephalitis and is treatable with intravenous acyclovir. Delay in treatment will increase the risk of poor outcome.
3. Fungal meningitis may present as a chronic, subacute, or acute condition. Both immunocompetent and immunocompromised patients may present with fungal meningitis. Given the prevalence of certain fungi in particular geographic regions, a travel history should be obtained to broaden the differential diagnosis and obtain more specific fungal serologies in the CSF.
4. Increased intracranial pressure is a common complication of cryptococcal meningitis and repeated lumbar punctures will be necessary over the course of inpatient treatment to relieve and monitor intracranial pressure and reduce the risks of complications such as blindness.
5. TB meningitis and fungal meningitis are common causes of basilar meningitis, resulting in cranial nerve dysfunction and hydrocephalus.

NEUROSYPHILIS

26. **What are the epidemiology and pathogenesis of neurosyphilis?**
Since the advent of penicillin, rates of syphilis infection have dropped sharply but have become concentrated among people with lower socioeconomic status and have continued to wax and wane in 10- to 15-year cycles. While neurosyphilis is not reported to the CDC, rates of primary and secondary syphilis increased from 2.9 to 5.3 per 100,000 between 2005 and 2013, with men being at much higher risk than women.
      Syphilis is due to infection with the spirochete *Treponema pallidum*. As in other organs, the pathology of syphilis in the CNS is related to inflammation and fibroblast proliferation in the walls of blood vessels leading to luminal stenosis and ischemia. Clinical manifestations vary based on the size of affected vessels.

27. **What are the typical clinical features of neurosyphilis and how is it diagnosed?**
Neurosyphilis is typically diagnosed by the combination of clinical presentation, routine CSF studies, and serologic tests, which can be divided into treponemal and nontreponemal. Neurosyphilis is not synonymous with late or tertiary syphilis, with a variety of forms occurring over the lifespan of infection. Common nontreponemal tests are the rapid plasma reagent and Venereal Disease Research Lab (VDRL) tests. While both become elevated early in the disease course, levels fall in later stages of the disease. A positive CSF VDRL is a highly specific but insensitive marker for diagnosis, with false positives due to pregnancy and a variety of infectious and autoimmune conditions.
      Treponemal tests include the fluorescent treponemal antibody (FTA) test, and *T. pallidum* hemagglutination assays (TP-HA) are highly sensitive but less specific. While the VDRL titer falls following treatment, FTA-ABS and TP-HA remain positive for life.
      Neurosyphilis can follow a variety of clinical syndromes:
1. Syphilitic meningitis: characterized by headache, meningismus, and possibly cranial nerve involvement. Typically occurs in the first 1 to 2 years of infection.
2. Meningovascular syphilis: patients present with signs and symptoms of both meningitis and ischemic infarctions resulting in focal neurologic signs such as hemiparesis as well as seizures and altered mental status. Typically occurs in the first 10 years of infection.
3. Parenchymatous neurosyphilis (general paresis of the insane): subacute to chronic dementing illness with impairment in memory, concentration, and potentially pain and ataxia due to tabes dorsalis. Late complication of untreated syphilis.
4. Tabes dorsalis: due to involvement of the dorsal columns of the spinal cord and the dorsal root ganglia presenting with sensory ataxia, tabetic gait, positive Romberg's sign, and lancinating pain. Late complication of untreated syphilis.

5. Gummatous neurosyphilis: symptoms are related to location of gummatous mass lesion; rarely encountered today. Late complication of untreated syphilis.

6. Asymptomatic: incidental finding upon lumbar puncture.

28. What is the differential diagnosis of neurosyphilis?
    • Syphilitic meningitis: viral or aseptic meningitis, *Cryptococcus* and TB meningitis should be considered in HIV-positive patients.
    • Meningovascular syphilis: other causes of stroke in the young such as either hypercoagulability or dissection.
    • Parenchymatous neurosyphilis: prion disease, autoimmune encephalitis, Hashimoto's encephalopathy, paraneoplastic encephalitis, neurodegenerative conditions such as frontotemporal dementia, corticobasal syndrome, Alzheimer's disease, dementia with Lewy bodies, and progressive supranuclear palsy.
    • Gummatous neurosyphilis: CNS tumors.

29. What are the expected CSF findings in neurosyphilis by manifestation and how is the infection treated?
    Regardless of symptomatic disease, the CSF of patients with neurosyphilis will likely show mildly elevated protein and mild lymphocytic pleocytosis. Glucose levels are often normal.
    Treatment of neurosyphilis consists of benzathine penicillin 4 million units intravenously every 4h for 10 to 14 days.

30. What are some important complications of neurosyphilis?
    Involvement of CN (cranial nerve) VII and VIII is common, as are optic neuritis, chorioretinitis, retinal vasculitis, neuroretinitis, and anterior or posterior uveitis. Patients with radiculitis may develop bowel and bladder dysfunction as well as lancinating pains. The Jarisch–Herxheimer reaction consists of fever, hypotension, tachycardia, headaches, and myalgias and may occur within 24h of initiation of treatment due to release of antigens from dead spirochetes.

31. What is the effect of coinfection with HIV on neurosyphilis?
    HIV infection is widely believed to increase the risk of developing neurosyphilis. Patients with HIV coinfection may be at increased risk of relapse despite appropriate treatment.

LYME AND NERVOUS SYSTEM

32. What are the epidemiology and pathogenesis of neuro-Lyme?
    The rate of Lyme disease reported to the CDC was 7.85 per 100,000 in 2005, with approximately 10% to 15% of these developing nervous system involvement. Peak incidence is in the summer months with an endemic area in the continental United States focused in the Northeast.
    The spirochete *Borrelia burgdorferi* is injected into the skin by the *Ixodes ricinus* tick and spreads hematogenously to affect other organs. The characteristic target-shaped erythema migrans rash appears at the site of inoculation as well as elsewhere on the body in the first few days to weeks following infection. Meningeal irritation and other neurologic symptoms develop after several weeks to months.

33. What are the typical clinical features of neuro-Lyme, and how is Lyme disease diagnosed?
    The most common clinical manifestations of neuro-Lyme are referred to as *Garin–Bujadoux–Bannwarth syndrome*, which consists of the triad of lymphocytic meningitis, cranial neuritis, and polyradiculitis. Meningitis typically follows a longer, more subacute course than viral etiologies. Cranial neuropathy typically affected CN VII, often bilaterally, with occasional involvement of CN III, IV, VI, and VIII. Polyradiculitis is difficult to distinguish clinically from mechanical compression and is characterized by dermatomal pain, weakness, and decreased reflexes.
    Two-tiered serologic testing is required to diagnose Lyme disease in the serum. Patients are screened with enzyme-linked immunosorbent assay (ELISA) for anti-*B. burgdorferi* antibodies. If positive, they are then tested for specific antigens by Western blot for both IgM and IgG antibodies. CNS involvement is confirmed when a patient has a typical neurologic neuro-Lyme syndrome and when CSF analysis reveals that the relative concentration of specific antibody in the CSF exceeds that in the serum.

34. **What is the differential diagnosis of neuro-Lyme?**
Neuro-Lyme disease can affect both the central and peripheral nervous system, and diagnostic considerations should be based according to presentation. Chronic meningitis may mimic tuberculous, syphilitic, lupus, or sarcoidosis meningitis. Cranial neuropathies typically involve the seventh nerve and may present similarly to idiopathic facial nerve palsy, Guillain–Barré syndrome, HIV, and basilar meningitides such as sarcoidosis, TB, or fungal infections. Radiculoneuritis develops subacutely to chronically and may mimic mechanical compression of the nerve root as well as a host of other toxic, metabolic, infectious, autoimmune, paraneoplastic, and neoplastic radiculoneuropathies.

35. **What are the expected CSF findings in neuro-Lyme?**
CSF findings are those of an aseptic meningitis with lymphocytic pleocytosis, typically <200 cells/μL, protein typically <150 mg/dL, and normal glucose.

36. **What are the appropriate antimicrobial agents for neuro-Lyme?**
Treatment typically consists of oral doxycycline for 2 to 4 weeks with intravenous ceftriaxone, cefotaxime, or penicillin G used in severe or refractory cases.

37. **What are some important complications of neuro-Lyme?**
Rarely, patients will develop inflammation of the brain parenchyma leading to acute encephalitis with MRI changes and hypermetabolism on positron emission tomography. Patients may develop "Lyme encephalopathy" with fatigue, cognitive slowing, and memory trouble. This entity is more likely due to systemic inflammation and is not associated with irreversible brain damage.

HIV AND THE NERVOUS SYSTEM: HAND, MYELOPATHY, AND NEUROPATHY

38. **What are the diagnostic criteria of HIV-associated neurocognitive disorder?**
HIV-associated neurocognitive disorder (HAND) is divided into three categories. Asymptomatic neurocognitive impairment (ANI) is characterized by poor performance (more than one standard deviation below the mean) in two or more domains of neuropsychiatric testing without note of symptoms by either patients or families. Patients are categorized as having mild neurocognitive disorder once performance falls more than one standard deviation below the mean in at least two domains and experience mild impairment in daily function. Patients have HIV-associated dementia (HAD) when performance falls at least two standard deviations below the mean in two or more domains and daily function is markedly impaired.

39. **What is the epidemiology of HAND and how has antiretroviral therapy (ART) affected this epidemiology?**
The advent of ART has markedly decreased the prevalence of moderate to severe HIV-associated dementia. However, milder forms of impairment remain very common, with some studies showing rates as high as 45%. It is believed that this may be related to low levels of viral replication causing chronic inflammation.

40. **What are the pathogenesis and treatments of HAND?**
Development of HAND is directly associated with CD4 nadir. Thus, early diagnosis and initiation of ART remains the mainstay of management. While some ART regimens have been shown to have better CNS penetration, there is no consensus as to whether ART drugs with higher CNS penetration lead to improved cognitive outcomes.

41. **What are the typical clinical features of HIV-associated vacuolar myelopathy?**
Patients experience a clinical picture similar to subacute combined degeneration seen in vitamin B12 deficiency. Affected spinal cord tracts include the dorsal columns and the corticospinal tract, resulting in spastic paraparesis without sensory level but with sphincter dysfunction along with sensory ataxia and impaired proprioception and vibration in the lower extremities. Reflexes are typically increased but may be diminished at the ankles due to concurrent HIV neuropathy.

42. **What are the epidemiology and pathogenesis of HIV-associated neuropathy?**
HIV-associated distal symmetric polyneuropathy (HIV-DSP) is a painful, small fiber sensory neuropathy and as such is diagnosed by skin biopsy rather than electromyography and nerve conduction studies.

It has remained remarkably common despite the introduction of ART, with prevalence >50%. HIV-DSP may be due either to side effects of ART or to direct neurotoxic effects of the virus itself.

43. What treatments are available for HIV-associated neuropathy?
Pain is commonly managed symptomatically with lamotrigine or topical capsaicin. Typical medications for neuropathic pain such as amitriptyline, pregabalin, or gabapentin have shown little effect.

44. What is the differential diagnosis for a ring-enhancing lesion in a patient with autoimmune deficiency syndrome (AIDS)?
While there are many causes of ring-enhancing lesions in both immunocompetent and HIV-infected individuals, the most important considerations in AIDS are toxoplasma, primary CNS lymphoma, tuberculoma, cryptococcoma, and bacterial abscess. Metastases and primary CNS neoplasms should also be considered. The differential diagnosis may be altered based on the degree of immunosuppression. Patients with CD4 counts >500/μL are more likely to have primary brain tumors or metastases, similar to immunocompetent hosts, whereas severely immunosuppressed patients with CD4 <200/μL are more likely to have opportunistic infections and AIDS-associated tumors.

45. What is the diagnostic algorithm for this type of patient?
Lesions can be broadly divided into those with and without mass effect on imaging. Those with mass effect include toxoplasma encephalitis, primary CNS lymphoma (PCNSL), and other infections such as bacterial abscesses, cryptococcoma, or syphilitic gummas. Those without mass effect include progressive multifocal leukoencephalopathy (does not typically enhance but may be due to in context of immune reconstitution inflammatory syndrome (IRIS)), HIV encephalopathy (does not typically enhance but may in the context of immune reconstitution syndrome), and cytomegalovirus (CMV) encephalitis (typically with ventriculitis and ependymal enhancement).
    Patients without focal signs or significant mass effect should undergo lumbar puncture with cell counts and basic chemistries as well as polymer chain reaction (PCR) for JC virus, Epstein–Barr virus, cytomegalovirus, and *Toxoplasma gondi* (PCR and serology). Workup should include blood cultures and full-body CT to assess for sources of bacterial infection or metastasis.

46. What are the typical clinical features, diagnostic findings, and treatment for toxoplasmosis encephalitis?
Toxoplasmosis encephalitis typically develops in patients with CD4 <200/μL and presents with focal neurologic signs that vary with the location of the protozoal abscess. However, it may also present with meningismus with fever, headache, and nuchal rigidity. Workup usually begins with neuroimaging, with MRI with contrast being more sensitive than CT for detection of multiple lesions. Characteristic imaging findings are multiple ring-enhancing lesions with mass effect, similar to a variety of other CNS infections and tumors. Diagnosis can be confirmed with serum antitoxoplasma IgG antibodies as well as PCR of the CSF. Ancillary imaging such as thallium SPECT (single-photon emission computed tomography), perfusion MRI, or MR spectroscopy may help distinguish toxoplasma encephalitis from PCNSL.
    Antimicrobial therapy typically involves induction with sulfadiazine 1500 mg four times daily and pyrimethamine 200 mg load followed by 75 mg daily for 6 weeks. Patients are then transitioned to maintenance therapy with one-half the dose of sulfadiazine and pyrimethamine until the patient has maintained CD4 >200/μL for at least 6 months. Leucovorin is coadministered to avoid pyrimethamine-induced hematologic toxicity.
    In the proper clinical context with consistent neuroimaging findings, patients should receive empiric treatment for 2 weeks with the antitoxoplasma regimen followed by repeat MRI brain with contrast to look for reduction in lesion size. If there is no treatment response after 2 weeks, the differential diagnosis should be reconsidered and a brain biopsy considered for definitive diagnosis.

47. What are the typical clinical features, diagnostic findings, and treatment for progressive multifocal leukoencephalopathy (PML)?
PML is an opportunistic infection of the CNS due to invasion of oligodendrocytes by the JC virus leading to demyelination. The JC virus latently infects over half the population but does not cause disease unless a person is immunocompromised due to HIV, lymphoreticular malignancy, or immunosuppressive drugs, most significantly natalizumab for the treatment of multiple sclerosis.
    Patients will present with deficits in the corticospinal tracts, gait abnormalities, memory or behavioral disturbance, or cortical sensory loss due to demyelination immediately below the cortex.

MRI shows T2 hyperintensity at the gray-white matter junction with little to no enhancement or mass effect. Lesions are common in the cerebrum but may be seen in the brain stem or cerebellum. Basic studies of CSF such as cell counts and chemistries are typically nonspecific, and diagnosis is made by imaging in conjunction with JC virus, PCR, or biopsy if PCR is negative.

Prognosis remains poor. The disease may carry as high as a 50% mortality rate when due to HIV, with little recovery of deficits among survivors. Management centers around immune reconstitution with cases due to AIDS optimized on ART and those due to natalizumab potentially undergoing plasma exchange to speed clearance of the medication. Cases not due to AIDS may benefit from cytosine arabinoside.

Immune reconstitution inflammatory syndrome (IRIS) may complicate the condition in those previously on natalizumab who have stopped treatment and AIDS patients newly on ART. PML IRIS may result in fulminant clinical deterioration and MRI findings of contrast enhancement and mass effect. Corticosteroids may be administered to reduce inflammation although the benefit is not clear.

48. What are the typical clinical features, diagnostic findings, and treatment for CMV infection?

CMV is a ubiquitous herpesvirus that rarely causes symptoms in normal hosts but may result in encephalitis with or without ventriculitis and myeloradiculitis in severely immunocompromised patients (CD4 <100 cells/μL).

Meningitis presents typically as headache, fever, and altered mental status and is commonly diagnosed by CSF PCR. CSF may show either a lymphocytic pleocytosis (ventriculitis) or a polymorphonuclear pleocytosis (myeloradiculitis) with protein elevation. Treatment typically consists of a 3-week course of ganciclovir and/or foscarnet.

Radiculitis presents as flaccid paralysis of the lower extremity with bowel and bladder symptoms due to characteristic involvement of the lumbosacral roots from caudal extension of meningitis. MRI shows spinal cord and nerve root edema as well as adherence of roots to the thecal sac. Treatment similarly involves ganciclovir and/or foscarnet. MRI in encephalitis may demonstrate a number of patterns, including subependymal ventricular enhancement.

49. What are the typical clinical features, diagnostic findings, and treatment for PCNSL in HIV-infected patients?

Presenting features of PCNSL vary based on location but frequently include focal signs, cognitive and personality changes, or increased intracranial pressure. It commonly appears as a single enhancing lesion on CT or MRI. Seizures are rare due to typical involvement of subcortical structures. It is overwhelmingly a diffuse, large B-cell lymphoma diagnosed by stereotactic biopsy, CSF cytology or cytometry, or vitrectomy if ocular involvement is noted.

Treatment involves induction with high-dose methotrexate in combination with a variety of other chemotherapy agents followed by consolidation with whole brain radiation and possibly other types of chemotherapies. Additionally, ART must also be initiated.

NEUROCYSTICERCOSIS

50. What is the most common infectious cause of epilepsy?

Neurocysticercosis (NCC) is the most common cause of infectious epilepsy and a major cause of acquired epilepsy globally. It is endemic throughout the developing world although incidence has increased in the United States and Europe in the past 30 years due to immigration. Almost 90% of patients diagnosed with NCC in the United States are immigrants from Mexico or South America.

51. Describe the four stages of NCC, including their appearance on neuroimaging.
- **Vesicular stage:** *Taenia solium* eggs are ingested, cross the intestinal wall, and enter the CNS via the bloodstream where they evolve into larvae (cysticerci) with a transparent membrane, clear vesicular fluid, and an invaginated scolex. Imaging shows small, rounded cystic lesions that are well demarcated due to lack of edema. Lesions have no surrounding enhancement because of the parasite's ability to secrete factors that make it undetectable to the human immune system. The scolex may be visualized as an interior hyperdense nodule on CT with a "hole-with-dot" appearance.
- **Colloidal stage:** Years after initial infection, the parasite begins to degenerate as it dies, resulting in host immunologic attack. As the cysticerci begin to involute, the vesicular wall thickens, vesicular fluid becomes turbid, and the scolex begins to undergo hyaline degeneration. The surrounding

tissue develops mononuclear inflammation. Lesions become more ill-defined on imaging due to development of edema and begin to show rim enhancement on contrast studies.

- **Granular stage:** Once the scolex is completely mineralized and nonviable, it is referred to as the *granular stage*. CT at this stage begins to show discrete, hyperdense nodular-enhancing lesions with variable levels of edema. On MRI, both T1- and T2-weighted images show areas of signal void with surrounding hyperintense rims due to gliosis.
- **Calcified stage:** This stage represents full calcification of the cyst with resolution of surrounding edema. In surrounding tissue, epithelioid cells coalesce to form multinucleated giant cells. CT shows small, hyperdense lesions without edema or enhancement. MRI has poor sensitivity for detection of calcified lesions.

52. **What is racemose neurocysticercosis?**
Lesions located within either the Sylvian fissures or basal cisterns achieve a large size and multilobulated structure referred to as the *racemose form*. These may behave as mass lesions that displace other structures and interfere with CSF flow and cause hydrocephalus. They may also result in an arteritis resulting in infarction.

53. **What are the diagnostic criteria for NCC?**
See Table 25-8.

Table 25-8. Diagnostic Criteria for Neurocysticercosis (NCC)

DIAGNOSTIC CRITERIA		DEGREES OF CERTAINTY	
Absolute	1. Histologic demonstration of parasite in the CNS 2. Direct visualization of parasite by fundoscopy 3. Evidence of cystic lesions showing scolex on CT or MRI	Definitive	1. One absolute criterion 2. Two major, one minor, and one epidemiologic criteria
Major	1. Imaging with cystic lesions without scolex, enhancing lesions, or typical parenchymal calcifications 2. Positive EITB for the detection of anticysticercal antibodies 3. Resolution of intracranial cystic lesions after treatment 4. Spontaneous resolution of small single enhancing lesions	Probable	1. One major and two minor criteria 2. One major, one minor, and one epidemiologic criteria 3. Three minor and one epidemiologic criteria
Minor	1. Imaging with hydrocephalus or abnormal enhancement of the leptomeninges and myelograms showing multiple filling defects 2. Clinical manifestations suggestive of neurocysticercosis 3. Positive CSF ELISA for anticysticercal antibodies or cysticercal antigens 4. Cysticercosis outside the CNS		
Epidemiologic	1. Evidence of household contact with *Taenia solium* 2. Prior residence in endemic area 3. History of frequent travel to endemic area		

CNS, Central nervous system; CT, computed tomography; MRI, magnetic resonance imaging; EITB, enzyme-linked immunoelectrotransfer blot; ELISA, enzyme-linked immunoassay.
From Del Brutto OH, Rajshekhar V, White AC Jr, et al.: Proposed diagnostic criteria for neurocysticercosis. *Neurology* 57(2):177-183, 2001.

54. How should NCC be treated?
See Table 25-9.

55. In addition to seizures, what are the other important clinical manifestations and complications of NCC?
Patients may develop headache, cognitive impairment, compressive myelopathy as well as lacunar infarcts as a result of occlusion of small vessels by surrounding inflammation or large vessel infarcts or focal neurologic signs due to local mass effects. Cysticercotic arachnoiditis may lead to entrapment and dysfunction of cranial nerves. Hydrocephalus may result from impaired CSF resorption or occlusion of the foramina of Luschka, Magendie, or Monro.

Table 25-9. Treatment of Neurocysticercosis (NCC)

Parenchymal Neurocysticercosis

Vesicular Cysts

Single cyst: use albendazole 15 mg/kg/day for 3 days or praziquantel 30 mg/kg in three divided doses every 2 hours. Corticosteroids are rarely needed. Use antiepileptic drugs (AEDs) for seizures.

Mild to moderate infections: use albendazole 15 mg/kg/day for 1 week or praziquantel 50 mg/kg/day for 15 days. Corticosteroids may be used when necessary. Use AEDs for seizures.

Heavy infections: use albendazole 15 mg/kg/day for 1 week (repeated cycles of albendazole may be needed). Corticosteroids are mandatory before, during, and after therapy. Use AEDs for seizures.

Colloidal Cysts

Single cyst: use albendazole 15 mg/kg/day for 3 days or praziquantel 30 mg/kg in three divided doses every 2 hours. Corticosteroids may be used when necessary. Use AEDs for seizures.

Mild to moderate infections: use albendazole 15 mg/kg/day for 1 week. Corticosteroids are usually needed before and during therapy. Use AEDs for seizures.

Cysticercotic encephalitis: cysticidal drugs are contraindicated. Use corticosteroids and osmotic diuretics to reduce brain swelling. Use AEDs for seizures. Perform decompressive craniotomies in refractory cases.

Granular and Calcified Cysticerci

Single or multiple: cysticidal drug therapy is unnecessary. Use AEDs for seizures. Use corticosteroids in patients with recurrent seizures and perilesional edema surrounding calcifications.

Extraparenchymal Neurocysticercosis

Small Cysts over Convexity of Cerebral Hemispheres

Single or multiple: use albendazole 15 mg/kg/day for 1 week. Corticosteroids may be used when necessary. Use AEDs for seizures.

Large Cysts in Sylvian Fissures or Basal CSF Cisterns

Racemose cysticercus: use albendazole 15 mg/kg/day to 30 mg/kg/day for 15-30 days (repeated cycles of albendazole may be needed). Corticosteroids are mandatory before, during, and after therapy.

Other Forms of Extraparenchymal Neurocysticercosis

Hydrocephalus: cysticidal drug therapy is unnecessary. Insert a ventricular shunt. Continual corticosteroid administration (50 mg three times a week for up to 2 years) may be needed to reduce the rate of shunt dysfunction.

Ventricular cysts: perform endoscopic resection of cysts. Albendazole may be used only in small lesions located in lateral ventricles. Ventricular shunt only needed in patients with associated ependymitis.

Angiitis, chronic arachnoiditis: cysticidal drug therapy is unnecessary. Corticosteroids are mandatory.

Cysticercosis of the spine: perform surgical resection of lesions. Anecdotal use of albendazole with good results has been reported.

From Del Brutto OH: Neurocysticercosis. *Continuum (Minneapolis, Minn.)* 18(6 Infectious Disease):1392-1416, 2012.

56. What is the clinical presentation of Creutzfeldt–Jakob disease (CJD)? What ancillary tests are useful in its diagnosis?

Early stages of CJD are characterized by behavioral change with hallucinations and agitation followed by ataxia and visual disturbance. The disease progresses rapidly over several weeks and almost invariably patients develop myoclonus triggered by startle response. Patients continue to deteriorate rapidly into stupor and coma.

Characteristic electroencephalogram (EEG) patterns initially show diffuse nonspecific slowing, which progresses to high-voltage slow and sharp wave complexes on an increasingly slow and low-voltage background. Imaging is of little diagnostic aid, and routine CSF and serum laboratory tests are normal. Although commonly used, the 14-3-3 protein is of uncertain sensitivity and specificity because it is elevated in many destructive lesions of the gray matter. MRI of the brain is more specific in the proper clinical context, showing restricted diffusion of the cortical ribbon and/or of the deep gray nuclei. Variant CJD may result in the "pulvinar" sign with restricted diffusion of the pulvinar nucleus of the thalamus.

57. What are the presenting symptoms for rabies? Who should receive rabies prophylaxis?

Rabies is transmitted by animal bites and is most commonly carried by bats in the developed world and by dogs in Africa and Southeast Asia, where the disease is far more prevalent. Patients may present with encephalitic rabies characterized by psychosis, autonomic instability, and pain following a prodrome of paresthesias at the site of inoculation. Some may present with "paralytic rabies," a clinical syndrome of acute flaccid paralysis followed by encephalopathy. Patients with either recent animal bites in developing countries or bat exposure in developed countries should receive postexposure prophylaxis with rabies immunoglobulin followed immediately by rabies vaccine, which is given in several doses over 2 to 4 weeks. While nearly universally fatal once symptomatic, this regimen is highly effective when administered promptly following exposure.

58. What are the common neurologic manifestations of leprosy?

Leprosy is one of the most common causes of peripheral neuropathy worldwide and may present as peripheral mononeuritis, mononeuritis multiplex, or polyneuropathy. Cranial nerve and autonomic neuropathy are less common.

59. Name three bacterial toxins that affect the peripheral nervous system and describe their presentations and mechanisms of action.

1. *Corynebacterium diphtheria* produces the diphtheria toxin. This toxin consists of two joined subunits, A and B, which are split after endocytosis, allowing A to inhibit protein synthesis. Patients develop inflammation of the throat after inhalation of the bacteria. Neurologic manifestations begin with palatal paralysis 1 to 2 weeks after symptom onset and then progress to ciliary body paralysis with loss of accommodation but preserved light reaction. Six weeks after initial infection the patient may develop a descending paralysis and require mechanical respiratory support. The illness will resolve if the patient does not succumb to cardiac and respiratory complications.

2. *Clostridium tetani* is introduced through a wound and produces tetanus toxin, a zinc-dependent protease that prevents release of gamma-aminobutyric acid by cleaving surface proteins on synaptic vesicles. Local tetanus involves local stiffness and muscle spasms around a wound, resolving in weeks to months. Generalized tetanus begins locally and generalizes over a few days to involve full body spasms including the pharyngeal, laryngeal, and respiratory muscles.

3. *Clostridium botulinum* is typically ingested through foods such as home-preserved items and produces the botulinum toxin. This toxin inhibits the release of acetylcholine from peripheral nerve endings at the neuromuscular junction. Symptoms develop in 12 to 36 hours and typically begin as diplopia due to extraocular movement paralysis with progression to other bulbar muscles, then the neck, trunk, limbs, and respiratory muscles.

KEY POINTS: INFECTIOUS DISEASES OF THE NERVOUS SYSTEM—PART 2

1. Neurosyphilis is not synonymous with tertiary syphilis and may have many manifestations over the lifetime of the infections including asymptomatic, meningitis, meningovascular disease, parenchymatous (general paresis), tabes dorsalis, and gummatous disease.

2. Neuro-Lyme disease has certain typical manifestations: lymphocytic meningitis, cranial neuritis (most typically involving CN VII), and polyradiculitis. Neuro-Lyme should be diagnosed in the proper clinical and geographical context (exposure history and consistent clinical syndrome), with CSF analysis revealing that the relative concentration of specific antibody in the CSF exceeds that in the serum.

3. HAND has three stages: ANI, MND, and HAD. ANI patients do not report cognitive difficulty but demonstrate mild impairment on neuropsychological testing, whereas MND patients report mild impairment and demonstrate such impairment on testing. HAD patients experience severe impairment affecting their independent functioning and have marked impairment on neuropsychological testing.

4. Ring-enhancing lesions on a gadolinium-enhanced brain MRI in a patient with AIDS may have multiple etiologies, with the most common being toxoplasmosis. Primary CNS lymphoma is an important mimic. Patients are typically treated empirically for 2 weeks with antitoxoplasmosis therapy. If there is either worsening or no improvement radiographically then a brain biopsy is indicated to exclude alternate diagnoses.

5. NCC is the most important infectious cause of epilepsy worldwide and is commonly seen in the United States. Patients' seizures should be treated with antiepileptic medications, but treatment of the infection depends on the stage of infection and location in the CNS.

6. CJD is a rapidly progressive dementia due to prion infection. In the proper clinical context, short of a brain biopsy, MRI brain is the most specific commonly available tool to support the diagnosis. MRI shows restricted diffusion of the cortical ribbon and/or of the deep gray nuclei. Variant CJD may result in the "pulvinar" sign, with restricted diffusion of the pulvinar nucleus of the thalamus.

 References available online at expertconsult.com.

WEBSITE

http://www.cdc.gov/tb/statistics

BIBLIOGRAPHY

1. Aksamit AJ: Progressive multifocal leukoencephalopathy. Continuum 18(6):1374-1391, 2012.
2. Centers for Disease Control and Prevention: Tuberculosis (TB). Available at:
   http://www.cdc.gov/tb/statistics/reports/2013/table1.html. Accessed September 2, 2015.
3. Del Brutto OH: Neurocysticercosis. Continuum (Minneapolis, Minn.) 18(6 Infectious Disease):1392-1416, 2012.
4. Del Brutto OH, Rajshekhar V, White Jr AC, et al.: Proposed diagnostic criteria for neurocysticercosis. Neurology 57(2):177-183, 2001.
5. Halperin JJ: Lyme disease: a multisystem infection that affects the nervous system. Continuum 18(6):1338-1350, 2012.
6. Irani DN: Cerebrospinal Fluid in Clinical Practice, Philadelphia, Elsevier, 2009.
7. Kranick SM, Nath A: Neurologic complications of HIV-1 infection and its treatment in the era of antiretroviral therapy. Continuum 18(6):1319-1337, 2012.
8. Patton ME, Su JR, Nelson R, et al.: Primary and secondary syphilis – United States, 2005-2013. MMWR 63(18):402-406, 2014.
9. Roos KL: Principles of Neurologic Infectious Diseases: Principles and Practice, New York, McGraw-Hill, 2004.

CHAPTER 26

NEUROGENETIC DISORDERS

Paolo Moretti

1. What are the different types of genetic changes and some of the mechanisms by which they can alter phenotype?
See Table 26-1.

Table 26-1. Types of Genetic Changes and Common Mechanisms by Which They Lead to Phenotypic Alterations

Chromosome abnormalities	Changes in the number or structure of chromosomes
DNA deletions	Deletions of DNA sequences
DNA insertions	Insertions of DNA sequences
Single Base Changes	
Missense	Single base substitutions leading to a change in amino acid sequence
Nonsense	Single base substitution leading to replacement of an amino acid codon with a stop codon
Splice site	Destruction or creation of a signal regulating the splicing of exons and introns
Synonymous	Substitution of one base for another that does not change the amino acid sequence of a protein coding gene. Some synonymous changes affect transcription, mRNA splicing/transport, or translation, leading to phenotypic abnormalities
Frameshift changes	Sequence variants (e.g., deletion, insertion, or splice site) leading to a change in the normal open reading frame of a protein coding gene
Regulatory changes	Sequence changes altering the level of gene expression
DNA expansion	Repeat sequences (e.g., triplet repeat disorders) that can change in size over time
Silent DNA changes	DNA changes occurring in either noncoding or coding regions of a gene that do not cause phenotypic changes

2. Describe some of the methods currently used for detection of different mutation types.
   - **Single nucleotide changes:** DNA sequencing. Other techniques more rarely used include single-strand conformation polymorphism, denaturing high-performance liquid chromatography and gel electrophoresis, restriction fragment length polymorphism, or hybridization analysis.
   - **Copy number variants (CNVs)** (for example, DNA deletions and duplications): array comparative genomic hybridization or chromosome microarray analysis, virtual karyotyping with single nucleotide polymorphism arrays, and in some instances next-generation sequencing. Other techniques more rarely used include cytogenetic techniques such as fluorescent in situ hybridization. DNA expansion mutations (for example, repeat sequences): polymerase chain reaction (PCR) and in some instances DNA sequencing techniques.

3. Explain the meaning of the terms *"variant of unknown significance"* (VUS) and *copy number variant* (CNV).

A VUS is an alteration in the normal or reference sequence of a gene that has no known effect on the gene function or no known association with disease risk. The significance of a VUS is unclear until additional studies clarify its biologic significance in a sufficiently large population. Gene sequencing studies such as whole exome sequencing often identify numerous allelic variants in many genes. A CNV is a form of structural variation of the genome that results in a change in the number of copies of one or more sections of DNA. CNVs range from about one kilobase (1000 nucleotide bases) to several megabases in size and can encompass a region containing only a fragment of a gene or a contiguous set of adjacent genes. The human genome contains both gains and losses of genetic material between different individuals. Although many CNVs are stable and heritable, de novo CNVs arise through a number of mechanisms at various stages of development. CNVs can increase or decrease the number of dosage-sensitive genes, leading to human phenotypic variability, complex behavioral traits, disease susceptibility, and highly penetrant diseases.

4. What are genome-wide association studies?

Genome-wide association studies consist of scanning DNA markers across the genome of many individuals in order to find the genetic variation associated with a particular disease. These studies are thought to be valuable in finding the genetic variation that contributes to more common and generally complex diseases as opposed to Mendelian disorders.

5. Describe three main mechanisms by which mutations can alter cellular function.

Loss-of-function mutations cause a reduction or absence of normal function in the product of a gene. When the mutant allele has a complete loss of function it is often called a *null allele* or an *amorphic allele*. Often, the phenotypes associated with loss-of-function mutations are recessive. However, in haploinsufficiency, a heterozygous loss-of-function mutation is sufficient to cause a phenotypic abnormality or disease. Gain-of-function mutations alter the gene in such a way that its product gains either a new or abnormal function. These mutations are usually associated with dominant phenotypes and are also called *neomorphic mutations*. Dominant negative mutations modify a gene in such a way that its product antagonizes the function of the normal wild-type allele. These mutations are also called *antimorphic* and cause alterations of molecular function, which generally lead to inactivation or gene function and are associated with dominant or semidominant phenotypes.

6. Discuss genetic anticipation, reduced penetrance, and variable expressivity in Huntington's disease and the molecular basis of these phenomena.

Anticipation is the term describing the earlier onset of signs and symptoms in successive generations of affected individuals in the same family. Its molecular basis lies in the expansion of the CAG trinucleotide repeat size as the altered huntingtin or *HTT* gene is passed from one generation to the next. Huntington's disease status (affected, unaffected, at risk) is associated with the size of the CAG trinucleotide repeat. In huntingtin, a normal repeat size corresponds to fewer than 26 CAG repeats. This size is not associated with increased risk of Huntington's disease in the allele carrier or his/her offspring. In contrast, a huntingtin copy containing 40 or more CAG repeats is classified as fully penetrant and is associated with 50% risk of disease in the offspring. A CAG repeat size ranging from 27 to 35 repeats is classified as intermediate, and it is associated with increased risk of disease in the offspring, but no increased disease risk in the carrier of the expanded allele. A repeat count of 36 to 39 is known to have reduced penetrance (the mutation carrier may or may not be affected) and 50% risk of disease in the offspring. Variable expressivity refers to the degree to which Huntington's disease is expressed in an individual. One example of this phenomenon is the association between CAG repeat size and age at onset of the disease. Individuals with huntingtin alleles containing 60 or more CAG repeats commonly have very young onset, before the age of 20 years.

7. Describe uniparental disomy (UPD) and name neurologic diseases in which it is involved.

UPD occurs when an individual carries two copies of a chromosome, or part of a chromosome, from the same parent and no copies from the other parent. UPD can be the result of heterodisomy or isodisomy. In heterodisomy, a pair of nonidentical chromosomes are inherited from the same parent, the result of a meiosis I error. Heterodisomy is essentially benign. In isodisomy, a single chromosome from one parent is duplicated during a meiosis II error. In contrast to heterodisomy, isodisomy may lead to the duplication of lethal or deleterious recessive mutations and has the potential to cause pathogenic phenotypes. Uniparental inheritance of imprinted genes can also cause phenotypical abnormalities. The best-known examples of neurologic diseases involving UPD include Prader–Willi syndrome and Angelman syndrome.

8. What are known inheritance mechanisms in mitochondrial disorders?
Maternal inheritance, autosomal recessive inheritance, X-linked recessive inheritance, and autosomal dominant inheritance.

9. Describe the spectrum of manifestations of a neurologic disorder that may initially present with a history of childhood diarrhea and bilateral juvenile cataracts.
A history of childhood diarrhea and bilateral juvenile cataracts is found in cerebrotendinous xanthomatosis (CTX), a recessively inherited metabolic disorder in which affected individuals have an abnormality of bile acid metabolism. CTX patients are homozygous or compound heterozygous for loss-of-function mutations in the *CYP27A1* gene, which encodes the enzyme sterol 27-hydroxylase. The patients are unable to synthesize normal amounts of chenodeoxycholic acid, leading to accumulation of its precursors in various tissues. One characteristic of CTX is the presence of tendon xanthomas. A variety of other signs and symptoms can be present including dementia, movement disorders, seizures, psychiatric symptoms, and spastic gait.

10. What are congenital disorders of glycosylation (CDG) and what neurologic manifestations can they cause?
CDG are a group of inherited conditions caused by abnormalities in protein glycosylation. A broad spectrum of clinical manifestations and abnormalities in multiple organ systems are associated with CDGs, including failure to thrive, chronic diarrhea, liver disease, abnormal subcutaneous fat distribution, retinitis pigmentosa, cutis laxa, developmental delay, hypotonia, and ataxia. The clinical presentation and course are highly variable, ranging from death in infancy to mild involvement in adults. Most commonly, the disorders begin in infancy. However, most types have been described in only a few individuals, and our understanding of the phenotypic spectrum of these disorders is limited.

11. Discuss genetic heterogeneity in the hereditary spastic paraplegias.
Genetic heterogeneity is defined by the presence of multiple genetic causes leading to a similar phenotype or the same disease. This phenomenon is common to many human diseases. Examples of neurologic diseases with marked genetic heterogeneity include spinocerebellar ataxia and hereditary spastic paraplegia (HSP). Clinically, HSP is a group of disorders characterized by progressive spasticity and weakness of the lower limbs associated with length-dependent distal axonal degeneration of the corticospinal tracts. Autosomal dominant, autosomal recessive, X-linked, and maternal inheritance have been described, and to date over 70 spastic gait disease loci and at least 55 spastic paraplegia genes have been identified. Moreover, a clinical and genetic overlap has been described between forms of HSP and other motor neuron diseases.

12. Is somatic mosaicism known to play a role in neurologic disease?
In addition to inherited DNA variation, disease-causing mutations can occur during mitotic cell divisions. Most cancer mutations are known to arise somatically. Mutations occurring during the mitoses that generate the embryo after fertilization and zygote formation may lead to mosaicism, a condition in which only a subset of the organism's cells harbor the mutation. Somatic mutations can also arise during the course of prenatal brain development and cause neurologic disease. Examples of neurodevelopmental disorders associated with somatic mosaicism in about 5% to 10% of patients include genetic disorders of neuronal migration caused by mutations in *LIS1* and *DCX*. Detection of somatic mosaicism may be challenging as the mutation may not be present in all tissues and cell types.

13. Explain the concept of contiguous gene syndromes.
Contiguous gene syndromes are caused by a deletion or duplication spanning multiple genes lying in close proximity to one another along a chromosome. The chromosome abnormality can involve as few as two genes and as many as dozens of genes. Contiguous gene syndromes may be associated with multiple clinical features caused by deletion or duplication of the multiple adjacent genes.

14. What are the main syndromic presentations of mitochondrial disorders and why are they important?
Manifestations of mitochondrial disease can occur in virtually any organ system. The clinical variability of these disorders can present a significant diagnostic challenge. Patients may demonstrate combinations of features that defy easy classification into known syndromes. However, knowledge

of recognized clinical syndromes found in mitochondrial disease can aid in the recognition of both common and less unusual presentations. Some of the main presentations of mitochondrial disease are shown in Table 26-2.

Table 26-2. Selected Neurologic and Nonneurologic Manifestations in Common Clinical Presentations of Mitochondrial Diseases

SYNDROME	NEUROLOGIC PHENOTYPES	NONNEUROLOGIC PHENOTYPES
Encephalopathy (MELAS; MERRF)	Dementia, epilepsy, myoclonus, stroke-like episodes, cerebellar ataxia	Lactic acidosis, pigmentary retinopathy, deafness, cardiac conduction defects, mild proximal weakness, diabetes mellitus, short stature
Myopathy (including exercise intolerance, myalgia, and myoglobinuria)	Mild to moderate limb girdle weakness	
PEO/PEO+/KSS	Insidious onset of ptosis and partial ophthalmoplegia, often asymmetric. Elevated CSF protein and ataxia (KSS)	
Mitochondrial neurogastrointestinal encephalopathy	PEO, demyelinating neuropathy, leukoencephalopathy	Hearing loss, progressive gut hypomotility, and cachexia
Leigh's syndrome	Early-onset loss of motor and verbal milestones, ataxia, emesis, strokes, elevated CSF lactate	Lactic acidosis, deafness
Neurogenic muscle weakness, ataxia, retinitis pigmentosa	Proximal neurogenic muscle weakness, sensory neuropathy, ataxia, learning difficulties, seizures	Pigmentary retinopathy
Leber's hereditary optic neuropathy	Subacute, usually painless optic neuropathy; occasionally dystonia, ataxia, neuropathy	Usually young adult males
Maternally inherited diabetes and deafness	Minimal or no other features	Minimal or no other features
Pediatric disease affecting multiple organ systems		Short stature, failure to thrive, anemia, cardiomyopathy, renal tubular acidosis

MELAS, Mitochondrial encephalopathy, lactic acidosis, and stroke-like episodes; *MERRF*, myoclonic epilepsy and ragged red fibers; *PEO*, progressive external ophthalmoplegia; *KSS*, Kearns–Sayre syndrome; *CSF*, cerebrospinal fluid.

15. Discuss the advantages and limitations of diagnostic tests used to evaluate individuals suspected of having a mitochondrial disorder.

The diagnosis of mitochondrial disease requires a detailed knowledge of the strengths and weaknesses of different diagnostic techniques. No single test or combination of tests can be used to confirm or exclude the diagnosis of mitochondrial disease in every patient. For instance, neuroimaging, and blood or CSF lactate may be useful in supporting a clinical suspicion of mitochondrial disease. However, lactic acidosis should not be considered either a prerequisite for diagnosis or a reliably sensitive and specific marker of mitochondrial dysfunction. Similarly, elevations of serum alanine, tricarboxylic acid cycle intermediates, or plasma acylcarnitine suggest the presence of mitochondrial dysfunction, but normal results do not exclude the diagnosis. In the muscle biopsy, mitochondrial proliferation in the form of ragged red fibers is suggestive of a mitochondrial respiratory chain defect. However, ragged red fibers may not be seen in early childhood and may be absent in patients with proven mitochondrial disease such as neurogenic muscle weakness, ataxia, and retinitis pigmentosa.

Ragged red fibers or cytochrome C oxidase deficiency may also be found in nonrespiratory chain defects and in normal individuals over 60 years of age. Respiratory chain enzymatic activity is an important aid in diagnosis, but partial deficiencies, secondary or compensatory effects, and nonstandardized methods of analysis may lead to results that are difficult to interpret. DNA-based testing is a powerful tool. Absence of mutations in certain tissues, presence of low-level heteroplasmy—the presence of more than one type of mitochondrial DNA within a cell or tissue—and sequence VUSs need to be considered in interpreting the results and remain important challenges.

16. A patient and his wife bring you results of genetic testing showing that he carries an *SMN1* deletion, whereas his wife does not. Another physician informed them that they are not at risk of conceiving a child with spinal muscular atrophy (SMA). Discuss this genetic counseling scenario.

Spinal muscular atrophy is a recessive disorder caused by either homozygous or compound heterozygous mutations in the *SMN1* gene. In about 95% to 98% of patients, both *SMN1* alleles carry a deletion of exon 7. In about 2% to 5% of SMA patients, one *SMN1* allele carries an exon 7 deletion, whereas the other allele contains a point mutation. The couple in the above example is still at risk of conceiving a child with SMA. *SMN1* sequence analysis should be performed in the parents. Moreover, because of complexities in carrier test interpretation (as opposed to diagnostic testing in an affected individual), formal genetic counseling should be considered.

17. A patient with progressive adult-onset cerebellar ataxia is tested using a panel for known dominant and recessive causes of ataxia. She is found to carry a heterozygous VUS in the *AFG3L2*, a gene linked to dominantly inherited SCA28. Is this variant the cause of her disease and how can this be demonstrated?

VUSs are DNA changes with unknown biologic consequences. In the above example, the available information is not sufficient to either demonstrate or exclude a pathogenic role for the VUS found in the patient. As SCA28 is dominantly inherited, the simplest approach either to demonstrate or exclude a pathogenic role of the VUS is to analyze other affected and unaffected individuals in the family. Identification of this VUS in multiple other affected individuals and the absence of this variant in unaffected family members would provide data in support of the role of this VUS in causing disease. Segregation of the same variant with disease in other ataxia pedigrees would further support a pathogenic role.

18. Describe an example of mutations in the same gene causing phenotypically different motor neuron diseases.

Selected genetic forms of motor neuron diseases offer examples of allelic disorders with overlapping phenotypes. For instance, mutations in the *ALS2* gene have been reported in juvenile amyotrophic lateral sclerosis (ALS), infantile-onset ascending hereditary spastic paralysis, and in familial juvenile primary lateral sclerosis. Mutations in the *VAPB* gene have been identified in ALS8 and in late-onset SMA. This phenotypic variability is not limited to motor neuron diseases and can present a significant diagnostic challenge, especially in very rare disorders.

KEY POINTS: DIAGNOSTIC TEST SELECTION

1. Sequencing technologies are used to identify sequence variants such as point mutations or deletions/insertions of a few to several nucleotides in length.
2. Identification of most insertions and deletions (CNVs) is generally accomplished using chromosome microarray technologies.
3. Measurement of repeat sequence length and identification of expansion mutations are based on the use of PCR and DNA fragment analysis by capillary electrophoresis.

KEY POINTS: INTERPRETATION OF DIAGNOSTIC TEST RESULTS

1. The presence of a sequence VUS in a gene previously associated with a disease phenotype is not sufficient to establish causality in a patient undergoing testing for the same disease.
2. Molecular testing for both copy number and sequence variants is necessary in dominant or recessive disorders known to be caused by these two molecular mechanisms.
3. Somatic mosaicism and heteroplasmy can be associated with failure to identify pathogenic mutations in individuals with genetic disorders in whom only blood is used as a source of DNA.

References available online at expertconsult.com.

WEBSITE

https://www.genetests.org/

BIBLIOGRAPHY

1. Valle D, Beaudet AL, Vogelstein B, Kinzler KW, Antonarakis SE, Ballabio A, et al., editors: The Online Metabolic and Molecular Bases of Inherited Disease. McGraw-Hill Education. Available at: http://ommbid.mhmedical.com.

CHAPTER 27

PAIN PROCESSING AND MODULATION

Everton A. Edmondson

1. **How is pain defined?**
   In 1994, thought leaders in the International Association for the Study of Pain defined pain as follows: "An unpleasant sensory and emotional experience associated with actual or potential tissue damage, or described in terms as such."

2. **Can pain occur without tissue injury or impending tissue damage?**
   Yes. While pain most commonly starts with a noxious or injuring stimulus, it may be initiated de novo in the central nervous system (CNS) without any stimulus. A noxious stimulus may occur at any tissue that triggers a cascade of physiologic events that should cause pain, but pain may not always be perceived.

3. **How can you have a painful stimulus or tissue injury yet not perceive pain?**
   The brain can evoke an inhibitory influence on ascending neural transmission. Emotional shock, decreased level of consciousness, and cerebral dysfunction are some examples of a disconnection between painful stimulus and pain perception.

4. **What are the emotional and cognitive aspects of pain perception?**
   If an individual recognizes a stimulus as painful but is emotionally indifferent to pain, then there is no sense of suffering—no distress, no anguish. The impact of the pain is largely nullified by a lack of an emotional, interpretive context.

5. **Describe the physiologic events from the time of painful stimulus to the actual perception of pain.**
   Using Fig. 27-1 one can track pain processing from the stimulus delivered at a finger to nerves ascending the somatosensory pathway from the peripheral nervous system to the brain. The depiction of a nail going through the fingertip is the pain stimulus. This painful stimulus first encounters the afferent nociceptors. Most nociceptors are bare nerve endings. Pain-conveying fibers are either C-fibers or A-delta nerve fibers.

6. **How does the noxious stimulus evoke a response at the nociceptor?**
   The noxious stimulus interacts with transduction channels at the nerve ending. Some channels respond to thermal stimuli (TRPV1), cold (TRPM1, TRPM8), and chemical/mechanical stimuli (TRPA1). Nociceptive stimuli activate these transduction channels and initiate the influx of a sodium and calcium current, thus causing depolarization and the propagation of current down the axon. This conversion of heat, cold, chemical, or mechanical energy to an electrical impulse at the nerve terminal is called *transduction*.

7. **What is a primary afferent?**
   The primary afferent is the peripheral nerve from the tissue where the stimulus is encountered. This afferent conveys a train of impulses toward the spinal cord. The afferent is essentially a sensory nerve transmitting impulses toward the CNS.

8. **What happens at the nerve terminal in the spinal cord?**
   The peripheral sensory nerve has its cell body at the dorsal ganglion. Its dendrites, which function as a nerve terminal, project into the spinal cord at lamina I and II. Neurotransmitters such as substance P, neurokinin-1 (NK-1), calcitonin gene-related peptide (CGRP), and glutamate are released at the terminal in the dorsal horn. All of these transmitters are excitatory. They provoke the influx of sodium and calcium into the cell of the second-order neuron. The second-order neuron is in lamina I (Lissauer's tract) or lamina II (substantia gelatinosa).

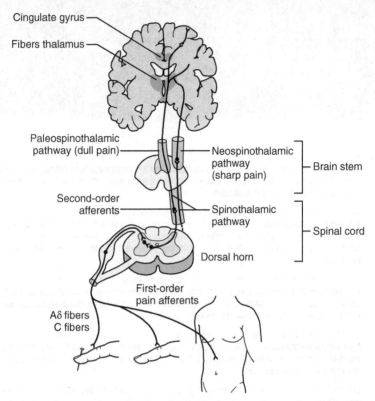

Figure 27-1. Ascending somatosensory pain pathway. Note that the stimulus provokes sensation at the fingertip; paleo- and neospinothalamic tracts relay to the thalamus (a major pain processing depot) and then to cortical structures such as the cingulate gyrus, providing emotive and interpretative processing of pain.

9. **How does the primary afferent synapse or interact with dorsal horn neurons?**
   There are interneurons that have intervening synapses between some of the primary afferents and neurons at deeper layers in the dorsal horn such as lamina V. Some of these lamina V neurons have long dendrites extending into lamina II and synapse directly with primary afferents. The dorsal horn is a very fertile territory for modulatory influences from descending nerves arising from higher centers as well as local interneurons. The interneurons are typically inhibitory. The preponderant influence from descending neural input is also inhibitory. See Table 27-1 for a summary of dorsal horn neurotransmitters or ligands.

10. **Once the primary afferent synapses with the second-order neuron, where does the second-order neuron project?**
    The axon of the second-order neuron projects as the spinothalamic tract. It descends to ventro-medial gray and crosses the midline through the anterior commissure and then ascends in the ventrolateral white matter of the cord as the spinothalamic tract (neospinothalamic). There is also a multisynaptic spinothalamic tract that ascends in the dorsomedial white matter of the spinal cord near the midline. This is called the *paleospinothalamic tract.* These tracts ascend to the brain stem, thalamus, somatosensory cortex, and limbic system (Fig. 27-2).

11. **How do the functions of the neospinothalamic and paleospinothalamic tracts differ?**
    The lateral spinothalamic tract (neospinothalamic tract) ascends to the thalamus and cortex with few synaptic connections. Therefore, sharp pain and the avoidance response can be evoked due to the

Table 27-1. Ligand–Receptor Interaction

RECEPTOR	DRUG OR NEUROTRANSMITTER	CHANNEL AND DIRECTION	EFFECT
GABA-A	GABA	Chloride influx	Inhibitory
GABA-B	GABA	Potassium influx	Inhibitory
Glycine	Glycine	Chloride influx	Inhibitory
Opioid	Opioids	Potassium influx	Inhibitory
μ, κ, σ	Opioids	Potassium influx	Inhibitory
α1, α2	Norepinephrine	Potassium influx	Inhibitory
SHT	Serotonin	Potassium influx	Inhibitory
AMPA	Glutamate	Sodium influx	Excitatory
NMDA	Glutamate	Sodium and calcium influx	Excitatory
NK-1	Substance-P	Sodium and calcium influx	Excitatory
NK-1,2	NK-1	Sodium and calcium influx	Excitatory
CCGP	CGRP	Sodium and calcium influx	Excitatory
GABA-B	Baclofen	Potassium influx	Inhibitory
GABA-A	Benzodiazepine	Chloride influx	Inhibitory
Gabapentinoid receptor	Gabapentin/Pregabalin	Blocks calcium, L-type	Inhibitory
α1, α2	SNRI	Potassium influx	Inhibitory
5-HT	SNRI	Potassium influx	Inhibitory
NMDA	Ketamine	Sodium and calcium influx	Excitatory
Conopeptide receptor	ω-Conopeptide	Blocks calcium, N-type	Inhibitory

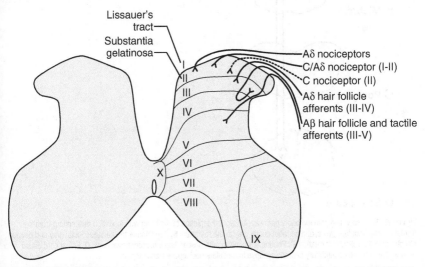

Figure 27-2. Rexed laminae in spine. Lamina I, a thin sliver of gray matter above lamina II with primary input A-delta and C-fibers; lamina II is the substantia gelatinosa; lamina III has A-delta hair follicle input; laminae III thru V, A-beta nonpainful tactile afferent information.

rapid transmission and perception of pain. In contrast, the dorsomedial thalamic tract (paleothalamic tract) synapses at multiple locations, including the recticular activating system, before reaching the thalamus and limbic system. Transmission along the paleothalamic system is slow and associated with more indolent visceral-autonomic and emotional/behavioral responses.

12. Describe the descending pain inhibitory system.
    From the prefrontal cortex, cingulate gyrus, and other limbic structures, inhibitory outflow descends to the thalamus and periaqueductal gray to the reticular region of the pons and medulla. From the brain stem nuclei, projections head to the spinal cord. There are serotonergic, noradrenergic, and opioidergic neurons that provide inhibitory pain input at the dorsal horn (Fig. 27-3).

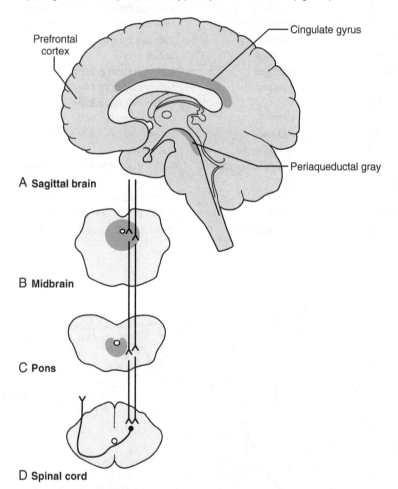

Figure 27-3. Descending pain inhibitory pathway. **A,** Sagittal depiction of the brain with inhibition descending from the frontal cortex, cingulate gyrus, and periaqueductal gray in the midbrain. **B,** Depiction of the periaqueductal gray and deeper structures in the reticular formation. **C,** Pontine tegmentum with descending inhibitory projections. **D,** Spinal cord dorsal horn where descending inhibitory neurons synapse to modulate nociceptive transmission.

13. Name some treatments that block pain transmission at the primary afferent level.
    Injection of anesthetic drugs like lidocaine blocks sodium channels at the nerve terminal and axon. This blockade prevents depolarization and transmission of impulses. Another approach is to deplete

substance P from the cutaneous nerve terminal with capsaicin. This depletion does not completely prevent pain transmission but reduces pain sensitivity at the cutaneous field supplied by the primary afferent.

14. **Describe pharmacologic interventions at the spinal cord and higher centers that inhibit pain.**

   Any drug or anesthetic approach that reduces excitatory input from primary afferents and second-order neurons results in analgesia. These drugs include opioids, serotonin–norepinephrine reuptake inhibitors (SNRIs), tricyclic antidepressants, N-methyl D-aspartate (NMDA) antagonists, calcium channel blocking drugs such as gabapentin for L-type channels, and Ziconitide® (omega-conopeptide) for N-type channels. Examples of these drugs are listed in Table 27-2.

Table 27-2. Equianalgesic Dose Conversions

DRUG	ORAL ROUTE	IV ROUTE	DURATION	HALF-LIFE
Morphine	30 mg	10 mg	3-4 hr	2 hr
Oxycodone	20 mg	—	4-6 hr	4.5 hr
Hydromorphone	7.5 mg	1.5-2 mg	4-5 hr	2-3 hr
Hydrocodone	30 mg	—	4-6 hr	3-4.5 hr
Codeine	200 mg	120 mg	4-6 hr	3 hr
Tapentadol	75-100 mg	—	4-6 hr	4-5 hr
Fentanyl	—	100 mcg	1-2 hr	1-2 hr
Buprenorphine	—	0.4 mg	6-12 hr	2.2 hr IV; 37 hr SL

Data from Knotkova H, Fine PG, Portenoy RK: Opioid rotation: the science and limitations of the equianalgesic dose table. *J Pain Symptom Manage* 38(3):426-439, 2009.

15. **How do antidepressants that inhibit norepinephrine and serotonin reuptake reduce pain?**

   These drugs work on the descending inhibitory pathways. They increase K^+ influx and block Ca^{++} influx at the second-order neuron in the dorsal horn. It should be noted, however, that this mechanism of action depends on the type of 5-HT receptor since some subtypes are excitatory rather than inhibitory.

16. **How are nociceptors sensitized?**

   After a burn of the skin, for example, inflammatory mediators are released at the injured tissue site. These include prostaglandins, bradykinin, protons, and cytokines. The local inflammatory milieu also triggers nociceptors to release substance P and calcitonin gene-related peptide (CGRP). These substances promote further vasodilation and facilitate the migration of inflammatory cells such as neutrophils and macrophages. Phosphorylation of the ionic channels makes these ionic channels more permeable to depolarizing ions like sodium and calcium, resulting in nerve hyperexcitability and nociceptor sensitization.

17. **How can this sensitizing process be blocked at the tissue level?**

   Some examples of peripheral desensitizing methods are antiinflammatory medications such as nonsteroidal antiinflammatory drugs and corticosteroids as well as direct neural blockade with anesthetics.

18. **What happens centrally in the spinal cord after tissue injury?**

   Tissue injury and inflammation result in locally released ligands that stimulate nociceptors and cause a barrage of electrical impulses from the primary afferent. Substance P, CGRP, and glutamate are released at the central nerve terminal of the primary afferent. These excitatory neurotransmitters trigger depolarization of the second-order neuron. Repeated depolarization activates G-protein-related second messengers, inducing a phosphorylation cascade and activation of transcription factors. The nerve may then upregulate its permeability to sodium and calcium and incorporate more ion channels in its membrane. Thus, the neuron becomes more sensitized to the incoming traffic of impulses.

19. Why is it that a blister burn becomes sensitive to light touch and stroking— stimuli that are not ordinarily painful?

This phenomenon occurs secondary to sensitization at the level of the dorsal horn. There, the C-fiber and A-delta nerve fibers conveying painful stimuli converge on second-order neurons that also receive input from A-beta fibers conveying light touch and stroking. Due to upregulation, the second-order neuron is now likely to depolarize in response to input from neurons conveying nonnoxious stimuli.

20. What is a wide-dynamic-range neuron?

A wide-dynamic-range neuron is the second-order neuron that receives input from primary afferents conveying impulses triggered by more than one type of stimulus modality—chemical, thermal, pressure, light touch, etc.

21. Are all second-order afferents wide-dynamic-range neurons?

Not necessarily. Some second-order neurons in lamina II (substantia gelatinosa) respond to only a specific type of noxious stimulus, and some may respond to multiple types of stimuli.

22. What is central facilitation?

Mendell and Wall determined that high-frequency C-fiber stimulation, not A-fiber stimulation, results in facilitating discharges from wide-dynamic range neurons. This phenomenon is called *wind-up*.

23. Define sensitization.

Sensitization is a left shift in the stimulus response curve such that a stimulus of lesser intensity is now able to evoke a painful response.

24. Define nociceptive pain.

Pain caused by stimulation of nociceptors by physical or chemical modalities such as pinch, crush, pressure, surgical incision, heat or extreme cold, or chemical irritation (such as exposure to acid or pepper).

25. What is neuropathic pain?

Pain caused by neuronal dysfunction, nerve injury, or disease.

26. What are the common features of neuropathic pain?

There may be hyperalgesia, allodynia, hyperpathia, dysesthesia, or lancinating jolts of pain. Nociceptive pain in the setting of sensitization may share some of these features. However, nociceptive pain is unlikely to be lancinating or associated with an electric jolt-like nature.

27. What is hyperalgesia?

Hyperalgesia is a painful reaction to a noxious stimulus that is perceived when the pain threshold is exceeded, at which point the painful response becomes exaggerated.

28. What is allodynia?

Allodynia is an exaggerated painful response to a nonnoxious stimulation such as light touch or stroking.

29. What is hyperpathia?

Hyperpathia is a general exaggerated response to painful stimuli, with no mention of threshold.

30. What is dysesthesia?

Dysesthesia refers to a painful, disagreeable sensation such as burning, icy-hot, prickly, itchy-prickly, intensely creepy-crawly, etc.

31. What is paresthesia?

Paresthesia is typically a nonpainful, tingling sensation.

32. What is deafferentation pain?

Deafferentation pain occurs in the setting of disruption of an afferent connection to the peripheral tissue. For example, this type of pain can occur in the setting of amputation, where nerves are transected and a limb or body part is missing, as well as brachial plexus avulsion injury and postherpetic neuralgia wherein the varicella zoster virus has destroyed the afferent input to second-order neurons.

33. What is central pain?
    Central pain arises from neuronal dysfunction within the CNS. The pain generator is not a peripheral nociceptor but a central population of neurons that spontaneously fire—delivering afferent traffic that is perceived as pain. Examples of central pain include spinal cord injury (which is both deafferentation and central), poststroke pain, and pain from a multiple sclerosis plaque.

34. How could central pain occur in the absence of peripheral tissue injury?
    As discussed above, neurons can become more readily depolarized and hence more sensitive because of a number of cellular changes. These include sustained exposure to excitatory transmitters like glutamate and substance P. Such activity may recruit cytokines, prostaglandins, and other inflammatory mediators. Activation of kinases promotes phosphorylation that may change the susceptibility of ion channels to depolarizing current and trigger a cascade to intracellular changes including the production of more sodium or calcium channels.

KEY POINTS: IMPORTANT NUANCES OF PAIN MODULATION

1. Nociception without emotional or cognitive/interpretative correlation is not perceived as harmful, disagreeable, or unpleasant, so protective behavior is often nullified.
2. C-fiber input drives the sensitization process and "wind-up" in the dorsal horn.
3. Preemptive blockade of nerve impulses quells the neuronal processes that result in sensitization.

PAIN SYNDROMES: RECOGNITION AND TREATMENT

NEUROPATHIES

35. Which of the common peripheral neuropathies are often painful?
    Examples include the following: diabetic polyneuropathy, diabetic mononeuritis multiplex, diabetic thoracoabdominal polyradiculitis, and the early phase of diabetic amyotrophy. Additionally, uremic neuropathy, ischemic neuropathy, toxic neuropathies such as arsenic poisoning, autoimmune deficiency syndrome (AIDS)-related polyneuropathy, nutritional deficiencies such as thiamine, pyridoxine, and folic acid deficiency.

36. How would you treat a painful diabetic neuropathy?
    Food and Drug Administration-approved drugs such as pregabalin and duloxetine are often employed. There are a large number of off-label anticonvulsants used including gabapentin, oxcarbazepine, valproate, or lacosamide. Tramadol is also effective in some cases. Tricyclic antidepressants can be employed, but the side effect profile is less favorable than that of duloxetine. In more severe cases, an opioid may have to be added to the pharmacologic cocktail.

37. How would you treat human immunodeficiency virus (HIV) neuropathy?
    Make sure the reverse transcriptase inhibitor used to treat the disease is not a provoking cause. Adding B vitamins, duloxetine, or pregabalin are often helpful.

38. Is there an advantage to using methylated folate and B12 products?
    Some individuals have a deficiency in methylene folate reductase activity in the CNS. The use of methylated folate is required to circumvent this problem. Pharmacogenetic testing is available to determine if an individual has this polymorphism (see the pharmacogenetic section of this chapter).

39. List entrapment neuropathies likely to present with pain.
    Carpal tunnel syndrome and ulnar nerve entrapment more commonly result in paresthesia and numbness, but painful symptoms are also quite common. Other entrapments include tarsal tunnel syndrome, lateral femoral cutaneous syndrome, suprascapular nerve entrapment, superior gluteal nerve entrapment, anterior interosseous syndrome, pronator teres syndrome, and radial tunnel syndrome.

40. How is carpal tunnel syndrome treated?
    Mild cases of carpal tunnel syndrome can be treated with a cock-up splint. Some orthopedists inject steroids into the carpal tunnel compartment under ultrasound guidance. More severe entrapment typically requires carpal tunnel release.

41. **How is ulnar entrapment treated?**
    The ulnar nerve may be entrapped at either the cubital tunnel in the elbow or Guyon's canal at the wrist. Avoiding pressure on the nerve at the level of the elbow is achieved by keeping the forearm on the volar side and avoiding rubbing the elbow on hard surfaces. Repetitive ulnar deviation and flexion at the wrist aggravates the ulnar nerve at Guyon's canal. Avoidance of such activities and use of nonsteroidal antiinflammatory drugs (NSAIDs) may help. Sometimes decompressive surgery is necessary.

42. **How is the diagnosis of tarsal tunnel syndrome made?**
    Clinically, there is pain, dysesthesia, and/or numbness in the medial foot and base of the foot including the big toe and adjacent three toes. The tendon sheath covering the nerve wraps over the medial malleolus down to the calcaneus. The nerve splits into three components, the calcaneal, medial, and lateral plantar nerves. Depending on the location of compression along this tunnel, the heel may be painful along with medial and lateral plantar nerve distribution.

43. **What intervention can be employed to reduce the discomfort of tarsal tunnel syndrome?**
    Conservative treatment includes steroid injection, physical therapy to mobilize the tibial nerve, and in recalcitrant cases surgery to decompress the tarsal tunnel is necessary.

44. **How do you determine if someone has lateral femoral cutaneous nerve entrapment (a.k.a. meralgia paresthetica)?**
    Typically, the patient presents with dysesthesia in the anteriolateral aspect of the thigh. There is often exquisite point tenderness at the region where the nerve traverses under the inguinal ligament. This area is at the lateral corner of the ligament near its attachment to the anterior superior iliac spine. Obesity, seatbelt trauma, and diabetes are relatively common causes for this syndrome.

45. **Discuss treatment options for lateral femoral cutaneous entrapment.**
    Corticosteroid injection near the vicinity of the nerve is often helpful. Weight reduction, if obesity is the source, is helpful. Avoiding recurrent trauma such as compression from a low-lying seatbelt buckle is advised. Surgery is not particularly helpful.

46. **How does a patient with suprascapular nerve entrapment present?**
    Typically, the patient has deep pain in the posterior shoulder along the muscles of the scapula—namely, supra-and infraspinatus muscles. Weakness in these muscles may occur, and in chronic cases, there may be atrophy. A relatively rare condition, this is increasing in prevalence from the use of backpacks.

47. **How is the above treated?**
    Steroid injections at the suprascapular notch, where the nerve passes under a ligament, can provide relief, but it may be temporary. Surgical decompression may be necessary.

48. **What is the anterior interosseous syndrome?**
    This syndrome is caused by entrapment of the anterior interosseous branch of the median nerve. It can be provoked by blunt trauma or repetitive flexion at elbow and wrist such as using an ice pick. The site of entrapment is between the tendinous origins of the pronator teres and the flexor digitorum superficialis. On occasion, it is caused by either a viral or inflammatory process. Symptoms include pain in the forearm and wrist. Easy fatigability and weakness in the distal flexors of the thumb and index finger are often noted. Creating a tight O-ring sign with the thumb and index finger is not possible; instead a flattened, weak pinch is made.

49. **What is the treatment?**
    Antiinflammatory medications, local steroid/anesthetic injection, pregabalin, gabapentin, duloxetine, or tricyclic antidepressants (TCAs) such as nortriptyline can be tried. If these fail, surgical decompression may be necessary.

50. **What is pronator teres syndrome?**
    The median nerve is entrapped in the proximal forearm by either the pronator muscle or its fibrous band, the lateral edge of the flexor digitorum superficialis, or the lacertus fibrosus. Symptoms include pain on forced pronation, chronic aching in the forearm, and weakness of the intrinsic muscles of the hand. A positive Tinel's sign may be elicited at the level of the proximal region of the pronator teres.

51. What is the treatment?

    Pronator teres syndrome is likewise treated conservatively with NSAIDs, TCAs, or pregabalin. If these fail, then steroid injections and surgical exploration if that fails.

52. What is radial tunnel syndrome?

    Radial tunnel syndrome is an entrapment of the posterior interosseous branch of the radial nerve at the proximal forearm. This may be due to an aberrant fibrous band, sharp tendinous margin, or a blood vessel. Symptoms include pain in the proximal and lateral forearm similar to tennis elbow. In fact, it is often mistaken for tennis elbow. It is a rare syndrome, and although tennis elbow is so common, radial tunnel syndrome should still be added to the differential diagnosis. Treatment is similar to the other entrapment syndromes.

    Note: Some of the pain syndromes in the above text are not uncommon.

NEURALGIFORM PAIN SYNDROMES OF HEAD AND NECK REGION

53. How common is trigeminal neuralgia?

    The estimated prevalence is 1 per 20,000 people suffer from this disorder.

54. What is the typical manifestation of trigeminal neuralgia?

    Typical manifestation is a paroxysmal pain that is described as either lancinating, boring, hot poker-like, or intense electrical "zap" in the trigeminal neural distribution.

55. Which division of the trigeminal nerve is most commonly affected?

    The maxillary division (V2) is affected most, then mandibular (V3), followed by the ophthalmic division (V1) in about 5% of cases. Bilateral involvement occurs in 10% of individuals. Involvement of all three divisions rarely occurs.

56. What is the etiology of trigeminal neuralgia?

    The most common cause is a tortuous vessel compressing the trigeminal ganglia. Other causes include aneurysm, tumor, and multiple sclerosis. It may also be idiopathic.

57. How is it treated?

    Anticonvulsant therapy is a mainstay. The drug of first choice is carbamazepine or its congener, oxcarbazepine. Other alternatives include phenytoin, valproate, baclofen, and lamotrigine. Lacosamide is a relatively new and promising addition to the armamentarium. If pharmacotherapy fails, then microvascular decompression (Janetta procedure) is the preferred step. Balloon compression, rhizotomy, and gamma knife therapy are other options.

58. What are the recommended diagnostic considerations?

    Magnetic resonance imaging (MRI) and magnetic resonance angiogram of the brain are suggested in order to exclude tumors, aneurysms, arachnoid cysts, multiple sclerosis plaque, or anomalous vasculature.

59. What is *tic douloureux*?

    Sometimes trigeminal neuralgia coexists with hemifacial spasms. This combination was originally called *tic douloureux*. Now *tic douloureux* is synonymous with trigeminal neuralgia, and *tic convulsif* is the term reserved for hemifacial spasms.

60. What is the typical clinical presentation of glossopharyngeal neuralgia?

    This syndrome is characterized by paroxysmal jolts or lancinating, sharp pain in the pharynx. Swallowing is often a trigger. This pain emanates from a dysfunctional cranial nerve IX (glossopharyngeal nerve). Some individuals experience syncope from the extreme pain and autonomic dysfunction.

61. What is the usual diagnostic workup?

    Evaluate the pharynx and hypopharynx by direct visualization to exclude tumor. Head and neck MRI study is the imaging of choice to evaluate the brain stem, palatine region, pharynx, and hypopharynx.

62. What is the treatment of glossopharyngeal neuralgia?

    The treatment is similar to trigeminal neuralgia. Try oxcarbazepine or carbamazepine as first line. Other anticonvulsants or baclofen may be tried. Anesthetic block of the glossopharyngeal nerve is short lived in efficacy. In recalcitrant cases, microvascular decompression may be pursued.

63. How does nervus intermedius neuralgia present?

This neuralgia is secondary to dysfunction of the nervus intermedius division of the facial nerve. The etiology could be viral, inflammatory, or vascular compression. When herpes zoster affects the nerve it is called *Ramsay Hunt syndrome*. The latter usually has a constant ear pain with superimposed paroxysmal pain. There are often vesicles in the external canal and/or on the tympanic membrane during the acute phase.

64. How is Ramsay Hunt syndrome treated?

Otic neuralgiform pain identical to nervus intermedius neuralgia may occur, but more typically there is a background of constant pain with superimposed jolts or paroxysmal lancinating pain in the ear. Vesicles are noted in the external canal, sometimes on the pinna or eardrum. Antiviral therapy with acyclovir and corticosteroids is administered along with opioids and anticonvulsant drugs such as oxcarbazepine and pregabalin.

65. How does red ear syndrome differ from Ramsay Hunt syndrome?

Red ear syndrome belongs in the trigeminovascular headache syndrome family of disorders. It is likened to sudden unilateral neuralgiform conjunctival injection and tearing (SUNCT). There are recurrent attacks of ear pain and temporal headache. The autonomic phenomenon is the paroxysmal onset of redness of the ear, but typically there is no tearing or rhinorrhea. The attack may last 15 seconds to 5 minutes, and there may be 20 to well over 100 attacks per day. This rare condition does not have a robust list of treatments. Anticonvulsants work modestly. Corticosteroids or C2,3 facet injections provide relief.

66. Elaborate on the clinical features of SUNCT.

SUNCT is a trigeminovascular headache syndrome characterized by stabbing, lancinating, shock-like, or piercing pain in the periorbital region radiating to the ear, cheek, and throat in some instances. The attacks last from 5 seconds to 4 minutes. It is unilateral and will rarely switch sides. It is associated with conjunctival redness/swelling and eye tearing. The headache responds to anticonvulsants such at carbamazepine. See Chapter 21 for more details on headache syndromes.

ACUTE HERPES ZOSTER AND POSTHERPETIC NEURALGIA

67. How can you distinguish an acute herpes zoster eruption from poison ivy or other blister-based eruptions?

The eruption follows a specific dermatomal pattern or a confluence of adjacent dermatomes.

68. Who is more prone to get shingles?

Individuals 60 years and older are more likely to get shingles, but it can occur at any age. Immunocompromised individuals such as cancer patients, patients with AIDS, and individuals with lupus and rheumatoid arthritis are not only more likely to get it, but they are also at risk for a disseminated form of the infection (multifocal or diffuse eruption of shingles).

69. At what age does the Centers for Disease Control (CDC) recommend that people be vaccinated for shingles?

Individuals 60 years and older are recommended to have the vaccine by virtue of the much higher risk of developing postherpetic neuralgia.

70. What is postherpetic neuralgia?

Both acute shingles and postherpetic neuralgia are severely painful. Itching or dysesthesia may precede the acute phase of zoster eruption. By the time the eruption becomes visible, the pain intensity is in full gear. The pain is lancinating, burning, constricting, or boring in quality. There is a background of constant pain and often a superimposed component of paroxysmal jabs. When the skin lesion heals, the pain begins to subside—indicative of concurrent healing of the nerve and reduction in its excitability. For some individuals this could occur within a month. For others it may extend into a second month. Those who have pain beyond this interval are said to have postherpetic neuralgia.

71. How long could postherpetic neuralgia last?

This condition varies in duration. The younger the individuals, the more likely they are to experience remission within weeks or a few months. By contrast, older patients may experience the pain indefinitely.

72. How likely is it to be permanent or last several years?

The incidence of postherpetic neuralgia among individuals under the age of 50 is less than 10%. By contrast, by the age of 60 the incidence jumps to 30% to 40%. Each decade above that has a higher and higher rate of getting postherpetic neuralgia for several years or permanently. For this reason, a preventive vaccine is recommended for those 60 years and older.

73. How do you treat acute zoster?

Prompt initiation of antiviral therapy is recommended. Some clinicians also add corticosteroids to the regimen, especially for individuals 50 years and older.

74. What is the antiviral regimen used to treat acute shingles?

Individuals with normal renal function can receive any of the following:

- Acyclovir 800 mg orally five times a day or IV 10 mg/kg every 8 hours for 7 to 10 days
- Famciclovir 500 mg three times daily for 7 days
- Valacyclovir 1 g three times daily for 7 days

Note: When prescribing, one needs to adjust dose in both the elderly and renally impaired patient for all the above listed anti-virals.

75. If early intervention with the above treatment was given, but the patient still crossed over into postherpetic neuralgia, what are the treatment options for such a patient?

The interventional pain management community argues that either sympathetic blockade or epidural blockage with anesthetic and steroids during the acute phase of the disease lessens the likelihood of getting postherpetic neuralgia. They extend this approach into the early phase of postherpetic neuralgia. Other interventions, later in the course of the disease, such as epidural spinal stimulation, receive mixed reviews. Pharmacologic measures such as topical lidocaine, IV lidocaine infusions during acute crises, and various formulations of gabapentin (topical compounding, or oral gabapentin, Gralise® or Horizant®) are often employed in this form of neuropathic pain. Regardless, in many instances successful treatment of postherpetic neuralgia is a daunting challenge.

SMALL FIBER NEUROPATHY-RELATED PAIN

76. What is small fiber neuropathy?

Small fiber neuropathy is a polyneuropathy isolated to the small nerve fibers, commonly the cutaneous unmyelinated fibers. The diagnosis can be confirmed with skin biopsy for analysis of nerve fiber density.

77. What are the clinical presentations?

The clinical presentations are quite varied. Some people present with fibromyalgia-like symptoms characterized by diffuse muscle aches. Others may have burning pain in the limbs or cutaneous insensitivity to painful stimuli. Some may concomitantly have visceral manifestations of the disease with gastroparesis, bladder dysfunction, chronic general dysmotility of the gastrointestinal tract, and/ or orthostatic hypotension secondary to autonomic dysfunction. Other syndromic manifestations include burning mouth syndrome.

78. Can small fiber neuropathy be mistaken for fibromyalgia?

Yes. Skin biopsy has uncovered small fiber neuropathy as the driver for symptoms thought to be secondary to fibromyalgia in some cases.

79. What is burning mouth syndrome?

Patients with this disorder present with either burning or hypersensitivity of the tongue. Others may have burning of the palate, gingiva, cheek, i.e., the soft tissues of the oral cavity. The most common presentation is burning and hypersensitivity of the tongue. The tongue may become smooth from atrophy of the papillae and taste may be affected. Patients often present to a dentist. Oral candidiasis, vitamin deficiencies, or chronic gingivitis must be ruled out. Typically, these diagnoses are excluded readily.

80. What are the causes of small fiber neuropathy?

Common causes include the following: diabetes or metabolic syndrome, Sjögren's syndrome, celiac disease, sarcoidosis, HIV disease, Lyme disease, alcoholism, and hypothyroidism. A sizable minority has an idiopathic source (40%). Less common causes include Fabry's disease. A disorder of the voltage-dependent sodium channel, Nav1.7, is noted in a significant number of "idiopathic" cases.

81. **What are the treatments for painful small fiber neuropathy?**
   Anticonvulsant adjuvant analgesics such as gabapentin, pregabalin, and acosamide can be used. Tricyclic antidepressants or duloxetine are also useful. In individuals with burning mouth syndrome, dry mouth is often a problem. Dry mouth precludes the use of tricyclic antidepressants. Since small fiber neuropathy has various causes, treating the underlying cause is necessary. If the neuropathy is from diabetes, good glycemic control is helpful. If it is autoimmune in origin, then either intravenous immunoglobulin or other immune-oriented treatment is needed. If it is hypothyroidism, correcting the deficiency is helpful. Supplementation with B vitamins is often an empiric addition.

ACUTE AND CHRONIC THORACOLUMBAR PAIN

Back pain is a very common condition, and most people have experienced back pain at least once during their lifetime.

82. **What are the common causes of acute pain of the mid-or lower back?**
   Common causes of acute nonspecific back pain include strain, myofascial dysfunction due to deconditioned state or poor posture, obesity, pregnancy, the perimenstrual state, and acute trauma.

83. **What is regarded as acute nonspecific back pain?**
   Nonspecific back pain refers to pain that is not associated with any radicular signs and evolves in the setting of a nonserious event and in the absence of warning signs such as fever or weight loss. The pain may be either nonmechanical (i.e., movement of the spinal segment does not provoke pain) or mechanical from disc disease, arthropathy, muscle or joint strain. The back pain may be referred pain such as menstrual-related back pain, constipation, or a disorder of the urinary tract.

84. **How do you treat acute nonspecific back pain?**
   The first duty is to make sure that a serious underlying pathology is not the cause of back pain. Thus, the history and physical examination findings are key. If a serious event such as either a major fall or motor vehicle accident has occurred, imaging is needed. If there is weight loss, fever, or neurologic deficits, the underlying pathology is no longer in the realm of benign nonspecific back pain, and imaging is mandatory. Acute, nonspecific back pain is treated conservatively with over-the-counter analgesics, muscle relaxants if there is muscle spasm, gentle back exercises, and as close to normal activity as the pain allows. If the back pain persists beyond 4 to 6 weeks, then diagnostic studies become warranted, and a change of therapeutic plan is in order.

85. **What do you do for a patient presenting with sciatica and lower back pain?**
   Such a patient needs diagnostic imaging with an MRI of the lumbar spine as first choice, and if MRI is precluded, computed tomography scan of the lumbar spine should be ordered. If the patient is free of neurologic deficits such as muscle weakness, a short tapering dose of steroids is reasonable. Other options if that fails to help include epidural steroid injection and neuropathic adjuvants such as gabapentin. In most instances conservative management will work, but lingering symptoms may warrant surgical consultation.

86. **How do you reconcile radicular symptoms in L5 distribution in a patient without nerve root compression from a small disc protrusion and no lateral recess or foraminal stenosis noted on MRI?**
   A leaky disc may be an alternative source of root inflammation rather than direct nerve root compression. If the patient has symptoms suggestive of sciatica, but there is no pain above the rim of the iliac crest, either piriformis syndrome as a source of sciatic compression or repeated compression from a bulky wallet should be considered.

87. **How would you approach a patient who presents with a history of severe, sharp pain in the mid-back after falling off a bar stool and landing on a concrete floor?**
   In the context of trauma, one is vertebral fracture. Most patients report severe, movement-elicited pain. Plain films of the thoracic spine and MRI are warranted. If fracture is confirmed, kyphoplasty may be an option if the patient is over 40 years old, the collapse is less than 80%, and there is no spinal stenosis from other causes.

88. **What is the prevalence of chronic back pain?**
   The prevalence ranges from 20% to 40% of the general population. An Internet-based survey study revealed that 30% of the general population has back pain lasting longer than 3 months, and about 50% of this population has chronic daily back pain.

89. **What are the common causes of back pain?**
The majority of patients with mechanical back pain suffer from either a myofascial syndrome or a poorly defined root cause. Other common causes include osteoarthritis, disc disease (herniation or degenerative), inflammatory arthritis such as inflammatory spondylitis, or rheumatoid arthritis.

90. **How do you treat chronic lower back pain?**
There is no simple or singular answer—especially in light of the fact that a large portion of back pain sufferers do not have a clearly identifiable source. Emphasis should be on improving function by way of physiotherapy and reconditioning measures. For nonspecific back pain the efficacy of interventional measures such as steroid injections is questionable. Opioid analgesics in this type of pain should be considered with extreme caution only. For osteoarthritic patients with pain correlating well with observed pathology, facet blocks or radiofrequency rhizotomy are reasonable approaches. Herniated disc and radicular pain may be treated with either epidural steroid injection or transforaminal root injections.

91. **Is a diagnostically based targeted approach feasible in the majority of chronic lower back pain sufferers?**
No. The majority of back pain sufferers may not have a diagnostically reliable source for their chronic pain. Back pain patients are a very heterogeneous population of patients. It makes study design a challenge when the precise source of pain is unclear. Nonetheless, there are a number of treatment measures that are generically broad spectrum in nature.

ACUTE AND CHRONIC NECK PAIN

92. **List common causes of neck pain.**
    - Cervical strain
    - Myofascial syndrome due to injury, overuse, malposturing, stress, or carrying a backpack or a heavy purse
    - Cervical spondylosis (common source of chronic neck pain)
    - Degenerative disc disorder—herniated or degenerative disc disease

93. **List serious causes of acute neck pain.**
    - Cervical trauma resulting in either fracture or subluxation
    - Cervical disc herniation resulting in myelopathic signs and symptoms
    - Acute neck pain associated with fever
    - Neck pain in a cancer patient associated with weakness, new-onset radicular numbness and/or pain or presence of a sensory level

94. **How do you treat acute cervical strain or nonspecific cervicalgia?**
Conservative treatment with NSAIDs with or without muscle relaxant is commonly employed. Most cases resolve within 2 to 6 weeks. If the pain lasts beyond this time, reevaluation is necessary. Sometimes there is lingering myofascial pain with reproducible trigger points. Trigger-point injection with either lidocaine and steroids or lidocaine alone is often helpful. Physical therapy should be considered for symptoms extending beyond 2 to 3 weeks.

95. **How do you approach the patient with fever and isolated neck pain?**
Fever and new-onset neck pain may be emanating from conditions such as cervical discitis, epidural abscess, or retropharyngeal abscess and should prompt emergent MRI of the cervical spine as well as complete blood count, erythrocyte sedimentation rate, and C-reactive protein.

KEY POINTS: THE LINK BETWEEN CLINICAL PRESENTATION AND TARGETED TREATMENT

1. Small fiber neuropathy may masquerade as fibromyalgia, burning mouth syndrome, or visceral autonomic dysfunction.
2. CDC recommends zoster vaccine for people at or over 60 years old due to higher incidence of postherpetic neuralgia.
3. Whatever the pain syndrome may be, think of pain processing mechanisms and how a drug, physical modality, or surgical intervention may alleviate the symptoms through targeted mechanisms.

MISCELLANEOUS ISSUES IN PAIN MANAGEMENT

96. What is pharmacogenetics?
Pharmacogenetics is the application of molecular genetics to decipher phenotype variations caused by genetic polymorphism or mutation.

97. Define polymorphism and mutation.
Polymorphism is a change in genotype that has an incidence of greater than 1% of the population. The most common cause of genetic variability is a single nucleotide change. In contrast, mutations occur in less than 1% of the population with higher occurrence of multisequence changes due to deletions, inversions, and duplications. The genotype/phenotype of the majority of a species population is called the *wild type*.

98. How may a polymorphism or mutation affect a patient's response to analgesics, anticonvulsants, and other pain-related pharmacotherapies?
Genetic variations exist at several levels: there are variants for transporters like P-glycoprotein for facilitation of absorption or distribution after a drug is consumed, metabolic enzymes such as cytochrome P450 enzymes affecting the conversion of the parent drug to active or inactive metabolites, and variants affecting enzymes responsible for enhancing excretion of a drug metabolite by making it more soluble for renal or fecal excretion through glucuronidation or sulfate conjugation. All in all, the response to a given drug may be enhanced, diminished, or made toxic or ineffective depending on the type of genetic polymorphism and influence any of the pharmacokinetic stages.

99. If a patient is receiving 2 mg of dilaudid intravenously every 3 hours, how much would that patient need when converted to oral dosing? Please look at the equianalgesic dosing table (see Table 27-2).
A reasonable dose would be about 8 mg every 3 hours according to the equianalgesic dose chart, but generally the conversion is factored down a bit to about 6 mg to start. The chart is just a general guideline, so individual variability must be taken into account.

100. Distinguish between tolerance and addiction.
Tolerance is the physiologic adaptation to a given drug such that the individual may develop faster metabolism and less of a physiologic response to the original dose. Addiction is the psychological dependence on a drug for nontherapeutic effects such as euphoria, sedation, or psychedelic experiences. In both instances, abrupt withdrawal of the drug may lead to withdrawal syndrome as is often seen with abrupt cessation of opioids, benzodiazepines, barbiturates, etc.

 References available online at expertconsult.com.

BIBLIOGRAPHY

1. Fishman SM, Ballantyne JC, Rathmell JP (eds): Bonica's Management of Pain, 4th ed. Philadelphia, Lippincott Williams and Wilkins, 2009.
2. Institute of Medicine: Relieving Pain in America: A Blueprint for Transforming Prevention, Care, Education, and Research. Washington, DC: National Academies Press, 2011.
3. Singh MK, Patel J, Gallagher M: Chronic Pain Syndrome, Medscape, 2014. Available at: http://emedwicine.medscape.com/article/310834-overview. [Accessed 25.06.15].

CHAPTER 28

PEDIATRIC NEUROLOGY

Angus A. Wilfong, James Owens

NORMAL NEUROLOGIC GROWTH AND DEVELOPMENT

1. In addition to the routine questions asked during a neurologic interview, what additional questions are important for a complete pediatric neurology history?
   - Antenatal history and risk factors
   - Perinatal history and risk factors
   - Neonatal history and complications
   - History of developmental milestones

2. List important features of the physical examination of infants and young children that may not be included in the examination of adults.
   - Measurement of the fronto-occipital circumference (FOC)
   - Palpation of cranial sutures and fontanelles if open
   - Dysmorphic facial features (such as hypertelorism, absence of philtrum, or low-set ears)
   - Limb asymmetries and malformations (including dermatoglyphics)
   - Abnormal skin lesions concerning for a neurocutaneous syndrome
   - Developmental reflexes

3. List the common developmental reflexes. When do you expect them to be present?
   See Table 28-1.

Table 28-1. Common Developmental Reflexes

REFLEX	APPEARS	DISAPPEARS
Lateral incurvation of trunk	Birth	1-2 months
Rooting	Birth	3 months
Moro	Birth	5-6 months
Tonic neck reflex	Birth	5-6 months
Palmar grasp	Birth	6 months
Crossed adduction	Birth	7-8 months
Plantar grasp	Birth	9-10 months
Extensor plantar responses	Birth	6-12 months
Parachute response	8-9 months	Persists
Landau reflex	10 months	24 months

4. What is the average FOC for a term newborn? What is the rate of growth over the first year?
   Average FOC of a term newborn is 35 cm. Average FOC growth is 2 cm per month for the first 3 months, 1 cm per month for the next 3 months, and 0.5 cm per month for the last 6 months. Adult head size averages approximately 57 cm.

PRENATAL DISEASES AND DEVELOPMENTAL DEFECTS

5. What is the Apgar score?
   The Apgar score is a clinical vitality rating scale applied to newborn infants in an attempt to identify those at risk for certain neonatal complications. Apgar is an eponym (Virginia Apgar, US obstetrical anesthesiologist), although it is often used as an acronym (Table 28-2).

Table 28-2. Apgar Score

	SIGN	Score		
		0	1	2
A	Appearance (color)	Blue, pale	Acrocyanosis	Pink
P	Pulse (heart rate)	Absent	<100	>100
G	Grimace (reflex irritability in response to nasal suctioning)	No response	Grimace	Cry
A	Activity (muscle tone)	Limp	Some flexion	Active motion
R	Respiration (respiratory effort)	Absent	Slow and irregular	Strong crying

Infants are routinely scored at 1 and 5 minutes after birth. Further scores may be made at 10 and 20 minutes if the infant appears to have been compromised.

6. **How is neonatal intraventricular hemorrhage (IVH) classified?**
   See Figure 28-1.

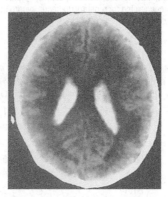

Figure 28-1. Unenhanced axial computed tomography (CT): grade III, intraventricular hemorrhage (IVH) in a premature newborn (32 weeks' gestation). Note acute ventricular distention with blood filling more than 50% of the ventricular volume. There is no parenchymal extension of the hemorrhage.

- Grade I: Localized subependymal hemorrhage into the germinal matrix
- Grade II: Subependymal hemorrhage with extension into the ventricles (less than 50% of the ventricular volume filled with blood)
- Grade III: Subependymal hemorrhage with extension into the ventricles and acute ventricular dilatation (greater than 50% of the ventricular volume filled with blood) (see Fig. 28-1)
- Grade IV (now referred to as a *periventricular hemorrhagic infarction*): Subependymal, intraventricular, and extension into the surrounding cerebral parenchyma

7. **What risk factors are thought to play a role in the genesis of IVH?**
   The most important risk factor for the development of an IVH is prematurity. While only about 10% of infants born at 28 weeks will develop a severe IVH, the risk for infants born at 24 weeks is closer to 25%. Birth weight (small, appropriate, or large for gestation age) is an independent risk factor. Other risk factors include mechanical ventilation, pneumothoraces, rapid expansion of intravascular volume (large or rapid IV infusions), rapid or wide fluctuations in blood pressure, hypoxic-ischemic injury, hypernatremia and hyperosmolality, and administration of certain medications such as indomethacin.

8. **What complications may arise secondary to an IVH?**
   The most common complications of IVH include posthemorrhagic hydrocephalus, seizures, and the parenchymal cerebral injury associated with periventricular hemorrhagic infarctions.

9. **Does the neurologic prognosis correlate with the different IVHs?**
   Generally, grades I and II IVH are relatively benign with some studies showing no long-term adverse developmental consequences. Grade III and periventricular hemorrhagic infarction (formerly grade IV) are consistently associated with adverse outcomes, with grade IV having by far the greatest likelihood of severe neurologic sequelae such as spastic quadriparesis, blindness, and cognitive impairment. Unilateral hemorrhages are associated with better neurodevelopmental outcomes than bilateral hemorrhages.

10. **What are the most common causes of a floppy baby? What are the least common?**
    By far the most frequent are the central causes involving the cerebellum, brain stem, basal ganglia, and cerebral hemispheres. The least common causes of infantile hypotonia afflict the peripheral nerves.

11. **What is the difference between macrocephaly and megalencephaly?**
    Macrocephaly refers to a large head, whereas megalencephaly refers specifically to a large brain.

12. **What is the differential diagnosis of macrocephaly in an infant?**
    - Hydrocephalus—obstructive or communicating
    - Extra-axial fluid collections
    - Thickened skull
    - Megalencephaly

13. **What is the differential diagnosis of megalencephaly?**
    - Toxic: cerebral edema from lead poisoning
    - White matter diseases such as Canavan's disease and Alexander's disease
    - Genetic disorders such as Sotos' syndrome

14. **Name genes commonly implicated in brain overgrowth syndromes.**
    - *PIK3CA*
    - *AKT1*
    - *AKT3*
    - *MTOR*
    - *PTEN*
    - *TSC1* and *TSC2*
    - *FGFR2* and *FGFR3*

    These genes are all part of the receptor tyrosine kinase (RTK)–phosphatidylinositol-3-kinase (PI3K)–AKT signaling pathway, which is an important regulator of cell growth.

15. **What is hemimegalencephaly? What clinical manifestations are commonly associated with hemimegalencephaly?**
    Hemimegalencephaly is a rare brain malformation associated with cortical overgrowth on one hemisphere. It is commonly associated with intractable partial seizures, significant developmental delay, and progressive hemiparesis. Several genetic causes have been discovered including *PIK3CA, PIK3R2, AKT3*, and *MTOR*. Surgical removal of the malformed hemisphere (hemispherectomy) may be necessary to achieve seizure control.

16. **In evaluating a child with microcephaly, what is the most important clinical feature?**
    Is the microcephaly congenital or acquired? Serial measurements of FOC are helpful. Is the FOC getting progressively worse (Rett's syndrome in girls), returning to normal (catch-up growth after a serious illness or prematurity), or remaining on the same percentile line (static process)? Review the antenatal history carefully for evidence of intrauterine infection. Did the infant appear healthy at birth? Any postnatal central nervous system (CNS) infections or trauma? Family history of microcephaly?

17. Which laboratory tests, if any, would you order in a child with microcephaly?
A head computed tomography (CT) scan allows assessment of the skull (for premature closure of the sutures) and also surveys for abnormal calcification (which may indicate infection with a toxoplasmosis, other agents, rubella, cytomegalovirus, herpes simplex [TORCH] agent, or earlier hypoxic-ischemic injury). A magnetic resonance imaging (MRI) scan gives greater anatomic detail of the brain parenchyma. In a neonate, TORCH titers may be measured if such an infection is suspected, and a chromosomal analysis—particularly a chromosomal microarray or targeted gene analysis depending on clinical suspicion—may be used to evaluate genetic causes. A basic metabolic screen (serum amino acids, urine organic acids, ammonia, and lactate) could be considered as well.

KEY POINTS: CAUSES OF INTRAUTERINE INFECTION

1. **TO** = **T**oxoplasmosis, **O**ther agents
2. **R** = **R**ubella
3. **C** = **C**ytomegalovirus
4. **H** = **H**erpes simplex virus

18. What are the most common complications of a lumbosacral myelomeningocele?
See Figure 28-2.

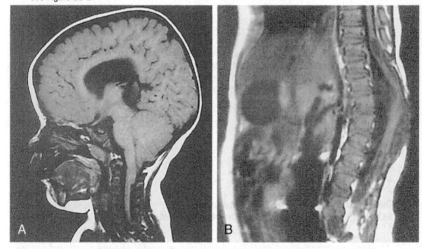

Figure 28-2. A, Unenhanced midsagittal T1-weighted magnetic resonance image (MRI) in a 6-month-old boy with type II Arnold–Chiari malformation. Note "herniation" or downward displacement of the cerebellar tonsils through the foramen magnum to the level of C2 and the associated obstructive hydrocephalus. **B,** Unenhanced midsagittal T1-weighted MRI lumbosacral spine: extensive thoracolumbar myelomeningocele associated with the Arnold–Chiari malformation in **A**. Note the dorsal kyphosis, absence of posterior elements of the vertebrae, and the malformed spinal cord at the level of the defect. A small syrinx in the cord is present above the defect.

- Type II Arnold–Chiari malformation resulting in hydrocephalus
- CNS infectious complications are common and devastating
- Renal failure due to chronic and repeated urinary tract infections and obstructive uropathy
- Seizures
- Progressive spasticity and weakness in the legs, worsening bladder and bowel function, progressive scoliosis, or increasing low back pain and stiffness due to a "tethered cord"

19. Classify the Arnold–Chiari malformations.
Type I: Downward displacement of the cerebellum with elongation of the medulla such that the cerebellar tonsils egress through the foramen.

Type II: Associated with lumbosacral myelomeningocele and numerous other nervous system malformations including:
- Small posterior fossa
- Cerebellar tonsil herniation through the foramen magnum
- Elongated and thinned medulla
- Characteristic beaking appearance of the quadrigeminal plate
- Hydrocephalus
- Syringomyelia and occasionally syringobulbia
- Interdigitation of gyri along the interhemispheric fissure

Type III: An occipital encephalocele with protrusion of cerebellar remnants into the overlying sac.

Type IV: Isolated hypoplasia of the cerebellum not associated with other nervous system malformations.

20. List the major developmental abnormalities of cortical development.
- Lissencephaly
- Holoprosencephaly
- Schizencephaly
- Polymicrogyria
- Pachygyria
- Double cortex syndrome (laminar heterotopia)
- Periventricular nodular heterotopia
- Focal cortical dysplasia

21. What is Down syndrome?
Down syndrome is a chromosomal anomaly with trisomy 21 characterized by marked infantile hypotonia with hyperflexibility of joints, cognitive impairment, brachycephaly with flat occiput, up-slanting palpebral fissures, late closure of fontanelles, flattened nasal bridge, epicanthal folds, speckling of iris (Brushfield's spots), fine lens opacities, small ears, hypoplastic teeth, short neck, brachydactyly with clinodactyly of fifth fingers, simian creases, wide space between first and second toes, congenital heart disease (in 40%), and hypogonadism.

22. A school-aged child is referred for evaluation of possible absence epilepsy because of constant "day-dreaming" and worsening grades. The mother and teachers relate a history of short attention span for schoolwork but not for television or video games, easy distractibility, impulsiveness, constant supervision needed to complete homework and chores, adventurous and risk-taking behavior, and constant physical activity (as if driven by a motor). What is the most likely diagnosis?
This is the usual presentation of a child with attention-deficit/hyperactivity disorder (ADHD). Some children have the attention deficit without the hyperactivity. Affected children have unusually short attention spans and are simply unable to concentrate for more than a few minutes for all but the most stimulating and enjoyable activities. Their constant distractibility and day-dreaming may be confused with the seizures of absence epilepsy.

23. What are the key diagnostic features of an autism spectrum disorder (ASD)?
- Deficits in social communication and social interaction
- Restricted, repetitive patterns of behavior, interests, or activities (such as repetitive movements, stereotyped speech, highly restricted interests, or very inflexible adherence to routines)
- Motor development is generally not affected though patients may be "clumsy"
- Symptoms are present from early in the developmental period
- Discrete categories such as "autistic disorder" and "Asperger syndrome" have now been replaced by one overarching diagnosis: ASD.

24. In addition to these key diagnostic features, name three common neurologic comorbidities of ASD.
- Sleep disturbance—particularly insomnia with difficulty initiating and/or maintaining sleep
- Epilepsy—which occurs at a much higher rate in ASD patients than in the general population
- ADHD—a disorder that may now be diagnosed in patients with an ASD

NEURODEGENERATIVE DISORDERS

25. **In general terms, how does a neurodegenerative disease affecting white matter present?**
Loss of motor skills, progressive spasticity, and ataxia. A disorder affecting the white matter is referred to as a *leukodystrophy*.

26. **In general terms, how does a neurodegenerative disease affecting gray matter present?**
Loss of intellectual skills (dementia), seizures, and blindness. A disorder affecting gray matter was once called a *poliodystrophy*.

27. **Name a neurodegenerative disorder that affects both the CNS and the peripheral nervous system.**
Krabbe's disease (globoid cell leukodystrophy) is an autosomal recessive enzyme defect in galacto-sylceramide beta-galactosidase that results in irritability, increased tone, optic atrophy, cortical blindness, and peripheral nerve segmental demyelination. Metachromatic leukodystrophy is an autosomal recessive lysosomal storage disorder caused by a mutation in arylsulfatase A that also affects both central and peripheral myelin.

28. **Which leukodystrophy is virtually always associated with a particular endocrinologic deficiency?**
See Figure 28-3. Adrenoleukodystrophy, an X-linked recessive disorder, is one of the peroxisomal disorders. It is characterized by impaired beta-oxidation of the very long-chain (C26) fatty acids, leading to their accumulation. In addition, patients also have adrenocortical insufficiency. Onset is usually between 4 and 6 years of age. An adult form of the disease called *adrenomyeloneuropathy* is characterized by progressive spastic paraparesis and peripheral neuropathy.

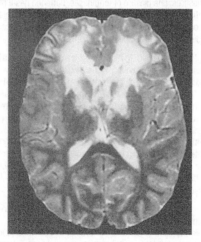

Figure 28-3. Unenhanced axial T2-weighted magnetic resonance image (MRI) in a 9-year-old boy with adrenoleukodystrophy. Note extensive dysmyelination involving the anterior centrum semiovale, subcortical white matter, genu of the corpus callosum, and internal capsule. The cerebral cortex, basal ganglia, and thalami are unaffected.

29. **How often does multiple sclerosis present in children?**
Approximately 3% to 5% of all patients with multiple sclerosis (MS) have onset of symptoms in childhood. The majority of affected children (more than 90%) are older than 10 years of age, but MS cases have been described in patients younger than 3 years of age.

30. **What is a cherry-red spot?**
Cherry-red spot is the bright red appearance of the fovea centralis of the eye as seen by funduscopy in children with certain gray matter storage diseases, classically Tay–Sachs disease. As the storage

material accumulates in the nerve fiber layer, the retina takes on a grayish-white appearance. Because there are very few fibers traversing the fovea, it retains its normal color and continues to reflect the bright red vascular choroid underneath.

31. What are the neuronal ceroid lipofuscinoses (NCL)?

NCL are a group of autosomal recessively inherited lysosomal storage disorders characterized by excessive neuronal accumulations of the lipid pigments, ceroid, and lipofuscin. They present as classic gray matter diseases with intractable seizures, progressive dementia, and blindness. Together they represent the most commonly diagnosed pediatric neurodegenerative disorder. The genetic basis of these diseases is increasingly understood with 13 genes presently implicated.

32. Which endocrinologic disorder may present as a gray matter neurodegenerative disease if it is missed on the newborn screening?

Congenital hypothyroidism (cretinism) is extremely difficult to detect clinically at birth, and the diagnosis may not be suspected until it is too late for replacement therapy to be maximally efficacious. Left untreated, these children develop prolonged jaundice, abdominal distention with umbilical hernia, large fontanelles, hypotonia, impaired bony development, large tongue, psychomotor retardation, seizures, spasticity, ataxia, and deafness.

33. What are ragged-red fibers?

In some of the mitochondrial cytopathies, mitochondria become clumped beneath the skeletal muscle sarcolemmal membrane. When the muscle biopsy specimen is prepared with modified Gomori's trichrome stain and viewed by light microscopy, the clumps of mitochondria stain red and give the muscle fibers a ragged appearance—hence the term *ragged-red fibers*.

NEUROCUTANEOUS SYNDROMES

34. What is the most common neurocutaneous syndrome?

Neurofibromatosis (NF) type I has an incidence of 1/3000 to 4000 of the population. Inheritance is autosomal dominant and the spontaneous mutation rate (chromosome 17) is very high (30% to 50%). Clinical characteristics include café-au-lait spots, neurofibromas, axillary/inguinal freckling, optic gliomas, megalencephaly, mental retardation, seizures, and characteristic bony lesions.

35. Which neurocutaneous syndrome is associated with infantile spasms and a hypsarrhythmia pattern on electroencephalogram?

Tuberous sclerosis (TS), an autosomal dominant disorder with genetic heterogeneity (similar phenotype with mutation on either chromosome 9 or 16). Incidence is 1/10,000 with a high-spontaneous mutation rate. Clinical features include mental retardation, seizures, adenoma sebaceum, ash-leaf spots, shagreen patches, café-au-lait spots, subungual and periungual fibromas (Koenen's tumors), gingival fibromas, dental enamel pits, retinal tumors (mulberry tumor of the optic disc), cardiac rhabdomyomas, renal angiomyolipomas, and CNS cortical tubers and subependymal hamartomas that calcify.

36. Of the more common neurocutaneous syndromes, which has no clear pattern of inheritance?

Sturge–Weber syndrome (encephalofacial angiomatosis), which is less common than NF or TS. Patients have a facial port-wine stain (nevus) that is usually unilateral involving the V_1 segment of the trigeminal nerve. The nevus may involve the ocular choroidal membrane, causing glaucoma. Arteriography reveals extensive arteriovenous malformation involving the ipsilateral cerebral hemispheric dura.

37. In addition to brain and skin involvement, which other neurocutaneous syndrome has an immune disorder and a high propensity for malignancy?

Ataxia-telangiectasia is an autosomal recessive disorder with an incidence of 1/100,000. Affected individuals develop telangiectasias by 2 to 4 years of age on exposed areas of skin and conjunctiva. Progressive cerebellar ataxia begins within the first few years of life. Patients have decreased or absent IgA and IgE and decreased IgG_2 and IgG_4. Defective cellular DNA repair leads to increased spontaneous and radiation-induced chromosomal aberrations, inducing various neoplasias. The disorder is caused by inactivation of the ataxia-telangiectasia-mutated protein kinase involved in detecting double-stranded DNA breaks and helping to coordinate repair.

INFECTIONS AND INFESTATIONS

38. **What are the most common bacterial pathogens for acute meningitis in neonates and children?**

Neonatal
- Group B beta-hemolytic streptococci
- *Escherichia coli*
- *Listeria monocytogenes*
- *Klebsiella pneumoniae*

Childhood
- *Haemophilus influenzae* type B
- *Streptococcus pneumoniae*
- *Neisseria meningitides*

While vaccination has largely eliminated *H. influenzae* type B, nontypable *H. influenzae* is still seen. Worldwide these three bacteria are responsible for approximately 90% of acute bacterial meningitis in childhood.

39. **What are the usual signs and symptoms of neonatal meningitis?**
- Lethargy
- Irritability
- Hypothermia or hyperthermia
- Poor feeding
- Bulging fontanelle (a later sign)
- Seizures

40. **What are the usual signs and symptoms of an older infant or child with acute meningitis?**
- Fever
- Headache
- Altered mental status
- Stiff neck
- Nausea and vomiting
- Seizures

41. **How does the presentation of tuberculous meningitis differ from acute bacterial meningitis?**

Tuberculous meningitis is difficult to diagnose in its earliest stages as the symptoms tend to be nonspecific, mild to moderate in severity, and persistent (weeks). Poor weight gain, low-grade fever, and listlessness may be seen in young children while older children may manifest headache and emesis. As the disease progresses the symptoms become more severe with obtundation and evidence of meningeal irritation. As tuberculosis tends to cause a basilar meningitis, cranial neuropathies are often seen in later stages. Cerebrovascular disease with ischemic strokes is also seen—likely due to the proximal anterior circulation passing through the inflammatory infectious exudate.

42. **A child from Central America presents with a prolonged partial motor seizure. Neurologic examination reveals no focal or lateralizing findings; however, funduscopic examination reveals early papilledema. CT scanning of the brain discloses a number of small, densely calcified lesions scattered along the gray–white junction of the cerebral hemispheres. What is the most likely diagnosis and how might you confirm your suspicions?**

The pork tapeworm, *Taenia solium*, is endemic in Central America. When a human (rather than the pig) becomes the intermediate host, he may develop neurocysticercosis. This occurs when the ingested *T. solium* ova become partially digested, releasing onchospheres that gain access to the circulation and are carried throughout the body. They then become larvae (cysticerci) in subcutaneous tissue, muscle, and brain where the majority die and become densely calcified. The diagnosis can be confirmed by serum or cerebrospinal fluid (CSF) antibody and antigen detection methods and in certain cases by tissue biopsy (Fig. 28-4).

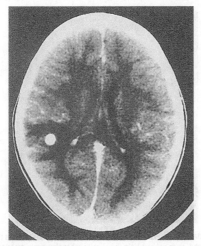

Figure 28-4. Enhanced axial computed tomography (CT): neurocysticercosis in a 7-year-old girl. Note the solitary, densely enhancing lesion with surrounding edema.

VASCULAR DISORDERS

43. **What is the most common hemoglobinopathy associated with cerebrovascular disease?**
    Approximately one-fourth of all patients with sickle cell disease experience cerebrovascular complications; the vast majority are children. When strokes occur in adults, they are more likely to be intracerebral hemorrhages as opposed to the infarctions that affect children. In addition to small vessel occlusion by sickled red cells, endothelial proliferation is also thought to be an important mechanism in the genesis of these strokes.

NEOPLASMS

44. **Where are brain tumors most common in infants, children, and adults?**
    In infants less than 1 year of age, supratentorial brain tumors predominate. In children older than 1 year, infratentorial tumors are more common. In adults, supratentorial tumors are again more frequently encountered. Brain tumors are the second most common malignancy in children.

45. **What are primitive neuroectodermal tumors (PNET)?**
    These are highly malignant, small, blue cell tumors. If a PNET is completely undifferentiated and is in the midline posterior fossa, it is often referred to as a *medulloblastoma*. PNET may show varying degrees of differentiation along different cell lines, including glial, ependymal, pineal, and neuronal (Fig. 28-5).

46. **A school-aged child complains of recurrent headaches and recent onset of marked polyuria and polydipsia. Examination reveals bitemporal homonymous hemianopsia and papilledema. Laboratory tests are consistent with diabetes insipidus. Where is the lesion?**
    The anatomic location of this lesion must be in the parasellar region. The visual field defect is produced by compression of the optic chiasm. The diabetes insipidus is produced by compression of the pituitary stalk (Fig. 28-6).

47. **What is the differential diagnosis of parasellar tumors in children?**
    - Craniopharyngioma
    - Germ cell tumor, including teratoma
    - Pituitary adenoma
    - Optic glioma

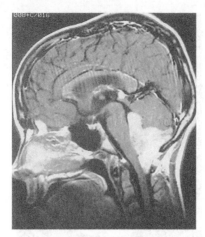

Figure 28-5. Enhanced midsagittal T1-weighted magnetic resonance image (MRI) reveals a posterior fossa primitive neuroectodermal tumor (PNET) in a 5-year-old boy. Note the brightly enhancing tumor mass extending upward through the fourth ventricle into the cerebral aqueduct and downward through the foramen magnum. There is compression of the medulla and marked displacement of the cerebellum. Early obstructive hydrocephalus is developing.

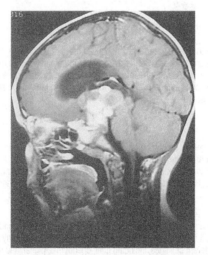

Figure 28-6. Enhanced midsagittal T1-weighted magnetic resonance image (MRI) demonstrates a craniopharyngioma in a 3-year-old girl. Note the large, multilobulated tumor extending from the parasellar region through the midbrain. The tumor has brightly enhancing solid areas and fluid-filled cysts. There is associated obstructive hydrocephalus.

- Hypothalamic glioma
- Chordoma of the clivus

48. Most posterior fossa tumors in children have a poor prognosis except for one, which has an excellent prognosis. What is it?
Juvenile cerebellar pilocytic astrocytoma has virtually a 100% 5-year survival rate. This tumor develops in the cerebellar hemispheres of school-aged children. Histologically, the tumor cells are hair-like (pilocytic). The tumor is classified as a grade 1 neoplasm, which is a well-circumscribed neoplasm without local invasiveness. Complete resection is curative.

49. An older child with medically intractable complex partial seizures has an MRI scan performed. The scan reveals a partially calcified mass in the right mesial temporal lobe without associated edema. What is the most likely diagnosis?

Gangliogliomas, oligodendrogliomas, and dysembryoplastic neuroepithelial tumors are slow-growing neoplasms whose only clinical signs may be intractable seizures.

INJURY BY PHYSICAL AGENTS AND TRAUMA

50. Does age have any effect on whether or not cranial irradiation would be considered as treatment for cancer?

Children who received cranial X-ray therapy (XRT) prior to 3 years of age have significantly reduced intelligence quotients later in life.

51. What are some of the other adverse effects that may be encountered in children who receive cranial XRT?

- Transient somnolence, headaches, and anorexia 6 to 8 weeks after initiation of XRT are common.
- Radiation necrosis (radionecrosis) may occur 1 to 3 years post-XRT and can mimic a mass effect, making it difficult to distinguish tumor recurrence from radionecrosis. Pathologically the lesion involves hyalinization of blood vessels with infarction and necrosis of brain tissue.
- Hypothalamic–pituitary dysfunction, which usually involves decreased production of growth hormone and thyroid-stimulating hormone.
- Formation of cataracts if the ocular globes were exposed to radiation.
- Induction of a second malignancy that may appear years later.

52. A 6-month-old infant presents with obtundation and recent seizures. Examination reveals no fever, anterior fontanelle slightly bulging, depressed level of consciousness, and hypotonia. On funduscopic examination, extensive, bilateral retinal hemorrhages and mild papilledema are observed. What is your leading diagnosis?

Child abuse, specifically the shaken-baby syndrome or nonaccidental trauma, needs to be first on the list of diagnostic possibilities. Because of the violent shaking of the body and head, these infants sustain subarachnoid hemorrhages and associated retinal hemorrhages. This commonly leads to seizures and may cause cortical infarctions as the cerebral vessels spasm.

53. What is a growing skull fracture?

This is a rather rare complication of linear skull fractures, usually occurring in children younger than 3 years of age. Because of brain and CSF pulsations, the opposing edges of bone along the fracture do not fuse. Resorption of bone along the edges occurs so that the fracture opening progressively enlarges, producing a "growing skull fracture."

SEIZURES AND OTHER PAROXYSMAL DISORDERS

54. What is a complex febrile seizure?

The seizure has focal features, lasts longer than 15 minutes or recurs within 24 hours, or occurs in a child younger than 6 months or older than 5 years of age.

KEY POINTS: SIMPLE FEBRILE SEIZURE

1. A generalized tonic or tonic–clonic seizure
2. Between 3 months and 5 years of age
3. Fever greater than 38° C not associated with a CNS infection
4. Lasting less than 15 minutes, no focal features, does not recur within 24 hours
5. No postictal neurologic abnormalities

55. Does having had a simple febrile convulsion increase the risk for later development of epilepsy (recurrent nonfebrile seizures)?

The risk is minimally elevated, if at all. At worst the risk rises from the background rate of 1% to a rate of 2% (meaning that 98% of patients with simple febrile seizures do not develop epilepsy). The risk for patients with complex febrile seizures is higher: 4% to 6%.

56. What is generalized epilepsy with febrile seizures plus GEFS+?

GEFS+ is an epilepsy syndrome with a highly variable phenotype. Within a single family some affected members may have febrile seizures alone, some may have febrile seizures and afebrile seizures, and others may have only afebrile seizures. The understanding of GEFS+ has been significantly advanced by the discovery of several associated genes including *SCN1A*, *SCN1B*, and *GABARG2*. Given that these genes encode ion channel or ionotropic receptor subunits, GEFS+ is presently considered a "channelopathy."

57. A 16-month-old child is being seen for difficult-to-control seizures. He was born at term with no neurodevelopmental concerns until a prolonged febrile seizure at 6 months of age. This febrile seizure was soon followed by another episode of febrile status epilepticus, and then the patient began having generalized tonic–clonic seizures as well as apparently focal seizures. Despite trials of several anticonvulsants he continues to have frequent seizures. His developmental trajectory, which was initially normal, has now slowed. What gene mutation does this patient most likely have?

The history of early prolonged febrile seizures followed by difficult-to-control afebrile generalized and focal seizures in a previously normal child would be consistent with Dravet syndrome, also called *severe myoclonic epilepsy* in infancy. The patient's acquired developmental delay would also be consistent. Patients go on to develop other types of seizures including atypical absence and myoclonic seizures. Approximately 70% to 80% of patients with Dravet syndrome have a mutation in the *SCN1A* gene, which codes for the neuronal type 1 alpha subunit of the voltage-gated sodium channel. Interestingly, mutations in this same gene can cause GEFS+, which is usually associated with a much better prognosis.

58. An 18-month-old child is referred for possible epilepsy. The mother relates a history of paroxysmal spells that have occurred over the past month. Each spell consists of the child turning red, then blue in the face, and then passing out with a few clonic jerks of the extremities. Immediately before each spell, the child had been startled, frightened, or frustrated and began crying. What is the probable diagnosis?

This is a typical history of blue breath-holding spells, a form of infantile syncope. Breath-holding spells occur in 4% to 5% of children; there is a positive family history in 25% of cases. Two-thirds have cyanotic or blue breath-holding spells, 20% have pallid breath-holding spells, and the remainder have a mixture of the two. The peak incidence is between 1 and 2 years of age and resolution usually occurs by 6 years of age. The spells follow minor injuries, fright, or frustration. Patients with a history of breath-holding spells are more likely to have symptomatic orthostatic syncope as adolescents.

HEAD PAIN

59. What are the clinical features of childhood migraine headaches?
- Migraine headaches in children are common (prevalence of 1% to 3% in 3- to 7-year-olds and almost 25% of adolescents).
- Fifty percent of all individuals who develop migraine had the onset of their attacks before 20 years of age.
- Boys are more frequently affected until puberty, after which time the incidence is considerably higher in girls.
- Younger children usually complain of a generalized, bifrontal, or bitemporal headache, rather than the hemicranial pain characteristically present in the older child or adult.
- Abdominal distress with nausea and sometimes vomiting is prominent.
- The child often appears pale and frequently stops all activities and lies down.
- Photophobia and phonophobia are usually present but may need to be inferred from behavior in younger children.
- If the child is able to fall asleep, the headache is usually gone upon awakening.
- Family history for migraine is positive in 70% to 90% of cases.

60. What are the different types of migraine headaches in children?
    - **Migraine without aura** (formerly common migraine): accounts for up to three-quarters of all migraine attacks. Clinical manifestations are those listed in the preceding answer.
    - **Migraine with aura** (formerly classic migraine): same as above except these individuals experience an aura just before the onset of the headache.
    - **Complicated migraine**: migraine headache associated with various transient neurologic phenomena. These include hemiplegic migraine, ophthalmoplegic migraine, vertebrobasilar migraine, and acute confusional migraine.
    - **Migraine variants or equivalents**: benign paroxysmal vertigo of childhood, paroxysmal torticollis, and cyclical vomiting of childhood are syndromes thought to be related to migraine.

61. What are the most important pharmacologic agents used in treating migraine?
    - **Symptomatic treatments**: Analgesics that have no action on the underlying cause of the migraine headache. Examples include aspirin, ibuprofen, acetaminophen, codeine, and meperidine. It is usually best to avoid narcotic preparations in the treatment of chronic illnesses if at all possible.
    - **Abortive therapies**: Vasoactive agents that modify the vasculature so that the migraine headache is aborted before becoming fully developed. Serotonin receptor partial agonists ("triptans") such as sumatriptan are most commonly used, though ergotamine derivatives are also sometimes employed, particularly in the management of prolonged or refractory headaches.
    - **Prophylactic medications**: Drugs that prevent the migraine headaches from occurring. Examples include beta-blockers, calcium channel blockers, antiepileptic medications (sodium valproate and topiramate), tricyclic antidepressants (amitriptyline), and cyproheptadine (an antihistamine that is also a serotonin receptor antagonist).

KEY POINTS: HEADACHES CONCERNING FOR AN INTRACRANIAL MASS

1. Recent onset of headaches or change in character of chronic headaches
2. Headaches that awaken the patient from sleep or are present on awakening in the morning
3. Association with altered mental status, vomiting, constriction of visual fields, or focal neurologic deficits

NEUROMUSCULAR DISORDERS

62. What protein is missing in Duchenne muscular dystrophy (DMD)?
    The missing gene product is a protein called *dystrophin*. Dystrophin is a structural protein that helps to link extracellular matrix proteins, via the sarcoglycan complex, with actin and myosin. It is important in several tissues, including skeletal muscle, cardiac muscle, and brain. Certain mutations of the dystrophin gene lead to essentially no dystrophin production and result in DMD. Other mutations allow for the production of some dystrophin and cause the less severe and late-onset Becker muscular dystrophy.

63. What are the clinical manifestations of DMD?
    Affected children are normal through the first year of life. The first clue is that the child may walk later than expected, but detectable weakness is not present until 3 to 4 years of age. The pelvic girdle weakens first and gives rise to the characteristic Gowers' sign. Soon widespread weakness is apparent, and relentless progression ensues. Most children become unable to walk by the end of their first decade. Once the patient is wheelchair bound, flexion contractures and progressive scoliosis develop. Cardiac involvement is invariable. Mild intellectual impairment is also common in these patients. Death from pulmonary infection, respiratory failure, or cardiac failure usually occurs by age 30 years.

64. What treatment is available for children with DMD?
    Treatment with daily oral corticosteroids from the time of diagnosis until the time the child requires a wheelchair appears to slow the course of DMD.

65. What are the most common congenital myopathies?
    - Central core disease
    - Centronuclear myopathy
    - Nemaline myopathy
    - Minimal change myopathy
    - Congenital fiber type disproportion

66. What are the clinical manifestations of myotonic muscular dystrophy type 1?
    - Myotonic dystrophy type 1 is caused by a trinucleotide (CTG) expansion in the *DMPK* gene. Myotonic dystrophy type 2 is less common and is caused by a tetranucleotide (CCTG) expansion in the *CCTG* gene.
    - Clinical manifestations of myotonic dystrophy type 1 usually begin in adolescence or early adult life with distal muscle weakness and myotonia. Given the phenomenon of anticipation the disease may manifest in childhood if the inherited repeat size is large.
    - Muscle wasting about the face and sternocleidomastoids, in combination with facial weakness, leading to the distinctive "hatchet-face" appearance
    - Partial ptosis, swan-like posture of the neck, enlarged paranasal sinuses, early prominent male-pattern balding in both sexes
    - Cataracts, cardiac conduction abnormalities, hypogonadism with testicular atrophy, and abnormal glucose tolerance

67. What is a common complication of neonates born to mothers with myotonic muscular dystrophy?
    Some newborns who have inherited the myotonic dystrophy gene from their mothers experience profound weakness, with respiratory failure and bulbar insufficiency requiring endotracheal intubation and mechanical ventilation. The mortality rate may be as high as 30% to 40%. Should the neonate survive, the weakness resolves spontaneously. The occurrence of the neonatal syndrome has no effect on the severity of the adult expression of the disease.

68. What are the two types of myasthenia that may affect the newborn or young infant?
    - **Transient neonatal myasthenia gravis**. Affected neonates are born to mothers with autoimmune myasthenia gravis. Because of transplacental transfer of maternal antiacetylcholine (ACh) receptor antibodies, newborns experience transient weakness and hypotonia, which may be severe and life threatening.
    - **Nonautoimmune congenital myasthenia syndromes**

69. Which types of myasthenia are not due to autoimmune production of antibodies against the ACh receptor?
    - Defects in ACh synthesis or mobilization
    - End-plate acetylcholinesterase deficiency
    - Slow-channel syndrome
    - End-plate ACh receptor deficiency

70. A school-aged child presents with a few days' history of progressive weakness in his legs. This "ascending paralysis" was first noted at his ankles and now has spread to involve his hips. List the differential diagnoses.
    - Guillain–Barré syndrome
    - Acute spinal cord lesion
    - Tick bite paralysis
    - West Nile virus
    - Poliomyelitis (usually asymmetrical weakness)
    - Periodic paralysis (usually episodic)
    - Acute cerebellar ataxia
    - Myasthenia gravis (usually waxing and waning)
    - Botulism (usually descending)

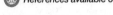 *References available online at expertconsult.com.*

BIBLIOGRAPHY

1. Dubowitz V: Muscle Disorders in Childhood, 3rd ed. Philadelphia, WB Saunders, 2001.
2. Fenichel GM: Clinical Pediatric Neurology: A Signs and Symptoms Approach, 7th ed. Philadelphia, Elsevier, 2013.
3. McMillan JA, Feigin RD, DeAngelis CD, Jones MD, (eds): Oski's Pediatrics, 4th ed. Philadelphia, Lippincott Williams & Wilkins, 2006.
4. Menkes JH, Sarnat HB, (eds): Child Neurology, 7th ed. Philadelphia, Lippincott Williams & Wilkins, 2005.
5. Swaimann KF, Ashwal S, Ferriero DM, Schor NF, (eds): Pediatric Neurology: Principles and Practice, 5th ed. Philadelphia, Mosby, 2012.
6. Volpe JJ: Neurology of the Newborn, 5th ed. Philadelphia, Saunders, 2008.

CHAPTER 29

PSYCHIATRY IN NEUROLOGY

Joshua J. Rodgers, Benjamin L. Weinstein

GENERAL PSYCHIATRY

1. When referring to brain dysfunction (neurologic and psychiatric disorders), why are the terms *focal* and *functional* preferred over *organic* and *inorganic*?
   Using the terms *organic* and *inorganic* to refer to neurologic and psychiatric disorders, respectively, follows from the dualistic (Cartesian) model—an antiquated model that regards mind and brain as two distinct entities, which somehow are unified. A modern neuroscience-based view is that mind is a verb; mind is what the brain does via the integration of mainly frontal and limbic cortical–subcortical circuits and distributed networks working in parallel processing. Disruption of the function of these circuits and networks underlies mental disorders.

2. What is the *Diagnostic and Statistical Manual for Psychiatric Disorders* (DSM)?
   In the United States, the DSM, now in its 5th edition (DSM-5), is the most widely used clinical diagnostic schemata for psychiatric disorders. While the earliest form of the DSM was intended solely as a research tool, it has since undergone revisions to improve the validity of its diagnostic constructs and, by incorporating developmental, medical, psychological, and psychosocial factors, expand in clinical utility and is used to inform treatment selection, patient education, and prognosis and to facilitate clinical communication.

3. Does the DSM describe specific diseases?
   Diagnoses in the DSM are based on sign and symptom clusters (phenomenology) involving cognitive, emotional, and/or behavioral dysfunction and are more akin to syndromes than diseases; the clinical presentation and course, rather than a specific etiopathology, defines the diagnosis. As such, there is often overlap among diagnostic criteria, and many disorders are considered to exist on a spectrum (and/or dimensions) ranging from normal experience/response to persistent and pervasive pathology (i.e., personality disorders).

4. At what point do symptoms (e.g., sad feelings) become a disorder (e.g., major depressive disorder) as defined in the DSM?
   Generally, to meet diagnostic criteria of a disorder the symptoms must result in distress and disruption of functional ability of the individual (e.g., interference with work). Allowances are made for culturally/religiously normative behaviors or sociopolitical deviance (DSM-5, p 20).

5. Why are psychiatric diagnoses generally "diagnoses of exclusion"?
   A multitude of etiopathologic origins can underlie psychiatric phenomenology. While the etiopathology may be known in some cases, psychiatric disorders are often complex and idiopathic. Care should be taken to evaluate for and exclude known medical causes of the phenomenology before a psychiatric diagnosis is made.

6. What are some interviewing techniques for eliciting sensitive information (e.g., sexual trauma history, suicidality, or current substance abuse)?
   - Start with open-ended questions and an empathic and nonjudgmental demeanor.
   - Consider follow-up with structured, systematic questions (employ structured interviews and/or screening tools as appropriate); straightforward questions are preferred.
   - Ease disclosure of sensitive information by use of normalization and symptom assumption (phrasing questions to imply a behavior is normal, understandable, or to be expected).

7. How can you foster patient alliance in difficult situations, e.g., patients with somatic symptom disorders (SSDs)?
   - Listen first and empathically and nonjudgmentally reflect the patient's understanding and concerns and validate the patient's experience of symptoms.
   - Avoid use of unnecessary stigmatizing labels or colloquial jargon (e.g., "it's all in your head") and empathize with the real experience of symptoms (e.g., psychogenic nonepileptic seizures are still seizures, they're just not caused by epilepsy).

- Find common goals (your goal should be the patient's improvement), and focus on these rather than convincing him or her of your diagnosis.
- Anchor proposed interventions in known or presumed pathophysiologic mechanisms as appropriate (i.e., use psychoeducation).
- Encourage use of a symptom diary, and focus on reduction rather than elimination of symptoms.
- Encourage frequent follow-up with a single provider (you if appropriate).
- Maintain vigilance for changing psychological, social, and biological factors (including routine health maintenance and screening for development of medical disorders).

8. What is motivational interviewing?
Motivational interviewing is a technique based on the Stages of Change Model developed initially to help patients with substance addiction address their ambivalence (mixed feelings) regarding their addiction and desire to quit. It has since been applied to a variety of situations in which fostering the intrinsic (within the patient) motivation to change is the goal (such as improving patient compliance with treatments).

9. What are the stages in the Stages of Change Model and are they clinically valid?
The Stages of Change Model, while heuristically valuable, has not been found to validly reflect any actual sequentially discrete sequence of change. The stages in the model are as follows:
- **Precontemplation:** characterized by denial and minimization
- **Contemplation:** characterized by thinking about change
- **Preparation:** characterized by making preparations to do something
- **Action:** characterized by actually implementing concrete actions directed at the problem
- **Maintenance:** characterized by implementing change-maintaining actions

10. What is the difference between classical and operant conditioning?
In classical conditioning, a conditioned stimulus (such as a bell ringing) is paired with a stimulus that is already hard-wired to evoke a response (such as food evoking salivation) until the conditioned stimulus evokes the same response. In operant conditioning, behavior is reinforced by reward and the best way to do this is with positive reinforcement given at an intermittent (variable) schedule (like how casinos reward gambling).

11. What are the major types of psychotherapies and which types may be better for patients with cognitive limitations?
Supportive therapy (Table 29-1) aims to bolster existing adaptive (healthy) coping skills and is well suited for nearly all patients, even those with cognitive limitations. Psychoeducation—teaching patients about brain function and the relevant aspects of their psychiatric disorder and treatments—is also appropriate for nearly all patients and can be empowering and facilitate adaptive coping. Psychotherapies that require higher levels of cognitive input on the part of the patient (as well as extensive training on the part of the therapist) include psychoanalysis, psychodynamic psychotherapy, interpersonal psychotherapy, cognitive behavioral therapy (CBT), dialectical behavioral therapy (DBT), and group and couples therapy.

Table 29-1. Select Supportive Therapy Techniques

Aim to enhance the patient's self-esteem; praise and encourage use of strengths.
Keep the therapy focused in a constructive direction rather than encouraging the patient to say whatever comes to mind.
Aim to allay any anxiety generated by the therapy itself.
Respond to the patient's questions with appropriate answers.
Make suggestions and give advice.
Use clarification and confrontation but generally avoid interpretation.

Adapted from Abernethy R, Schlozman S. An overview of the psychotherapies. In Stern TA, Fava M, Wilens TE, Rosenbaum JF, editors. *Massachusetts General Hospital Comprehensive Clinical Psychiatry.* London, Elsevier, p. 104 (Box 10-4), 2016.

12. What basic workup is recommended for patients presenting with psychiatric signs and symptoms and what additional exams or tests may be considered? See Table 29-2.

Table 29-2. Laboratory Tests and Other Studies Useful for Psychiatric Symptom Workup

TEST	PURPOSE/CLINICAL SITUATION/WHEN TO CONSIDER
*Physical exam: including complete neurologic exam, vital signs, height and weight (BMI), waist circumference	All patients; observe for focal deficits; exclude medical problems; establish a baseline; monitoring
Basic labs: *CBC, *BMP, *calcium, *phosphorus, *LFTs, lipids, *UA, pregnancy test, hemoglobin A1c, *vitamin B12, *folate, vitamin D, blood alcohol level, *thiamine, *urine toxicology screen	Routine evaluation of most psychiatric complaints (evaluate for medical illness and substance use) and baseline and routine monitoring of pharmacologic treatments
*Prescription drug levels	Sub- or supratherapeutic effects (e.g., toxicity)
Medication levels	Sub- or supratherapeutic effects (e.g., toxicity); especially for medications with narrow therapeutic windows such as lithium, valproate, clozapine, and tricyclic antidepressants
*Thyroid function tests (TFTs)	Mood or anxiety symptoms, dementia, lithium monitoring
Serology for *HIV, *syphilis (FTA-Abs), hepatitis C, and Lyme	Routine screening; suspicion of infectious etiology
*ESR, *antinuclear antibodies, consider other serum or CSF antibody studies (e.g., anti-NMDAR antibodies)	Evaluate for inflammatory, autoimmune, and paraneoplastic disorders
*Ceruloplasmin	Evaluate for Wilson's disease
Genetic analysis	Rule out a genetic disorder (e.g., Huntington's disease). Pharmacology selection (identification of cytochrome P450 or COMT hyper- or hypometabolizers)
Electrocardiogram (ECG)	For monitoring of QT interval effects of medications and arrhythmias contributing to panic symptoms
Chest X-ray (CXR)	Delirium and paraneoplastic workup
Lumbar puncture (LP)	CNS infections, autoimmune encephalopathy; consider in delirium and psychosis workup
Neuroimaging (CT, *MRI, PET, etc.)	Evaluate for CNS pathology (e.g., stroke, tumor, demyelination, atrophy, proteinopathies, etc.)
Electroencephalography (EEG)	Confusion, history, or clinical suspicion for seizure, narcolepsy, or head injury
Polysomnography (sleep study)	Sleep apnea, restless legs syndrome, etc.
Neuropsychologic testing	Assess intelligence, memory, language, executive function, and better characterize psychiatric diagnosis

Bolded items are recommended for general workup for most psychiatric symptoms, baseline, and treatment monitoring.
*Recommended in the routine workup of first-break psychosis.
BMI, Body mass index; CBC, complete blood count; BMP, basic metabolic panel (including electrolytes, glucose, blood urea nitrogen, creatinine); LFTs, liver function tests; UA, urinalysis; HIV, human immunodeficiency virus (e.g., immunoassay); CSF, cerebrospinal fluid; ESR, erythrocyte sedimentation rate; FTA-Abs, fluorescent treponemal antibody absorption (RPR is insufficient); NMDAR, N-methyl-D-aspartate receptor; COMT, Catechol-O-methyltransferase; CNS, central nervous system; CT, computed tomography; MRI, magnetic resonance imaging; PET, positron emission tomography.
Data from American Psychiatric Association: Psychiatric evaluation of adults, 2nd ed. Am J Psychiatry 163(6 Suppl):3–36, 2006; Freudenreich O, Schulz S, Goff DC. Initial medical work-up of first-episode psychosis: a conceptual review. Early Interv Psychiatry 3(1):10–18, 2009.

13. **What is the biopsychosocial model?**

    In the biopsychosocial model, one of several frameworks used for psychiatric case formulations, biological (e.g., genetic, medical, pharmacologic), psychological (e.g., abuse history, coping strengths or weaknesses, adaptive and maladaptive defenses), and social (e.g., relationship or work stressors and supports) factors, are considered as contributors to the clinical presentation and as potential avenues for intervention.

14. **What is the typical age of onset for major psychiatric disorders and how might this knowledge change management?**

    Psychiatric disorders typically begin to manifest in adolescence to early adulthood, with roughly 75% of cases having a first onset before age 24 years. For example, the typical age of onset of schizophrenia is between 15 and 35 years of age, and onset after 45 years of age is rare. Increased diagnostic suspicion and keeping a lower threshold for further workup to rule out other (neurologic or medical) causes is necessary before diagnosing a psychiatric disorder in a patient presenting outside of the typical age range.

MENTAL STATUS EXAM

15. **How is the mental status exam (MSE) performed and what are its main components?**

    The MSE is continuously performed throughout the encounter via observation of the patient. You can always perform an MSE; it is not appropriate to document "unable to perform" a MSE as this means the patient was not observed. If the patient does not participate in the encounter (due to disordered consciousness, refusal, or other reason), then that is an important observation to note as part of the MSE (Table 29-3).

16. **What is the difference between mood and affect?**

    The terms *mood* and *affect* are sometimes used to represent the patient's subjective (reported emotional feelings) and objective (observed emotional expression), respectively. However, the DSM describes both mood and affect as emotional feelings with objective and subjective

Table 29-3. The Main Components of the Mental Status Exam (MSE)	
Appearance and	Apparent age, body habitus, appropriateness of dress, grooming, hygiene, and distinguishing features
Behavior	Demeanor, posture/position, level of distress, degree of eye contact, attitude, psychomotor activity, gait, abnormal movements
Speech and	Coherence, rate, rhythm, volume, tone, and prosody
Language	Fluency, repetition, comprehension, naming
Mood and affect	Subjective and objective components of each, quality and range
Thought process and	Logicality, linearity, goal-directedness (inferred from speech)
Thought content	Suicidality, homicidality, delusions, obsessions, and usually also including perceptions: illusions and hallucinations)
Sensorium and	Level of consciousness and its stability
Cognition	Orientation, attention, concentration, intelligence, abstraction, executive function, construction (visuospatial)
Memory and	Registration and immediate, delayed, and autobiographical recall
Fund of knowledge	In relation to sociocultural and educational background
Insight and	Awareness of problems/behaviors including causes and ramifications; motivation to change
Judgment	Rationality of decisions made based on careful thought

Note: A variety of component headings and subcomponents are used in clinical practice, and this list is a suggestion of components and is not intended to be exhaustive.
From American Psychiatric Association: Psychiatric evaluation of adults. 2nd ed. *Am J Psychiatry* 163: (6 Suppl):3–36, 2006.

components and differentiates them temporally—whether the emotion is persistent (days to weeks) or temporary (seconds to hours), respectively. Thus, mood is the persistent "emotional climate," and affect is the transient "emotional weather." This use more appropriately describes the phenomenology of emotion and helps to distinguish mood disorders from affect disorders. For example, the colloquial "mood swings" occurring over seconds to hours are better described as affective lability.

17. **What are some psychiatric or neurologic conditions associated with disordered affect?**
Affective lability may be one feature of some mood disorders (e.g., bipolar disorders) and personality disorders (e.g., borderline personality disorder), but *these disorders should not be diagnosed on the basis of this feature alone*. Pathologic laughing and crying (also called *pseudobulbar affect*) can result from disruption of afferents (especially brain stem [i.e., bulbar] serotonergic afferents) to paralimbic regions by various disorders including amyotrophic lateral sclerosis, multiple sclerosis, traumatic brain injury, Alzheimer's disease, and others. Witzelsucht (pathologic punning) is associated with frontal lobe injury. Ictal laughing (gelastic epilepsy) or crying (dacrystic or quiritarian epilepsy) are associated with complex partial seizures.

18. **Name and describe some abnormal thought processes and the dysfunction or disorders associated with each.**
See Table 29-4.

Table 29-4. Abnormal Thought Processes and Associated Disorders

THOUGHT PROCESS	DESCRIPTION	ASSOCIATED DYSFUNCTION
Tangential	Logical and linear but not goal directed	Impaired attention and memory
Circumferential or circumstantial	Talking around a topic, overinclusive; gets to the point eventually	Executive dysfunction
Preservation	Repetition of words or phrases; stuck on a theme or idea; difficulty shifting set	Autism, catatonia, frontal lobe injury
Flight of ideas	Generally logical but nonlinear and not goal directed (like the seemingly erratic flight of a bird); often seen with uninterruptible, "pressured" speech	Bipolar mania
Loosening of associations	Statements are not logically connected to each other; the listener has to "connect the dots"	Psychotic disorders
Derailment	The logical link between trains of thought is suddenly and completely disconnected	Psychotic disorders
Thought blocking	A sudden prolonged pause as though the thought was blocked perhaps by some other internal stimuli	Psychotic disorders
Clang associations	Excessive alliteration or rhyming; words are linked by sounds rather than meaning	Psychotic disorders, Tourette syndrome

19. **Why use screening tools, rating scales, and structured interviews?**
Screening tools, rating scales, and structured interviews can help guide the evaluation, ensure important screening questions are asked, and facilitate patient report that might not have spontaneously volunteered. Some are validated measures of symptom severity and help anchor the diagnosis and treatment response to quantifiable data (rather than just clinical impressions) and may be used for research purposes as well. Some (e.g., Patient Health Questionnaire-9 [PHQ-9], and the Neuropsychiatric Inventory-Q [NPI-Q]) are self-report measures and can be filled out by the patient prior to the visit. Some require a clinician to administer and may be brief and focused (e.g., Beck Depression Inventory) or long and thorough (e.g., the Structured Clinical Interview for DSM-5 Disorders [SCID-5]).

20. Name some examples of bedside screening tools and structured interviews.
    See Table 29-5.

Table 29-5. Select Screens, Rating Scales, and Structured Interviews

General diagnostic instruments	SCID-5	Structured Clinical Interview for DSM-5 Disorders
	MINI	Mini-International Neuropsychiatric Interview
	SCAN	Schedules for Clinical Assessment in Neuropsychiatry
	NPI-Q	Neuropsychiatric Inventory (brief self-assessment version)
Mood disorders	HAM-D	Hamilton Depression Rating Scale
	MADRS	Montgomery–Asberg Depression Rating Scale
	BDI	Beck Depression Inventory
	Y-MRS	Young Mania Rating Scale
Anxiety disorders	HAM-A	Hamilton Anxiety Rating Scale
	BAI	Beck Anxiety Inventory
	Y-BOCS	Yale–Brown Obsessive Compulsive Scale
	BSPS	Brief Social Phobia Scale
	CAPS	Clinician Administered PTSD Scale
Psychotic disorders	PANSS	Positive and Negative Syndrome Scale
	BPRS	Brief Psychiatric Rating Scale
	AIMS	Abnormal Involuntary Movement Scale
	BARS	Barnes Akathisia Rating Scale
Substance use disorders	CAGE	CAGE questionnaire
	DAST	Drug Abuse Screening Test
Cognitive and executive function screens	MMSE	Mini-Mental State Examination
	CDT	Clock-Drawing Test
	DRS	Dementia Rating Scale
	FAB	Frontal Assessment Battery

Adapted from Roffman JL, Mischoulon D, Fava M. Diagnostic rating scales. In Stern TA, Fava M, Wilens TE, Rosenbaum JF, editors. *Massachusetts General Hospital Comprehensive Clinical Psychiatry*. London, Elsevier, p. 64 (Table 6-1), 2016.

21. What combination of assessments is recommended for cognitive disorder screening?
    The Mini Mental State Exam (MMSE) with age- and education-normative corrections and supplemented with measures of spatial function (e.g., Clock-Drawing Test) and executive function (e.g., Frontal Assessment Battery [FAB]) form a reasonable cognitive screening battery recommended by the American Neuropsychiatric Association.

CAPACITY

22. What is capacity, who evaluates for capacity, when is it evaluated, and how is it different from competency?
    Capacity—the patient's ability to make a medical decision—is evaluated by the physician who is rendering the intervention and its evaluation should be part of every informed consent process (i.e., every medical decision) to varying degrees, based on the complexity and potential consequences of the decision. The patient may have capacity for some simple decisions (e.g., starting an antidepressant) but lack capacity for more complicated decisions (e.g., surgical interventions). In contrast, competency is a legal term for the ability to participate in legal proceedings (e.g., stand trial) and is determined by a judge, sometimes based on evaluations by physicians.

23. What are the essential components of capacity?

    The essential components of capacity (all of which are required) and special situations are recalled by the mnemonic **CURVES**: the patient must be able to **C**ommunicate a **C**hoice and express an adequate **U**nderstanding of the risks, benefits, alternatives, and consequences, and the choice must logically follow (i.e., be **R**easonable) from this understanding and the patient's expressed **V**alue system. In **E**mergency situations when no **S**urrogate decision maker is available, life- or limb-saving interventions may be performed for a patient who lacks capacity.

24. If the patient is found to lack decision-making capacity, who makes the decision(s)?

    If an advanced directive document (e.g., living will, health care power of attorney, physician orders for life-sustaining treatment, legal guardian, etc.) outlining the patient's wishes for care and/or selection of surrogate decision maker is not available, then the duty of surrogate decision maker generally defaults to the next of kin in a hierarchy that varies somewhat by state but typically has the patient's spouse at the top followed by adult children, then parents, then siblings and other family members.

25. Is being psychotic grounds enough for involuntary hospitalization? What are the general civil involuntary commitment criteria?

    Having a mental illness alone is not grounds for involuntary hospitalization. In the United States, each state government defines the criteria for involuntary hospitalization in its mental health code, and these usually follow the American Psychiatric Association's Model that requires six criteria to be met: (1) the patient has a mental illness that (2) is treatable by hospitalization, (3) poses a danger to others or self (including severe decompensation), (4) does not voluntarily consent, (5) lacks capacity, and (6) hospitalization is the least restrictive treatment. Involuntary (court-mandated) outpatient treatment is also possible.

SUICIDE

26. What are the major risk factors for suicide?

    Some major risk factors for suicide are presented in Table 29-6. The strongest risk factor for suicide is the presence of a psychiatric disorder, especially a mood disorder (~50% of all suicides). Other

Table 29-6. Risk Factors for Suicide

Psychiatric illness (major depression [comorbid anxiety raises risk], bipolar disorder, drug dependence, alcoholism, schizophrenia, personality disorders, panic disorder)
Neurologic disorders (Huntington's disease, epilepsy, multiple sclerosis, stroke, TBI)
Race (Caucasian and Native American)
Marital status (widowed, divorced, or separated; especially divorced men)
Living alone
Recent personal loss
Unemployment
Financial/legal difficulties
Comorbid medical illness (having chronic illness, pain, or terminal illness)
History of suicide attempts or threats
Male gender
Advancing age
Family history of suicide
Recent hospital discharge
Firearms in the household
Hopelessness

TBI, Traumatic brain injury.
Adapted from Weintraub BR, Brezing C, Lagomasino I, et al. The suicidal patient. In Stern TA, Fava M, Wilens TE, Rosenbaum JF, editors. *Massachusetts General Hospital Comprehensive Clinical Psychiatry*. London, Elsevier, p. 590 (Box 53-1), 2016.

risk factors include access to firearms (~50% of suicides are by use of firearms), age in a bimodal fashion (15 to 24 years and 65+), and Caucasian and Native American race. Men are more likely to complete suicide though women make more attempts. Roughly one-quarter of suicide completions are in the context of alcohol intoxication. The presence of severe anxiety, panic attacks, insomnia, and major psychosocial loss increase the risk for imminent suicide. Prior suicide attempt is the best predictor of future suicide attempts.

27. **What psychiatric diagnoses carry the highest risk for suicide completion? What about suicide attempts and suicidal gestures? What about neurologic disorders?**
The suicide completion rates are highest for depression (~15%) and schizophrenia (~10%). The presence of anxiety, mixed-manic state, or eating disorder (especially anorexia nervosa) elevates the risk. Persons with borderline personality disorder frequently engage in "parasuicidal gestures" and are also at high risk for suicide completion (4 to 10%). Suicide is common in Huntington's disease (8% to 20%) and may be predicted in at-risk individuals with soft neurologic signs. Suicide risk is also increased for neurocognitive disorders (delirium and dementia), stroke, traumatic brain injury, multiple sclerosis (up to 7×), and epilepsy (~5×)—especially temporal lobe epilepsy and complex partial seizures (up to 25×).

28. **How do you screen for suicide and safety?**
Direct, straightforward, and empathic questioning regarding suicidal and homicidal ideation and intent and other safety issues is recommended. Several reliable and valid structured instruments are available to facilitate the suicide risk assessment. These include the Beck Scale for Suicidal Ideation (BSS), Beck Hopelessness Scale (BHS), Reasons for Living Inventory (RFL), and the Columbia-Suicide Severity Rating Scale (C-SSRS).

29. **How do you manage suicide risk?**
Table 29-7 presents some essential components of suicide risk management.

Table 29-7. Management of Suicide Risk

Stabilize the medical situation
Create a safe environment
- Remove potential means for self-harm
- Provide frequent supervision (hospitalize involuntarily if necessary)
Identify and treat underlying mental illness
Identify and modify other contributing factors

Adapted from Brendel RW, Brezing C, Lagomasino I, et al. The suicidal patient. In Stern TA, Fava M, Wilens TE, Rosenbaum JF, editors. *Massachusetts General Hospital Comprehensive Clinical Psychiatry.* London, Elsevier, p. 590 (Box 53-1), 2016.

30. **What two psychotropic medications have the best evidence to support their role in reducing suicide risk?**
Lithium (in patients with bipolar disorder) and clozapine (in patients with schizophrenia or schizoaffective disorder) have been shown to significantly reduce the risk of suicide and, despite their reputations for adverse effects, actually result in prolonged survival. Clozapine even has a Food and Drug Administration (FDA) indication for reducing suicide risk in patients with schizophrenia or schizoaffective disorder.

31. **Why did the FDA issue a black box warning for an increased risk of suicidality for antiepileptic drugs (AEDs)? Do AEDs increase the risk for depression and suicide in epilepsy?**
The FDA's black box warning is based on a 2008 meta-analysis finding of a nearly twofold increase in suicidal ideation or behavior associated with AED use. This issue has remained controversial due to the study's limitations and the fact that epilepsy itself increases the risk for depression and suicide. A more recent systematic review and large population-based study found that AED use may actually decrease the risk of suicide for people with epilepsy. However, AED use was associated with increased risk of suicide-related behavior for people with depression or other disorders (but not bipolar disorder). Several AEDs (e.g., barbiturates, felbamate, levetiracetam, tiagabine, topiramate, vigabatrin, zonisamide) may be particularly prone to inducing depression. The best predictor of suicide in epilepsy is comorbid depression, and this necessitates routine screening and treatment for patients with depression.

OTHER PSYCHIATRIC EMERGENCIES

32. **What are the potentially life-threatening causes of delirium and how can they be recalled?**
    The potentially life-threatening causes of delirium are outlined in Table 29-8 and can be recalled by the mnemonic WHHHHIIMPS.

Table 29-8. Potentially Life-Threatening Causes of Delirium

CONDITION	DIAGNOSTICS	TREATMENT
Wernicke's encephalopathy	Clinical triad: change in mental status, gait instability, ophthalmoplegia	Thiamine 500 mg IM (may see improvement over the course of hours)
Hypoxia	Oxygen saturation/ABGs	Treat etiology
Hypoglycemia	Blood glucose	PO/IV administration of glucose, dextrose, sucrose, or fructose
Hypertensive encephalopathy	Blood pressure	Antihypertensive medication
Hyperthermia/hypothermia	Temperature	Cooling or warming interventions
Intracerebral hemorrhage	MRI/CT	Per hemorrhage type/location
Infectious process (e.g., sepsis, bacteremia, subacute bacterial endocarditis)	Infectious workup	Treat infectious agent/site
Meningitis/encephalitis	LP, MRI	Antibiotic medication
Metabolic (e.g., chemical derangements, renal failure, hepatic failure, thyroid dysfunction)	Laboratory investigations	Per derangement
Poisoning/toxic reaction (e.g., environmental exposures, medications, alcohol, illicit substances)	Toxicology panel	Per toxin
Status epilepticus	EEG	IV benzodiazepines and/or anticonvulsants

ABGs, Arterial blood gases; CT, computed tomography; EEG, electroencephalogram; IM, intramuscular; IV, intravenous; LP, lumbar puncture; MRI, magnetic resonance imaging; PO, oral (per os).
Adapted from Prager LM, Ivkovic A. Emergency psychiatry. In Stern TA, Fava M, Wilens TE, Rosenbaum JF, editors. *Massachusetts General Hospital Comprehensive Clinical Psychiatry.* London, Elsevier, p. 943 (Table 88-1), 2016.

33. **What are some of the core features of catatonia and malignant catatonia?**
    Catatonia is a peculiar syndrome of seemingly opposite features such as severe psychomotor retardation (stupor) or agitation; excessive and strange activity such as grimacing, odd mannerisms; repetitive, nongoal-directed stereotypies; maintenance of postures spontaneously (posturing), or with passive induction (catalepsy) that may be altered even with resistance from the examiner (waxy flexibility), or resisted with equal and opposite force (gegenhalten); or withdrawal from interaction (negativism) or communication (mutism), or the mimicking of movements or speech (echopraxia and echolalia). Catatonia is denoted as malignant when autonomic lability (fever, widely variable heart rate or blood pressure) is present.

34. **How is neuroleptic malignant syndrome (NMS) related to catatonia and how are these conditions treated?**
    NMS is considered to be a drug-induced form of malignant catatonia. These are medical emergencies with high fatality rates if not treated quickly. Electroconvulsive therapy (ECT) is the treatment of choice of these conditions. While arranging for ECT, discontinue use of any dopamine blocking agents (neuroleptics), initiate treatment with benzodiazepines, provide supportive treatment (e.g., hydration, antipyretics, and antihypertensives), and monitor vitals and creatine kinase levels.

35. **How does serotonin syndrome (SS) develop? What features differentiate SS from catatonia?**

    SS symptoms can emerge in the setting of serotonergic medication overdose, use of two or more serotonergic agents (e.g., selective serotonin reuptake inhibitors [SSRIs] with monoamine reuptake inhibitors, tramadol, or other agents that alter serotonin synthesis, release, catabolism, or reuptake), or when tumors (e.g., carcinoid, small-cell carcinoma) secrete serotonin-like substances. SS shares some features with catatonia but gastrointestinal (GI) symptoms (diarrhea), tremor, myoclonus, ocular clonus, and hyperreflexia set it apart.

PERSONALITY DISORDERS

36. **What are defense mechanisms?**

    All people employ defense mechanisms to cope with internal and external conflicts and stressors. Some of these mechanisms are adaptive (promote functioning and strengthen relationships) while others are maladaptive. The clinician should remember that people (the clinician included) are generally trying to do the best they can with the ego resources and skills that they have.

37. **Briefly describe some common defense mechanisms. Which defense mechanism may interfere with delivery of care (i.e., which are maladaptive)?**

    Generally maladaptive (immature and neurotic) defense mechanisms:
    - Reaction formation—substitution of diametrically opposite thoughts, feelings, behaviors
    - Projection—attribution to others (may be to a delusional extreme)
    - Projective identification—feelings are misattributed as justifiable and attributed also to others often to the point of inducing projected feeling in others
    - Splitting—"black and white thinking"; compartmentalizing positive and negative attributes rather than integrating them into a cohesive whole
    - Idealization—regarding others as perfect or better than they really are
    - Acting out—unconscious expression in action of a wish or impulse
    - Dissociation—transient loss of or alteration of identity
    - Denial—rejection of reality
    - Displacement—redirection of impulses to a safer target

    Generally adaptive (mature) defense mechanisms:
    - Altruism—vicarious gratification through service to others
    - Anticipation—feeling in advance and considering consequences and alternative solutions
    - Humor—finding the humor in a stressful situation
    - Identification—modeling aspects of oneself after another's example
    - Sublimation—feelings are converted or channeled into more socially acceptable forms
    - Suppression—difficult feelings are intentionally avoided to cope with the present reality
    - Others—mindfulness, acceptance, respect, tolerance

38. **What constitutes a personality disorder as defined in the DSM-5?**

    "A personality disorder is an enduring pattern of inner experience and behavior that deviates markedly from the expectations of the individual's culture, is pervasive and inflexible, has an onset in adolescence or early adulthood, is stable over time, and leads to distress or impairment" (DSM-5, p 645).

    The diagnosis of personality disorders should be avoided while the patient is in a crisis; avoid throwing around pejorative labels for difficult patients.

39. **What are the major types, shared characteristics, and clusters of personality disorders?**

    Paranoid, schizoid, and schizotypal personality disorders share odd or eccentric characteristics and are grouped together in cluster A. Borderline, histrionic, narcissistic, and antisocial personality disorders share dramatic, emotional, or erratic features and make up cluster B. Dependent, avoidant, and obsessive–compulsive personality disorders share anxious or fearful features and are grouped together in cluster C (DSM-5, p 646).

40. **How are personality disorders treated?**

    Psychotherapies, including DBT (mainly used for borderline personality disorder), CBT, and psychodynamic therapy, as well as group therapy are the mainstay of treatment of personality disorders. Pharmacotherapy, if used, is typically symptom focused.

41. What personality characteristics may be associated with temporal lobe epilepsy?

    Classically, the temporal lobe epilepsy personality was described as humorless, hyposexual, overly concerned with religious questions, "sticky" in interpersonal relationships, and hypergraphic. This classic description has not reliably held up and is only occasionally found in patients with temporal lobe epilepsy.

GENERAL PSYCHOPHARMACOLOGY

42. What are the major indications for antidepressants?

    Under the label of "antidepressants" falls a broad range of medications with diverse mechanisms of action and clinical utility beyond simply the treatment of depression. Table 29-9 lists some of these indications.

Table 29-9. Possible Indications for Antidepressants

- Major depressive disorder and other unipolar depressive disorders, including secondary to a general medical condition (including poststroke, posttraumatic brain injury, etc.)
- Atypical depression (e.g., monoamine oxidase inhibitors)
- Depression with psychotic features (in combination with an antipsychotic drug)
- Bipolar depression (in combination with a mood stabilizer)
- Seasonal affective disorder
- Pathologic laughing and crying and other affect disorders (e.g., SSRIs)
- Panic disorder
- Social anxiety disorder
- Generalized anxiety disorder
- Posttraumatic stress disorder (sertraline and paroxetine)
- Impulse-control disorders (e.g., SSRIs)
- Obsessive–compulsive disorder (e.g., clomipramine and SSRIs)
- Bulimia nervosa (avoid bupropion due to seizure risk)
- Neuropathic pain (tricyclic drugs and SNRIs)
- Insomnia (e.g., trazodone, amitriptyline)
- Enuresis (imipramine best studied)
- Attention-deficit/hyperactivity disorder (e.g., desipramine, bupropion)
- Poststroke motor recovery (e.g., fluoxetine)
- Smoking cessation (bupropion)

SNRIs, Serotonin norepinephrine reuptake inhibitors; *SSRIs,* selective serotonin reuptake inhibitors.
Data from Fava M, Papakostas GI. Antidepressants. In Stern TA, Fava M, Wilens TE, Rosenbaum JF, editors. *Massachusetts General Hospital Comprehensive Clinical Psychiatry.* London, Elsevier, p. 490 (Box 43-1), 2016; Chollet F, Tardy J, Albucher JF, et al. Fluoxetine for motor recovery after acute ischaemic stroke (FLAME): a randomized placebo-controlled trail. *Lancet Neurol* 10(2):123–123, 2011; Wortzel HS, Oster TJ, Anderson CA, et al. Pathological laughing and crying: epidemiology, pathophysiology, and treatment. *CNS Drugs* 22:531– 545, 2008.

43. What class of antidepressant is generally considered as the first-line therapy?

    The SSRIs, because they are generally effective (but not necessarily more effective than other options) and generally better tolerated than other options, are considered first-line therapy for a number of psychiatric disorders including major depressive disorder, affect disorders, anxiety disorders, obsessive–compulsive disorder (OCD), and eating disorders.

44. What are the most common adverse effects of SSRIs? What is the most common reason for discontinuation of SSRIs?

    GI side effects (e.g., nausea, loose stools) are the most common side effect of SSRIs, but these features usually resolve within the first weeks of starting treatment. The most common reason for discontinuation of treatment with SSRIs is sexual dysfunction (e.g., decreased libido, anorgasmia).

45. Which SSRI has the most anticholinergic activity? What other antidepressants are anticholinergic and what problems may patients experience as a result of this effect?
Paroxetine (Paxil) is an SSRI that, unlike the other SSRIs, can have anticholinergic effects similar to the tricyclic antidepressants (TCAs). This can result in significant cognitive impairments even at therapeutic doses.

46. What are the advantages and disadvantages of bupropion compared to the SSRIs?
Bupropion does not generally cause the sexual dysfunction, GI symptoms, weight gain, or sedation that can occur with SSRIs, and it can help with smoking cessation. It may also help with attention-deficit/hyperactivity disorder symptoms (non-FDA-approved indication). Bupropion is associated with increased risk of seizure, especially at higher doses and in patients with eating disorders.

47. What is the mechanism of action of mirtazapine and how might the side effects of this medication be used therapeutically?
Mirtazapine is an antidepressant that acts as an inhibitor of presynaptic alpha-2-noradrenergic receptors and causes an increase in release of serotonin and norepinephrine. It also blocks serotonin (5-HT2, 5-HT3), and histamine (H1) and as a result can improve nausea, stimulate appetite, and treat insomnia.

48. What medications generally increase the concentration of TCAs (e.g., amitriptyline) and what other drug–drug interactions are important to consider with TCAs?
Antipsychotics, methylphenidate, SSRIs, quinidine, antifungals, macrolide antibiotics, verapamil, cimetidine, and thiazide diuretics all increase TCA levels. Other sedative, anticholinergic, antihypertensive, and cardiotoxic drugs can have additive effects with TCAs. TCAs in combination with SSRIs can cause SS and/or prolong QTc and induce torsades de pointes.

49. What common medications when used in combination with lithium increase lithium levels (and the possibility of toxicity) or cause idiosyncratic neurotoxicity?
Medications that increase lithium levels include nonsteroidal anti-inflammatory drugs (NSAIDs) such as naproxen and ibuprofen (aspirin has no effect on lithium levels), thiazide diuretics, angiotensin II receptor antagonists, angiotensin-converting enzyme inhibitors, and some antibiotics (tetracycline, spectinomycin, and metronidazole). Calcium channel blockers and antipsychotics with lithium can cause idiosyncratic neurotoxicity, and the latter combination can increase the risk for NMS.

50. What are some common adverse effects and signs of toxicity of lithium treatment and at what serum lithium levels may they be seen?
Common adverse effects of lithium at therapeutic levels (~0.6 to 1.0 mEq/L) include acne, weight gain, edema, changes in the glomerular filtration rate, hypothyroidism (necessitates monitoring thyroid-stimulating hormone levels when on lithium), tremor, GI (nausea, diarrhea, cramping), and cognitive complaints. Initial signs of lithium toxicity typically begin to manifest when serum lithium levels are above 1.5 mEq/L, but can be present above 1.0 mEq/L. Visual changes (blurring), slurring of speech, hyperreflexia, dysarthria, ataxia, confusion, fever, autonomic instability, leukocytosis, and limb rigidity can develop. Arrhythmias, seizures, and coma can develop at levels above 2.5 to 3 mEq/L.

51. For what phases of bipolar disorder (mania, depression, and maintenance) is lithium an effective treatment?
Lithium is an effective and first-line treatment of all bipolar disorder phases.

52. What AEDs are effective for bipolar disorder and for which phases are they effective?
See Table 29-10.

Table 29-10. Antiepileptic Drugs (AEDs) for Bipolar Disorder

	ACUTE MANIA	ACUTE DEPRESSION	MAINTENANCE
Valproate	+	−	−
Carbamazepine	+	−	−
Lamotrigine	−	+/−	+

From Ostacher MJ, Hsin H. The use of antiepileptic drugs in psychiatry. In Stern TA, Fava M, Wilens TE, Rosenbaum JF, editors. *Massachusetts General Hospital Comprehensive Clinical Psychiatry*. London, Elsevier, p. 536 (Table 48-1), 2016.

53. What are the important adverse effects associated with valproate?

Valproate is associated with a relatively high rate of teratogenicity (neural tube defects, increased risk of autism) as well as polycystic ovarian syndrome and is not recommended for use in women of childbearing age. Common adverse effects include weight gain, headache, lethargy, tremor, nausea, dyspepsia, and blurred vision. Valproate commonly (in up to 44% of users) causes a transient hepatic transaminitis (elevated liver enzymes), and liver failure is possible and can be fatal. Stevens–Johnson syndrome and other severe dermatologic reactions, as well as pancreatitis and multiorgan failure, are much less common but possible adverse effects of valproate.

54. What psychotropics have a relatively high potential for lowering seizure threshold?

While epileptic seizures have been reported during treatment with nearly all psychotropics, some, mainly antidepressants and antipsychotics, are associated with a higher risk, and the risk increases in a dose-dependent fashion and depending on other health factors (e.g., electrolyte imbalances in persons with eating disorders or dehydration). Bupropion, clomipramine, maptroline, chlorpromazine, and clozapine carry a higher risk.

55. What are the dosage equivalents of the commonly used sedative hypnotics?

Table 29-11 provides approximate equivalencies for commonly used sedative hypnotics. It is important to note that there can be significant differences in metabolism of and sensitivity to these agents for each individual.

Table 29-11. Sedative–Hypnotic Dose Equivalents

GENERIC NAME	DOSE EQUIVALENTS (mg)
Benzodiazepines	
Clonazepam	0.25-0.5
Alprazolam	0.5
Lorazepam	1
Diazepam	5
Chlordiazepoxide	12
Barbiturates	
Phenobarbitol	30
Pentobarbitol	100

Adapted from Renner R Jr., Ward E. Drug addiction. In Stern TA, Fava M, Wilens TE, Rosenbaum JF, editors. *Massachusetts General Hospital Comprehensive Clinical Psychiatry.* London, Elsevier, p. 303. (Table 27-3), 2016.

56. What are the main dose-limiting side effects of the second-generation (atypical) antipsychotics (SGAs)?

Sedation (especially with clozapine, quetiapine, olanzapine, asenapine) and extrapyramidal symptoms (e.g., akathisia, dystonia, parkinsonism; especially for risperidone, asenapine, lurazidone) are common dose-limiting side effects of SGAs. Anticholinergic effects, orthostatic hypotension, and seizures are a concern with increasing clozapine dose. Metabolic effects of SGAs (e.g., weight gain, dyslipidemia, hyperglycemia, and potentially diabetes) may be present at any dose and result in significant morbidity. The rare but potentially lethal agranulocytosis that can be induced by clozapine is also possible at any dose and necessitates the close monitoring involved with the use of this drug.

57. What are some common psychotropic medications or medication classes listed on the American Geriatric Society 2012 Updated Beers Criteria for Potentially Inappropriate Medication Use in Older Adults?

- Antipsychotics (all antipsychotics carry an FDA black box warning regarding association with increased mortality when used in the elderly with dementia)
- TCAs (amitriptyline, clomipramine, doxepin, etc.—due to anticholinergic effects)
- Barbiturates (increased risk of dependence and overdose)
- Antihistamines, anticholinergics, benzodiazepines, and other sedative hypnotics (cause cognitive impairments, delirium, falls)
- Bupropion, clozapine, olanzapine, maprotiline (lower seizure threshold)

58. What baseline labs/measures should be obtained prior to starting an antipsychotic?
    - Height and weight (body mass index—BMI)
    - Waist circumference
    - Baseline Abnormal Involuntary Movement Scale (AIMS)
    - Blood pressure
    - Electrocardiogram (for QTc monitoring)
    - Fasting lipid profile
    - Fasting plasma glucose
    - Complete blood count with differential (weekly initially for clozapine)
    - Consider a pregnancy test

SCHIZOPHRENIA SPECTRUM AND OTHER PSYCHOTIC DISORDERS

59. What does the term *psychosis* mean?
    Psychosis refers to a deficit in reality testing—the ability to differentiate self-generated stimuli (e.g., thoughts, imagery, and feelings) from external stimuli (i.e., perceptions) and assign appropriate meaning to experiences—with a lack of insight regarding the deficit.

60. What are the five major domains of impairment in schizophrenia spectrum and other psychotic disorders?
    1. Perception (hallucinations—perceptions without stimuli)
    2. Belief (delusions—fixed false beliefs despite conflicting evidence)
    3. Thought (disorganized thinking/speech; e.g., loosening of associations, derailment)
    4. Motor (disorganized motor behavior; e.g., catatonic behavior)
    5. Emotion (negative symptoms; e.g., flattened affect, alogia, avolition, anhedonia, asociality)
    The assessment of each of these domains, as well as cognition, mood (depression or mania), and historical elements (onset and time course) are critical in differentiating the psychotic disorders from medical condition- and substance-induced psychoses (DSM-5, pp 87, 113).

61. What is meant by positive and negative symptoms of schizophrenia and which account for greater impairment in overall functioning?
    Hallucinations and delusions are considered *positive* symptoms because they are experiences in *addition* to normal experience, whereas *negative* symptoms ("the 5 As": diminished or flattened **a**ffective expression, **a**volition, **a**logia, **a**nhedonia, and **a**sociality) denote a *deficit* of experience. Negative symptoms are prominent in schizophrenia and are thought to account for greater functional impairment in persons with schizophrenia and greater burden for their caretakers (DSM-5, p 88).

62. Is the catatonia syndrome only associated with schizophrenia?
    No. Roughly 15% of cases of catatonia are associated with psychotic disorders. Among psychiatric disorders, mood disorders, primarily bipolar disorder, account for most catatonia cases (~30%). Perhaps nearly half of the time catatonia is in the context of a medical condition.

63. What is the difference between a hallucination and an illusion?
    Hallucinations are sensations (visual, auditory, olfactory, gustatory, or tactile) without stimuli and are contrasted with illusions that are misperceptions of actual stimuli (e.g., perceiving a shadow on the wall as a snake).

64. What are some of the major causes of hallucinations?
    Hallucinations can be caused by a multitude of etiologies, but the essential common theme is aberrant activation of the primary sensory cortex. Examples include focal epilepsy, toxic (including hallucinogenic substances) and metabolic encephalopathy (including delirium, interictal and postictal hallucinations), rapid eye movement (REM) sleep intrusion (including parahypnagogic and parahypnopompic hallucinations—considered normal), and release phenomena (e.g., Charles Bonnet syndrome, sensory deprivation). The presence of hallucinations should prompt workup to rule out these known causes. Hallucinations may be part of the phenomenology of schizophrenia, but schizophrenia is a syndrome and should not be thought of as a *cause* of hallucinations.

65. In what sensory modalities may hallucination occur and does the modality suggest a particular syndrome or etiology?

Hallucinations may be experienced in any sensory modality—visual, olfactory, gustatory, tactile, and somatic, proprioceptive, equilibroceptive, nociceptive, thermoceptive, and chronoceptive (Table 29-12).

Table 29-12. Hallucination Modalities and Associated Syndrome or Etiology

MODALITY	ASSOCIATED SYNDROME/ETIOLOGY	COMMENT
Auditory	Schizophrenia and related psychotic disorders (SaRPD), mood disorders with psychotic features	Rare to have other types in the absence of auditory in SaRPD
Visual	Delirium, migraine, REM-intrusion (narcolepsy, sleep deprivation) Substance intoxication/withdrawal Dementia with Lewy bodies, epilepsy, Charles Bonnet syndrome, midbrain (peduncular) pathology	Hypnagogic and hypnopompic hallucinations are considered normal Insight is more likely retained
Olfactory and gustatory	Seizure disorder (temporal lobe epilepsy), schizophrenia, migraines, Parkinson's disease	Typically unpleasant odors (e.g., feces) in schizophrenia
Tactile	Substance (e.g., stimulants), alcohol and benzodiazepine withdrawal, delusional parasitosis	Formication is the sensation of insects crawling on the skin
Somatic	Schizophrenia, limbic, and temporal lobe epilepsy, anti-Parkinson's medications, multiple sclerosis, thalamic pain syndrome	Typically unpleasant (e.g., feeling organs rotting) in schizophrenia
Chronoceptive	Substance use (e.g., stimulants, psychedelics)	

Freudenreich O, Brown HE, Holt DJ. Psychosis and schizophrenia. In Stern TA, Fava M, Wilens TE, Rosenbaum JF, editors. *Massachusetts General Hospital Comprehensive Clinical Psychiatry*. London, Elsevier, p. 314 (Box 28-3), 2016.

66. What is a delusion?

A delusion is a fixed, false belief that persists despite evidence to the contrary. Culturally or religiously normative beliefs are not considered delusions.

67. What are characteristics of delusions associated with schizophrenia, delusional disorder and dementia, and delirium?

In schizophrenia and delusional disorder, delusions are typically well systematized and paranoid. In advanced dementia, delusions of infidelity or jealousy that are not very well systematized are typical. Delusions are common in delirium but they are generally fleeting, fluctuating, and not well systematized.

68. What workup should be completed for a first-episode ("first-break") psychosis before a diagnosis of a primary idiopathic psychiatric disorder diagnosis (such as schizophrenia) can be made?

See Table 29-12.

69. What percentage of first-break psychosis presentations is due to a medication effect?

Up to a quarter of first-break psychosis presentations are due to a substance or medication effect (DSM-5, p 113).

70. What substances, medications, or toxins may cause psychosis?

The following is a partial list of potentially psychotogenic substances divided by category:
- **Substances:** alcohol, sedatives, hypnotics, and anxiolytics (intoxication or withdrawal), hallucinogens (e.g., phencyclidine), inhalants
- **Medications:** anesthetics and analgesics, anticholinergic agents, antihistamines, anticonvulsants, antiparkinsonian medications, chemotherapeutic agents (e.g., cyclosporine, procarbazine), corticosteroids, muscle relaxants, phenylephrine, pseudoephedrine, disulfiram
- **Toxins:** anticholinesterase, organophosphate insecticides, sarin and other nerve gases, carbon monoxide, carbon dioxide, and volatile substances such as fuel or paint (DSM-5, p 113).

71. Both Huntington's disease and schizophrenia complicated by tardive dyskinesia (TD) may present with psychosis and chorea-like movements. How are these distinguished?

Genetic testing will of course identify the Huntington's disease gene, but clinically in TD the movements are generally more localized, stereotyped, and repetitive and only rarely involve the forehead or gait. Keep in mind that patients with chorea treated with antipsychotics may also develop TD.

72. Describe the prodromal phase of psychotic disorders. What treatments at this stage may change outcomes (i.e., reduce risk of development of a psychotic disorder)?

The development of full-syndrome schizophrenia and related psychotic disorders can be preceded by many months by a prodrome of social withdrawal and isolation, cognitive difficulties, suspiciousness and other attenuated psychotic symptoms, and suicidality. Patients are frequently (mis)diagnosed with a depressive disorder during this phase. Treatment during this phase with psychoeducation, psychosocial interventions (e.g., stress reduction), CBT (psychosis-specific CBT programs have been developed), and neuroprotective agents (including omega-3 fatty acids) has been shown to reduce the rate of transition to first-break psychosis as much as or more than medications and is preferred by patients.

73. What are the pharmacologic treatment options for acute psychosis?

First-line agents include potent typical (e.g., haloperidol, perphenazine) and second-generation (e.g., risperidone, olanzapine, quetiapine, ziprasidone, or aripiprazole) antipsychotics with the selection depending on previous response, side-effect profiles and patient preference, and other pharmacodynamic and kinetic considerations. The availability of risperidone, olanzapine, aripiprazole, and haloperidol in multiple preparations (e.g., oral, intramuscular, long-acting injectable, etc.) makes these preferred agents for many situations. Adjunctive use of benzodiazepines, if not contraindicated, may be helpful for the agitated psychotic patient. SGAs (many of which have antidepressant effects) alone or in combination with a mood stabilizer or an antidepressant can treat comorbid mood and psychotic symptoms (e.g., schizoaffective disorder).

74. Is the use of combinations of antipsychotics evidence based?

The use of combinations of antipsychotics, while popular, is not supported by evidence or guideline recommendations.

BIPOLAR AND RELATED DISORDERS

75. What is the core diagnostic feature and supporting symptoms for a manic episode? (Hint: the mnemonic DIGFAST may help.)

A manic episode is the polar opposite of depression (hence, the name *bipolar disorder*), and the core feature is a *significant shift in mood persisting at least a week* (4 days for hypomania) characterized by elation, expansivity, or irritability *and* abnormally increased goal-directed activity or energy. Functioning must be impaired and the possibility of contributing substance intoxication or withdrawal (e.g., cocaine) or medical conditions (e.g., delirium, behavioral variant frontotemporal degeneration, hyperthyroidism) must be ruled out. Other supporting features include:
- **D**istractibility
- **I**ndiscretion (e.g., spending beyond means, sexual promiscuity, or foolish investing)
- **G**randiosity
- **F**light of ideas/racing thoughts
- **A**ctivity: increased goal-directed activity
- **S**leep: reduced *perceived need* for sleep
- **T**alkative: increased rate and amount (i.e., pressured speech) (DSM-5, pp 123–125)

76. What are the best (most efficacious and well-tolerated) pharmacotherapeutic options for acute mania?

Meta-analyses have found that the antipsychotics haloperidol, risperidone, and olanzapine (in that order) are more effective than mood stabilizers, and olanzapine and risperidone (in that order) are better tolerated as well. Lithium may be the most effective mood stabilizer but may not be as well tolerated as valproate. Quetiapine is about as effective as lithium and about as well tolerated as valproate. For severe acute mania, the American Psychological Association guidelines recommend the combination of lithium or valproate with an antipsychotic (such as olanzapine) with consideration for benzodiazepine adjunctive therapy. Monotherapy with a mood stabilizer may be possible following treatment of the acute episode.

77. Why should antidepressants not be used in isolation (without a mood stabilizer) for bipolar depression?

    Unchecked, antidepressants may precipitate a manic episode in susceptible patients (i.e., patients with an underlying bipolar disorder). This is one reason close follow-up of patients starting an SSRI for a first depressive episode is important.

78. How quickly do mood episodes switch in bipolar disorder with rapid cycling?

    Bipolar disorder with rapid cycling is defined by manic/hypomanic, mixed, or depressed episodes (which meet full criteria for such episodes) occurring four or more times in a year. The concept of ultrarapid cycling (URC) has been proposed to describe episodes alternating every several days or weeks, but URC was not included in the DSM-5. It is important to reiterate that affective lability/instability ("mood swings" throughout the day or from day to day) alone does not constitute a bipolar mood disorder (DSM-5, pp 150-151). The effects of substances of abuse, personality disorders, or other affect disorders should be considered in the differential of affective lability/instability.

DEPRESSIVE DISORDERS

79. What is the diagnostic minimum and average length of a major depressive episode?

    For the diagnosis of major depressive disorder (MDD) the episode must be at least 2 weeks long. On average, depressive episodes are 30 weeks long. In severe cases, symptoms may be treated prior to meeting full criteria for a major depressive disorder.

80. What are the core diagnostic features for MDD? (Hint: the mnemonic SIG: E CAPS may help.)

    There must be a pervasive and persistent depressive mood (or irritable mood in children and adolescents) and/or loss of interest/pleasure (anhedonia) for ≥2 weeks and ≥4 of the following symptoms (recalled with the mnemonic for the prescription of energy pills: "SIG: E CAPS"): S: sleep disruption; I: reduced interests/pleasure; G: feelings of guilt/worthlessness; E: reduced energy/fatigue; C: concentration/decision-making ability diminished; A: appetite/weight loss or increase; P: psychomotor agitation/retardation; S: suicidal ideation or attempt.

81. What is the basic pathophysiology of mood disorders?

    Mood disorders are heterogeneous clinically, a variety of pathoetiologies are possible, and the specific pathophysiology is not well understood. Most models of depression involve catecholamine (serotonin, dopamine, and norepinephrine) imbalances and involve dysfunctional medial frontal–subcortical networks.

82. How is depression distinguished from apathy, dementia, or delirium?

    Apathy (indifference or lack of concern) is not depression (a persistently low mood) but may be a feature of depression. Depression is often comorbid with dementia and may itself cause cognitive problems ("pseudodementia"), but again a persistently low mood is not characteristic of dementia. Hypoactive delirium can be distinguished from depression by its (typically) acute onset, fluctuating course, and impaired environmental awareness. (Delirium is discussed further below.)

83. What is the most effective treatment of MDD? What are the treatment options?

    Electroconvulsive therapy (ECT) is by far the most effective treatment of MDD, especially MDD with psychotic features. Other interventions include lifestyle modifications (e.g., improved sleep hygiene, diet, and exercise), psychotherapy (e.g., CBT), and pharmacotherapy (e.g., SSRIs), and combinations of these interventions are more effective than any of them alone. Repetitive transcranial magnetic stimulation, deep brain stimulation (of the anterior cingulate gyrus), and vagal nerve stimulation are other options that may be effective.

84. What are the contraindications for ECT?

    There are no absolute contraindications for ECT. Relative contraindications include increased intracranial pressure (mass effect), recent intracranial hemorrhage, thromboembolic stroke, or myocardial infarction, unstable angina, heart failure, or vertebral fracture. ECT is safe in pregnancy and may be preferred to pharmacotherapy in this setting. ECT is safe in epilepsy, and the use of ECT as a treatment for refractory status epilepticus has been described in case reports.

85. **Besides mood disorders, for what other disorders is ECT effective?**
Schizophrenia (especially when catatonic features or affective symptoms are present), schizoaffective disorder, catatonia in other settings (including NMS), refractory Parkinson's disease (reduces motor symptoms; especially if "on/off" phenomenon is present), intractable epilepsy (especially when mood disorders, which are highly comorbid with Parkinson's disease and epilepsy, are present), and some endocrinopathies.

86. **What is seasonal affective disorder (SAD) and how is it treated?**
SAD is a disorder of mood (not an affect disorder) characterized by persistent depressive symptoms with an onset related to environmental changes in day–night length—short days and long nights—the incidence of which is more common farther from the equator. SAD treatments include appropriately timed bright light therapy and melatonin.

ANXIETY DISORDERS

87. **What group of mental health disorders are the most common in the United States?**
In the United States, the most common mental health disorders are the anxiety disorders (including phobias, generalized anxiety disorder, panic disorder, and others), with 12-month and lifetime prevalence of about one in five and one in three, respectively. (Major depressive disorder followed by alcohol dependence are the most common individual disorders.)

88. **What role does psychotherapy have in the treatment of anxiety disorders? Name and briefly describe some cognitive–behavioral interventions for anxiety disorders.**
Psychotherapies, of which CBT is best supported by evidence, are the mainstay of treatment of anxiety disorders, with pharmacotherapies serving mostly as augmentative therapy.
- Psychoeducation—pathophysiology education and building of therapeutic alliance
- Distress tolerance—learning to tolerate rather than avoid anxiety
- Cognitive restructuring—challenging and changing maladaptive thinking
- Modeling—the patient observes others exposed to and tolerating the feared stimulus
- Exposure and response prevention—imaginal or direct exposure to the feared stimulus or to the associated symptoms and learning to prevent the avoidance of the stimulus or symptoms
  - Graduated exposure—exposure to and tolerance of a less-to-most-feared stimulus hierarchy
  - Flooding—the patient is exposed directly to the feared stimulus until symptoms abate

89. **What are the main pharmacotherapy options for treatment of anxiety disorders in the short term and long term?**
SSRIs, typically starting at a low dose, are the first-line pharmacologic treatments of choice for many anxiety disorders including panic disorder and generalized anxiety disorder. Though they may take 3 to 4 weeks to have a noticeable effect, they are effective and safe long-term treatments for anxiety disorders. Other long-term options include SNRIs and TCAs, and there is also some evidence for use of buspirone and beta-blockers (e.g., propranolol). Benzodiazepines, such as lorazepam and clonazepam, have a role as augmentative therapy in the short term for reduction of acute severe anxiety symptoms, but long-term use of these agents is associated with worsening of anxiety symptoms and developing tolerance and dependence.

90. **What are some limitations to the use of alprazolam (Xanax) for panic disorder?**
The rapid onset advantage of alprazolam is offset by its high potency (leading to the development of tolerance) and short duration of action (leading to withdrawal symptoms that mimic panic symptoms and may lead to more frequent use).

91. **What are some medical causes of panic symptoms?**
Panic disorder is highly comorbid with psychiatric and medical disorders, and some disorders can directly mimic the symptoms of severe anxiety or a panic attack. These medical panic mimics include hyperthyroidism, pulmonary embolism, asthma, chronic obstructive pulmonary disease, obstructive sleep apnea (mimic of nocturnal panic), arrhythmias and mitral valve prolapse, pheochromocytoma (adrenaline and noradrenaline secreting tumor), and caffeine or other stimulant overuse.

OBSESSIVE–COMPULSIVE AND RELATED DISORDERS

92. What is the basic pathophysiology (neurologic basis) of OCD?

The perseveration of motor and/or thought processes in OCD is thought to be mediated by overactive, inadequately inhibited, cortical–subcortical (basal ganglia including caudate) circuits. Specifically, in OCD, the caudate nucleus, as well as the medial and orbitofrontal and anterior cingulate cortex, and to some extent the thalamus, is hypermetabolic on functional imaging.

93. What are the known effective pharmacologic interventions for OCD?

Clomipramine is a serotonin reuptake inhibitor (SRI), with a side-effect profile similar to TCAs (anticholinergic, antihistaminergic, alpha-blocking) and also including SSRI-like anorgasmia, which has established efficacy in OCD. Several SSRIs (fluoxetine, fluvoxamine, paroxetine, and sertraline) are FDA approved for OCD, and other SSRIs and SNRIs have evidence to support their use in OCD.

TRAUMA- AND STRESSOR-RELATED DISORDERS

94. Must a person be directly exposed to trauma to develop posttraumatic stress disorder (PTSD)? What are the core symptoms of PTSD?

No, PTSD may develop following direct or indirect (e.g., witnessing or learning about trauma done to others) exposure to traumatic events, defined in the DSM-5 as "actual or threatened death, serious injury or sexual violation." The core symptoms of PTSD, which must be present for at least 1 month for the diagnosis, include intrusive memories, nightmares, or dissociations; avoidance of these intrusive experiences or external reminders of the trauma; mood and/or cognition alterations; and hyperarousal symptoms (DSM-5, pp 271-272).

95. What are the recommended first-line therapies for PTSD? What pharmacotherapeutic options are FDA approved for treatment of PTSD? What medications may be effective at reducing the nightmares associated with PTSD?

PTSD treatment guidelines typically recommend prolonged exposure therapy, cognitive processing therapy, and/or trauma-focused CBT as first-line treatments with pharmacotherapy as adjunctive. The FDA has approved only two medications, sertraline and paroxetine, both SSRIs, for the treatment of PTSD. Prazosin, an alpha-1 antiadrenergic, has been shown to reduce nightmares and sleep disruption in patients with PTSD.

DISSOCIATIVE DISORDERS

96. What historical elements may be common in dissociative disorders such as dissociative identity disorder, dissociative amnesia, and depersonalization/derealization disorder?

A history of severe childhood physical, sexual, and emotional abuse, or a history of traumatic wartime or natural disaster experiences is common in these disorders. Dissociation or depersonalization can be part of the normal experience during extreme situations, but for people with dissociative disorders the symptoms are severe, persistent, and disabling.

97. Dissociative amnesias and the amnesia of dementia (e.g., Alzheimer's disease) can be distinguished by what features?

While personality can change in some dementias, dissociative amnesias involve loss or alteration of identity. Furthermore, dissociative amnesia is retrograde (as opposed to the typically anterograde—deficit of new learning—amnesia of dementia), isolated to personal information, and associated with a traumatic event.

SOMATIC SYMPTOM AND RELATED DISORDERS

98. The diagnosis of somatoform disorder in DSM-IV has been replaced with somatic symptom disorder (SSD) in DSM-5. What is the difference?

The new diagnostic scheme focuses on the *presence of symptoms* and the excessive distress and abnormal/maladaptive emotional, cognitive, and behavioral *responses* to the symptoms rather than the *absence* of a medical explanation. Indeed, SSD is highly comorbid with medical disorders (DSM-5, p 309). As an example, patients with known neuropathologically based movement disorders commonly also have conversion disorder (functional neurologic disorder) features/symptoms (altered sensory or motor function incompatible with known neurologic disorders)—these are not mutually exclusive.

99. What are some major factors that are thought to contribute to SSDs?
    - Genetic and biological susceptibilities (e.g., decreased pain tolerance)
    - Childhood trauma (e.g., physical, sexual, and emotional abuse)
    - Operant conditioning—learning (i.e., somatic complaints gain attention)
    - Sociocultural norms (e.g., if somatic complaints are valued over emotional complaints)

100. SSDs are differentiated from factitious disorder and malingering by what key feature(s)?
    In SSD, symptoms are not intentionally (consciously) produced. Symptoms produced intentionally to assume the sick role (i.e., "primary gain") or without obvious external reward are characteristic of factitious disorder. Symptoms produced intentionally for monetary or other "secondary gain" are consistent with malingering. Reporting to the appropriate legal authorities may be necessary in cases of malingering (considered fraud) and factitious disorder imposed on another (a.k.a. Münchausen syndrome by proxy).

101. What treatment for SSD has been shown to decrease rates of hospitalization and reduce patient's health care spending by 50%? What additional strategies should be employed?
    Individual and group psychotherapy. Additional strategies include scheduling frequent follow-up visits with a single provider (establishing a "medical home") and following a collaboratively developed treatment plan. Use of psychotropic medications for SSD is generally not helpful and may be problematic due to the compliance issues typical in this population.

FEEDING AND EATING DISORDERS AND ELIMINATION DISORDERS

102. What are some important complications of anorexia nervosa and bulimia nervosa?
    Eating disorders are among the most debilitating and potentially lethal mental health disorders due to the accompanying malnutrition and vitamin deficiencies, electrolyte imbalances, and potential for seizures.

103. What exam findings are associated with eating disorders?
    Emaciated or low-weight patients may exhibit bradycardia, hypotension, orthostasis, hypothermia, acrocyanosis (bluish discoloration of the extremities due to poor circulation), lanugo (especially fine, soft body hair), murmur of mitral valve prolapse, and flattened affect. Patients who induce vomiting may exhibit erosion of dental enamel, Russel's sign (calluses on the knuckles of the hand due to repeated contact with the incisors when inducing vomiting), and hypertrophy of the parotid and/or salivary glands.

DISRUPTIVE, IMPULSE-CONTROL, AND CONDUCT DISORDERS

104. What is unique about the emotional and behavioral outbursts that characterize the disruptive, impulse-control, and conduct disorders (including intermittent explosive, oppositional defiant, and antisocial personality disorders, pyromania, kleptomania, and others) that may help distinguish them from outbursts in other disorders such as delirium, substance intoxication/withdrawal, or autism spectrum disorders?
    They are purposeful, frequent, persistent actions causing harm to self or violations of the rights of others and/or societal norms, occur with pervasiveness across situations, and are disproportionate to provocation (DSM-5, pp 461, 469).

105. What is the difference between an impulsive and a compulsive act?
    Impulsive reactions to internal or external stimuli are purposeful but happen quickly without foresight of consequences and may relieve a tense feeling but often result in feelings of guilt and remorse. Compulsions are typically rule-bound, repetitive, stereotyped behaviors engaged in as a response to unwanted, intrusive thoughts (obsessions), which then relieve the guilt or anxiety associated with the obsession.

106. What are the pharmacotherapeutic options for impulse control disorders (ICDs)?
    ICDs include a broad range of disorders of similar but complex pathophysiologies involving systems that incorporate most of the major neurotransmitters. Possible therapeutic options include mu opioid antagonists (to interrupt the reward reinforcement of ICD behaviors), SSRIs, atypical antipsychotics, beta-blockers, stimulants, anticonvulsants, and other agents. Nearly half of patients with intermittent explosive disorder attained full (29%) or partial (17%) remission of criterion A (outbursts with dyscontrol of aggressive impulses) with fluoxetine treatment. Reducing or discontinuing medications that may be contributing (e.g., dopaminergic treatments of parkinsonism) should also be considered.

SUBSTANCE-RELATED AND ADDICTIVE DISORDERS

107. Describe the time course of signs and symptoms of alcohol withdrawal.
    See Table 29-13.

Table 29-13. Time Course and Associated Signs and Symptoms of Alcohol Withdrawal

TIME COURSE: ONSET*/DURATION	SIGNS AND SYMPTOMS
Early: 6 hr/2 days	Anxiety, tremor, palpitations, nausea, anorexia
6-48 hr/3 days	Seizures
12-48 hr/2 days	Alcoholic hallucinosis (visual, auditory, tactile hallucinations with intact sensorium)
Late: 48-96 hr/5 days	Delirium tremens (deficit in awareness and attention (impaired sensorium); often with agitation, tremor, hallucinations, autonomic hyperactivity, and abnormal movements (parkinsonism, chorea, dystonia, myoclonus) and catatonia

*Onset is time since last drink.
Adapted from Tetrault JM, O'Connor PG. Substance abuse and withdrawal in the critical care setting. *Crit Care Clin* 24(4):767–788 (Table 2), 2008; Brust JCM: Acute withdrawal: diagnosis and treatment. In Sullivan EV, Pfefferbaum A, editors. *Handbook of Clinical Neurology*, vol. 125 (3rd series) Alcohol and the Nervous System, Elsevier BV; pp. 123–131. 2014.

108. What are the major signs and symptoms of intoxication and withdrawal for common substances of abuse (cocaine, benzodiazepines, marijuana/synthetic cannabinoids, opiates, nicotine, and amphetamines) and what treatment may be required?
    See Table 29-14.

109. What substances (or metabolites) can be detected in the urine at the following times after consumption? What about hair follicle testing?
    • Up to 2 to 4 weeks? Long acting barbiturates, marijuana (if use was heavy)
    • Up to a week? Phencyclidine (PCP), methaqualone
    • Up to 4 days? Cocaine metabolites
    • Up to 72 hours? Marijuana (occasional use), morphine, heroin, methadone, benzodiazepines
    • Up to 48 hours? Amphetamines, codeine, propoxyphene
    • Less than 12 hours? Alcohol, cocaine
    Most of these substances can be detected for up to 90 days in hair follicles.

110. What are some commonly abused and technically legal to purchase substances that can cause severe psychiatric symptoms that will not show up in routine urine toxicology screens?
    Synthetic cannabinoids (a.k.a. "K2" or "spice"), "bath salts," and some cough syrups (when consumed in excess) can result in severe psychiatric symptoms, but these substances are not screened for in standard urine toxicology.

111. What are the common neurotransmitter and CNS nuclei involved in the development of addiction to drugs of abuse?
    The mesolimbic reward system—involving mainly dopaminergic projections from the ventral tegmental area to the nucleus accumbens and other regions—is primarily disrupted by addictive substances. This results in disruption of networks mediating conditioned learning, mood regulation, and control of inhibition, motivation, and drives.

Table 29-14. Select Substances of Abuse and Features of Intoxication and Withdrawal and Associated Treatments

SUBSTANCE	INTOXICATION	WITHDRAWAL
Cocaine	Myocardial ischemia, stroke, rhabdomyolysis, hyperthermia, seizures, hypertension, insomnia Tx: supportive; consider benzos, avoid beta-blockers	Dysphoria (depressed affect), fatigue, sleep disturbance, vivid dreams, psychomotor retardation or agitation Tx: supportive
Amphetamines/ methamphetamines	Diaphoresis, hypertension, tachycardia, insomnia, agitation, psychosis Tx: consider benzos and antipsychotics as needed	Fatigue, irritability, anxiety, insomnia, psychosis Tx: supportive; consider benzos as needed
GABA-R agonists (alcohol, barbiturates, benzodiazepines)	Slurred speech, unsteady gait, impaired memory or attention, confusion, stupor, coma Tx: supportive; consider flumazenil	Tremors, anxiety, irritability, autonomic hyperactivity, seizures, delirium Tx: supportive; substitution of long-acting benzo taper
Marijuana and synthetic cannabinoids	Euphoria, anxiety, panic attacks, paranoia, depersonalization, derealization, psychosis Tx: supportive; consider benzos and antipsychotics as needed	Anger, aggression, anxiety, irritability, dysphoria, insomnia Tx: supportive
Opioids	Euphoria, anesthesia, pinpoint pupils, somnolence, respiratory suppression Tx: supportive; consider naloxone	Autonomic hyperactivity, restlessness, irritability, pupil dilation, tremor, lacrimation, rhinorrhea, nausea, vomiting, diarrhea, myalgias, arthralgias Tx: supportive symptomatic care; consider methadone or buprenorphine-naloxone
Nicotine	Enhancement of alertness and concentration, variably calming or anxiety provoking, appetite suppression, tachycardia, vasoconstriction Tx: supportive	Sweating, frequent urination, gastrointestinal disturbances, drowsiness, bradycardia Tx: supportive; nicotine replacement
Hallucinogens	Hallucinations, derealization, pupillary dilation, tachycardia, palpitations, sweating, blurred vision, tremors, discoordination. Tx: supportive; consider antipsychotics as needed	Anxiety, dysphoria, flashbacks Tx: urinary acidification, supportive care

Tx, Treatment considerations; Benzos, benzodiazepines.
Adapted from Tetrault JM, O'Connor PG. Substance abuse and withdrawal in the critical care setting. *Crit Care Clin* 24(4):767–788 (Table 4), 2008.

DELIRIUM

112. **What is the cardinal feature of delirium and what are other core features?**
Impaired *environmental awareness and ability to direct, sustain, and/or appropriately shift attention* defines the delirium syndrome (DSM-5, p 599). This impairment is typically of acute onset and waxes and wanes in severity (usually worse at night ["sundowning"]) but there are chronic forms of delirium as well. Emotional, cognitive, psychomotor, circadian rhythm, and sleep–wake disturbances

are also common in delirium. Use of the Delirium Rating Scale-R-98 (DRS-R-98) and other rating scales can assist the diagnoses of delirium and track response to treatment.

113. **How is delirium distinguished from dementia, depression, and other psychiatric disorders?**
In dementia there is typically a chronic, progressive decline in one or more cognitive domains, and attention and awareness are generally unaffected until late in the disease process.
Likewise, in depression, concentration may be impaired but attention and awareness are not affected.

114. **In general, what is the pathophysiology (neurotransmitter disturbance) of delirium and how does this generalization help guide empiric treatment while investigations are under way to uncover the underlying cause?**
In general, the delirious state is relatively *hyperdopaminergic* and *hypocholinergic*. Thus, dopamine-blocking antipsychotics (especially haloperidol, risperidone, olanzapine, and quetiapine), usually at low doses, are a well-established recommended intervention and procholinergic agents (especially physostigmine in anticholinergic-induced delirium) may be of use, though the evidence base is mixed. This is in addition to other supportive measures. Polypharmacy (especially with anticholinergics) is a common cause of delirium, and regimen simplification (especially removal of anticholinergics, opiates, and other sedatives) is a very important intervention.

115. **What abnormal cardiac rhythm is (rarely) associated with intravenous haloperidol?**
QTc prolongation and torsades de pointes. Telemetry and close monitoring of potassium and magnesium are recommended. Remember that all antipsychotics may prolong the QTc interval.

116. **If delirium is diagnosed, what other psychiatric disorders can be diagnosed?**
None!

117. **What is delirium tremens (DT) and what can guide the management of DT?**
DT is a special type of delirium that generally manifests about 3 days into withdrawal from heavy use of gamma-aminobutyric acid agonists (e.g., alcohol, benzodiazepines, barbiturates). Features of DT include tremors, autonomic hyperactivity (fever, hypertension, tachycardia, diaphoresis), disorientation and confusion, and visual, auditory, or tactile hallucinations. Untreated, seizures and even status epilepticus may follow, and the potential for mortality is high. The Clinical Institute Withdrawal Assessment for Alcohol is a useful scale that quantifies the severity of withdrawal symptoms and helps to guide appropriate benzodiazepine administration.

118. **Which benzodiazepines are metabolized by glucuronidation and may be preferred in situations in which liver function may be compromised (such as alcoholic cirrhosis)?**
Lorazepam, temazepam, and oxazepam are metabolized by glucuronidation and not by the hepatic CYP450 system.

119. **Describe the general approach to the severely agitated patient in the acute setting?**
First, ensure caretaker safety. A quiet, low-stimulation, safe environment (i.e., free of movable objects and sharp edges) should be sought for the agitated patient. Evaluation should include consideration of potentially contributory medications (e.g., anticholinergics), substances (e.g., cocaine), pain, infection, or other underlying medical problems. Emergency medications should be considered.

120. **What emergency medications should be considered for severe agitation in the acute setting?**
A commonly used emergency treatment of agitation (sometimes called the *B52 cocktail*) is a combination of diphenhydramine (Benadryl) 50 mg (for dystonia prophylaxis) per os or intramuscularly, haloperidol 5 mg, and lorazepam 2 mg. Olanzapine 10 mg intramuscularly and other newer parenteral alternatives are also available. Quetiapine or clozapine may be preferred in patients with Parkinson's disease and delirium. The doses suggested above should be decreased considerably for patients with increased sensitivity to psychotropics such as those with developmental disorders or brain injuries and the elderly.

121. **How long does it take for delirium to resolve?**
Even after resolution of the underlying cause of delirium and normalization of laboratory values it can take some time for the CNS to return to homeostasis. In many cases it can take weeks or months for delirium to resolve. In some vulnerable populations (e.g., patients with advanced dementia) the delirium may never resolve, even with appropriate care.

122. Describe the "ABC" approach for managing problematic behavior.

The antecedents–behavior–consequences (ABC) method approaches behavior from a classical and operant conditioning perspective—i.e., behavior is either conditioned to occur due to particular stimuli (antecedents) and/or is reinforced by reward (consequences). Avoiding the stimuli, deconditioning the response, or manipulating the consequences can eliminate, reduce, or redirect problematic behavior.

KEY POINTS: PSYCHIATRY IN NEUROLOGY

1. Psychiatric diagnoses, as described in the *Diagnostic and Statistical Manual*, 5th Edition (DSM-5), are generally idiopathic diagnoses of exclusion based on sign and symptom clusters (i.e., phenomenology-based syndromes) that cause "clinically significant distress or impairment in social, occupational, or other important areas of functioning."
2. Rather than categorically exclusive, mental illnesses, including personality disorders, exist on a spectrum and are multidimensional.
3. Many psychiatric disorders may be described as "functional" disorders as they generally involve dysfunction cortical–subcortical circuits and distributed neuronal networks.
4. Psychiatric disorders and neurologic disorders are interrelated and often comorbid, and many neurologic disorders may present first with psychiatric symptoms.
5. All patients should be screened for psychiatric disorders and suicidality.
6. An elevated suicide risk is associated with depressive disorders, anxiety disorders, schizophrenia, and some neurologic disorders (e.g., Huntington's disease).
7. Clozapine and lithium are associated with a reduction in suicide in certain populations.
8. Psychiatric problems generally respond very well to treatment; the best approach is generally combinations of psychotherapy, pharmacotherapy, lifestyle modification, and strengthening social supports.
9. Supportive therapy and psychoeducation are appropriate for most patients and can be empowering and bolster healthy coping and resilience.
10. Clinicians can foster alliance by first listening and empathically and nonjudgmentally reflecting the patient's understanding and concerns and validating the patient's experience of symptoms.
11. The mental status exam is performed by observation throughout the patient encounter.
12. The cardinal feature of delirium is impaired attention and awareness, which may wax and wane. No other psychiatric disorder can be diagnosed in the context of delirium.
13. A patient's capacity for medical decision making is assessed by the treating physician as part of the informed consent process to some degree for every medical decision.
14. Catatonia, neuroleptic malignant syndrome, and serotonin syndrome are emergencies that overlap considerably in their pathophysiology, phenomenology, and treatment.
15. Psychiatric disorders typically manifest before the fourth decade, and new onset outside of this range should raise diagnostic suspicion and consideration of additional workup.
16. Routine evaluation of psychiatric signs and symptoms includes a physical exam and basic laboratory workup. Additional tests may be necessary depending on the clinical presentation.
17. Mood is the persistent "emotional climate" and affect is the transient "emotional weather," and both have subjective and objective components.
18. Bipolar disorder is defined by persistent (lasting many days to weeks) and extreme shifts in mood, not transient affective lability.
19. SSRIs are first-line therapies for a broad range of disorders due to their efficacy and tolerability.
20. Second-generation "atypical" antipsychotics are associated with lower rates of extrapyramidal symptoms but higher rates of metabolic adverse effects than "typical" antipsychotics.
21. Psychosis describes a deficit in reality testing but psychotic disorders typically also involve impairments in thought, beliefs, motor function, and emotional regulation.
22. Electroconvulsive therapy is by far the most effective treatment of major depressive disorder.
23. Exposure and response prevention is a mainstay of treatment for anxiety disorders.
24. Eating disorders are among the most debilitating and potentially lethal mental health disorders.
25. The ABC approach is an effective intervention for managing problematic behavior.
26. Alcohol and sedative hypnotic withdrawal can be lethal.

References available online at expertconsult.com.

WEBSITE

http://psychiatryonline.org/guidelines

BIBLIOGRAPHY

1. American Psychiatric Association: Diagnostic and Statistical Manual of Mental Disorders (DSM-t), 5th ed. Washington, D.C., American Psychiatric Association, 2013.
2. Arciniegas DB, Anderson CA, Filley CM (eds): Behavioral Neurology & Neuropsychiatry, New York, Cambridge University Press, 2013.
3. Daroff RB, Bradley WG (eds): Bradley's Neurology in Clinical Practice, Philadelphia, Elsevier, 2012.
4. Gabbard GO (ed): Gabbard's Treatments of Psychiatric Disorders, Washington, D.C., American Psychiatric Publishing, 2014.
5. Jeste DV, Friedman JH (eds): Psychiatry for Neurologists, Totowa, NJ, Humana Press, 2006.
6. Mesulam MM (ed): Principles of Behavioral and Cognitive Neurology, 2nd ed. New York, Oxford University Press, 2010.
7. Sadock BJ, Sadock VA, Belkin GS (eds): Kaplan & Sadock's Pocket Handbook of Clinical Psychiatry, 5th ed. Philadelphia, Lippincott Williams & Wilkins, 2010.
8. Spiegel JC, Kenny JM: Psychiatry Test Preparation and Review Manual, London, Elsevier, 2013.
9. Stern TA, Fava M, Wilens TE, Rosenbaum JF (eds): Massachusetts General Hospital Comprehensive Clinical Psychiatry, London, Elsevier, 2016.

CHAPTER 30

NEURO-OTOLOGY

Helen S. Cohen, Jonathan Clark

1. **What are the primary behaviors mediated by the vestibular system?**
   The vestibular system mediates four kinds of behaviors.
   1. It controls the vestibulo-ocular reflex (VOR), an eye movement that compensates for head movement by moving the eye in the direction opposite to the head in order for the individual to see clearly during movement. If you stare at this page and move your head back and forth, you will be able to see the text clearly because you have a functional VOR. People with decreased or absent vestibular function complain of blurry vision and avoid moving their heads.
   2. Vestibular input contributes to balance. In the light, on a flat surface you can stand and walk well without any vestibular function. Decrease the light, or make the surface uneven or unstable, however, and you will rely on your vestibular function to help you maintain balance. Think of the time that you slipped on a wet floor or on ice and almost fell but pulled yourself upright. Think of the time that you learned to skate on ice or roller blades, or used a skateboard. You were able to perform those skills using vestibular function. People with decreased or absent vestibular function complain of imbalance or they walk with wide-based, ataxic gaits.
   3. Vestibular function contributes to spatial orientation—to the sense of being upright, the sense that you are moving or stationary, and your sense of how much and how far you have turned. When you took the elevator to a different floor, even though the elevator was an enclosed box and no visual cues were available to you, you could sense the motion of the elevator. Think of the time that you flew in an airplane and did not look out the window, yet you knew when the plane was turning or slowing to land. You knew those things because you used your vestibular function. Ice skaters, dancers, skiers, and skateboarders all use vestibular function to know when they are upright or upside down in the air. Pilots use their vestibular function to help them stay oriented in conditions of reduced visual information. People with reduced or absent vestibular function may not be able to perform those skills. They may feel or look tilted and they may have either a constant sense of motion, known as *vertigo*, or a sense that the rest of the world is moving, known as *oscillopsia*. Oscillopsia may be mimicked clinically by closing one eye and moving the open eye with a finger on the eyelid, causing an oscillatory movement of the visual image.
   4. Vestibular function helps to modulate some vasovagal responses. When you ran a race, such as the 50-yard dash in school, you used vestibular function to modulate your heart rate, breathing, sweating, and other autonomic functions to increase blood to your muscles and oxygen to your lungs, to cool off your body, and to stop digesting your food. An acute attack of vertigo may be characterized by nausea or vomiting, increased heart rate and respiration, and sometimes the need to urinate or defecate.

2. **What are the primary structures of the vestibular labyrinth?**
   The membranous vestibular labyrinth sits in the bony canals and vestibule of the inner ear in the temporal bone. The labyrinth floats in perilymph, a fluid that is similar to cerebrospinal fluid (CSF) and has a high sodium:potassium ratio. Perilymph communicates with CSF via the cochlear aqueduct. By contrast, the fluid that fills the labyrinth, the endolymph, has a high potassium:sodium ratio. The labyrinth has three, orthogonal semicircular canals, each of which has two names: *superior* or *anterior*, *horizontal* or *lateral*, and *inferior* or *posterior*. The superior and posterior semicircular canals are joined at the common crux. The common crux and one end of the lateral canal end in the utricle, which is one of the two sacs. The utricle (approximately in the horizontal plane) is joined to the other sac, the saccule (approximately in the vertical plane).

   Each semicircular canal has an enlargement at one end, the crista ampullaris, or ampulla. Within the ampulla is the crista, or tiny hillock that runs across the width of the canal, on three sides of which are cilia that are the apical ends of the hair cells. The cilia project into a gelatinous cupula, or cup. These mechanical structures transduce rotational motions of the head by bending the cilia when the endolymph moves due to movement of the head. The base of the chalice-shaped Type 1 hair cell and the columnar-shaped Type II hair cells emit neurotransmitters that are picked up by the vestibular

nerve. Each Type I hair cell is encapsulated by a single afferent vestibular nerve ending, but that afferent ending can have multiple efferents. Type II hair cells communicate with multiple afferent nerve endings and efferents. Hair cells have muscarinic acetylcholine receptors. The afferent vestibular nerve fibers in cranial nerve XIII, however, express glutamate and histamine.

The two sac-like otoliths, the utricle, and saccule each has a slightly curved sensory surface on one wall, known as a *macula*, in which the hair cells are located. The macular surfaces are approximately orthogonal to each other, oriented to detect linear motion of the head, including the constant force of gravity, in any plane in space. In the macula the cilia are covered with a layer of calcium carbonate crystals 2.7 times more dense than endolymph, known as *otoconia*, imbedded in a protein matrix membrane. When the head moves in a linear direction, for example, forward, the inertia of the otoconia causes the otoconial membrane to lag behind the motion of the head for a fraction of a second, bending the underlying cilia and, if the cell membrane depolarizes, releasing neurotransmitters.

The superior portion of the vestibular nerve innervates the anterior and horizontal semicircular canals, most of the utricle, and a small portion of the saccule. The inferior portion of the vestibular nerve innervates the posterior semicircular canal, most of the saccule, and a small portion of the utricle.

The adequate stimulus to every part of the system is acceleration or deceleration of the head: a change in the rate of speed of the head. When the head is moving at a constant velocity or is at rest (0 velocity) the system does not detect head movement. The mechanical properties of the labyrinth change the signal so that the signal that ascends the vestibular nerve to the vestibular nuclei represents head velocity.

3. What are the central vestibular pathways?

The vestibular nerve projects to the vestibular nuclei in the rostral medulla. From there, vestibulospinal tracts descend to cervical, thoracic, and lumbosacral levels of the spinal cord. Therefore, vestibular signals are involved in mediating balance during standing and walking. Note, however, balance is not only controlled by the vestibular system. It is a multifactorial function. In particular, visual signals have been recorded in the vestibular nuclei. Vision is known to have a strong influence on balance, and patients with vestibular impairments may be particularly sensitive to both real and apparent visual motion.

From the vestibular nuclei pathways project to the several regions of the cerebellum: the dentate nuclei, flocculus, nodulus, and ventral uvula. Inhibitory pathways project back to the vestibular nuclei. Those pathways are largely involved in mediating eye movements, especially the VOR, controlled by projections from the vestibular nuclei via the medial longitudinal fasciculus to the nuclei of cranial nerves III, IV, and VI.

Pathways also project rostrally via the medial geniculate and ventroposterior inferior nuclei of the thalamus to the small vestibular cortex in the parieto-insular cortex and posterior lateral sulcus. That area is probably involved in spatial orientation. Pathways from the vestibular nuclei also project to the nucleus tractus solitarius, the parabrachial complex, and the vagus nerve to mediate vasovagal responses.

4. What is the basis for the arterial circulation to the inner ear?

The arterial supply to the entire inner ear—the cochlea and vestibular labyrinth—derives from the internal auditory artery, a branch of the anterior inferior cerebellar artery. The internal auditory artery forms two branches: (1) the anterior vestibular artery, which supplies the anterior semicircular canal, the horizontal semicircular canal, and the utricle, and (2) the internal auditory artery, which forms the common cochlear artery. The common cochlear artery divides into (1) the vestibulo-cochlear artery to supply the posterior semicircular canal and saccule as well as the basal turn of the cochlea, and (2) the main cochlear artery, which supplies the rest of the cochlea.

5. What are the primary symptoms of acute vestibular impairment?

The Committee for Classification of Vestibular Disorders of the Barany Society published the vestibular symptom classification scheme in 2009 (Table 30-1). Vestibular symptoms can include vestibulo-ocular, vestibulo-spinal, and vestibulo-autonomic symptoms and may include disequilibrium, vertigo, oscillopsia, nausea, nystagmus, diaphoresis, increased heart rate, and respiration. Disequilibrium, or poor balance, is caused by the decrease in signal to the vestibulo-spinal tracts. Vertigo, the illusion of self-motion, may be perceived as angular (spinning, whirling, or gentle rocking) or linear (to and fro, side to side). Vertigo is probably caused by decreased signals to the vestibular cortex. Oscillopsia, a related sensation, is the illusion of motion in the visual world around the individual and is probably caused by nystagmus. The primary characteristics of the symptom history include symptom onset and duration, time course (constant or episodic), specific triggers and other aggravating or alleviating factors, associated symptoms, and family history of similar episodes.

Nystagmus is the rapid, involuntary, back-and-forth motion of the eyes. In the acute period quick phases beating away from the involved side alternate with slow phases moving toward that side,

Table 30-1. International Classification of Vestibular Disorders I (ICVD-I) Classification of Symptoms v1.0 (January 2009)

1. Vertigo
   - Spontaneous vertigo
   - Triggered vertigo
     - Positional vertigo
     - Head-motion vertigo
     - Visually-induced vertigo
     - Sound-induced vertigo
     - Valsalva-induced vertigo
     - Orthostatic vertigo
     - Other triggered vertigo
2. Dizziness
   - Spontaneous dizziness
   - Triggered dizziness
     - Positional dizziness
     - Head-motion dizziness
     - Visually-induced dizziness
     - Sound-induced dizziness
     - Valsalva-induced dizziness
     - Orthostatic dizziness
     - Other triggered dizziness
3. Vestibulo-visual symptoms
   - External vertigo
   - Oscillopsia
   - Visual lag
   - Visual tilt
   - Movement-induced blur
4. Postural symptoms
   - Unsteadiness
   - Directional pulsion
   - Balance-related near fall
   - Balance-related fall

From Bisdorff A, von Brevern M, Lempert T, Newman-Toker DE: Classification of vestibular symptoms: towards an international classification of vestibular disorders, *J Vestib Res* 19(1-2):1-13, 2009.

usually horizontal with a torsional component. The nystagmus has greater amplitude when vision is absent (prevents the ability to fixate visually), such as when the patient is tested with Frenzel lenses or infrared video oculography (VOG). In peripheral lesions the nystagmus is more intense when the patient looks toward the direction of the quick phases, i.e., away from the involved side; this phenomenon is known as *Alexander's law*. Alexander's law is not usually true of central lesions.

The patient has oscillopsia because higher centers, which have not given movement commands, do not expect visual feedback from movements of the eyes. When the individual makes a movement that the brain has planned, theoretically the brain plans to expect certain sensory feedback arising from that movement and a copy of the motor command may be sent elsewhere in the brain to await that feedback. (The copy is known as *efference copy* or *corollary discharge*. If the expected feedback is received after the movement the individual knows that he has moved and can use that feedback to determine if the movement was successful or if the motor command should be adjusted on the next trial. If the movement was not successful the individual can use the feedback to adjust the motor command on the next trial. This movement–feedback loop is the theoretical basis for motor learning.) In an individual who has a vestibular disorder and whose subcortical oculomotor system is generating nystagmus, no efference copy will be received by some higher center in expectation of receiving visual feedback. Therefore, the motion of the visual image across the retina will be misinterpreted as motion of the world around the person rather than motion of the eyes and, therefore, the patient will experience oscillopsia.

Patients may have nausea, diaphoresis, and cardiovascular signs because of vestibulo-autonomic projections of the vestibular nuclei to several nuclei such as the parabrachial nucleus, nucleus of the solitary tract, nucleus ambiguous, and dorsal nucleus of the vagus nerve.

6. **What are the primary symptoms of chronic vestibular impairment?**
Chronic vestibular dysfunction is characterized by fewer vasovagal symptoms but patients may have impairments of the motor functions influenced by the vestibular system. Therefore, they often describe having vertigo, disequilibrium, stomach awareness or nausea, blurred vision, and sensitivity to visual motion. These symptoms are usually less intense than during an acute attack. Patients may have anxiety about their condition. They may limit their activities at home, at work, and in the community as a result of their symptoms.

7. **What distinguishes peripheral from central causes of vestibular dysfunction?**
Most patients with peripheral vestibular dysfunction have more severe vertiginous symptoms, while those with central nervous system etiology usually do not have severe vertigo. Patients with peripheral vertigo may have short episodes, lasting seconds (benign positional vertigo), minutes (Ménière's disease), or hours (vestibular neuritis). Auditory symptoms (hearing loss, tinnitus, and aural fullness) are more frequently associated with peripheral vestibular disease. Position changes associated with vertigo are more often related to peripheral causes. Central causes of vestibular dysfunction have a more variable presentation, which may be described as tilting to one side, or nonspecific lightheadedness or clumsiness. Associated symptoms of diplopia, such as dysphasia, dysarthria, hemiparesis, cephalgia, seizures, memory loss, or sensory findings, suggest central etiology. In central vestibular dysfunction, the nystagmus is usually more prominent than symptoms and may be disconjugate. Visual fixation suppresses peripheral nystagmus and increases amplitude of the central nystagmus. See Table 30-2.

Table 30-2. Peripheral versus Central Vestibular Disorders' Characteristics

PERIPHERAL	CENTRAL	BOTH	NOTES
Alexander's law	No Alexander's law	Vertigo	
Visual suppression at least partly	No visual suppression	Disequilibrium	
Positional, classical D–H	Not positional	Nausea	
Normal saccades, pursuit, OKN	Possible abnormal saccades, pursuit, OKN	Hearing loss	
	Possible: hoarseness, difficulty swallowing, mixed sensory loss characteristic of lateral medullary syndrome	Sudden onset of symptoms	
Minor skew deviation	Large skew deviation		
No gaze-evoked nystagmus	Gaze-evoked nystagmus is present		
Possible impaired C-VEMP	Possible impaired O-VEMP		Details still unclear in this new area
Bithermal caloric weakness	No caloric weakness		If rotatory chair is impaired and caloric weakness is not present the problem may still be peripheral
Rotatory chair VOR decreased gain but intact phases	Rotatory chair decreased gain and abnormal phases	Both caloric impairment and rotatory impairment may be present in either central or peripheral	

D–H, Dix–Hallpike; OKN, optokinetic nystagmus; C-VEMP, cervical vestibular evoked myogenic potentials; O-VEMP, ocular evoked myogenic potentials; VOR, vestibulo-ocular reflex.

8. **Can medications affect the function of the vestibular labyrinth?**

A patient having an acute attack of vertigo, nausea, and vomiting, suggesting the onset of labyrinthitis or vestibular neuronitis, may be treated palliatively with promethazine or prochlorperazine for nausea/vomiting (many patients may not be able to tolerate oral medications at this stage so suppositories may be necessary) and with steroids, such as prednisone, dexamethasone, or methylprednisolone, to reduce inflammation.

Pharmacologic intervention for Ménière's disease (endolymphatic hydrops) is initially vestibular suppressant medications such as the antihistamine meclizine or the benzodiazepine lorazepam. If those medications are ineffective the use of diuretics may reduce fluid fluctuations in the inner ear. For example, medications such as hydrochlorothiazide may be tried.

Some medications such as the antineoplastic cisplatin, and aminoglycoside antibiotics, notably gentamicin, are highly toxic to hair cells. Large doses of either drug will cause permanent damage to hair cells and, therefore, permanent bilateral vestibular and hearing losses. Therefore, intratympanic gentamicin is used as a last-resort treatment for Ménière's disease, when destroying vestibular function on one side may be therapeutic to help the patient overcome debilitating attacks of vertigo that do not respond to pharmacologic intervention.

9. **What is the most common major peripheral vestibular disorder and what are the characteristics?**

The most common cause of episodic vertigo and peripheral vestibular disorder is benign paroxysmal positional vertigo (BPPV). It is probably caused when particles of otoconia become fractured or displaced from the otoconial membrane, enter the common crus, and, in over 95% of cases, fall into the posterior canal, attaching themselves to the membranous wall of the canal and/or the cupula of ampulla. Based on studies of in vitro frog labyrinths but not live humans, these two subtypes are (1) canalithiasis and (2) cupulolithiasis, respectively. In rare cases BPPV may affect the anterior semicircular canal or the horizontal canal. The symptoms of BPPV of the posterior canal are vertigo elicited by pitch (up or down) rotations of the head and then a stationary position for several seconds, for example, looking upward toward the ceiling or a high shelf, looking downward toward the floor or under a bed, lying down in bed and rolling onto the affected side, or sitting up and transferring out of bed. The vertigo elicited in these situations is characterized by a delay to onset of a few seconds from moving the head into the stimulus position to the onset of vertigo. It is often intense but lasts only a few seconds.

The standard clinical test for posterior canal BPPV is the Dix–Hallpike maneuver. In this test the patient sits with her legs in front of her. The clinician turns the patient's head 45° to the side to be tested, if possible, and then pitches the head back so that at the end of the motion the patient lies supine, so that at the end of the motion the neck is hyperextended approximately 30° if possible. For a patient with cervical limitations or other musculoskeletal limitations the test can be adapted by having the patient lie partly supine on the ipsilateral scapula or even lie on the ipsilateral side but facing contralaterally away from the test side, in the side lying test.

Nystagmus elicited by the Dix–Hallpike maneuver is pathognomonic if the nystagmus has the following characteristics: beating (quick phases) upward in the vertical plane, ipsilateral to the test side in the horizontal plane, and torsion of the eye also beating ipsilateral to the test side. So, the quick phases act like an arrow pointing to the affected side. The nystagmus appears 2 to 30 seconds after the head has been moved into the test position. It waxes and wanes, with a few small beats, larger beats, and then smaller beats again. During Dix–Hallpike testing patients will complain of vertigo with the delay to onset and the same duration as the nystagmus. They may become diaphoretic or anxious and may have nausea during the test and afterward. After seconds to minutes the nausea subsides.

Nystagmus is inhibited with visual fixation, so the best way to perform the Dix–Hallpike maneuver is with fixation-occluding magnifying lenses over the eyes. Traditional evaluation included high plus or magnifying lenses (Frenzel lenses) that magnify the eyes and prevent the patient from focusing on a pattern. Frenzel lenses have been largely replaced with infrared video-oculography, in which small infrared video cameras imbedded in goggles are placed over the patient's eyes. The image is then either recorded on a laptop computer or viewed on a screen. The alternative, older recording technique is electronystagmography (ENG), also known as *electro-oculography*, in which electrodes placed around the eyes record the corneoretinal potential.

BPPV of the anterior canal and horizontal canal is possible, but unusual. To test the patient for anterior canal BPPV, use the reverse side lying test: while the patient sits on the side of the treatment table, turn her head 45° to face the test side. Rapidly place the patient nose downward and have her lie on the ipsilateral shoulder. Wait for the onset and cessation of nystagmus. To test the patient for lateral canal BPPV have the patient lie supine with the neck pitched forward (downward) approximately 30° to bring the horizontal canal into alignment with earth vertical. Rotate the head to either side, waiting several seconds to observe nystagmus.

Approximately half of BPPV patients complain of disequilibrium and have balance impairments. They may fail Romberg testing. Therefore these patients complain of difficulty walking, particular difficulty ascending and descending stairs, and particular difficulty walking on unstable surfaces.

The recurrence rate for BPPV is high; at least 30% of patients have a recurrence. The disorder is twice as common on the right as on the left and twice as common in women as in men. The first onset often occurs in the late 40s or early 50s and becomes more common with advancing age. Comorbidities include mild head trauma for which the patient may not have sought medical attention or more severe head trauma, smoking, diabetes, upper airway inflammatory disease such as cold, flu, allergies or sinus infection, and any other vestibular impairment.

10. What is the treatment for BPPV?

Medication is not effective in the treatment of BPPV. The standard of care for treatment of BPPV of the posterior canal is to manipulate the head to attempt to move the otoconia backward through the semicircular canal to return to the utricle. Several repositioning maneuvers have been developed to do this. The most common maneuver, the canalith repositioning maneuver (Epley maneuver), puts the patient in the Dix–Hallpike test position, then rotates the head contralaterally during supine lying, and then holds the head facing contralaterally while the patient sits up. An alternative maneuver, the liberatory maneuver (Semont maneuver), puts the patient in the side lying position on the ipsilateral side but with the head facing contralaterally—so the nose is pointed diagonally upward. Then the patient is moved rapidly through a 180° arc to lie nose downward on the contralateral side. Note that the last stage of the canalith repositioning and liberatory maneuvers are the same. Three to five trials are often needed, and one to three treatment sessions on different days are often needed. The two maneuvers are equally effective. Vibration of the head is not needed, has been shown to be ineffective, and will probably annoy the patient. Special instructions to sleep sitting up, limit head movement, or wear a cervical collar have also been shown to be ineffective.

Repositioning exercises that are similar to the repositioning maneuvers, three times per day, five repetitions per session, for at least 1 week are also effective, although somewhat less effective than the repositioning maneuvers themselves. Practicing repositioning exercises after successful treatment, however, does not prevent the recurrence of another episode.

Repositioning treatments for lateral canal and anterior canal BPPV are also available. To treat lateral canal BPPV the log-rolling maneuver is used. Have the patient lie supine. Rotate the head contralateral to the involved side, then, keeping the head still, have the patient roll contralaterally away from the involved side onto the contralateral shoulder, then rotate the head and body into prone lying, and then into side lying on the ipsilateral side. The patient will have rolled 270°. Then have the patient sit up. Repeat three or four times if needed. To treat anterior canal BPPV use Semont's maneuver in reverse: turn the face 45° toward the involved side, have the patient lie on that side; wait until the vertigo subsides, and then briskly move the patient 180° to the contralateral shoulder with the face looking upward. After the vertigo has subsided, keep the head facing toward the ipsilateral side and have the patient sit up. Three or four trials may be needed.

A surgical procedure, canal plugging, is available but rarely used since most patients respond well to repositioning maneuvers and exercises.

11. What are other peripheral vestibular disorders? How are they treated?

1. Labyrinthitis or vestibular neuronitis, caused by inflammation from viral influence or possibly microvascular ischemia or compromise, is common. Patients have acute or gradual onset of vertigo, disequilibrium, and nausea and may have other vasovagal signs. They are likely to have decreased responses to bithermal caloric testing and low-frequency rotational tests of the VOR in darkness, impaired balance, impaired sense of the visual vertical, or they may sit with the head tilted to one side chronically. Patients tend to seek medical care when they have difficulty reading, doing chores around the house, exercising, driving, or have had falls.

In the acute phase, use of steroids such as methylprednisolone may be useful. Medications are not useful in patients with chronic symptoms. Meclizine and scopolamine are widely used but are not very effective and the sedative effects can be disabling. The current standard of care is to refer these patients for vestibular rehabilitation exercises, which use head movements to increase the patient's tolerance for movement and decrease vertigo gradually over 1 to 4 weeks. In addition, balance therapy exercises may be indicated. Since many patients need specific instructions and coaching, as well as advice about how to function while they are having symptoms, these patients are best referred to occupational therapy or physical therapy with a trained therapist.

2. Ménière's disease (endolymphatic hydrops) is well known but not as common. It is characterized by fluctuating but progressive, low-frequency sensorineural hearing loss, tinnitus, fullness in the affected ear, and a sudden, unprovoked episode of vertigo lasting minutes to hours. It is thought to be caused by a buildup of endolymph that is not resorbed normally. These patients have normal balance and minimal or no vertigo in between Ménière's attack so that by the time they arrive at the clinic their vestibular function often appears to be normal. The disorder itself may cause BPPV or labyrinthitis.

    The first line of treatment is dietary modification with a low-sodium diet. Since many patients may not understand the concept of using no salt at all or may have difficulty meal planning, counseling with a nurse, occupational therapist, or dietician may be useful. If dietary management alone is not therapeutic, the patient should be managed with diuretics, such as hydrochlorothiazide. Antiemetics, such as promethazine, may also be useful. In most cases, patients may function well on such a regimen. Some patients progress to profound hearing loss and attacks of vertigo so intense that they cannot function. In those cases, treatment with intra-tympanic gentamicin may be used to destroy the hair cells of the affected vestibular labyrinth. This procedure should be performed by an otoneurologist or neurotologist who has had subspe-cialty training and has experience with this disorder. After gentamicin injections the patient may still have some residual vertigo. These patients often do well with vestibular rehabilitation for vertigo habituation exercises.

    Several surgical procedures are available although, with the advent of gentamicin treat-ment, these procedures have become less widely used, mostly as a last resort if the patient fails gentamicin injections. Endolymphatic sac surgery is controversial and is no longer widely used. Similarly, endolymphatic shunts were widely used in the past but are now rarely performed. Vestibular labyrinthectomy can be performed but vestibular nerve section may be preferred as the less complex procedure that is likely to be just as reliable. These procedures often result in chronic vertigo and disequilibrium. Patients who fail to compensate completely after surgical procedures should be referred for vestibular rehabilitation.

3. Bilateral vestibular impairment or loss is rare but can occur. It is most often due to the use of aminoglycosides or due to autoimmune disorders, but it may be idiopathic or may be related to meningitis or polyneuropathy. Typical autoimmune disorders that can cause bilateral vestibular loss are rheumatoid arthritis, systemic lupus erythematosus, Cogan's syndrome, and Sjögren's syndrome. Patients present with disequilibrium and oscillopsia and may have had falls. They may also have vertigo if some vestibular function remains.

    Depending on the pathophysiology, some patients may benefit from use of corticosteroids. When suspected of autoimmune disorders patients should be referred to rheumatology. Patients with bilateral vestibular loss may benefit from vestibular rehabilitation for balance exercises, vertigo habituation if vertigo is present, and from functional skills training.

4. Acoustic neuroma, a schwannoma of the vestibular nerve, is rare. It is often diagnosed with mag-netic resonance imaging (MRI) when the patient has unexplained hearing loss. These tumors grow slowly, over many years. Therefore, older patients may benefit from watchful waiting. Treatment with medication and rehabilitation is not effective. Two surgical procedures are available: (1) surgi-cal resection of the tumor or (2) stereotactic radioablation (gamma knife). Although gamma knife is reputed to spare residual hearing, it may not spare hearing in individual cases. With a small tumor a surgical resection may be able to spare hearing in some cases depending on the approach. After surgery some patients compensate well within 2 months. Other patients may benefit from vestibu-lar rehabilitation if they are still symptomatic after the acute phase of recovery.

5. Perilymph fistulas are rare. They occur when the bony semicircular canal of the anterior semi-circular canal, or the oval or round window of the middle ear, has been breached. Superior canal dehiscence (SCD) occurs when the arcuate eminence, which contains the superior semicircular canal, erodes over time, presumably due to minute changes in intracranial pressure over the course of a lifetime as the individual coughs or strains. These patients complain of vertigo elicited by loud sounds and may even have nystagmus (Tullio's phenomenon). Sometimes these patients speak very softly because the sound of their own voices elicits vertigo. The clinical diagnostic test for SCD is the cervical vestibular evoked myogenic potential. The follow-up in suspected SCD is

computed tomography (CT) scan in the plan of the anterior semicircular canal. The treatment is surgical intervention to patch the area.

Other types of fistulas are rare and are most often caused by head trauma. They can also be caused by otic barotrauma from diving accidents. Diagnosis, although difficult, may be aided with the use of computerized dynamic posturography (computerized Romberg testing) in the condition with eyes closed and movable support surface given with and without a puff of air to the impaired ear to observe for increased postural sway. The surgical intervention involves middle ear exploration and patching if necessary.

12. **What are the common central vestibular impairments?**
    1. Vestibular migraine or migrainous vertigo, previously called *migraine-associated vertigo* or *migraine-related vestibulopathy*, is the most common central nervous system vestibular disorder and occurs in 1% of the general population and 11% of patients in specialized dizziness clinics. It is an underrecognized cause of episodic vertigo and may affect a third of migraine patients. For a diagnosis of vestibular migraine there are at least five episodes of moderate or severe intensity vestibular symptoms lasting 5 minutes to 72 hours, current or previous history of migraine with or without aura, and migraine features during half of the vestibular episodes and not better accounted for by another vestibular or headache diagnosis. Another related condition, basilar-type migraine, commonly has vertigo, but requires at least two posterior circulation manifestations lasting between 5 and 60 minutes for the diagnosis. Basilar-type migraine is not synonymous with vestibular migraine. An early manifestation, benign paroxysmal vertigo of childhood, requires five episodes of severe vertigo, occurring without warning and resolving spontaneously within minutes to hours with a neurologic exam and tests between episodes. Vestibular migraine may present with positional vertigo, mimicking BPPV. The nystagmus in vestibular migraine during the acute phase is usually persistent and not aligned with a single semicircular canal. Treatment includes the same medications used to treat migraine (triptans, beta-blockers, membrane channel agents, or acetazolamide) and control of dietary triggers, as well as vestibular rehabilitation for those with gait and balance complaints.
    2. Multiple sclerosis (MS) can affect vestibular function, particularly when it affects brain stem tracts or nuclei. True vertigo is estimated to occur in 20% of MS patients. Lesions affecting the vestibular nuclei and/or the root entry zone of cranial nerve VIII represent the most common locations where demyelinating activity can provoke vertigo in patients with MS. However, other causes of vertigo should be explored in MS patients in order to avoid unnecessary treatment with corticosteroids and vestibular suppressants. One study of new onset vertigo in an MS population found that BPPV was the most common cause of vertigo in MS patients. The patients diagnosed with BPPV were treated successfully with particle repositioning maneuvers, and the remaining patients were treated with conventional therapies appropriate for the specific diagnosis. Multiple sclerosis of the brain stem often results in internuclear ophthalmoplegia affecting the medial longitudinal fasciculi or neighboring tracts, which can affect visual vestibular interaction (pursuit, cancellation, and vestibular smooth eye movements).
    3. Seizures can cause vertigo if the vestibular cortex and other projection areas are involved, and have been called *vertiginous epilepsy* or *epileptic vertigo*. Vertigo can occur as part of the aura of temporal lobe seizures, but there are other associated aura symptoms and the patient is amnestic during the seizure. Seizures involving the posterior insula (parieto-insular vestibular cortex), superior temporal gyrus, and temporoparietal cortex have been observed to result in vertigo. Seizures involving the paramedian precuneus are involved in processing of static and dynamic vestibular otolithic information, hence the vertigo may be linear (to and fro or side to side) rather than rotatory. Disequilibrium (epileptic dizziness) without vertigo has also been observed in aura from temporal lobe epilepsy. Nystagmus has been observed in association with seizures or epileptiform discharges originating from the cortical areas involved in the generation of smooth pursuit and fast eye movements.
    4. Cerebellopontine angle tumors such as acoustic neuroma mentioned above may present with a peripheral nerve lesion or central lesion if nearby brain stem structures are compromised.
    5. Cerebrovascular disease including vertebrobasilar insufficiency can present with vertigo and vestibular impairment. Acute vestibular syndrome is often due to vestibular neuritis but may result from posterior fossa (vertebrobasilar) stroke or ischemia affecting either brain stem or cerebellum. Misdiagnosis of posterior fossa stroke in the emergency department is common. The three-step bedside oculomotor examination (HINTS: head-impulse, nystagmus, test-of-skew) may reliably

identify stroke in acute vestibular syndrome. The presence of normal horizontal head impulse test, direction-changing nystagmus in eccentric gaze, or skew deviation (vertical ocular misalignment) was 100% sensitive and 96% specific for stroke. Skew deviation is associated with brain stem lesions. Lateral medullary syndrome may cause vertigo, disequilibrium, nausea, and nystagmus as well as hoarseness, difficulty swallowing, and mixed sensory loss. Strokes (embolic, ischemic, and hemorrhagic) involving the vestibular cortex have resulted in vestibular symptoms including vertigo. Acute rotatory vertigo has been seen following a small hemorrhage in the left medial temporal gyrus, presumably affecting the vestibular cortex. Pusher syndrome is less common, but can result from a cerebrovascular accident (CVA) affecting the vestibular cortex. Patients often feel they are being propelled or pushed. They may have impaired sense of subjective visual, vertical, ocular torsion, and skew deviation. This condition usually resolves quickly. Although the acute symptoms may resolve quickly some patients have residual vertigo and disequilibrium. If so, those patients may be helped with vestibular rehabilitation.

13. What are nonpathologic causes of vestibular impairments?
    1. Mal de debarquement, literally sickness disembarking, is a rare disorder that may occur after an intense motion experience. Patients complain of vertigo and a sense of swaying or rocking and they may be observed to rock or sway while sitting quietly. It is most often reported after a voyage on a cruise ship but may occur after flying in turbulence, as a pilot or passenger. It is more common in women than men and can last for months to years. It recurs when the individual is re-exposed to the initial stimulus. Benzodiazepines may be helpful. Vestibular suppressants such as meclizine and scopolamine are not helpful. Vestibular rehabilitation is contraindicated. Patients should be advised to avoid intense motion experiences until the symptoms subside, including head-shaking exercises, running, use of elliptical machines for exercise, and long car, train, or airplane rides.
    2. Motion sickness, often during a boat or car ride but also during sea voyages, air travel, and the initiation of space travel, probably occurs due to visual–vestibular conflict or, in the case of space travel, due to reinterpretation of signals from the otolith organs. In land-based travel individuals may feel better by using a visual reference to confirm the sense of motion, such as looking at an object on the horizon. Motion sickness often causes nausea, vomiting, other vasovagal symptoms, decreased concentration, and difficulty thinking. Medications that are useful include antihistamines, anticholinergic antimuscarinics, 5-HT3 serotonergic receptor antagonists, and stimulants. Antihistamines are the most common medication for treating motion sickness, have a longer duration of action, and are relatively safe. Oral forms are used for prevention, while parenteral administration is used for treatment of motion sickness. Medications with mixed anti muscarine and antihistamine effects include diphenhydramine and promethazine. Scopolamine is one of the most effective drugs to prevent motion sickness at dosages of 0.3 to 0.6 mg orally. Intranasal scopolamine may be rapidly administered as a rescue therapy for motion sickness. Stimulants, such as D-amphetamine or ephedrine, often in combination with scopolamine, are effective in preventing motion sickness. Dextroamphetamine (5 to 10 mg) has been used effectively in combination with promethazine (Phen-Dex) or scopolamine (Scop-Dex) and can counter some of the sedating effects of antihistamines. The 5-HT3 serotonergic receptor antagonists, such as ondansetron or granisetron, may be effective at preventing motion sickness and have few side effects.
    3. Presbystasis, or disequilibrium of aging, is a multifactorial problem. During the aging process the vestibular labyrinth loses hair cells, the otoconia may fracture and change shape, the vestibular nerve loses fibers, and the vestibular nuclei lose cells. In addition the brain shrinks and proprioception and tactile senses decrease. A diagnosis of presbystasis is often given to a patient complaining of nonspecific dizziness who is over 65 years old when no specific cause is identified. Although the patient may not have true vertigo, he or she may have slips, trips, and even falls. This problem is compounded by polypharmacy, sleep disturbance, peripheral neuropathy, musculoskeletal problems including foot deformities, hip and knee pain and arthritis, visual decline (cataracts, age-related macular degeneration), and cognitive decline. Patients may benefit from a review of medications and if possible decreased medication usage. They should have a through visual work-up by ophthalmology or optometry to improve vision with better eyeglasses and treatment of cataracts and other problems. They should be worked up for foot deformities and counseled by podiatry about use of proper footwear. Evaluation by orthopedics for hip and knee pain may be beneficial. Evaluation of cognitive function by neuropsychology and hearing function by audiology

may be beneficial. Referral to occupational therapy and physical therapy will be beneficial for functional assessment, functional skills training, strength training, assessment of need for home modifications, and training to avoid falls and how to deal with falls if they occur. Social service intervention may also be needed.

14. **What are nonneurologic causes of dizziness?**
Patients complaining of dizziness often have subjective descriptions that are unreliable and inconsistent. A patient complaining of vertigo does not mean the cause is a vestibular disorder, and a patient who denies vertigo may have a vestibular disorder. Lightheadedness is a very nonspecific symptom, but if accompanied by a near-loss of consciousness, suggests diminished cerebral blood flow, possibly cardiac in origin. Many patients have hyper- or hypotension that can cause lightheadedness, cardiac arrhythmias, imbalance, and difficulty walking. Lightheadedness can be seen with metabolic disorders, medication side effects, or drug interactions, hence all patients should be evaluated for polypharmacy. Hypoglycemia may cause dizziness in severe diabetics. Many older people limit their fluid intake to avoid frequent bathroom trips and then become dehydrated. Dehydration may cause lightheadedness due to loss of volume. Severe rhinosinusitis can cause dizziness that the patient may interpret as positional vertigo, if the problem is exacerbated by positional changes.

15. **What are common comorbidities with vestibular disorders?**
Vestibular disorders are seen in the population in middle and older age, so aging processes are related to the developing of these impairments. Vestibular disorders are also associated with diabetes mellitus, smoking, alcoholism, vascular disorders, autoimmune disorders, and head trauma. Peripheral vestibular disorders are common after upper airway inflammatory disorders such as a cold, flu, or sinus infection. Use of ototoxic medication can cause vestibular impairment. Migraine can cause vestibular disorders. Multiple sclerosis can cause a central vestibular impairment.

16. **What tests should be used for screening and for objective diagnostic testing?**
Most but not all tests assess the VOR. In the clinic the head impulse test, in which the head is rapidly rotated 20° to either side while the patient fixates on a central target, might show an abnormality. Look for one or two compensatory saccades. The test is only reliable if the patient is elderly, can relax enough to allow the clinician to perform the test, and has a large decrease in VOR function. Head shaking might be useful to elicit vertigo, but it has not been shown to be reliable.
　　The Dix–Hallpike maneuver is pathognomonic for BPPV, if the patient has a classical pattern of nystagmus beating upward in pitch, and ipsilaterally in horizontal and roll directions. For a patient who cannot perform the Dix–Hallpike maneuver, side lying may be used instead. For either test, expect to see a delay of a few seconds followed by a burst of nystagmus lasting several seconds.
　　Tandem walking for 10 steps with eyes open is not reliable; tandem walking for 10 steps with eyes closed might be useful if the patient has no other neurologic deficit, peripheral neuropathy, musculoskeletal deformities, or weakness. Standing balance testing with the Romberg test, with eyes closed on an unstable surface such as compliant foam, is reliable, unless the patient has peripheral neuropathy, musculoskeletal deformities, or weakness. Patients under the age of 55 years should be able to perform the test for 25 seconds. Patients aged 60 to 79 years should be able to perform the test for 9.5 seconds. Patients aged 80 years and older should be able to perform for 4 to 5 seconds. The most reliable screening test, however, is a history of true vertigo, as opposed to lightheadedness, nausea, or some other form of dizziness.
　　The objective diagnostic battery of tests assessing the vestibular system, often referred to as *ENG* for the original recording technique of electro-oculography, includes cervical vestibular evoked myogenic potentials (C-VEMP), ocular evoked myogenic potentials (O-VEMP), low-frequency rotational tests in darkness in a rotatory chair, Dix–Hallpike maneuvers, and bithermal caloric tests. In C-VEMP a tone is played in the ear while the ipsilateral sternocleidomastoid muscle is recorded with electromyography as it is stressed by lifting the head against gravity or pushing against a hand. A very slight relaxation of the muscle should be observed in response to sound as indicated by the response at the p13–n23 waveform. If the patient is responsive to sound at a very low threshold, however, the response might be consistent with superior canal dehiscence. VEMP is also considered a test of saccular function. The absence of a C-VEMP response might be consistent with loss of inferior vestibular nerve function, if a response is absent. This response is inhibitory, uncrossed, descending, and sacculocollic.
　　In O-VEMP electrodes are placed on the face around the eyes and are used to measure a tiny response to auditory stimulus or tap in the contralateral eye muscles, primarily the inferior oblique,

as the patient looks upward to stress the eye muscles. The response is seen at n10. This response is excitatory, crossed, ascending, and utriculo-ocular. Impaired O-VEMP responses may indicate superior vestibular nerve impairment or central impairment. The uses of these evoked potentials are still being worked out.

In the rotatory chair the VOR and other eye movements—saccades, smooth pursuit, and optokinetic nystagmus—are usually recorded with VOG. If, however, VOG is not available or the patient cannot tolerate the goggles, ENG can be used. Saccades, pursuit, and optokinetic responses are used to test the integrity of the brain stem and cerebellar mechanisms that control eye movements including the VOR. Impaired saccades and other eye movements may be an early indicator of multiple sclerosis. These eye movements and the VOR should be conjugate. Disconjugate eye movements may indicate internuclear ophthalmoplegia or some other central deficit. Patients should also be observed for the presence of spontaneous nystagmus and gaze-evoked nystagmus.

The rotatory chair can be used for low- or high-frequency testing. It is most comfortable and least disturbing for the patient when used for low-frequency testing. The VOR is linear in the range of 0.1 to 7.0 Hz. Therefore, testing is usually performed below and above 0.1 Hz, such as 0.0125, 0.05, and 2.0 Hz with sinusoidal stimuli ±60°. Higher-frequency tests with steps of velocity, rather than sinusoids, are useful when bilateral vestibular impairment is suspected. Patients who are claustrophobic may become stressed during testing. Therefore, technical staff must be supportive but firm in convincing such a patient to complete the test. Other patients may become drowsy. For that reason patients are usually asked to play word games during testing to maintain consistency of eye movements.

For objective diagnostic testing Dix–Hallpike maneuvers should be performed using VOG or ENG and recorded on the computer for later analysis. Other positional tests such as side lying can also be performed.

Bithermal caloric testing uses changes in the temperature of the external ear and tympanic membrane to cause a change in the temperature of the middle ear and eventually inner ear, causing flow of the endolymph in one labyrinth only. Caloric testing is highly reliable in detecting unilateral peripheral vestibular loss. The alternate binaural bithermal caloric test is usually performed while the patient is lying supine with the neck flexed 30° to bring the lateral canal into the earth vertical position. Then, each lateral canal can be tested separately. Typically irrigations are performed at 30° C and 44° C in each ear, using water for the best stimulus, or air if the patient has a perforated tympanic membrane. Cold and warm caloric stimuli elicit opposite current flows and therefore opposite responses. Remember the side of stimulation and the response using COWS: cold, opposite, warm, same. So, for example, left cold irrigation elicits right-beating nystagmus and left warm irrigation elicits left-beating nystagmus. To perform the test correctly the patient must have all four irrigations. The four measures are combined in the Jonkees formula, shown below, to calculate relative weakness of one side using the velocity of the slow phase of nystagmus, which represents the VOR, where RC, RW, LC, and LW indicate the peak slow-component velocity of nystagmus from right cool, right warm, left cool, and left warm irrigations.

$$100 \times [(LC + LW) - (RC + RW) / (LC + LW + RC + RW)] = \% \text{ caloric paresis}$$
$$100 \times [(LC + RW) - (RC + LW) / (LC + LW + RC + RW)] = \% \text{ directional preponderance}$$

A weakness of 25% or greater is usually considered to be abnormal and indicative of impaired peripheral vestibular function. Directional preponderance of greater than 30% indicates an abnormal asymmetry between right-beating nystagmus (right warm and left cool) and left-beating nystagmus (left warm and right cool) evoked by the caloric irrigations. Directional preponderance is a nonspecific sign of vestibular dysfunction. A total eye velocity of less than 30° may indicate a bilateral impairment or loss. The bithermal caloric test response approximates the low-frequency response in the rotatory chair, to frequencies below 0.1 Hz, but the two tests elicit different characteristic patterns of nystagmus and should be used to complement each other. The disadvantage of caloric testing is interindividual variability of caloric vestibular responses.

Computerized dynamic posturography measures the integrity of the vestibulo-spinal tracts and the use of visual–vestibular interaction. It is not a purely vestibular test but may give some insight into the patient's status and may be informative if a patient has intact VOR responses, such as an elderly person who is subsequently diagnosed with presbystasis. The test battery, which is the computerized version of the clinical Romberg test, has the patient stand on a movable force platform that measures the change in postural sway under the patient's feet. The patient is tested under six conditions: eyes open (control condition), eyes closed with stationary force platform, eyes open but with movement of the visual surround in phase with postural sway (sway referenced) to "fool" the system and make visual information useless, eyes open with sway-referenced force platform motion, eyes closed with sway-referenced force platform motion, and eyes open with sway-referenced motion of the force platform and of the visual surround. In normals performance decreases across the different conditions. In patients significantly decreased performance on conditions five and six is most likely to be consistent with a vestibular impairment. Normal performance on conditions five and six but abnormal performance on conditions one or two might be consistent with malingering.

CT scans (high resolution fine cuts of temporal bones) are essential for diagnosis of superior canal dehiscence syndrome but not useful for diagnosis of other disorders. MRI is the gold standard test for diagnosis of acoustic neuroma, multiple sclerosis, cerebrovascular infarct or hemorrhage, intracranial tumor, and cerebellar or brain stem degeneration. Other peripheral vestibular disorders are not diagnosed with imaging technologies.

17. **Can alternative medicine strategies decrease the symptoms of vestibular disorders?**
Common alternative medicine strategies used by people with vertigo and balance problems are pressure points with wrist bands, acupuncture, massage, yoga, taking extra vitamins, and, less commonly, hypnosis. Many people eat peppermint candies, take ginko biloba, eat ginger cookies, or drink herbal teas to decrease nausea. Some patients try chiropractic manipulations. No evidence supports the use of any of these interventions. Limited evidence, however, suggests that using high potency ginger extract is more likely to ensure an effective treatment. This type of treatment may be useful with patients for whom standard antiemetic medications are contraindicated, such as pregnant woman and some cancer patients.

Dietary modification has been proven to be beneficial for patients with Ménière's disease, as a low-sodium diet may reduce the frequency and intensity of Ménière's attacks. Migraine trigger diet elimination may benefit patients with vestibular migraine. Dietary modification has not been shown to be useful for treating other vestibular disorders.

18. **Does diet affect vestibular disorders?**
For patients with Ménière's disease use of a low-sodium diet may be therapeutic to reduce the buildup and fluctuating levels of endolymph that putatively causes Ménière's disease. Patients should be counseled not to add salt to their food and to avoid high-salt prepared foods. No evidence supports the use of dietary restrictions for any other vestibular disorders. Migraine and hence vestibular migraine is often associated with dietary triggers that are specific to the individual. Dietary management would include elimination of foods or chemical additives associated with precipitation of migraine. Typical dietary management of migraine includes eliminating food additives (MSG, aspartame sweeteners), tyramine foods (red wine, beer, avocados, aged cheese, soy-based foods, processed meats, nuts, chocolate), and tannin foods (coffee, tea, chocolate, red wine, apple juice).

19. **Do patients with vertigo and balance disorders have mental health problems?**
Having vertigo and/or a balance problem can produce some anxiety in even well-adjusted individuals due to the sense of being out of control of the body and not well grounded with reference to gravity. This kind of problem is relatively common. Particular situations where visual acuity is reduced can be problematic such as driving in rain, snow, or fog. Some patients feel uncomfortable in open areas without useful visual verticals or in areas with real or virtual visual motion such as large screen theaters or moving escalators. In some cases patients are so distressed that the anxiety prevents them from functioning. Depersonalization and derealization symptoms have been seen in significantly greater rates in patients with vestibular disorders than in the controls.

Counseling by a licensed mental health care provider, such as a masters- or PhD-level psychologist, can be beneficial in reducing the anxiety caused by having the symptoms of vestibular disorders. Therefore, particularly anxious patients should be referred for counseling. Focused behavioral therapy, in particular, has been shown to be effective.

20. **Can mental health problems cause dizziness?**
Anxiety, in particular, can cause psychogenic dizziness, but rarely causes true vertigo (the sensation of self-motion). These patients may appear normal on objective diagnostic tests but may

describe lightheadedness when asked to hyperventilate. If given some time during the initial visit the patient may express anxiety about a particular life event or about life issues in general. The patient might express concern about health problems or may describe the occurrence of specific stressors. Anxiety disorders commonly present with chronic continuous dizziness and patients may not appreciate the relationship of dizziness and anxiety symptoms. Anxiety patients may describe their symptoms as an out-of-body experience, floating, or an internal spinning sensation without visualizing the environment spinning. These psychophysiologic symptoms represent a combination of psychiatric and physiologic factors. Some patients, particularly patients with migraine, are chronically sensitive to motion (self and surround). Anxiety disorders may last for days and may be precipitated by stress, complex visual motion (large screen theater), and con fining spaces with large crowd movement. Anxiety-related dizziness is best managed by standard anxiety therapy.

Stress has been shown, in several objective studies, to exacerbate vertigo. Therefore, take the patient seriously when she or he describes having stress. A mild vestibular impairment may be present but the effects may be magnified by the stress, either in the patient's personal/family life or in the patient's professional/work life. Therefore psychogenic dizziness may be one component of a more complex picture.

Psychogenic dizziness may be situational, i.e., related to specific events or places, such as having an MRI if the individual is claustrophobic, going to the workplace when the patient is having some problems with coworkers, going to court during divorce proceedings, or being in crowds if the individual has posttraumatic stress disorder.

The clinical picture in these patients includes short-term, variable episodes of dizziness, with or without true vertigo, shortness of breath or a sense of "blacking out," sudden vasovagal signs when the individual is sitting still and not moving his head, paresthesias, or symptoms that become worse in the presence of the spouse or significant other.

These patients should be treated for the vestibular disorder, if one is present. They may benefit from sensible advice and information about the nature of the vestibular disorder and the possible relationship of dizziness to stress or anxiety. They may benefit from meeting with a qualified mental health professional for counseling with cognitive behavioral therapy or other forms of psychotherapy as appropriate to the patient's mental health problem. The same patients may benefit from judicious use of medications, but beware of the side effects of medications, including dizziness! They may also benefit from working with an occupational therapist on redesigning or modifying the patient's lifestyle to reduce stressors.

21. **What are the guidelines to determine if a patient should not operate heavy equipment, drive a car, or pilot a boat, aircraft, or spacecraft?**
   The Physician's Guide to Assessing and Counseling Older Drivers, 2nd edition (American Medical Association and National Highway Transportation Safety Administration, 2010) states that physicians should screen for red flags such as medication use, ask about new-onset impaired driving behaviors, assess driving-related functional skills, treat underlying causes of functional decline, refer patients who require driving evaluation or specialized training to a certified driver rehabilitation specialist, counsel patients about safe driving, and follow up to see if patients have followed through on recommendations.

   Patients with vertigo do not necessarily have to avoid driving. In general people with vertigo have no greater rate of accidents than the rest of the population, probably because many of them limit their driving out of caution. A patient who has acute vertigo should be counseled not to drive or fly an airplane. A patient who is in remission or whose vertigo has ceased or is under control should be advised not to drive if vertigo recurs. Patients should also be counseled to avoid or limit driving under conditions of reduced visibility, such as darkness, rain, fog, sleet, or snow, and under conditions of reduced road safety such as ice, snow, or a light rain that may cause hydroplaning. Patients who must drive for long distances should be counseled to take frequent breaks in case of vertigo and to pull off the road immediately in case of an attack of vertigo.

   Patients who take centrally acting medications, like antiemetics, antihistamines, or benzodiazepines, should be counseled to avoid driving after taking these medications. In general five half-lives are required to eliminate active metabolites. Red flags for the physician include acute and chronic medical conditions that affect motor or sensory function, sensorimotor integration, or cognitive function (decision-making, spatial navigation). Such conditions include CVA, seizure, vertigo, arrhythmia, syncope, sleep disorders, dementia, some psychiatric disorders in which the patient may be a danger to himself or others, chronic renal failure, severe respiratory disease requiring oxygen, and some cancers that require treatment with chemotherapy.

If you advise a patient not to drive or not to operate other vehicles, then you should determine if the patient has alternate forms of transportation, such as a bus service for disabled people. If the patient lives in a region with inadequate public transportation then he or she may choose to drive a vehicle regardless of the physician's advice because the patient has no other way to run errands, make clinic visits, and perform other essential activities outside of the home. In that case, referral to social services may assist the patient in finding other resources for transportation. Individuals with concern about their condition who still drive may want to use vehicle safety enhancement technologies, which include collision avoidance braking, night vision displays, and lane change warning. One caution to potentially vestibular impaired drivers is to have them take a clinic or office equivalent of a field sobriety test, which has components of vestibular assessment, including ocular stability, gait, balance, and coordination. If they could not pass the test then a routine police road stop could generate a driving under the influence (DUI) or driving while impaired (DWI) citation.

Individuals who must maintain especially good alertness and good spatial orientation, such as pilots and professional drivers, should be reassessed before being released to drive. If the physician needs evidence that a patient is, or is not, safe to drive, assessment by a certified driving rehabilitation specialist (CDRS), most of whom are occupational therapists, may be indicated. To find a CDRS see the website for the Association of Driver Rehabilitation Specialists (www.aded.net).

Similar concerns affect the physician's assessment for operating heavy machinery, flying airplanes and spacecraft, climbing ladders, and handling potentially dangerous equipment and materials. Some simple guidelines can be considered. For example, a patient with active benign paroxysmal positional vertigo should not climb a ladder or perform other tasks that require looking upward or downward, until the BPPV has resolved. Patients with vertigo and disequilibrium should not be required to run, jump, move around the environment quickly, walk on unstable surfaces, or perform tasks that may disorient them. Pilots should avoid flying if they are prone to vertigo, especially if the episodes are recurrent, unpredictable, incapacitating, or impede performance of any pilot duties. Generally such individuals would have an FAA Aviation Medical Examiner physical and specialty evaluation.

KEY POINTS: NEURO-OTOLOGY

1. The vestibular system detects head movement and uses that information to control the VOR and to contribute to optokinetic responses, spatial orientation, postural control, and vasovagal responses.
2. Acute and chronic disorders of the vestibular system are characterized by disturbances in the behaviors mediated by the vestibular system, e.g., blurred vision, vertigo, impaired balance, nausea, and temporary changes in cardiovascular measures.
3. Standard objective tests of the vestibular system assess the VOR, other eye movements, and postural responses. Screening tests assess the VOR, vertigo, and balance.
4. Most vestibular disorders can be treated. Some disorders are best treated with exercise and other aspects of rehabilitation; other disorders are best treated with medication and/or surgery.
5. The effects of vestibular disorders can be somewhat disabling and may affect safety. The physician should carefully consider whether the individual patient is safe to drive, fly, or operate heavy machinery.

WEBSITES

www.vestibular.org
www.baranysociety.nl
www.nidcd.nih.gov
www.entnet.org
www.texasneurologist.org
www.lesvertiges.com
www.aded.net

References available online at expertconsult.com.

BIBLIOGRAPHY

1. Baloh RW, Kerber KA: Baloh and Honrubia's Clinical Neurophysiology of the Vestibular System, 4th ed. Oxford, Oxford University Press, 2011.
2. Bisdorff A, von Brevern M, Lempert T, Newman-Toker DE: Classification of vestibular symptoms: towards an international classification of vestibular disorders. J Vestib Res 19(1-2):1-13, 2009.
3. Bronstein A: Oxford Textbook of Vertigo and Imbalance. Oxford, Oxford University Press, 2013.
4. Committee on Hearing and Equilibrium Guidelines for the Diagnosis and Evaluation of Therapy in Meniere's Disease. American Academy of Otolaryngology-Head and Neck Foundation, Inc. *Otolaryngol Head Neck Surg* 113(3):181-185, 1995.
5. Goldberg JM, Wilson VM, Cullen KE, et al.: The Vestibular System: A Sixth Sense. Oxford, Oxford University Press, 2012.
6. Guide for Determining Driver Limitation Texas Medical Advisory Board, Texas Department of State Health Services, EMS Certification and Licensing, 2014.
7. Physician's Guide to Assessing and Counseling Older Drivers, 2nd ed. American Medical Association and US Department of Transportation/National Highway Traffic Safety Administration, 2010.

1. **What is believed to be the source of the electrical activity recorded by scalp electrodes in the electroencephalogram (EEG)?**
   The best available evidence indicates that surface-recorded and scalp-recorded electrical activity results from extracellular current flow associated with summation of excitatory postsynaptic potentials and inhibitory postsynaptic potentials.

2. **What are the different frequencies recorded from the scalp EEG?**
   Four frequency bands are recorded: delta, ≤4 Hz; theta, 4 to 7 Hz; alpha, 8 to 13 Hz; and beta, ≥13 Hz.

3. **What are the features of an EEG in an awake, normal adult?**
   The EEG reveals a dominant rhythm in the occipital leads bilaterally. The frequency of this rhythm in most adult individuals is between 9 and 11 Hz. This rhythm is variously referred to as the *occipital dominant rhythm*, the *occipital dominant alpha rhythm*, or simply the *alpha rhythm*. The occipital dominant rhythm is best seen when the individual has his or her eyes closed and is relaxed. This rhythm usually attenuates when the eyes are opened. In the anterior regions, alpha frequency activity is also present but is lower in voltage and generally less continuous than that in the posterior regions. There is also low-voltage 18- to 22-Hz activity present in the anterior leads (Fig. 31-1).

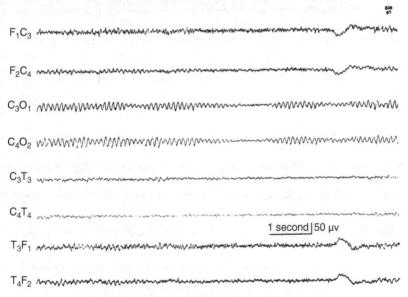

Figure 31-1. Normal waking electroencephalogram (EEG) in an adult.

4. **What are the EEG features of the various sleep stages in the adult?**

NONRAPID EYE MOVEMENT (NREM) SLEEP

Stage 1: The first change in the EEG as an individual becomes drowsy is the disappearance of the occipital dominant alpha rhythm, followed by increasing amounts of theta frequency activity in all regions. During stage 1, diphasic sharp waves also appear in the EEG, occurring maximally at the vertex. These sharp waves are referred to as *vertex transients* (Fig. 31-2, *A*).

Stage 2: The onset of stage 2 NREM sleep is characterized by the appearance of sleep spindles. Sleep spindles consist of bursts of 12- to 14-Hz activity, maximally expressed over the central regions of the head. These bursts generally last less than 2 seconds in the adult. The background activity during stage 2 sleep consists of relatively low-voltage, mixed frequency EEG background activity, with delta activity comprising less than 20% of the sleep period (see Fig. 31-2, *B*).

Stage 3: As the patient enters deeper NREM sleep, the amount of delta activity increases in voltage and quantity. During stage 3 NREM sleep, the amount of delta activity comprising the record varies between 20% and 50%. Sleep spindles persist into stage 3 sleep (see Fig. 31-2, *C*).

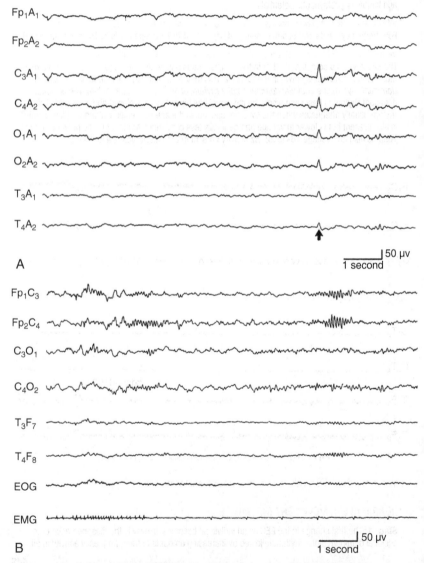

Figure 31-2. A, Stage 1 NREM sleep. Arrow denotes vertex transient. **B,** Stage NREM sleep.

Stage 4: During stage 4 NREM sleep, the amount of delta activity comprises more than 50% of the record. Spindles persist into stage 4 NREM sleep (see Fig. 31-2, *D*).

RAPID EYE MOVEMENT (REM) SLEEP

This state is also referred to as *paradoxical sleep*. The EEG during REM sleep reveals a generally lower voltage record similar in appearance to stage 1. However, in some individuals, runs of alpha frequency activity may appear in the occipital leads identical to the alpha rhythm in the awake tracing. During this stage of sleep, the individual has spontaneous rapid eye movements and tonic motor activity is suppressed (see Fig. 31-2, *E*).

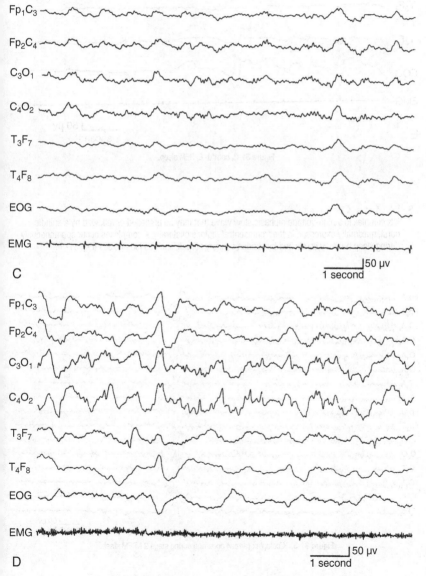

Figure 31-2, cont'd **C,** Stage 3 NREM sleep. **D,** Stage 4 NREM sleep.

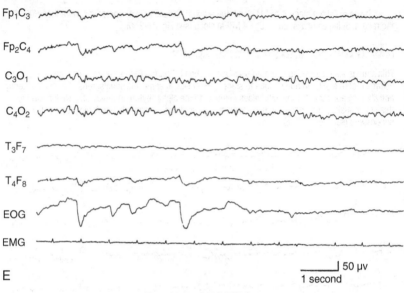

Figure 31-2, cont'd E, REM sleep.

5. What is a K complex?

A K complex is a high-voltage diphasic slow wave that may be preceded or followed by a spindle burst, maximally expressed in the frontocentral regions bilaterally. K complexes occur spontaneously during sleep but may be elicited by sudden sensory stimuli, such as loud noises (Fig. 31-3).

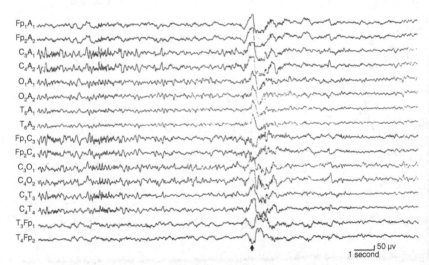

Figure 31-3. K complex (*arrow*) occurring during stage 2 NREM sleep.

6. **What is the *tracé discontinu* pattern?**
   Tracé discontinu refers to the EEG pattern seen in premature infants. When the brain's electrical activity first appears, it is discontinuous, with long periods of quiescence or flattening. Initially, it is present in all states of waking and sleep. In early prematurity (24 to 26 weeks), the periods of flattening may last up to 60 seconds. As age increases, the periods of inactivity shorten, and at 30 weeks' conceptional age, the EEG activity becomes continuous during REM sleep. At about 34 weeks, the EEG activity becomes continuous in the awake state. Continuity appears last in NREM, or quiet sleep, at about 37 to 38 weeks (Fig. 31-4).

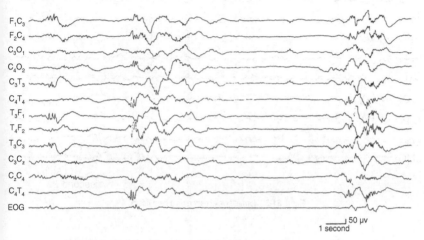

Figure 31-4. *Tracé discontinu* pattern and beta–delta complexes in a premature infant.

7. **What does the EEG show in an awake term infant?**
   The typical awake pattern in a term infant is characterized by a mixture of alpha, beta, theta, and delta frequencies and is often referred to as a *polyfrequency record* or *activité moyenne* (Fig. 31-5).

8. **What is the *tracé alternant* pattern? At what age is it seen?**
   The *tracé alternant* pattern is seen from about 37 to 38 weeks' conceptional age to about 5 to 6 weeks postterm. This pattern occurs during NREM sleep and is characterized by bursts of slow waves mixed with low-voltage sharp activity, separated by episodes of generalized voltage attenuation lasting from 3 to 15 seconds but not absolute quiescence (Fig. 31-6).

9. **What are beta–delta complexes in the premature infant?**
   Beta–delta complexes, also referred to as *brushes*, are considered an EEG hallmark of prematurity. They are characterized by slow waves with bursts of superimposed fast activity (see Fig. 31-6). They first appear in the EEG at about 26 weeks' conceptional age in the central regions, and their abundance reduces with age.

10. **At what age do vertex transients appear in the EEG? At what age are these transients synchronous? At what age are they symmetric?**
    Vertex transients first appear in the EEG at 6 to 8 weeks postterm. They are synchronous and symmetric from the time they first appear.

11. **At what age do sleep spindles first appear in the EEG? At what age are they synchronous? At what age are they symmetric?**
    Like vertex transients, sleep spindles first appear in the EEG at 6 to 8 weeks postterm. From the time they first appear, they are symmetric on the two sides; however, spindle synchrony does not occur until about 12 months of age.

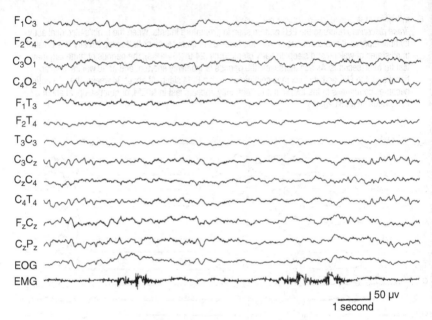

Figure 31-5. Normal awake pattern in a term infant.

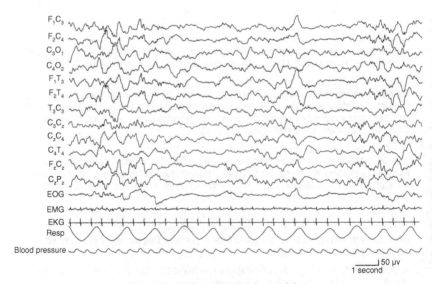

Figure 31-6. *Tracé alternant* pattern in a term infant.

12. At what age does the occipital dominant rhythm first appear? At what age does the occipital dominant rhythm attain a frequency of 8 Hz?

   At approximately 3 months of age, a rhythm that blocks with eye opening and disappears with drowsiness appears in the occipital leads bilaterally. The frequency of this rhythm when it first appears is 3 to 4 Hz. At 1 year of age, the occipital dominant rhythm is approximately 6 Hz. It does not reach 8 Hz until the age of 3 years.

13. What are the differences in the EEG of an awake child or young adolescent compared with an adult?

   - The background activity in the child's EEG is usually higher in voltage.
   - The occipital dominant rhythm in children is mixed, with slower fused waveforms referred to as *slow waves of youth.*
   - There is more theta frequency activity in the anterior leads of a child's EEG (Fig. 31-7).

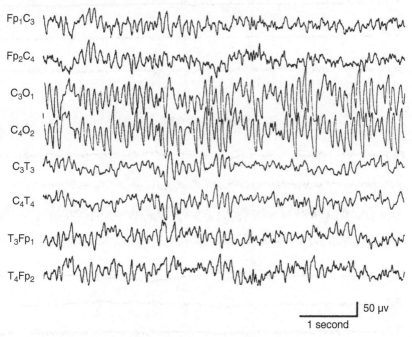

Figure 31-7. Normal waking EEG in a 9-year-old child.

14. What is the mu rhythm?

   The mu rhythm is a normal central rhythm of alpha-activity frequency, usually in the range of 8 to 10 Hz, that occurs during wakefulness. This rhythm is detectable in about 20% of young adults but is less common in older individuals and children. The mu rhythm is blocked or attenuated by movement or thought of movement of the contralateral extremity (Fig. 31-8).

15. What is a breach rhythm?

   A breach rhythm typically refers to a high-voltage, sharply contoured rhythm appearing over an area of a skull defect. It is important to realize that this is an accentuated normal rhythm and should not be reported as a focal abnormality (Fig. 31-9).

16. What is the most common finding in pseudotumor cerebri?

   Although there may be a variety of nonspecific findings in patients with pseudotumor cerebri, the EEG is usually normal.

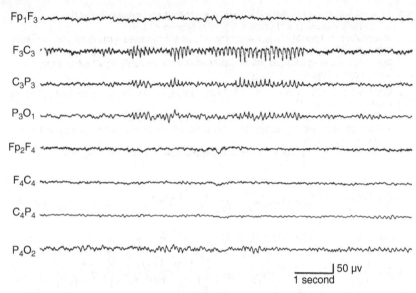

Figure 31-8. Mu rhythm.

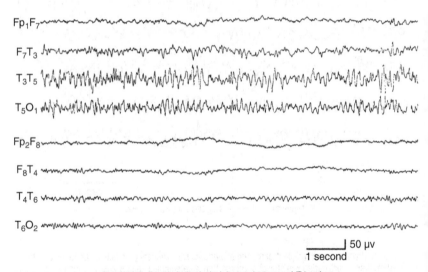

Figure 31-9. Breach rhythm in the left posterior temporal (T$_5$) region.

17. If you were recording the EEG at the time a patient experienced a middle cerebral artery infarction, what would be the sequence of EEG changes you would expect to see?

The initial change following an ischemic episode is depression of the background rhythms over the ipsilateral hemisphere, followed by the appearance of continuous polymorphic slow activity over this hemisphere, maximally expressed in the temporofrontal region (Fig. 31-10).

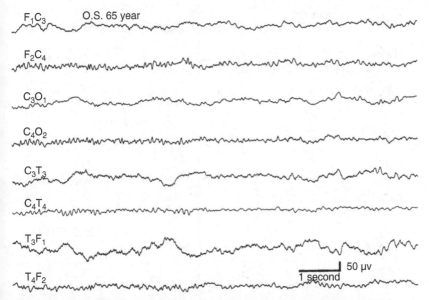

Figure 31-10. EEG of a patient with a left middle cerebral artery infarction. Note depression of activity over the left hemispheric leads and left temporal slowing.

18. **An EEG is obtained 3 years after a person has experienced a hemispheric infarction. What EEG findings may be seen in this patient?**
As in the acute state, the EEG recorded years after a hemispheric infarction may continue to show depression of background activity over the ipsilateral hemisphere. Focal slow-wave activity may also continue ipsilaterally. However, the focal slow-wave activity is not as continuous as it is in the acute state. The patient may continue to show depression of the occipital dominant rhythm on the side of the infarct. However, in many patients, the amplitude of the occipital dominant rhythm returns to normal ipsilaterally, and in some patients, the occipital dominant rhythm becomes enhanced on the side of the infarction (called the *paradoxical enhancement of the alpha rhythm*). A small number of patients may reveal a spike focus ipsilaterally. Finally, a large percentage of patients will show a normal EEG years after a hemispheric infarction.

19. **What are the typical EEG changes seen with a small lacunar infarct?**
Small lacunar infarcts usually produce no change in the background EEG activity; the EEG in such infarcts is usually normal.

20. **What types of EEG findings may be seen with a subdural hematoma?**
Depression of background activity over the ipsilateral hemisphere or focal slow-wave activity over the ipsilateral hemisphere are the findings most frequently seen with a subdural hematoma. Episodic bifrontal slow activity may also occur. However, it is important to remember that the EEG may be normal.

21. **A 6-year-old child presents with headache and ataxia. A posterior fossa tumor is suspected. What EEG findings suggest this diagnosis?**
The most common EEG finding associated with posterior fossa tumors in children is paroxysmal biocipital delta activity (Fig. 31-11).

22. **What is the significance of triphasic waves in the EEG?**
Triphasic waves usually appear in the EEG when there has been diffuse slowing of background rhythms. Although triphasic waves may be seen with a variety of encephalopathies (e.g., infectious, toxic, postanoxic), they most often are associated with metabolic encephalopathies, most commonly hepatic or renal (Fig. 31-12).

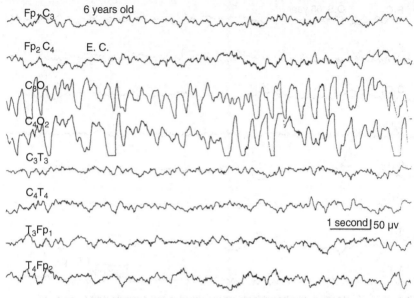

Figure 31-11. Rhythmic occipital slow activity in a child with a posterior fossa tumor.

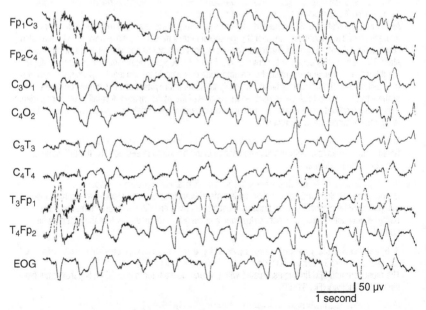

Figure 31-12. EEG in metabolic encephalopathy demonstrating triphasic waves in the frontal regions.

23. **What is the relationship between clinical improvement and EEG improvement in children with various encephalopathies?**
Although in older individuals with various types of encephalopathies, clinical and EEG improvement usually occur simultaneously, in children the clinical status of the patient may improve more rapidly than the EEG.

24. **What is the usual progression of EEG changes in Alzheimer's disease (AD)?**
During the early stages of AD, the EEG may be normal. As the disease progresses, the EEG initially shows slowing of the occipital dominant rhythm, which, in turn, is followed by increasing amounts of theta-frequency activity and then by the appearance of bifrontal and, in some patients, biocciptal delta activity. Occasional sharp waves may appear in the frontal and posterior head regions in severely demented patients; however, these sharp waves never develop the periodic character of the sharp waves seen with Creutzfeldt–Jakob disease. Marked asymmetries of the background activity and focal slow-wave activity are not features of AD. While these findings may be present in those with AD, they are not considered specific to the disorder and may be present in cerebral disorders due to other etiologies.

25. **What are the major differences between the periodic pattern seen with Creutzfeldt–Jakob disease and that seen with subacute sclerosing panencephalitis (SSPE)?**
See Table 31-1 and Fig. 31-13, *A* and *B*.

Table 31-1. Creutzfeldt–Jakob Disease versus Subacute Sclerosing Panencephalitis

	CJD	**SSPE**
Complex morphology	Diphasic or triphasic	Slow waves or groups of slow waves; may have sharp component
Period	Classically, 1 second	4-14 second
Distribution	Generalized, but may begin focally or lateralized to one hemisphere	Usually generalized but maximal in frontocentral leads
Background activity	Diffusely slow when complexes first appear	May be normal when complexes first appear

CJD, Creutzfeldt–Jakob disease; *SSPE*, subacute sclerosing panencephalitis.

26. **What is the EEG pattern associated with Creutzfeldt–Jakob disease and what other disease processes may produce a periodic pattern similar to that seen with Creutzfeldt–Jakob disease?**
The periodic pattern consisting of generalized, high-voltage diphasic and triphasic sharp waves recurring with a period of 1 second is highly suggestive of Creutzfeldt–Jakob disease. However, a pattern indistinguishable from that seen in Creutzfeldt–Jakob disease may occur in the postanoxic state. Also, a similar type of pattern may be seen with lithium intoxication.

27. **What is the significance of periodic lateralizing epileptiform discharges (PLEDs)? What is the most common etiology?**
Periodic lateralizing epileptiform discharges signify the presence of a large destructive lesion involving one hemisphere. They may be seen with a variety of lesions, including tumors, abscesses, hematomas, and herpes simplex virus encephalitis. However, the most common cause of PLEDs is acute cerebral infarction (Fig. 31-14).

28. **What classes of drugs produce increased amounts of voltages of beta activity in the EEG at therapeutic doses?**
The most common classes of drugs that produce increased fast activity in the EEG are the sedatives, anxiolytic agents, central nervous system (CNS) stimulants, and antihistamines. Antidepressants may

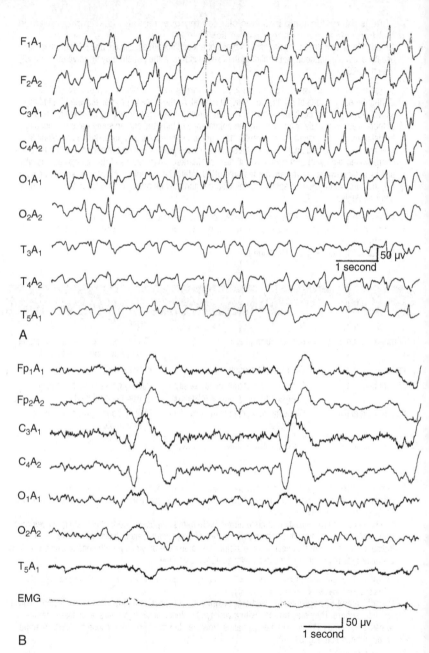

Figure 31-13. A, Periodic pattern in Creutzfeldt–Jakob disease. **B,** Periodic pattern in subacute sclerosing panencephalitis (SSPE).

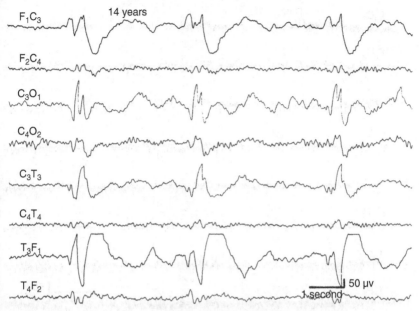

Figure 31-14. Periodic lateralizing epileptiform discharges (PLEDs).

increase the amount of beta activity in the EEG at therapeutic doses but also result in an increase in the amount of theta-frequency activity (Fig. 31-15).

29. **What is hypsarrhythmia?**
    Hypsarrhythmia is the interictal EEG pattern usually seen in infants who experience infantile spasms. The pattern consists of random, high-voltage slow waves mixed with high-voltage, multifocal spike and sharp waves arising from all cortical regions. The triad of infantile spasms, hypsarrhythmia, and mental retardation is often referred to as *West's syndrome* (Fig. 31-16). In assessing EEGs suspected of hypsarrhythmia it is important to consider the voltage calibration of the recording, which will indicate the amplitude of waveforms and allow the designation of high voltage.

30. **What are the characteristics of the three-per-second spike and slow-wave pattern?**
    This pattern is bilateral, symmetric, and usually maximally expressed in the frontocentral regions. In some patients, however, the bursts of three-per-second spike and wave activity may be restricted to or maximally expressed in the occipital regions. The discharges appear and disappear suddenly. The frequency of the spike and wave complexes may vary slightly during the bursts. The first few complexes of the bursts may occur at a frequency of 3.5 to 4.0 Hz, whereas the last few may slow to 2.5 Hz. As soon as the 3-Hz spike and wave bursts stop, the EEG returns to its interictal state immediately with no postictal depression or slowing (Fig. 31-17).

31. **A 10-year-old girl with staring spells is referred for an EEG. What routine activating procedures should be performed on this patient?**
    The common activating procedures usually performed on patients with suspected seizures are hyperventilation, photic stimulation, and sleep. Generalized spike and wave activity may be activated by any of these three activating procedures, whereas focal spikes are usually activated only by sleep.

32. **Which two normal patterns are frequently confused with generalized spike and wave activity in children?**
    The first is hypnagogic hypersynchrony. This pattern appears at 3 to 4 months of age and persists until 10 to 12 years of age. It consists of paroxysmal rhythmic 3- to 5-Hz activity, maximally expressed in

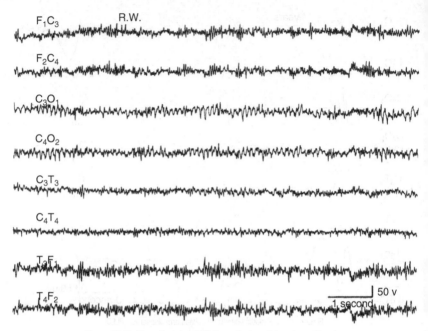

Figure 31-15. Excessive beta activity in a patient receiving a benzodiazepine.

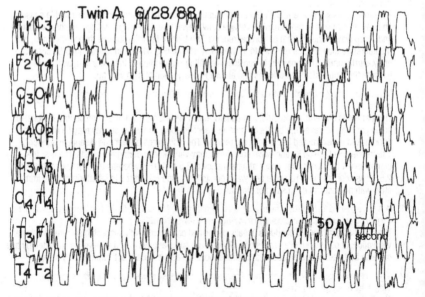

Figure 31-16. Hypsarrhythmia.

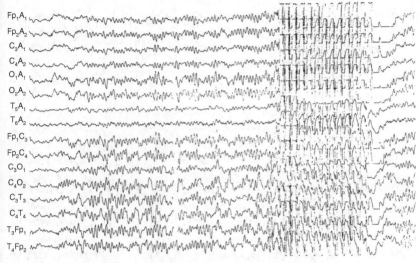

Figure 31-17. Three-hertz spike and wave in a child with absence seizures.

the central and centrofrontal regions. This activity may occur in long runs; however, it may also appear in brief paroxysms. Faster components may be mixed with the paroxysmal slower activity. The second pattern often confused with generalized spike and slow-wave activity is the normal hyperventilation response. Children, particularly between the ages of 5 and 15 years, often show a buildup of high-voltage, frontal-dominant, generalized 3- to 4-Hz activity. This high-voltage, rhythmic slow activity may be continuous or occur in a paroxysmal fashion while the child is deep breathing. This pattern may be easily confused by the novice electroencephalographer with the 3-Hz spike and slow-wave pattern, which may also occur during hyperventilation in children (Fig. 31-18, *A* and *B*).

33. **What are the characteristics of focal epileptiform spikes?**
A spike is an EEG transient with a duration of less than 70 ms. The transient may occur alone, but frequently a slow wave follows, forming a spike and slow-wave complex. The duration of the slow wave may last from 150 to 350 ms. The spike transient may be monophasic or polyphasic. The polarity of most focal epileptiform spikes recorded at the scalp is surface negative. Surface-positive spikes rarely occur in patients with epilepsy (Fig. 31-19).

KEY POINTS: ELECTROENCEPHALOGRAPHY

1. The normal adult EEG, relaxed with eyes closed, is characterized by 9 to 11 cycles per second activity in the back of the brain (occipital lobes) called the *alpha rhythm.*
2. Each stage of sleep has a very characteristic EEG pattern.
3. PLEDs on an EEG imply an acute, large lesion involving one hemisphere, such as a stroke or focal encephalitis.
4. The three-per-second spike and wave pattern on an EEG is usually seen in patients with absence seizures.
5. The finding on an EEG that is most suggestive of focal epilepsy is a very brief (less than 70 ms) transient deflection called a *spike.*

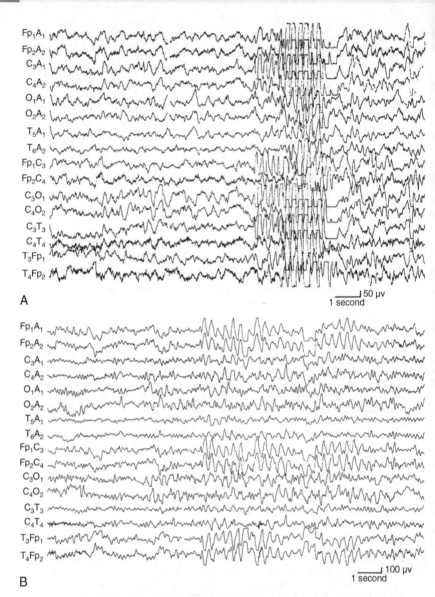

Figure 31-18. A, Hypnagogic hypersynchrony. **B,** Hyperventilation response in a child.

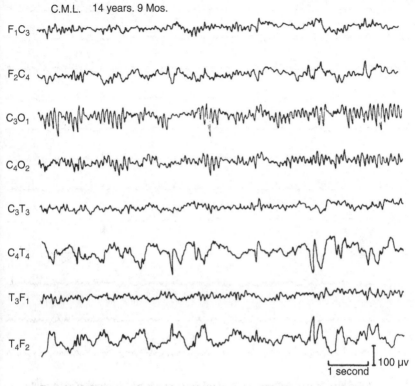

C.M.L.   14 years. 9 Mos.

F_1C_3

F_2C_4

C_3O_1

C_4O_2

C_3T_3

C_4T_4

T_3F_1

T_4F_2

1 second   100 μv

Figure 31-19. Right temporal spikes mixed with slow waves in a child with complex partial seizures.

34. Which three normal EEG patterns may be confused with focal epileptiform spikes in the EEG?
    1. Vertex transients—synchronous diphasic sharp waves that appear at the vertex
    2. Lambda waves—multiphasic spikes that appear in the occipital leads, with eyes open, and are associated with saccadic eye movements when looking at geometric patterns
    3. Positive occipital sharp transients of sleep—positive sharp waves that appear in the occipital leads during NREM sleep (Fig. 31-20, *A* to *C*)

35. What are the typical clinical characteristics of a patient whose EEG shows bursts of generalized 2-Hz spike and slow-wave activity?
    This generalized spike and slow-wave activity is characterized with frequencies ranging from 1 to 2.5 Hz. Those with this pattern have varying degrees of developmental and mental retardation. These patients experience multiple types of seizures, most commonly atonic, tonic, atypical absence, and generalized tonic–clonic. Partial seizures may also occur. These seizures are generally refractory to anti-epileptic drug therapy, are often treated with polytherapy, and have been more amenable to newer anti-epileptic drug and stimulation therapies. This constellation of clinical and EEG features is often referred to as the *Lennox–Gastaut syndrome* (LGS), or *slow-spike and slow-wave syndrome* (Fig. 31-21). An additional EEG feature of LGS is paroxysmal fast activity during sleep, which consists of diffuse, anterior dominant, bilaterally synchronous bursts of 15- to 20-Hz activity, which last for several seconds.

36. What are the usual effects of NREM and REM sleep on interictal generalized or focal epileptiform discharges?
    In general, NREM sleep greatly enhances the frequency of interictal generalized spike and wave or focal spike activity, particularly the first NREM sleep episode of nocturnal sleep. On the other hand, REM sleep is usually associated with a marked attenuation or total abolishment of epileptiform activity.

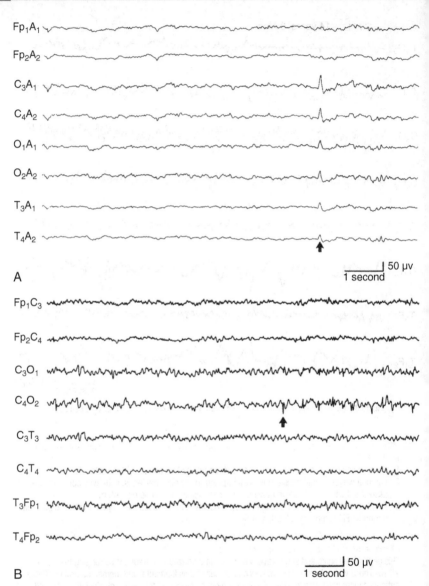

Figure 31-20. A, Stage 1 NREM sleep. Arrow denotes vertex transient. **B,** Lambda waves (*arrow*) in the occipital leads in an individual looking at a geometric design.

37. **What types of EEG changes may be seen postictally?**
   Immediately after a generalized tonic–clonic seizure, there is marked depression of background activity in all regions, followed by an increase in the voltage and frequency of the background activity and a gradual return to the baseline state. Focal slowing may also occur postictally in a patient who has experienced a generalized tonic–clonic seizure. Following a partial seizure, the EEG frequently shows regional or hemispheric depression of the background activity over the ipsilateral hemisphere

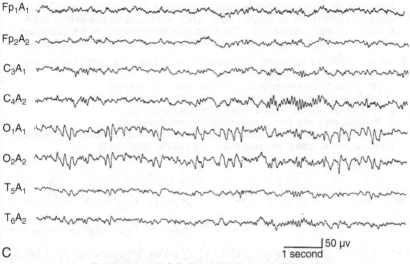

Fp₁A₁
Fp₂A₂
C₃A₁
C₄A₂
O₁A₁
O₂A₂
T₅A₁
T₆A₂

C

⎯⎯⎯⎯⎯ ⏌50 µv
1 second

Figure 31-20, cont'd **C,** Positive occipital sharp transients of sleep.

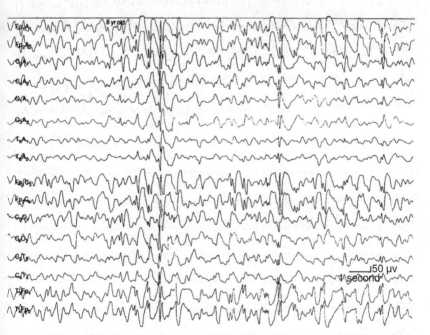

Figure 31-21. Two-hertz spike and slow-wave activity in a patient with Lennox–Gastaut syndrome.

and/or focal slow-wave activity over the ipsilateral hemisphere. The duration that the postictal changes will persist in the EEG is highly variable. In general, the longer the duration of the seizure, the longer the postictal changes persist. This is particularly true in children, who may show diffuse or focal postictal changes for days following a prolonged seizure or an episode of status epilepticus.

38. What four EEG patterns with an epileptiform morphology are classified as patterns of uncertain diagnostic significance?
   1. The 14- and 6-Hz positive bursts (14- and 6-per-second positive spikes)
   2. The rhythmic temporal theta bursts of drowsiness (psychomotor variant pattern)
   3. The 6-Hz spike and wave pattern (phantom spike and wave pattern)
   4. The small, sharp spike pattern (benign epileptiform transients of sleep)

   The 14 and 6-per-second positive burst pattern is a pattern of childhood and adolescence, whereas the remaining three patterns are usually seen in adulthood (Fig. 31-22, A to D).

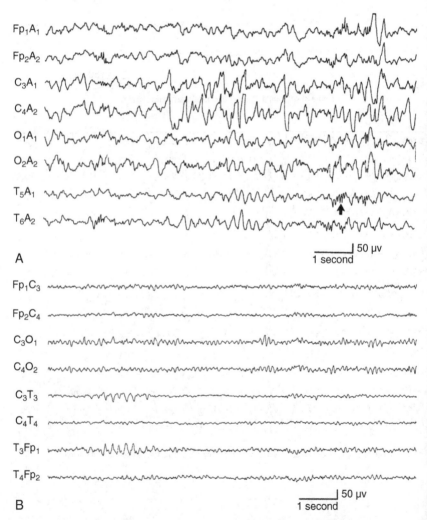

Figure 31-22. A, 14- and 6-per-second positive spike pattern. **B,** Psychomotor variant pattern.

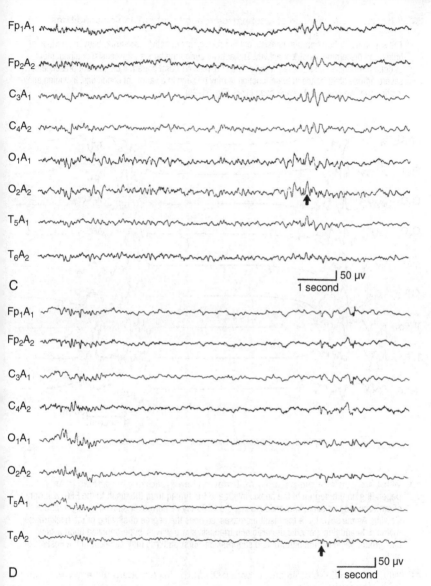

Figure 31-22, cont'd **C,** Phantom spike and wave pattern. **D,** Small sharp spike pattern.

39. What is the significance of a suppression-burst pattern? Which conditions may produce this pattern?

The suppression-burst pattern consists of brief paroxysms of activity occurring between periods of little or no discernible electrical activity. The activity during the bursts may consist of alpha, theta, or delta frequencies and/or sharp waves. The suppression-burst pattern indicates the presence of a severe diffuse disturbance in brain function. It may be seen in a variety of conditions, including anoxic insult, drug overdose, and severe head injury (Fig. 31-23).

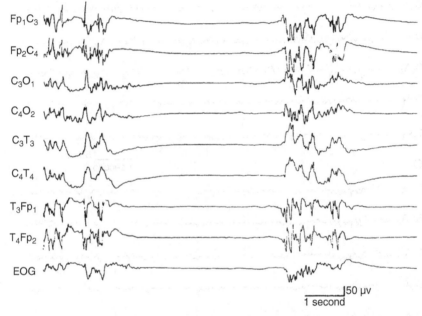

Figure 31-23. Suppression-burst pattern in a comatose patient.

40. What are some of the patterns that may be seen following an anoxic insult?

Depending on the degree of the anoxic insult and the timing from the insult to the EEG, a variety of patterns may be seen. With mild insults, the EEG may be normal or show only slight diffuse slowing. As the severity of the insult increases, so does the degree of slowing of the background rhythms. In addition, periodic diphasic and triphasic sharp waves, superimposed upon a slow background, alpha coma pattern, and suppression-burst patterns may all occur in the postanoxic state.

41. What are the three brain stem coma patterns? Which pattern generally has the best prognosis?

Alpha coma, spindle coma, and theta coma. Of these, spindle coma usually carries the best prognosis (Fig. 31-24, *A* to *C*).

42. What are the major criteria for EEG recording in a case of suspected brain death?
- A minimum of eight scalp electrodes and reference electrodes to cover the major brain areas.
- The interelectrode impedances should be under $10,000\,\Omega$ but over $100\,\Omega$.
- The interelectrode distances should be at least 10 cm, which will enhance amplitudes.
- The sensitivity should be changed from 7 to $2\,\mu V/mm$ during most of the recording with inclusion of appropriate calibrations to distinguish electrocerebral silence from a low-voltage EEG.

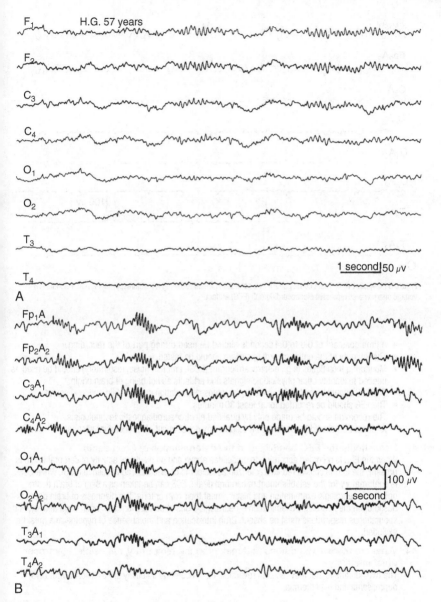

Figure 31-24. A, Alpha coma pattern in a comatose patient following a brain stem infarction. Note alpha-frequency activity in frontal deviations. **B,** Spindle coma pattern in a comatose patient following a midbrain contusion.

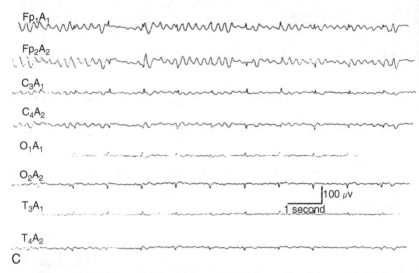

C

Figure 31-24, cont'd C, Theta coma pattern in a comatose patient following a cardiorespiratory arrest. Periodic low-voltage sharp waves represent electrocardiograph (ECG) artifact.

- A time constant of 0.3 to 0.4 seconds should be used during part of the recording.
- The integrity of the entire recording system should be tested.
- Monitoring techniques (e.g., electrocardiogram [ECG], ambient noise, respiratory) should be used as needed to identify other physiologic signals and artifacts as not being of brain origin.
- The EEG should be tested for reactivity by intense stimulation such as pain and loud sound.
- The EEG should be recorded for at least 30 minutes.
- The recording should be made only by qualified electroneurodiagnostic technologists.
- A repeat EEG should be performed if there is any doubt about electrocerebral silence.

43. **How should the EEG be utilized in the determination of brain death?**
    When the EEG is recorded according to guidelines above and no electrical activity of cerebral origin is present, the EEG is considered characterized as isolectric or electrocerebral silence (ECS). While ECS is confirmatory for the establishment of cerebral death, ECS can be taken as a sign of brain death only if the neurologic examination and history meet their own criteria. The diagnosis of brain death is based upon the neurologic examination—neurologic signs of cortical function, brain stem activity, and spontaneous respirations must be absent. Drug intoxication and the absence of hypothermia must be excluded.

44. **What are the two conditions that may produce temporary, reversible, electrocerebral inactivity?**
    The two conditions that may result in reversible electrocerebral inactivity are overdoses with CNS depressants and hypothermia.

 References available online at expertconsult.com.

BIBLIOGRAPHY

1. Blume WT, Holloway GM, Kaibara M, Young GB: Blume's Atlas of Pediatric and Adult Electroencephalopathy, Philadelphia, Wolthers Kluwer Health/Lippincott Williams & Wilkins, 2011.
2. Ebersole JS (ed): Current Practice of Clinical Electroencephalography, 4th ed. Philadelphia, Wolters Kluwer Health, 2007.
3. Fisch B (ed): Fisch and Spehlman's EEG Primer: Basic Principles of Digital and Analog EEG, New York, Elsevier, 2006.
4. Hrachovy RA: Development of the normal electroencephalogram. In Levin KH, Lüders HO (eds): Comprehensive Clinical Neurophysiology, Philadelphia, Saunders, 2000, pp 387-413.
5. Schomer DL, Lopes da Silva L (eds): Neidermeyer's Electroencephalography: Basic Principles, Clinical Application, and Related Fields, 6th ed. Philadelphia, Wolters Kluwer Health/Lippincott Williams & Wilkins, 2011.

CHAPTER 32

ELECTROMYOGRAPHY

James M. Killian

1. **What is an electromyogram (EMG)? How is it recorded?**
   An EMG is an electrical recording of resting and voluntary muscle activity transmitted from a needle electrode through a preamplifier and amplifier to a loudspeaker and digital visual display. When an EMG is ordered as part of the overall electrodiagnostic examination, motor and sensory nerve conduction studies are included with the needle recording.

2. **What are the clinical indications for ordering an EMG?**
   An EMG is usually ordered to determine the localization and severity of neurogenic disorders and to differentiate them from myogenic disorders. Focal neurogenic lesions are localized using the same logic used in the clinical muscle examination, but important subclinical information can be determined, especially in muscles with variable weakness. Myogenic disorders are separated into inflammatory (myositis) and noninflammatory (myopathy).

3. **What are the characteristics of normal voluntary motor unit potentials?**
   Normal voluntary muscle potentials appear as waveforms with a duration of 5 to 15 ms, two to four phases, and amplitudes of 0.5 to 3 mV (depending on the location and size of the muscle).

4. **What are polyphasic units? When are they seen on EMG?**
   Polyphasic units are voluntary motor units with more than four phases. They are seen in both myogenic and neurogenic disorders.

5. **What are the characteristics of abnormal voluntary motor unit potentials?**
   Abnormal motor unit potentials are classified as either neurogenic or myogenic. Neurogenic motor units appear of longer duration and higher amplitude than normal potentials and are usually polyphasic. Myopathic potentials are just the opposite, with shorter durations and smaller amplitudes than normal potentials. They are also usually polyphasic.

6. **What are the EMG characteristics of fasciculation potentials?**
   A fasciculation is an involuntary firing of a single motor neuron and all its innervated muscle fibers. It is displayed by EMG as a single motor unit and, if close to the surface, is visible as a brief irregular undulation of muscle.

7. **What is the significance of fasciculations? When are they nonpathologic?**
   Fasciculations may be associated with pathology in the anterior horn cells, motor roots, or the cramp-fasciculation syndrome. However, fasciculations may be present with no evidence of any nerve or muscle disease and then are termed *benign fasciculations*.

8. **What are the EMG characteristics of fibrillation potentials?**
   Fibrillations are involuntary contractions of single muscle fibers and cannot be seen through the skin. Electrically, they appear as regular or irregular, short, small action potentials that sound like static or cooking bacon. Fibrillations are always abnormal and indicate loss of innervation of a single muscle fiber from a variety of causes.

9. **What is the importance of insertional activity?**
   Insertional activity is the discharge of single muscle fibers during insertion of an EMG needle and does not indicate abnormality. The discharges look like fibrillations on the EMG. Increased insertional activity is the brief continuation of these discharges after needle movement stops. This finding may indicate irritable muscle fibers, such as in early denervation, but it is often nonspecific.

10. **What are positive sharp waves?**
    Positive sharp waves are spontaneous discharges from groups of denervated muscle fibers. They are larger than fibrillation potentials but have the same pathologic implication (i.e., denervation). They appear on the EMG screen as downward monophasic wave formations that indicate a positive polarity—hence the name.

11. **What electrical activity can be measured from the endplate?**
High-frequency, short-duration potentials can be seen when the EMG needle is close to or in the motor endplate. They are called either *endplate activity* or *endplate noise*. This activity is not pathologic but may be confused with fibrillation potentials.

12. **What are the two types of myotonia? Describe their appearance on an EMG.**
Myotonia refers to a delayed relaxation of muscle after contraction or needle insertion. The two types of myotonia are true and pseudo. True myotonia occurs in the myotonic dystrophies and myotonia congenita and is seen as rapid firing muscle action potentials that vary in amplitude ('dive bombers'). Pseudomyotonia has a more stable firing frequency that resembles an airplane in steady flight, with abrupt termination. Pseudomyotonia occurs in both muscle and nerve disorders, including myositis, glycogen storage diseases, hyperkalemic periodic paralysis, root disease, and anterior horn cell disorders.

13. **What is meant by the term *myokymia*?**
Clinical myokymia is observed as irregular undulation of focal superficial layers of muscle, which represents underlying involuntary irregular contraction of groups of muscle fibers. This usually is a result of chronic proximal root abnormalities but also can be seen in focal nerve or muscle lesions and under certain circumstances is not associated with any pathology (orbicularis oculi myokymia).

14. **What are three types of electrical myokymia noted by EMG sampling?**
   - Groups of involuntary motor discharges (doublets or triplets)
   - Continuous discharges of motor units in a steady unchanging frequency ("marching soldiers") often called continuous repetitive discharges
   - High-frequency continuous runs of short motor units ("racecars") called *neuromyotonia*. These are associated with muscle cramping and pain in the extremities and can be either focal or generalized and considered of autoimmune ion origin called *Isaacs' syndrome*.

15. **What are the EMG characteristics recorded in a myopathy?**
In myopathy, the individual motor unit potentials are smaller and shorter because of a reduction in the size of the muscle fibers. The discharging motor unit firing rate is unchanged; therefore, a full pattern of muscle activity on effort ("interference pattern") is still seen on the EMG screen.

16. **What are the EMG characteristics of activity recorded from a denervated muscle?**
Fibrillations and positive sharp waves begin in resting muscles 7 to 14 days after the onset of axonal denervation. When partially denervated muscle is voluntarily contracted, clinical weakness from axonal transmission loss is seen on the EMG as a reduction in motor unit firing patterns proportional to the amount of axonal dysfunction.

17. **How soon do electrical changes develop after a nerve is transected?**
Transection of a nerve is followed immediately by loss of voluntary activity; therefore, no electrical motor units are seen with attempted contraction. Spontaneous abnormal EMG activity consisting of fibrillation and positive sharp waves begins 7 to 10 days later and reaches maximum level at about 14 to 21 days.

18. **After nerve transection, what happens to nerve conduction in the distal segment?**
Nerve conduction in the distal segment is retained for up to 3 days after proximal transection of the nerve, but conduction is immediately lost across the transected nerve. Wallerian degeneration of the affected axons rapidly interferes with nerve conduction, and after 3 to 5 days all conductibility is lost.

19. **How do recruitment patterns differ in normal muscles, myopathies, and neurogenic disorders?**
The pattern of motor activity on effort does not differ between normal muscles and those with myopathic abnormalities because all motor units are intact and fire normally. However, neurogenic abnormalities result in a dropout of motor units, which reduces the recruitment pattern according to the severity of axonal loss. In severe cases, the pattern on effort consists of only two to three units firing at rates of >25/s.

20. **What are the clinical indications for ordering nerve conduction velocities (NCV)?**
NCV are ordered to demonstrate either presence or absence of focal lesion or generalized abnormalities of the peripheral motor and sensory nerves, to assess the severity of peripheral nerve abnormalities, and to determine whether the nerve pathology is axonal or demyelinating.

21. What is the normal NCV?

    Normal motor NCV in the arm is above 50 m/s and in the leg above 42 m/s. Distal latencies vary with the nerve studied as do sensory nerve conduction measurements.

22. What is a normal compound motor action potential (CMAP)?

    A CMAP is the muscle contraction resulting from stimulation of a motor nerve and is a measure of the functioning motor axons in that nerve. The amplitude varies with the muscle that is stimulated. In the hand it is above 6 mV, and in the foot it is above 1 mV.

23. What is a normal sensory nerve action potential (SNAP)?

    A SNAP measures the compound surface potentials from skin electrodes over the conducting sensory axons after nerve stimulation. Proximal velocities are similar to motor conduction in the arms (50 m/s) but slower than motor conduction in the legs (35 m/s). The SNAP amplitude depends on the size of the nerve (numbers of axons) studied, but it may range from 10 to 100 µV, which is small compared with the amplitude of CMAPs in millivolt.

24. What is the H reflex? How is it used clinically?

    The H reflex is the electrical counterpart of the ankle jerk; it gives clinical information about any pathology in the S1 afferent–efferent reflex arc. Submaximal stimulation of the proximal tibial nerve is transmitted afferently to the spinal nerve, eliciting an efferent motor nerve discharge to the gastrocnemius muscle. The H reflex may be either prolonged or absent in neuropathies, S1 radiculopathies, or sciatic mononeuropathies. The H reflex in the arm can also be measured in the median nerve.

25. What is the F wave? How is it useful clinically?

    After motor nerve stimulation, the F wave is seen as a late motor action potential that follows the initial compound muscles' action potential (M wave). Retrograde (antidromic) transmission of stimulated motor axons causes a discharge of the motor neurons in the spinal cord, resulting in a late discharge of the distal muscle. An F wave usually is tested on the median, ulnar, peroneal, and tibial motor nerves. The F wave gives information about abnormal conductibility across both proximal and distal nerve segments and is useful in acute and chronic demyelinating neuropathies.

26. What is repetitive nerve stimulation (RNS)? How is it used clinically?

    RNS measures the motor responses to slow rates of motor nerve stimulation. RNS is used as a diagnostic test for myasthenia gravis (MG) and Lambert–Eaton myasthenic syndrome (LEMS).

27. What does RNS show in a patient with MG?

    About 65% to 85% of patients with MG show an abnormal (>10%) decremental motor response to slow repetitive stimulation of a motor nerve at 2 to 3 Hz. The highest yield is in the proximal muscles, such as the trapezius, when the spinal accessory nerve is stimulated in the neck. The facial nerve may also be tested and has a higher yield in MG, but the results are often technically unsatisfactory because of patient discomfort. Prolonged renal clearing of neuromuscular blockade medications in intensive care patients may result in findings similar to MG.

28. What does RNS show in a patient with LEMS?

    Repetitive stimulation in LEMS shows preexercise low-amplitude compound muscle action potentials in distal muscles because of reduced release of acetylcholine (ACh) at the motor nerve terminal. The muscle potentials will double or triple in size after exercise because of increased release of ACh at the motor nerve terminal (postexercise facilitation). Decremental responses similar to MG often are superimposed on the facilitated motor units. Botulism may show RNS findings similar to LEMS.

29. What is the clinical utility of single-fiber EMG?

    Single-fiber EMG measures the difference in transmission time (jitter) between two individual muscle fiber discharges from the same motor unit. A delay beyond normal, known as *prolonged jitter*, indicates an abnormality in neuromuscular transmission at the motor endplate. Special needles and recording equipment are necessary for the procedure. Single-fiber EMG is used mainly in the diagnosis of early cases of MG, with a sensitivity of 90% to 95%. However, it is a nonspecific measurement and may show abnormal results in motor neuron disease and other neurogenic disorders.

30. Define neurapraxia and conduction block. How do they differ from axonal damage?

    Neurapraxia is a reversible diffuse or focal physiologic nerve lesion or early compressive lesion seen after either trauma or inflammation. If the lesion is focal, motor conduction distal to the lesion is normal but conduction proximal to the lesion is either absent or slowed for up to 4 to 6 weeks. Recovery is the rule because there is no axonal loss, and no actual reinnervation must occur. In contrast, focal axonal lesions require a longer period for recovery because the actual axons have been damaged and have undergone wallerian degeneration. Thus, recovery in axonal damage requires actual reinnervation. Conduction block is a focal lesion of myelin with no axonal pathology. In early stages, conduction block manifests only as a decreased CMAP with proximal stimulation compared with a normal distal CMAP. Motor conduction velocities are normal. Conduction block is often seen in demyelinating neuropathies of various causes. As it progresses to involve more myelin, motor nerve conductions slow significantly.

31. How can the EMG and nerve conduction studies help differentiate a demyelinating peripheral neuropathy from an axonal peripheral neuropathy?
Demyelinating neuropathies show moderate to severe slowing of motor conduction (>20% of normal) with temporal dispersion of the CMAP, normal distal and reduced proximal amplitudes (conduction block), and delayed distal latencies and F waves. Axonal neuropathies show a milder or borderline slowing in conduction velocity, with generally low CMAP amplitudes at both proximal and distal sites of stimulation because of axonal loss. The EMG shows denervation abnormalities early in axonal neuropathies and later in demyelinating neuropathies, when axons begin to degenerate from loss of myelin.

32. What does the EMG show in polymyositis?
Myopathic motor units, fibrillations, and pseudomyotonia are the classic triad of EMG findings in polymyositis.

33. Can inclusion body myositis (IBM) be differentiated from polymyositis by EMG?
Proximal myopathic and myositic abnormalities may be seen in both conditions, but the EMG findings in IBM may show a concentration of focal myositic abnormalities in the forearm flexors and quadriceps muscles. IBM also often shows mixed neurogenic and myopathic motor units in proximal muscles, confusing the diagnosis with conditions such as motor neuron disease.

34. Describe the EMG findings in spastic (upper motor neuron) paresis.
No abnormal findings are noted if the anterior horn cells and roots are normal. EMG patterns on attempted maximum effort are nonspecifically reduced according to the level of spasticity because of a lack of upper motor neuron control.

35. What EMG findings confirm the diagnosis of amyotrophic lateral sclerosis (motor neuron disease)?
The EMG should show widespread proximal and distal denervation with fasciculations and/or giant units in at least two extremities, plus denervation in either the tongue or thoracic paraspinous muscles. Cervical and lumbar spondylosis may show similar abnormalities in the extremities but normal tongue and thoracic paraspinous muscles.

36. What do EMG and nerve conduction studies show in Guillain–Barré syndrome? What is their prognostic utility?
In early Guillain–Barré syndrome, the EMG simply shows reduction in motor unit firing patterns, depending on the degree of paralysis. Motor conduction may be normal with only delayed distal latencies and F waves. After 14 to 21 days, the development of spontaneous denervation activity (fibrillations and positive sharp waves) will evolve in severe cases indicating wallerian degeneration (axonal loss). The EMG is useful prognostically because the presence of axonal loss generally implies longer recovery time. Motor conduction velocities show marked slowing in proximal and distal motor conduction, delayed distal latencies, and other changes of demyelination, beginning 3 to 5 days after onset. Severe slowing may be delayed for 7 to 14 days, limiting early diagnosis. Sensory conduction studies often show normal results, but the earliest sign is loss of H reflexes. Some cases may also show low median SNAP with normal sural SNAP.

37. How is EMG useful in brachial plexus lesions?
The main value of the EMG is in delineating both the presence and degree of denervation in the arm muscles and thus localizing damage to the roots, trunks, cords, or distal branches of the brachial plexus. The amount of axonal damage (fibrillations and positive sharp waves) determines prognosis. When the plexopathy is diffuse, motor and sensory conduction studies in the arm can be severely abnormal but may be relatively spared in many cases.

38. What is the role of EMG and nerve conduction studies in evaluating a patient with a suspected radiculopathy from cervical or lumbar disc disease?

EMG can confirm the root distribution of muscle weakness noted on clinical examination and give information about muscles that were not examined completely because of either pain or lack of full effort. Nerve conduction studies have limited value unless multiple cervical or lumbar roots are chronically affected, but such studies can either identify or exclude other focal peripheral nerve lesions.

39. Describe carpal tunnel syndrome (CTS).

CTS causes nocturnal hand paresthesias from compression of the median nerve at the wrist by thickening of the flexor retinaculum, possibly in conjunction with congenital narrowing of the carpal tunnel or, rarely, in association with other conditions that cause either thickening or pressure on the median nerve.

40. What is the best test for an electrical diagnosis of CTS?

SNAP latencies of the median nerve at the wrist are delayed twice as often as motor latencies. CTS is diagnosed electrically by a delay in sensory conduction latencies from the index finger or midpalmar area to the wrist. The most sensitive is the palmar distal latency. Needle EMG is of limited value but can indicate denervation of the thenar muscles in more advanced cases.

41. What other conditions are associated with median nerve entrapment at the wrist?

The differential diagnosis of CTS includes the following: (1) fluid retention secondary to pregnancy, (2) hypothyroidism, (3) diabetes, (4) amyloid deposits, and (5) hereditary hypertrophic neuropathies (Charcot–Marie–Tooth type 1A and hereditary neuropathy with liability to pressure palsies).

42. How is CTS treated?

Wrist splints at night may be helpful for mild to moderate cases that show mainly sensory abnormalities on nerve conduction studies. More severe, persistent cases require surgical sectioning of the transverse carpal ligament (flexor retinaculum), which should be decompressed from the wrist to the distal margin of the ligament in the upper palm region.

43. What are the most common causes of ulnar nerve entrapment at the elbow (cubital tunnel syndrome)?

External pressure over the flexed nerve in a shallow groove, repeated flexion dislocation of the nerve over the medial epicondyle, and compression of the nerve as it enters the aponeurosis of the flexor digitorum (cubital tunnel syndrome) may cause ulnar nerve lesions at the elbow. Arthritis from an old fracture (tardy ulnar palsy) and rheumatoid arthritis are less common causes. Diabetes with neuropathy often has subclinical focal elbow lesions from postural pressure, especially from wheelchairs.

44. Describe the role of EMG and nerve conduction studies in diagnosing ulnar nerve entrapment at the elbow.

Motor and sensory conduction studies can confirm focal ulnar nerve entrapment at the elbow in 60% to 80% of cases, with the EMG indicating the distribution and degree of denervation in the ulnar-innervated hand and forearm muscles.

45. Which is the best conduction test for diagnosis of ulnar nerve entrapment at the elbow?

Both motor and sensory conduction studies are helpful. The motor conduction across the elbow segment may show the earliest motor delay or conduction block. The proximal elbow amplitude and velocity of ulnar sensory conduction may be affected more than motor slowing. In early cases, studies may be normal.

46. What is the best therapy for ulnar nerve entrapment at the elbow?

Therapy varies according to the underlying mechanism of entrapment. Elbow protectors are helpful for both mild and early moderate pressure lesions, but surgery is indicated for more persistent, severe entrapments. Surgery may involve either sectioning of the flexor digitorum aponeurosis in cubital tunnel syndromes or a medial epicondylectomy in flexion nerve dislocations and tardy ulnar palsies. Translocation of the nerve over the anterior forearm muscles may be necessary in some cases.

47. How is a lesion in the C8 root differentiated from either a plexus or ulnar nerve lesion?

- For a lesion in the C8 root, the EMG should show denervation in either all or some of the following muscles: (1) extensor carpi ulnaris (radial C8), (2) abductor pollicis brevis (median C8T1), (3) first dorsal interosseous, abductor digiti quinti, and flexor carpi ulnaris (ulnar C8), and (4) C8 paraspinous muscles (but not always reliable). Motor and sensory conductions are normal in the ulnar and median nerves unless multiple roots are involved.

- A lesion in the plexus (lower trunk or medial cord) involves denervation in all of the above muscles, except for normal C8 paraspinous muscles. Sensory conduction studies are abnormal in the ulnar and medial antebrachial cutaneous forearm nerves. Motor conduction is normal or minimally slow unless atrophy is severe.
- In ulnar nerve lesions, the EMG is normal in the radial and median-innervated C8 muscles but shows denervation in the ulnar-innervated muscles of the forearm and hand. Motor and sensory ulnar conduction studies also are abnormal, but the medial antebrachial cutaneous nerve is normal.

48. What is the key muscle in differentiating a radial nerve palsy from a C7 radiculopathy?

Flexor carpi radialis is a C7 muscle but is innervated by the median nerve. Thus, an abnormality detected in that muscle indicates a root lesion.

49. How is a radial nerve palsy differentiated from a brachial plexus posterior cord lesion?

Abnormalities in the deltoid muscle (axillary nerve) in addition to radial-innervated muscles indicate a lesion in the posterior cord of the brachial plexus.

50. How is a suprascapular nerve lesion differentiated from a C5–C6 radiculopathy?

Preservation of the deltoid, biceps, and rhomboid muscles, with abnormalities in the supraspinatus and infraspinatus muscles, indicates a suprascapular nerve lesion. A rotator cuff tear will show normal EMG of all the shoulder muscles.

51. Describe the difference between a long thoracic nerve palsy and a C5–C6 radiculopathy.

A long thoracic nerve palsy causes winging of the scapula with the arms outstretched because of weakness of the serratus anterior muscle. However, C5–C6 shoulder and arm muscles (e.g., deltoid, biceps, supraspinatus) will remain normal. The serratus anterior muscle is not routinely studied by EMG. Long thoracic nerve conduction is either slow or nonconductible when performed 3 days after onset.

52. How is a peroneal nerve palsy differentiated from an L4–L5 radiculopathy?

The invertors of the foot (posterior tibial muscle) are abnormal in L4–L5 radiculopathies and spared in peroneal nerve lesions.

53. How does a femoral nerve lesion differ from an L3 radiculopathy?

Abnormalities in the hip adductors in addition to the quadriceps muscles are present in L3 radiculopathies.

54. How does a femoral nerve lesion in the pelvis differ from a lesion at the inguinal level?

Weakness and denervation in the iliopsoas in addition to the quadriceps muscle indicate a femoral nerve lesion in the pelvis.

55. What is the value of motor conduction velocities in Bell's palsy?

Facial nerve conduction studies 3 to 5 days after the onset of Bell's palsy may indicate the prognosis. Normal latencies and amplitudes at 5 days indicate an excellent prognosis for recovery, unless the underlying nerve lesion is still evolving. Loss of nerve conductibility at 3 to 5 days indicates the onset of wallerian degeneration with a prognosis of slow incomplete or nonrecovery. EMG is not of prognostic value until 2 to 3 weeks when signs of spontaneous axonal denervation activity can be seen.

56. Describe the role of EMG and nerve conduction studies in critical care patients who develop neuromuscular weakness.

These studies help to distinguish critical illness polyneuropathy (CIP) from critical illness myopathy (CIM) and prolonged neuromuscular blockade.

57. How does CIP differ from CIM (acute quadriplegic myopathy)?

CIP is an axonal polyneuropathy associated with sepsis. Nerve conduction testing shows abnormal motor and sensory conduction. EMG shows distal denervation, more in the legs than arms. Results of direct muscle stimulation and repetitive nerve stimulation are normal. CIM is a muscle membrane disorder usually seen with use of nondepolarizing blocking agents and corticosteroids. EMG findings are limited by profound weakness. Some cases may show spontaneous fibrillations from fiber necrosis.

Motor nerve conduction studies and direct muscle stimulation are both nonconductible, indicating proximal muscle lesions.

58. **Which tests are used to diagnose neuromuscular blockade in the intensive care unit?**
    Prolonged neuromuscular blockade occurs in patients with abnormal renal function who have been treated with nondepolarizing blocking agents. Repetitive nerve stimulation shows decrement similar to MG and distinguishes these patients from patients with polyneuropathy or myopathy.

59. **Which drugs can cause myopathic EMG changes with chronic use?**
    Myopathic EMG abnormalities can be seen with long-term use of steroids, statin drugs and other cholesterol-lowering agents, chloroquine, amiodarone, and colchicine. The findings are usually mild but indistinguishable from other types of myopathies and are slowly reversible after cessation of the drug.

60. **What is the role of neuromuscular ultrasound as an adjunctive to EMG and nerve conduction studies in nerve and muscle disorders?**
    Neuromuscular ultrasound can complete the EMG diagnosis in motor neuron disease by demonstrating multiple areas of the limbs and tongue with deep muscle fasciculation and atrophic muscle areas not accessible by needle or visual inspection. Primary muscle disease can show hyperechoic muscle changes. Measurement of nerve size circumferences can be important in neuropathies with enlarged nerves such as chronic inflammatory demyelinating polyneuropathy and Charcot–Marie–Tooth type 1A. Focal nerve enlargement can be seen in CTS and ulnar nerve elbow lesions and excludes cysts, masses, and vascular lesions.

KEY POINTS: ELECTROMYOGRAPHY

1. Fasciculations (the involuntary firing of a single motor unit) by themselves are often benign.
2. Myotonia, a delayed relaxation after muscle contraction, is most common in myotonic muscular dystrophies but can be seen in other conditions.
3. Muscle disease on EMG shows full contraction patterns of all muscles but with short small amplitude motor units.
4. Nerve disease on EMG shows a dropout of motor units and reduction in muscle contraction pattern, with prolonged, large amplitude motor units.
5. Patients with myasthenia gravis often show a decremental response to repetitive stimulation in proximal muscles greater than distal muscles.

 References available online at expertconsult.com.

WEBSITE

www.aanem.org

BIBLIOGRAPHY

1. Pease WS, Lew HL, Johnson E: Practical Electromyography, 5th ed. Philadelphia, Lippincott Williams & Wilkins, 2010.
2. Preston DC, Shapiro BF: Electromyography and Neuromuscular Disorders, 3rd ed. Boston, Butterworth-Heinemann, 2013.
3. Stewart JP: Focal Peripheral Neuropathies, 4th ed. Philadelphia, Lippincott Williams and Wilkins, 2010.

CHAPTER 33

NEUROPATHOLOGY

Matthew D. Cykowski

BASIC TERMINOLOGY AND LABORATORY PROCEDURES

1. **What are the two major disciplines in the field of pathology?**
   The two disciplines of pathology are anatomic pathology and clinical pathology. Pathologists commonly use the shorthand "AP" and "CP" to refer to these fields. To become certified by the American Board of Pathology in AP/CP in the United States requires a 4-year residency, whereas standalone AP or CP certifications typically require a 3-year residency.

2. **What does anatomic pathology entail? How does this relate to neurologic and neurosurgical practice?**
   Anatomic pathology deals with the examination of tissues and fluids from patients (living, sometimes deceased) in order to make a diagnosis. Examination may involve microscopic examination of a biopsy specimen from an enhancing brain tumor, examination of a resection specimen from a dural-based mass, or examination of a cytology specimen prepared from the cerebrospinal fluid of a patient with primary central nervous system (CNS) lymphoma or medulloblastoma (looking for leptomeningeal dissemination). Least commonly, but every bit as important, anatomic pathology involves the performance of an autopsy.

3. **What does clinical pathology entail? How does this relate to neurology and neurosurgical practice?**
   Neurologists, surgeons, and other physicians work more often with the clinical pathology laboratory than with the anatomic pathology lab even though they may not be aware of this. Clinical pathology deals with the examinations of patient tissues and fluids (whole blood, serum) to assist clinicians in making a diagnosis. In a hospital, the clinical pathology lab reports routine laboratories such as chemistry panels. Clinical pathologists must oversee the function of blood banks, clinical chemistry and hematopathology laboratories, and clinical microbiology and molecular pathology laboratories, among other divisions.

4. **Where do samples go to when they go "to the lab"?**
   When neurologists send a specimen "to the lab," it is important to know the basic divisions between AP and CP as described above. By knowing this, you will make sure the appropriate individuals are notified if there is an issue in how the specimen should be submitted (for example, a cerebrospinal fluid sample) or if there is an unexpected result.

5. **What is a neuropathologist?**
   Neuropathologists are physicians who have certification in AP, occasionally in CP, and who have undergone two additional years of fellowship training in neuropathology. Typically these individuals have subspecialty certification in neuropathology, as well as certification in AP and even CP. In a hospital-based practice, it is common for neuropathologists to handle AP testing on nervous system tissues, including autopsy, as well as neuromuscular pathology and even ophthalmic pathology.

6. **What is a frozen section?**
   This term refers to the intraoperative consultation performed on unfixed, fresh tissue. Relative to the neurologic patient, this occurs when a neurosurgeon is asked to obtain tissue to facilitate diagnosis when other methods are not specific enough to render an appropriate treatment. At the time of surgery, the neurosurgeon contacts the AP frozen section laboratory and places an order for a frozen section. The neuropathologist is notified and prepares to receive the fresh tissue. Typically, the patient remains under anesthesia so that the frozen section diagnosis can guide surgical treatment as needed (infiltrating versus circumscribed glioma) or rebiopsy can be performed if the tissue is not diagnostic.

7. **What decisions are made during intraoperative consultation/frozen section? What are the goals?**
First and foremost, the goal is not to render a final diagnosis. Instead, the neuropathologist must decide at frozen section how the tissue is to be triaged in consultation with the neurosurgeon. These decisions include whether tissue should be sent sterilely to the microbiology lab, sent fresh to the flow cytometry lab in order to rule out lymphoma or other hematopoietic malignancy, frozen for future molecular and/or research studies, or even placed in glutaraldehyde fixative for electron microscopy. It is crucial to understand that once a piece of tissue is fixed in formalin, it is forever lost to a number of possible studies that require unfixed tissue. This may mean a definitive diagnosis is not possible because the triaging of tissues was inappropriate (this is fortunately rare).

8. **How is an intraoperative consultation actually performed?**
With these triaging issues settled (or at least under way), the pathologist often makes a cytologic preparation, typically by smearing a small piece of tissue on a slide and staining the slide to examine the cellular characteristics of the tissue. A portion of the tissue is then rapidly frozen in a cryostat at about −25° C and thinly sectioned at 5 to 7 μm. This rapidly frozen and sectioned tissue is typically stained with hematoxylin and eosin (H&E) and examined microscopically in the frozen section room by the pathologist. The frozen section process is a caricature of the routine process of fixing, embedding, and staining tissues and as such the quality is never that of permanent sections (see below).

9. **Is the frozen section diagnosis the final diagnosis for a patient?**
Not usually. In conjunction with the cytologic preparation, and with knowledge of the clinical examination and radiologic findings, the pathologist renders a preliminary diagnosis or "frozen section diagnosis." Rarely, this may be a specific and definitive diagnosis (myxopapillary ependymoma or pituitary adenoma). More commonly, this is a diagnostic category (high-grade glioma) or a descriptive diagnosis (reactive gliosis with perivascular lymphocytic and plasmacytic inflammation; no tumor identified).

10. **What happens to the tissues after the frozen section is complete?**
The unfrozen tissue is submitted in formalin, which fixes the tissue. Frozen tissue is thawed to room temperature and also submitted in formalin for routine histologic processing (the artifacts introduced by freezing this tissue will remain in the permanent sections, however). Overnight and the following morning, routine histologic processing is performed and a definitive and final diagnosis is ideally made from this formalin-fixed tissue.

11. **How do pathologists refer to the formalin-fixed, unfrozen tissue they rely on to make a final diagnosis?**
These are called *permanent sections*, or in pathology jargon, *permanents*. Rarely, an intraoperative consultation yields a diagnosis of "lesional tissue present; defer to permanents," which means that any further classification of the lesion requires processing of the formalin-fixed tissue.

12. **Why do results in anatomic pathology take so long to obtain (>24 hours or even days in some cases)?**
It is important to keep in mind that tissues for pathologic analysis are fixed in formalin, sampled and submitted by a pathologist and undergo processing steps on machines that dehydrate the tissues to allow them to be penetrated by paraffin (a wax). The same tissues are embedded in a block, sectioned on a microtome, placed on a slide, and stained with H&E, special stains (e.g., Luxol fast blue for myelin), or immunostains (glial fibrillary acidic protein, or GFAP, to demonstrate glial differentiation in a tumor). The slides of an individual case must then be cover-slipped and ordered together with the relevant requisition forms for delivery to the pathologist, sometimes over multiple iterations if special studies are performed. This process is akin to an assembly line and requires many skilled technical personnel prior to the pathologist even receiving slides that are sufficient to render a final diagnosis.

13. **What are some of the clinical indications for a frozen section?**
Frozen sections are ideally performed if this information would guide the surgical approach or medical treatment. An example would be the differential diagnosis of ependymoma versus diffuse glioma in the spinal cord, with the former being amenable to gross total resection and the latter not. Likewise, if a preliminary diagnosis would immediately impact the treatment strategy (e.g., confirming a suspected diagnosis of pineal region germinoma) or triaging of tissues (for cultures, flow cytometry), intraoperative consultations may be appropriate. However, microscopic examination of formalin-fixed tissues is always preferable to frozen section as fixed tissues have preserved anatomic detail and can be used for special studies. If a frozen section neither guides surgical approach nor immediately

impacts either treatment or triaging of the tissues, it is not indicated and may cause critical diagnostic tissue to be expended in the form of a suboptimal histologic preparation.

14. **What are special stains? What are immunostains?**
Special stains, or "specials," are histochemical stains neuropathologists utilize to identify some specific feature of a tissue. Examples include silver-based stains to identify neurofibrillary tangles, periodic acid–Schiff stains to identify glycogen in various tissue types such as tumor cells, muscle fibers, and basement membrane material in capillaries. Special stains do not rely on an antigen–antibody reaction. In contrast, immunohistochemistry relies on dilutions of polyclonal and monoclonal antibodies (immunostains or "immunos") and their reactions to specific tissue and tumor antigens. The binding of antibodies in tissue is visualized using a secondary antibody reaction. Pathologists use the presence/absence, distribution, and intensity of immunostaining to assist in making a diagnosis (for example, to demonstrate neuronal differentiation in a tumor).

CELLULAR REACTIONS TO INJURY AND VASCULAR NEUROPATHOLOGY

15. **What is lipofuscin? Where in the brain is this commonly identified?**
Lipofuscin is a pigment that accumulates with aging in the normal nervous system. Examples of neurons with prominent lipofuscin pigment include those of the dorsal thalamus, inferior olive, subiculum of the hippocampal formation, lateral geniculate nucleus, motor neurons of both the primary motor cortex and ventral horn of the spinal cord, and dentate nucleus of the cerebellum.

16. **What is central chromatolysis?**
This process takes place when there is axonal damage distal to the neuronal cell body. In central chromatolysis, the nucleus becomes eccentrically placed, the normal, granular, basophilic Nissl substance dissipates, and the cytoplasm becomes distended like a balloon.

17. **What is a cellular inclusion? Name some examples.**
This is a nonspecific term referring to the accumulation of abnormal material in either the nucleus or cytoplasm of a cell, either glial or neuronal, recognized on either H&E or special studies. Important examples include (1) the globular cytoplasmic deposits of alpha-synuclein in the substantia nigra with a surrounding clear halo (*Lewy bodies*), (2) the violaceous intranuclear inclusion of a patient with herpes encephalitis and bilateral hemorrhagic necrosis of the temporal lobes (*Cowdry type A inclusions*), (3) the intranuclear inclusions of a patient with Huntington's disease, a trinucleotide repeat disorder, (4) the eosinophilic, cytoplasmic bodies of a patient with rabies (*Negri bodies*), (5) the eosinophilic, refractile cytoplasmic rods in the pyramidal neurons of the hippocampus in an older patient with Alzheimer's disease (AD) neuropathology (*Hirano bodies*), and (6) the small, round, lightly eosinophilic inclusions in the ventral horn motor neurons of a patient with amyotrophic lateral sclerosis (ALS) (*Bunina bodies*).

18. **What is the significance of a "red" neuron?**
Red neurons (also called *ischemic* or *acidophilic neurons*, *eosinophilic neuronal necrosis*) indicate acute hypoxic/ischemic damage with neuronal death. The "red" in the name refers to the dense staining of eosin in the cytoplasm of these neurons. Simultaneously, the nuclei of these cells shrink in size and their chromatin condenses (these nuclei are said to be "pyknotic"). The nuclei eventually fragment in a process called *karyorrhexis*.

19. **What is dark cell change? Are all dark neurons in a brain specimen indicative of hypoxic/ischemic injury?**
No. "Dark" cell change may be an artifact in brain tissues that are manipulated either during biopsy or shortly after death (at autopsy). Distinguishing dark cell change from red neurons is not always easy. In general, the nuclei of neurons truly undergoing hypoxic injury are shrunken and their chromatin condensed (they appear pyknotic).

20. **What is reactive gliosis?**
This term is nonspecific and indicative of some injury to the nervous system, which may imply a reactive proliferation of astrocytes, oligodendroglia, or even microglia. Typically, however, pathologists use reactive gliosis to imply one of two situations: either *reactive astrocytosis* (increased number of nonneoplastic astrocytes) or *astrogliosis* (increased ramification of astrocytes). Reactive astrocytes are conspicuous on H&E stain as they appear larger than resting astrocytes and have dense eosinophilic cytoplasm and star-shaped astrocytic processes.

21. How does granular ependymitis look microscopically and what does it indicate?

Ventricular spaces in the nervous system are lined by columnar cells with intercellular tight junctions and apical microvilli and cilia. These are the ependymal cells. Whenever there is injury to the ventricular lining due to hydrocephalus, intraventricular hemorrhage, or infections with a predilection for the ventricular lining (e.g., cytomegalovirus), there is loss of ependymal cells. A small nodule of reactive gliosis without overlying ependyma is formed and this is termed *granular ependymitis*. Often seen by the neuropathologist long after the initial insult, the presence of granular ependymitis indicates that the aforementioned mechanisms of ependymal injury must be considered.

22. Where in the nervous system does Bergmann gliosis occur? What does it represent?

Bergmann gliosis is a proliferation of the normal resting Bergmann glia (astrocytes) of the cerebellar cortex. This typically occurs in response to hypoxic injury with loss of ischemia-susceptible Purkinje cells but may also be seen in degenerative diseases that involve the cerebellar cortex with Purkinje cell loss (e.g., multiple system atrophy). This pathologic process is typically apparent on H&E.

23. What normal structures in the aging brain may be mistaken for fungi or even Lafora bodies?

These structures are corpora amylacea, which accumulate in astrocytic processes adjacent to periventricular regions, blood vessels, around the base of the orbitofrontal cortex, and within the olfactory bulb. They represent normal aging in most brains, similar to lipofuscin pigment. Corpora amylacea are basophilic, round structures on H&E stain that may appear to have multiple concentric rings. These structures appear similar to encapsulated fungi or to the polyglucosan bodies that may be see in Lafora disease and type IV glycogen storage disease.

24. What is an infarct?

Infarction occurs when there is frank tissue necrosis and cell death. This may be due to either hypoperfusion (e.g., cardiogenic or septic shock) or vessel occlusion due to an embolic event or thrombus formation (e.g., hypercoagulable state).

25. How long does it take for red neurons to appear following acute hypoxic/ischemic injury?

The best answer is that this estimate varies widely in both the literature and among knowledgeable observers. A safe answer is approximately 6 hours following an ischemic event. In reality, this is not a hard and fast rule and shorter intervals have been reported in autopsy studies.

26. What is the other form of neuronal cell death besides the formation of red neurons? What takes place in this process?

Apoptosis with the formation of apoptotic bodies. This may be seen in ischemic injury (particularly in infant brains where red neurons are rarely formed), infection, and neurodegenerative disease. Similar to red neurons, the nuclear chromatin condenses in apoptotic cells and then fragments (termed karyorrhexis). These nuclear fragments are seen as multiple, small, densely basophilic fragments called *apoptotic bodies*. This process is not unique to neurons that have been injured, since apoptosis with formation of apoptotic bodies is characteristic of some high-grade tumors, including primary CNS lymphoma and small blue cell tumors of childhood such as medulloblastoma and retinoblastoma.

27. How is a subacute infarct differentiated from an acute infarct?

Subacute infarcts demonstrate reactive vascular proliferation, gliosis, and may begin to demonstrate accumulation of macrophages to clear necrotic debris. Axonal retraction balls may also begin to form. The boundaries are not absolute, however, and red neurons may still be present in infarcts that otherwise appear to be subacute.

28. How do infarcts appear macroscopically and how are these separated from hemorrhagic contusions?

The appearance of an infarct may vary greatly by location, age, and whether it has been reperfused. The characteristic appearance, however, is a dusky discoloration of the cerebral cortical ribbon in the depths of cerebral sulci with variable amounts of hemorrhage. Unlike contusions, the pial surface and molecular layer of the cortex are spared (contusions disrupt these layers).

29. **What is a lacunar infarct?**
These are small infarcts that typically involve the basal ganglia, cerebral white matter, and brainstem in patients with a history of hypertension.

30. **What is a "watershed" zone?**
These are brain regions positioned at the periphery of the zones of perfusion for two or more vessels (hence the use of the term *arterial border zones*). Blood flow to these areas is less than other brain regions, which explains their selective vulnerability for hypoxic/ischemic injury. For example, the cerebral convexity in the lateral parietal area is a watershed zone for the anterior and middle cerebral arteries.

31. **What neuronal populations are particularly susceptible to hypoxic/ischemic injury?**
The most notable sites to examine for hypoxic/ischemic injury include sector CA1 of the hippocampus, the Purkinje cell layer of the cerebellar cortex, and the middle laminae of the cerebral cortex. Sector CA2 of the hippocampus, unlike CA1, is particularly resistant to hypoxic injury and is thus referred to as the *dorsal resistant zone*.

32. **What is the end stage of any necrotizing lesion in the brain (infarct, contusion)?**
If the patient survives such an insult, these lesions become cystic cavities with a rim of gliotic brain tissue. Macrophages infiltrate the lesion to remove the necrotic debris and may persist for a long time following the insult. In the case of cerebral infarcts, the necrotic tissue is resorbed, the red neurons are no longer present, and a cavity with a glial scar is all that remains (residual macrophages may be present).

33. **What is the characteristic macroscopic appearance of a venous infarct?**
These infarcts result from dural venous sinus thrombosis and produce hemorrhagic necrosis that is parasagittal, bilateral, and may appear symmetrical. These involve both white matter and cortex of the affected regions. Associated clinical conditions include hypercoagulability, dehydration, and meningitis.

34. **What are the major causes of intraparenchymal hemorrhage?**
These include (1) trauma with massive contusion and laceration of the brain surface, (2) chronic hypertension with small vessel disease (subcortical hemorrhage following rupture of the lenticulostriate arteries), (3) cerebral amyloid angiopathy (typically as cerebral lobar hemorrhage), (4) tumor-associated hemorrhage (most often with melanoma, glioblastoma, and metastases of highly vascular tumors), (5) infectious etiologies (mycotic aneurysms, angioinvasive fungal infections), (6) reperfusion of an infarct, and (7) rupture of a vascular malformation.

35. **Describe the histologic appearance of an arteriovenous malformation (AVM).**
On H&E examination, AVMs comprise thick-walled, aberrant vascular channels with intervening gliotic brain tissue. Some of the large vessels will be arterial, which is demonstrated by the presence of an elastic lamina on H&E stain and special stains that highlight the elastic lamina (e.g., Movat pentachrome or Verhoeff–Van Gieson stains).

36. **What process may be seen in the cortex adjacent to an AVM or any vascular malformation?**
Cortical dysplasia may be present. Dysplasia consists of cortex containing dysmorphic neurons that are abnormally shaped, maloriented, enlarged, and possibly multinucleated, with an atypical columnar/vertical and laminar/horizontal organization of cortex. In any setting, cortical dysplasia may range from very mild to severe and a variety of grading schemes for this pathology have been proposed.

37. **Describe the histologic appearance of cavernous hemangioma (cavernoma)?**
Cavernous hemangioma has *no* intervening brain tissue (at least for the purposes of a board exam!) and consists of venous channels, including thick-walled, muscularized veins without an elastic lamina. These lesions often have a rim of tissue with gliosis and hemosiderin-laden macrophages, the latter giving rise to the famous "ferruginous penumbra" on T2-weighted MRI sequences.

38. **What are the most common locations of hypertensive intraparenchymal hemorrhage?**
Basal ganglia (specifically the putamen), basis pontis/brainstem, and cerebellum.

39. An elderly patient with lobar hemorrhage and cognitive impairment may have what combination of findings? What genetic features predispose to this (in nonfamilial AD)?

In cerebral amyloid angiopathy (CAA), amyloid deposits in the vessel walls of leptomeningeal and cortical capillaries and small arterioles, giving them a rigid appearance often likened to "lead pipes." CAA often goes hand in hand with other AD neuropathology and is a major risk factor for cerebral lobar hemorrhage. When CAA is severe, there may be fibrinoid necrosis of the vessel wall, luminal occlusion, and a foreign body-type giant cell reaction. In contrast to arterioles and capillaries, which are affected by CAA, cerebral veins, venules, and white matter vessels typically are *not* affected. Both CAA and AD neuropathology are significantly associated with the presence of an apolipoprotein E epsilon 4 (ApoE ε4) allele.

40. Which ApoE allele is thought to be protective against cerebral amyloid angiopathy and AD neuropathology?

Apolipoprotein E epsilon 2 (ApoE ε2).

41. What is Wallerian degeneration and how does it look microscopically?

This is a secondary axonal degeneration that follows neuronal death proximally (e.g., infarct, ALS) or following tract/axonal destruction (e.g., in diffuse axonal injury). This appears microscopically as atrophy of the involved white matter structure with accumulation of macrophages. In the case of axonal damage with transection this may induce bulbous swellings of the axon termed *axonal "retraction balls."* It may take 1 week or more for these changes to become apparent on routine microscopy.

TRAUMA AND FORENSIC NEUROPATHOLOGY

42. How does cerebral edema look macroscopically? What herniation syndromes may result from severe edema?

Cerebral edema is characterized by a "heavy" brain (subjectively assessed first by handling the brain at autopsy and then objectively by weighing the brain). There is typically effacement of the normal sulcal spaces. Gyral contours may be flattened as the cerebral hemispheres press up against the skull and on serial sections the ventricular spaces often appear slit-like. If the brain has been formalin fixed, there may be pink discoloration of brain tissue due to the fact that formalin could not easily penetrate into the effaced sulcal spaces. If the edema is severe enough, there may be downward displacement of the cerebellar tonsils into the foramen magnum (tonsillar herniation) and/or of the mesial temporal lobes over the edge of the tentorium cerebelli (uncal herniation).

43. If a patient has a significant ischemic injury in the cerebrum with subsequent cerebral edema and unilateral uncal herniation, they may develop Duret hemorrhages. Who was Duret and what are Duret hemorrhages?

Henri Duret was a French surgeon who trained in part with the famed neurologist Jean-Martin Charcot and was active in the late nineteenth century. The hemorrhages named after Duret (also called *secondary brainstem hemorrhage*) occur in the brainstem following cerebral edema with herniation. These are thought to be due to the rupture of small penetrating vessels, particularly into the central portions of the midbrain, pons, and medulla.

44. If the same patient demonstrated a Kernohan's notch, what does that refer to?

This is observed as disruption and hemorrhage of the cerebral peduncle opposite the side of uncal herniation and thus opposite the side of a space-occupying hemispheric lesion (hematoma, intracerebral hemorrhage). It arises when the cerebral peduncle is forced up against the "sharp" edge of the tentorium as the uncus of the opposite hemisphere herniates.

45. How does a Kernohan's notch create a false localizing sign?

In a patient with a right-sided epidural hematoma, the right uncus would herniate and the left cerebral peduncle would develop the destructive lesion known as *Kernohan's notch.* Since the motor fibers within the affected peduncle have yet to decussate, the motor deficits would appear largely on the right side of the body. Thus, motor deficits would be paradoxically ipsilateral to the hemispheric lesion rather than contralateral.

46. Who was Kernohan?

James Kernohan was an Irish-born neuropathologist who worked for many years at the Mayo Clinic in Rochester, Minnesota.

47. How does an epidural hematoma arise?
Epidural hematoma arises following laceration of the middle meningeal typically, which courses in the superficial-most aspect of the dura. This typically follows skull fracture. After the artery is torn, blood accumulates between periosteal dura and skull. Formation of the hematoma is limited by the sutures, resulting in an elliptical hematoma that compresses brain parenchyma as it expands.

48. How and where does subdural hematoma arise? Why is this region susceptible?
Subdural hematoma occurs when hemorrhage begins in the border cell layer of the dura (innermost part of dura adjacent to arachnoid) due to tears in cortical bridging veins. This is a good location for hematomas to form due to the paucity of tight junctions between cells of this layer.

49. How does a subdural hematoma progress?
As the hematoma expands, the dura responds by forming granulation tissue, which comprises fibro-blastic and capillary proliferation. This may result in further hemorrhage into the hematoma within the potential "subdural" space. As a result, many subdural hematomas have some combination of recent and remote hemorrhage, the latter being characterized by blood breakdown products (e.g., hemosiderin) and degenerated erythrocytes.

50. What are the "membranes" of a subdural hematoma, where do these begin forming, and why are they important?
Subdural membranes begin on the dural side (where fibroblasts reside). In the first week after the hematoma develops, a membrane of fibroblasts, collagen, and capillaries is formed on the dural side to "wall off" the hematoma while clot lysis is under way. In the second week, fibroblasts, collagen, and capillaries of granulation tissue grow along the arachnoid side of the hematoma from the dural side. If the hematoma is stable, over many months the clot will resorb and only the inner and outer hematoma membranes remain. This is why examination of the dura at autopsy will always include an evaluation for membrane formation on the inner aspect of the dura, even if the blood clot is not visible grossly.

51. How do chronic subdural hematomas further expand?
Particularly with slowly developing, chronic hematomas, the granulation tissue formed contains cap-illaries susceptible to further hemorrhage. These are termed *microbleeds* and may further expand the hematoma.

52. In subdural hematoma over a convexity, how does the contralateral hemisphere appear?
Often the contralateral cerebral hemisphere will be smooth surfaced with loss of normal gyral contours. This is due to the mass effect caused by the hematoma with shifting of the uninvolved cerebral hemisphere up against the skull.

53. Define the term *extramedullary hematopoiesis*. Why does this happen (though rarely) in subdural hematoma?
Extramedullary hematopoiesis is when blood precursor cells typically found in bone marrow (erythroblasts, megakaryocytes, myeloid precursors) accumulate outside of the bone marrow. This is an uncommon but curious finding in chronic subdural hematoma. The mechanisms underlying this are not understood.

54. List several mechanisms by which subarachnoid hemorrhages may form.
Ruptured berry aneurysm within the circle of Willis (the vast majority in the anterior circulation), traumatic brain injury, iatrogenic causes (e.g., a very rare complication of stereotactic brain biopsy), and bleeding from vascular malformations (e.g., arteriovenous malformations).

55. Describe a contusion of the brain and how this is formed.
Contusions are hemorrhagic lesions of the brain surface, which are essentially brain "bruises." When these take place in the cortex (mesial temporal lobes) they result in disruption of the molecular layer and pial surface. These typically form either when the brain is displaced against a bony surface (temporal tips against the petrous ridges or orbitofrontal surface of the brain against the sphenoid wings), or alternately, when a depressed fracture displaces bone inward to disrupt the brain surface.

56. What is a coup contusion?
Coup contusions result from a traumatic closed head injury to a head that is not in motion. True coup contusions are not common. Much more common are countercoup contusions, as seen when the temporal tips slide against the petrous ridges after falling backward and hitting the back of the head, or fracture contusions (see previous answer).

57. **Infarcts of the brain and contusions both have what shape? How might these be distinguished?**
Both of these may be wedge-shaped, hemorrhagic lesions involved the gray matter. The base of the wedge is at the pial surface, and its apex points toward the white matter. Contusions hemorrhage due to laceration of vessels. Infarcts may hemorrhage as dead tissue is reperfused. However, infarcts, unlike contusions, have an intact pial surface and molecular layer.

58. **Contusive brain injuries are very rare in infants and very young children. Therefore, what should be considered when countercoup contusion hemorrhages are identified in the brain of a small child?**
Nonaccidental head injury.

59. **What triad of findings is characteristic of nonaccidental head injury in infants?**
Retinal hemorrhage, subarachnoid hemorrhage, and subdural hematoma. These may be present even in the absence of skin and scalp bruising or skull fracture.

60. **What is diffuse axonal injury (DAI)?**
DAI is a pathologic processes thought to mediate the cognitive disturbance following severe head trauma. DAI follows rapid acceleration–deceleration head injuries that generate rotational forces on the brain. This pathologic process may be subtle on autopsy examination yet result in very significant cognitive impairment or even death.

61. **How might DAI be recognized macroscopically?**
DAI is observed as punctate or linear hemorrhage in the white matter and brainstem of a patient with head trauma.

62. **What is the microscopic correlate of DAI?**
In DAI, axonal swellings form in various brain locations, including the dorsolateral brainstem (tectal plate), corpus callosum, and other sites. These axonal swellings may be followed by axonal disruption with formation of bulb-like structures termed *retraction balls* (these are visible on H&E stain). Neuropathologists may perform an immunohistochemical evaluation with amyloid precursor protein (APP), which highlights DAI.

63. **Along with DAI, what other two components form a triad that is common in closed head injury?**
Subarachnoid hemorrhage and subdural hemorrhage may also be seen with DAI in patients with closed head injury.

64. **What is a "gliding contusion" and what does it indicate?**
Gliding contusions are indicative of DAI and significant head trauma following closed head injury. Their macroscopic correlate is punctate and linear hemorrhages in the bilateral parasagittal white matter of the frontal and parietal lobes.

65. **What are the respective patterns of injury in methanol and carbon monoxide toxicities?**
Methanol toxicity results in bilateral putaminal necrosis. Carbon monoxide poisoning causes bilateral, internal segment of globus pallidus necrosis.

66. **What is the macroscopic appearance of a brain affected by bilirubin deposition (kernicterus)?**
The subcortical nuclei (basal ganglia), cranial nerve nuclei, olives, and periventricular regions of the brainstem have bright yellow pigmentation in hyperbilirubinemia. The microscopic correlate of these findings is neuronal necrosis due to the toxic nature of the unconjugated bilirubin.

NEUROPATHOLOGY OF NEURODEGENERATIVE DISEASE

67. **What is the role of tau in normal cells?**
Tau is a protein involved in the stabilization of microtubules. Microtubules have a critical role in stability of the cytoskeleton.

68. **Describe the differences between pathologic and normal tau in brain cells.**
Normal tau is a microtubule-associated protein (MAP). This protein is soluble, nonphosphorylated, and naturally has a range of isoforms (up to six) that result from variations in mRNA splicing.

In contrast, pathologic tau is hyperphosphorylated, insoluble, and cannot have its normal interaction with microtubules. The accumulation of this insoluble form of pathologic tau is detected on H&E examination as basophilic, flame-shaped or globose tangles, or by special techniques (e.g., silver-based stains or antibodies to phosphorylated tau).

69. **Describe the role of *MAPT* in the production of tau.**
    MAPT resides on the long arm of chromosome 17 (17q21-22) and is a large gene comprising 16 exons (or coding regions). Alternative splicing in three exons (E2, E3, and E10) results in six different forms of normal tau protein. These isoforms are further subdivided into 3-repeat (3R) and 4-repeat (4R) tau (also see the next question). *MAPT* mutations result in an autosomal dominant form of frontotemporal dementia characterized by both dementia and parkinsonism.

70. **How do 3R and 4R tauopathies differ?**
    These differ in the number of microtubule-binding repeats contained in the final tau protein. 3R tau isoforms contain three such repeats, whereas 4R tau isoforms contain four.

71. **Which neurodegenerative diseases are associated with the accumulation of pathologic tau in brain cells?**
    These include AD and also progressive supranuclear palsy (PSP), corticobasal degeneration (CBD), argyrophilic grain disease (AGD), frontotemporal lobar degeneration (FTLD) with tau inclusions (FTLD-tau), and chronic traumatic encephalopathy (CTE), among others.

72. **Which of these tauopathies are characterized by accumulation of 3R tau? 4R tau? Both 3R and 4R?**
    AD tangle pathology consists of both 3R and 4R tau isoforms. PSP, AGD, and CBD are all 4R tauopathies, whereas FTLD-tau (Pick's disease) is a 3R tauopathy. FTDP-17 resulting from *MAPT* mutations may contain either 3R or 4R tau.

73. **What is the characteristic macroscopic (gross) appearance of the brain affected by severe AD neuropathology?**
    The brain may be profoundly atrophic with hydrocephalus *ex vacuo* (expansion of the ventricular system secondary to tissue volume loss), marked thinning of the cortical ribbon, bilateral hippocampal atrophy, and widening of the cerebral sulci.

74. **What two cardinal pathologic features characterize AD?**
    AD is characterized by the accumulation of pathologic forms of intracellular hyperphosphorylated tau in the form of neurofibrillary tangles and extracellular deposits of parenchymal amyloid in the form of plaques.

75. **Describe the amyloid plaque pathology of AD.**
    Amyloid-β (Aβ) deposition in brain parenchyma may occur as multiple isoforms generated from proteolysis of amyloid precursor protein (APP). The deposition of Aβ occurs as either extracellular diffuse or dense cored plaques visualized with immunostains to Aβ/APP and special stains like Congo red and thioflavin-S. Dense cored plaques are also visible on H&E stain.

76. **What is a neuritic plaque?**
    A dense-cored plaque surrounded by a rim of silver or tau-positive dystrophic neurites.

77. **What is the Thal staging system for amyloid plaque pathology?**
    The Thal staging system describes the extent and progression of Aβ parenchymal deposition in five progressive phases. This evaluation may be based on Aβ immunohistochemistry as well as a silver stain. The first phase is deposition of extracellular amyloid in the six-layered isocortex with progressive extension to the mesial temporal lobe (phase 2), basal ganglia and diencephalon (phase 3), brainstem (phase 4), and, less commonly, cerebellar cortex (phase 5).

78. **Is neurofibrillary tangle pathology ever encountered outside of AD?**
    Neurofibrillary tangles are frequent pathologic findings in cognitively normal older patients. Further, neurofibrillary tangles are among the diagnostic features of other tauopathies including PSP, FTLD-tau, CBD, and CTE. Tau inclusions are also seen in a wide range of other degenerative diseases (e.g., ALS/motor neuron disease) and in nondegenerative brain diseases as well (e.g., subacute sclerosing panencephalitis following measles infection).

79. **What is the CERAD system for estimating the likelihood of AD?**
The CERAD system was established in 1991 and uses a neuritic plaque score based on semiquantitative estimation of plaque density as sparse, moderate, and frequent in cortex. CERAD stands for the Consortium to Establish a Registry for Alzheimer's disease. CERAD criteria propose that a neuritic plaque score is assigned for a given brain to make a determination of "normal," "definite AD," "probable AD," and "possible AD" in conjunction with the patient's age, presence/absence of clinically defined dementia, and other lesions likely to contribute to dementia.

80. **In what forms does pathologic tau accumulate in AD?**
Filamentous, hyperphosphorylated tau accumulates as intracytoplasmic neurofibrillary tangles, neuropil threads, and dystrophic neurites within neuritic plaques. These may be identified by either silver-based stains (e.g., Bielschowsky, Gallyas) or immunohistochemistry. On H&E, tangles can be identified as basophilic, flame-, or crescent-shaped inclusions in neurons of the cortex and hippocampus, whereas in subcortical and brainstem neurons these form globose tangles. Unlike more "pure" tauopathies, tau in AD does not typically accumulate within glia.

81. **What are "pretangles"? What are "ghost tangles"?**
"Pretangles" are tau-positive, perinuclear, and nonfibrillary structures in the neuronal cytoplasm thought to represent an incipient version of a mature neurofibrillary tangle. "Ghost" tangles are disintegrating extracellular neurofibrillary tangles identified after the involved neurons are lost.

82. **What is the Braak and Braak staging system for AD neuropathology?**
This is a six-stage system for recording the hierarchical distribution of neurofibrillary pathology. Stage I shows neurofibrillary tangles within the transentorhinal cortex straddling the rhinal sulcus in the anteromedial temporal lobe. Stage II is characterized by involvement of the transentorhinal cortex and also the superficial entorhinal cortex. Stage III is characterized by involvement of stage I and II areas but with more extensive and deeper involvement of the entorhinal cortex and additional neurofibrillary pathology in the hippocampal formation and temporal isocortex (sparse). Stage IV has involvement of the preceding regions as well as tangle pathology in cingulate and insular cortices; rare isocortical tangles may be present in stage IV. Stages V and VI are characterized by diffuse isocortical involvement with stage VI distinguished by significant involvement of primary sensory cortices.

83. **How do the 2012 National Institute on Aging/National Institutes of Health (NIA/NIH) criteria bring together CERAD score, Thal phase, and the Braak staging scheme?**
These criteria suggest that an "ABC" score be provided, which describes AD neuropathologic changes associated with Aβ deposition and neurofibrillary tangle pathology. The score incorporates the Thal phase of the extent of amyloid deposition ("A"), the Braak and Braak neurofibrillary stage ("B"), and the neuritic plaque density score of the CERAD system ("C"). For example, a brain with Thal phase 1 or 2 amyloid pathology, Braak stage 1 or 2 neurofibrillary pathology, and a CERAD neuritic plaque score of "sparse" would be A1 B1 C1 in the 2012 NIA/NIH criteria. The final ABC scores are assigned one of four levels of AD neuropathologic change as "not," "low," "intermediate," and "high." These values are correlated with the clinical level of cognitive impairment to determine whether the AD neuropathologic change provides an adequate explanation for the clinical findings. The recommendations also encourage the reporting of Lewy body pathology, vascular pathology, TAR DNA binding protein 43-kDa (TDP-43) protein deposition, and hippocampal sclerosis.

84. **What differentiates the tau pathology of AD from age-related neurofibrillary tangle pathology?**
Age-related neurofibrillary pathology may be seen in cognitively normal patients or in patients with mild cognitive impairment. Likewise, mild neocortical amyloid plaque pathology is a very frequent finding in normal aging. What differentiates AD from non-AD pathology is the extent and density of tau pathology, which very frequently involves a six-layered neocortex (isocortex). AD patients also typically have more abundant amyloid plaque pathology in the form of diffuse and neuritic plaques.

85. **Can a neuropathologist confidently diagnose AD from autopsy material alone?**
No. The final diagnosis of AD requires a correlation of premortem clinical findings and postmortem pathologic findings. Because of this requirement, current guidelines from the NIA/NIH provide a "likelihood" estimate of whether the pathologic findings observed would have contributed to a clinically recognized dementia.

86. **What differentiates the tau pathology of AD from that seen in other tauopathies?**
These diseases differ in the (1) the spatial distribution of tau pathology, (2) the relative extent of amyloid pathology (typically far less severe than seen in AD), (3) the number of repeats in the tau isoform accumulating in cells (3R vs 4R), and (4) in some diseases, the presence of glial cytoplasmic inclusions.

87. **Which of the non-AD tauopathies have accumulation of pathologic tau in glial cells?**
These include AGD, CBD, FTLD-17, and PSP. In the diseases both neurons and glial cells accumulate the pathologic tau. Glial inclusions are also seen in diseases with accumulation of TDP-43 (FTLD TDP-43 and ALS) and alpha-synuclein (multiple system atrophy, discussed below).

88. **What is the neuropathologic basis of "Pick's disease"?**
Pick's disease is a type of FTLD with tau-positive inclusion (FTLD-tau). These patients have a severe dementing illness with prominent frontal executive dysfunction and disinhibition. Macroscopically there is pronounced frontotemporal atrophy with "knife-edge," sharp-appearing gyral crests. The parieto-occipital regions are spared in contrast (Note: AD may have a similar macroscopic appearance so frontotemporal atrophy is not pathognomonic for FTLD or Pick's disease.) These patients have eosinophilic, globular inclusions that are tau and silver-stain positive termed *Pick bodies*. Unlike AD, amyloid pathology is not typically prominent.

89. **What is AGD?**
AGD is a non-AD tauopathy occurring in elderly patients and is thought to account for 5% of all dementias. The original pathologic descriptions were in clinically demented patients without significant AD pathology (not as incidental autopsy findings).

90. **How is AGD diagnosed pathologically?**
First, most patients lack the profound atrophy seen in AD brains on gross examination. Second, on microscopic examination, AGD brains demonstrate short, stubby, and spindle-shaped threads in the neuropil that are positive on tau immunostain and silver special stain ("argyrophilic"). These "grains" have been likened to grains of rice and appear dot-like on cross-section. These patients also have tau accumulation in glial cells in the form of oligodendroglial coiled bodies. Mild AD pathology (Braak stage ≤III) is very common in these patients and does not make their diagnosis AD.

91. **Where do "grains" in AGD frequently occur?**
These are most abundant within the mesial temporal lobe (superficial entorhinal cortex, amygdala, and hippocampus). Much like AD, these lesions progress over time to involve other limbic regions (anterior cingulate) and neocortex.

92. **Since AGD also features neurofibrillary tangle pathology and occurs in elderly patients, why isn't this just considered AD neuropathology?**
First and foremost, AGD is a 4R tauopathy, unlike the mixture of 3R and 4R tau isoforms seen in AD. Second, unlike AD, AGD has no significant association with the frequency of the apolipoprotein E epsilon 4 (ApoE ε4) allele. However, AD and AGD pathology can coexist on neuropathologic examination. In fact "low stage" AD-type neuropathology is present in many non-AD disorders, particularly those of older patients (e.g., ALS, multiple system atrophy [MSA], dementia with Lewy bodies). Third, AGD brains demonstrate both the hallmark "grains" of the disease as well as glial cytoplasmic inclusions (see above).

93. **What is MSA? How old are typical MSA patients?**
MSA is a sporadic, progressive alpha-synucleinopathy characterized by (1) dysautonomia, (2) cerebellar dysfunction, and/or (3) parkinsonism. These features correspond to the earlier clinical designations of Shy–Drager syndrome, olivopontocerebellar atrophy, and striatonigral degeneration. Patients may also experience stridor (due to vocal cord palsy), dysphagia, rapid eye movement sleep disturbance, cognitive impairment, and upper motor neuron signs. Onset in the sixth or seventh decade of life is most typical, and patients rarely live beyond 10 years after diagnosis.

94. **What neuropathologic finding is the core diagnostic feature of MSA?**
In life, "possible" and "probable" MSA diagnoses may be made using clinical and laboratory criteria. However, the clinical findings of MSA may overlap those of atypical Parkinson's disease, corticobasal degeneration, and progressive supranuclear palsy. Therefore, a definitive diagnosis requires

demonstration of alpha-synuclein immunoreactive glial cytoplasmic inclusions (GCIs) that are the hallmark of MSA. These GCIs also react on silver stains (they are "argyrophilic"), as well as ubiquitin, and the ubiquitin pathway-related protein, p62.

95. **In the literature, what is the difference between the clinicopathologic findings of MSA in US and Western European populations versus those in Japan?**
   US and European studies report a clear predominance of MSA with predominant parkinsonian features, or MSA-P (~60%). In the Japanese literature, the vast majority of patients have MSA with predominant cerebellar symptoms, or MSA-C (>80%). The reasons for these differences are not clear.

96. **What four alpha-synucleinopathies may have significant clinical symptoms of dysautonomia with pathologic involvement of structures involved in autonomic function (e.g., intermediolateral cell column, peripheral ganglia, hypothalamus)?**
   MSA, Parkinson's disease, dementia with Lewy bodies, and primary autonomic failure.

97. **What do glial cytoplasmic inclusions in MSA consist of? Are they seen in other alpha-synucleinopathies?**
   Granulofilamentous material with filaments having a diameter of 20 to 40 nm. Rare reports of glial inclusions in non-MSA alpha-synucleinopathies exist, but these are uncommon. MSA patients may also have pleomorphic neuronal inclusions and alpha-synuclein-positive processes or neurites.

98. **What is the neuropathologic process underlying primary autonomic failure?**
   Loss of postganglionic sympathetic nerve fibers with Lewy body formation and neuronal loss in autonomic ganglia. In contrast, MSA patients have pathologic involvement of preganglionic neurons in the intermediolateral cell column, within Onuf's nucleus of S2–S4 that controls urinary continence, within the hypothalamus, and within catecholaminergic and serotonergic neuron groups of the brainstem.

99. **What is the characteristic macroscopic appearance of MSA? How might this overlap with that of Parkinson's disease?**
   MSA-P patients show findings of striatonigral degeneration, which results from massive neuronal loss, volume loss, and gliosis within the dorsolateral putamen, caudate nucleus, and substantia nigra pars compacta with relative sparing of globus pallidus. The putamen in these patients is often slit-like and discolored. Pallor within the substantia nigra and locus ceruleus, reflecting loss of pigmented catecholaminergic neurons, is also common. The loss of pigmentation in brainstem nuclei overlaps with a key gross feature of Parkinson's disease. However, Parkinson's disease patients are not expected to have profound striatal degeneration.

100. **What is the key macroscopic finding in patients with a predominant olivoponto-cerebellar atrophy form of MSA, or MSA-C?**
   These patients experience severe neuronal loss with volume loss and gliosis in the basis pontis and inferior olives, as well as loss of pontocerebellar and olivocerebellar fibers, and severe atrophy of the middle cerebellar peduncle and cerebellar white matter. The cerebellar cortex is usually atrophic with Purkinje cell loss. Unlike patients with dementia with either Lewy bodies or AD, cortical atrophy in MSA patients is not common.

101. **What is the characteristic neuropathology of ALS?**
   ALS neuropathology is characterized by motor neuron loss and gliosis in the frontal cortex, spinal cord, and brainstem somatic motor nuclei (though sparing the nuclei of cranial nerves III, IV, and VI). Ubiquitinated inclusions of transactivating responsive sequence (TAR) DNA-binding protein 43 kDa (TDP-43) are also present in both neurons and glia.

102. **What is the most common genetic risk factor identified to date in both sporadic and familial ALS?**
   Hexanucleotide expansion of *C9orf72*. This results from an expansion of a noncoding GGGGCC hexa-nucleotide repeat in the *C9orf72* locus at chromosome 9p21, leading to the accumulation of small nuclear RNA fragments and accumulation of 25-kDa C-terminal TDP-43 fragments that become phosphorylated and cytotoxic to the cell.

TUMOR NEUROPATHOLOGY: GLIAL TUMORS

103. What is a glioma?

A glioma is a neoplasm comprising tumor cells with glial characteristics (on cytology, H&E examination, and/or immunohistochemistry). The three major "flavors" of glial tumors are astrocytic, oligodendroglial, and ependymal.

104. Do glial tumors simply arise from mature glial cells?

Probably not. Glial tumors are very complex and cannot always readily be classified as being astrocytic, oligodendroglial, or ependymal in origin. Other tumors may have neoplastic glial elements and neoplastic ganglion cells (i.e., ganglioglioma). Among the infiltrating, or diffuse, gliomas, tumors with concomitant astrocytic and oligodendroglial features on histology are not uncommon. This suggests the possibility that these tumors arise from cells capable of showing both astrocytic and oligodendroglial-type differentiation. For this reason, molecular classification is paramount in infiltrating gliomas—in other words, microscopic analysis *alone* is not always sufficient and may lead to diagnostic errors and assumptions that result in patient mismanagement.

105. What are the two fundamental classes of glioma?

Infiltrating (diffuse) gliomas and circumscribed gliomas. Of these two, infiltrating gliomas cannot be cured by surgery alone since removal of all tumor cells is not possible. Infiltrating gliomas will recur in nearly all instances and may progress to higher-grade tumors.

106. What is the difference between diffuse and circumscribed gliomas?

Diffuse gliomas are capable of infiltrating normal brain elements (cortex, white matter, subcortical structures, brainstem, spinal cord, etc.). Circumscribed gliomas do not infiltrate and typically have a sharp margin with respect to surrounding brain tissue.

107. What are the infiltrating gliomas?

Infiltrating gliomas are World Health Organization (WHO) Grades II–IV tumors, including diffuse astrocytoma (WHO Grade II), anaplastic astrocytoma (WHO Grade III), oligodendroglioma (WHO Grade II), anaplastic oligodendroglioma (WHO Grade III), and glioblastoma (WHO Grade IV).

108. Why do glial (or any brain tumors) have WHO Grades?

WHO grading of tumors provides guidance to neuropathologists, neuro-oncologists, and other physicians as to the potential for a tumor to recur, transform into more malignant forms, and ultimately lead to the patient's death. The grades range from WHO Grade I (e.g., pilocytic astrocytoma) to WHO Grade IV (e.g., medulloblastoma, glioblastoma).

109. Who decides how brain tumors should be graded?

A consensus of experts in tumor neuropathology and neuro-oncology makes these decisions based on their collective understanding of the literature and extensive personal experience in dealing with brain tumors. The document arising from this gathering of experts is the WHO classification of tumors of the CNS. However, it is important to understand that these "grades" and rules are not fixed in stone and are amenable to change over time as more data are collected on various tumor types.

110. What are some examples of circumscribed gliomas?

Pilocytic astrocytoma, ependymoma, subependymoma, angiocentric glioma, pleomorphic xanthoastrocytoma.

111. **What are the cardinal morphologic features of diffuse astrocytomas, WHO Grade II?**
Diffuse astrocytomas, which are WHO Grade II tumors, are characterized by infiltrating atypical glial cells with neither perinuclear cytoplasmic haloes nor typically calcification within the tumors. There is greater nuclear pleomorphism than is typically seen with oligodendroglioma.

112. **What are the hallmark morphologic features of oligodendroglioma, WHO Grade II?**
Oligodendrogliomas are characterized by tumor cells with round, monotonous nuclei and perinuclear haloes that infiltrate brain parenchyma (this combination is rarely seen in diffuse astrocytoma). Typically, oligodendrogliomas appear vaguely nodular at low-power magnification and demonstrate frequent calcifications. Secondary structures (of Sherer) may be seen, which include perivascular aggregation of tumor cells, perineuronal satellitosis, and subpial spread.

113. **As described in the preceding question, who was Scherer of the "secondary structures of Scherer"?**
Hans-Joachim Scherer was a European neuropathologist who was born in modern-day Poland in 1906 (then part of Western Prussia). He described the cytologic and architectural features of infiltrating gliomas and many of these principles remain diagnostically valuable. There is controversy regarding the use of his name along with the term *secondary structures* as he was affiliated with the Nazi regime during his career.

114. **What are the histologic features of an anaplastic astrocytoma, WHO Grade III?**
These tumors have the features of diffuse astrocytoma, but additionally they have mitotic activity, hypercellularity, and greater nuclear pleomorphism. They lack necrosis and microvascular proliferation since either of these features would equate to glioblastoma.

115. **What makes an anaplastic oligodendroglioma, WHO Grade III?**
These tumors have the features of oligodendroglioma, but they additionally demonstrate significant mitotic activity, nodules of hypercellularity, microvascular proliferation (corresponding to enhancement on MRI), and even necrosis.

116. **What makes a glioblastoma, WHO Grade IV?**
Glioblastomas are defined as any infiltrating glial tumor with either necrosis or microvascular proliferation (only one is required). The necrosis does not have to be pseudopalisading necrosis, and any necrotic foci are sufficient. Mitotic figures and significant nuclear pleomorphism are typical in glioblastoma. (Note: "multiforme" is no longer used in WHO terminology although the term "GBM" is still often used clinically.)

117. **What are the two mainstay molecular tests in diffuse glioma diagnosis?**
The two essential markers in the diagnosis of diffuse glioma are testing for whole arm deletion of chromosomes 1p and 19q, as well as mutation analysis of the isocitrate dehydrogenase 1 (*IDH1*) and *IDH2* genes.

118. **Which is the more favorable finding in a diffuse glioma: *IDH* mutation or wild-type *IDH1/IDH2* genes?**
IDH mutations are prognostically favorable features of diffuse gliomas. Identification of an *IDH* mutation by either sequencing analysis or immunohistochemistry may also be helpful to identify a lesion as a tumor rather than gliosis which would be negative for an IDH mutation or that tumor does not represent a diffuse glioma.

119. **Are *IDH* mutations identified in other brain tumors besides diffuse gliomas?**
No. They have been identified in other systemic malignancies (e.g., some leukemias), but in the brain these indicate diffuse glioma.

120. **What about the 1p/19q status of a tumor?**
Whole-arm 1p and 19q codeletion in a tumor typically goes hand in hand with *IDH* mutation, and together these are nearly always diagnostic of oligodendroglioma. An infiltrative glioma with *IDH* mutation and whole-arm codeletion of chromosomes 1p and 19q is the best possible combination of molecular events in a glioma. Nonetheless, even this "ideal" entity remains a malignancy.

121. **How do pathologists evaluate tissues for *IDH* mutations and 1p/19q codeletion?**
IDH mutations can be identified in the molecular pathology laboratory by sequencing, or alternatively, in the anatomic pathology laboratory by immunohistochemistry (antibodies are made to the most

common form of mutant IDH1 protein, R132H). Codeletion of 1p and 19q is most frequently identified using fluorescence in situ hybridization.

122. **Pathologists may also examine diffuse gliomas for nuclear staining of p53. What is the role of p53 immunostaining? What are they looking for?**
Strong nuclear expression of p53 protein in tumor cells is much more common in diffuse astrocytomas and is less common in oligodendrogliomas. Mutations in *TP53* are very common events in the early initiating events that lead to the formation of diffuse astrocytomas. However, p53 protein expression is not a perfect proxy for *TP53* mutation status and must be interpreted with that caveat.

123. **Which circumscribed gliomas have the "cyst with an enhancing mural nodule" appearance?**
These include pilocytic astrocytoma and ganglioglioma, pleomorphic xanthoastrocytoma (or "PXA"), and hemangioblastoma. All of these tumors may present as solid, noncystic tumors, and conversely, glioblastoma, metastases, pituitary adenomas, and other typically solid tumors may be cystic!

124. **Describe the characteristic histologic appearance of ependymoma.**
Ependymoma is a circumscribed glial tumor whose tumors cells may have long fibrillary processes on cytology preparations and salt-and-pepper nuclear chromatin reminiscent of neuroendocrine tumors. On permanent sections, these tumors have perivascular pseudorosettes, where tumor cells aggregate around blood vessels and send their cell processes toward the vessel basement membrane. If you are fortunate, you may see "true" ependymal rosettes, where tumor cells aggregate around a true lumen (not a vessel) in an attempt to recapitulate an ependymal-lined canal.

125. **What immunostains are helpful in ependymoma?**
These tumors are usually GFAP positive but the most helpful stain is one for epithelial membrane antigen (EMA). The staining pattern is very unique, showing perinuclear dots of EMA staining, representing intracellular small lumina with microvilli and cilia, and accentuation of staining at the luminal border of true ependymal rosettes.

126. **What is a myxopapillary ependymoma?**
Myxopapillary ependymoma, WHO Grade I, is classically a heterogeneously enhancing, boxcar-shaped mass in the lumbar cistern. Tumor nuclei are typically bland and perivascular rosettes are often very pronounced. Unlike conventional ependymoma, these tumors frequently have mucin-filled microcysts, which can be highlighted by the special stain Alcian blue. Some tumors may be densely hyalinized.

127. **List three entities commonly in the differential of a lumbar cistern/filum terminale mass.**
Schwannoma, myxopapillary ependymoma, and paraganglioma (of the filum terminale).

128. **What does hyalinized mean and what tumors have this feature?**
Hyalinized refers to a quality of the collagen within a tumor, in which it takes on a glassy and densely eosinophilic appearance. The prototypical example occurs around the vessels of schwannoma. However, meningiomas and myxopapillary ependymomas may be densely hyalinized, which can make diagnosis challenging! Like eosinophilic granular bodies and Rosenthal fibers, hyalinization is not a histologic finding expected in high-grade tumors.

129. **What are subependymomas?**
These are circumscribed gliomas with ependymal-type cytology. Unlike ependymoma, however, these tumors have alternating acellular fibrillary zones (appearing "pink" on H&E where no nuclei are present) with clusters of nuclei (appearing "blue" on H&E). Mucin-filled microcysts may also be present, particularly when these tumors arise in the lateral ventricle (as enhancing, circumscribed masses).

130. **Where else might subependymomas occur?**
These also occur in the fourth ventricle, and rarely, in the spinal cord.

131. **Describe the characteristic histology of pilocytic astrocytoma.**
Pilocytic astrocytomas are noninfiltrating tumors with biphasic "loose" (microcystic) and "dense" (fibrillary, non-cystic) histology whose tumors cells have long, hair-like, or "piloid," processes. These tumors may contain thick, tortuous Rosenthal fibers and eosinophilic granular bodies, which are both reassuring findings in any neoplasm.

132. What is the molecular "signature" of pilocytic astrocytoma?
A *KIAA1549-BRAF* gene fusion. This is not seen in any other brain tumors and is most typical of pilocytic astrocytomas of the posterior fossa.

133. What other nervous system tumor classically shows biphasic (loose/dense) histology?
Schwannoma.

134. What seemingly worrisome features of pilocytic astrocytoma may be seen that are accepted by neuropathologists as not being particularly worrisome?
Pilocytic astrocytomas may show bizarre, degenerative-type nuclear atypia, including multinucleated cells. Cytologically, these tumors may have extensive regions of oligodendroglial cytology including perinuclear haloes. They may also show low-level mitotic activity and invasion of leptomeninges if they are superficial (in the cerebellar cortex). Worse still, microvascular proliferation is accepted in the spectrum of WHO Grade I pilocytic astrocytoma where this would make a WHO Grade IV glioblastoma in an infiltrating glioma!

135. A tumor in the temporal lobe of a patient with seizures looks identical to a pilocytic astrocytoma. However, abnormal ganglion cells are present, some of which contain coarse Nissl substance and others that contain multiple nuclei (not something normal ganglion cells have). What is the best diagnosis?
Ganglioglioma, WHO Grade I. This tumor has neoplastic ganglion cell and glial elements. A much less common tumor would be a ganglion cell tumor, which has only neoplastic ganglion cells and no glial component.

136. A different patient with a long history of seizures has a cystic and solid mass resected from their temporal lobe. The tumor cells are very pleomorphic and bizarre appearing. However, you cannot find mitoses, and there is neither necrosis nor microvascular proliferation. Other cells have cytoplasm that appears vacuolated ("bubbly") and rare cells look like atypical ganglion cells. The tumor does not infiltrate the adjacent brain parenchyma. Special stains and immunostains demonstrate that the tumor cells have pericellular reticulin and label with both neuronal and glial markers. What is the best diagnosis?
Pleomorphic xanthoastrocytoma, or PXA, WHO Grade II.

137. Where other conditions are Rosenthal fibers seen in?
Rarely these are seen within and adjacent to other tumors, most classically in the wall of a craniopharyngioma. They may be seen next to nonneoplastic cystic or expanding lesions in nervous system parenchyma (e.g., pineal cysts). Finally, they are a diagnostic feature of the genetic/metabolic syndrome Alexander's disease, which has a mutation in the glial fibrillary acidic protein gene (*GFAP*).

138. Where else are eosinophilic granular bodies seen?
Eosinophilic granular bodies may be seen in multiple settings, but for practical purposes it is convenient to remember the "big three": pilocytic astrocytoma, ganglioglioma, and pleomorphic xanthoastrocytoma.

TUMOR NEUROPATHOLOGY: NONGLIAL TUMORS

139. What are the possible WHO grades of meningioma?
There are three grades of meningioma, which are WHO Grade I (the typical meningothelial meningioma), WHO Grade II (atypical meningioma and two select histologic variants), and WHO Grade III (anaplastic meningioma and two more select histologic variants).

140. In the broadest sense, how are meningiomas graded?
Meningiomas are graded on the basis of (1) architectural/cytologic features, (2) brain invasion, and (3) other atypical histologic features including mitotic activity.

141. What is the most common grade of meningioma?
Meningiomas are frequently WHO Grade I, arising as enhancing, dural-based masses that impinge upon but do not invade brain parenchyma. Their histology may vary widely, but the prototypical Grade I meningioma has lobules and sheets of bland meningothelial-type cells with psammoma bodies (concentric calcifications), whorls of tumor cells, and nuclear pseudoinclusions.

142. What makes a meningioma WHO Grade II, or "atypical"?
There are several ways to get to atypical meningioma, WHO Grade II, and these include: (1) any meningioma with brain invasion (harder to determine sometimes than you would think!), OR (2) any meningioma with four or more mitotic figures in 10 high-power microscopic fields, OR (3) meningiomas with predominant choroid or clear cell histology. In addition, a meningioma is WHO Grade II if it has three or more of the following five features: necrosis, small-cell change (cells look like lymphocytes), hypercellularity, prominent nucleoli, and loss of pattern with "sheeting" architecture.

143. Why is brain invasion alone a criterion for WHO Grade II?
This is based on the increased likelihood of recurrence in meningiomas with brain invasion independent of their other histologic features.

144. What makes a meningioma WHO Grade III, or "anaplastic"?
These include (1) 20 or more mitoses in 10 high-power microscopic fields, (2) predominant papillary or rhabdoid histology, or (3) sarcoma-like, melanoma-like, or carcinoma-like histology. In the absence of conventional meningioma histology somewhere in the tumor, a meningioma that looks like anaplastic carcinoma is a metastatic carcinoma to the dura (breast cancer loves to do this in particular) until a primary site is ruled out clinically.

145. What patients typically develop bilateral vestibular schwannomas?
Neurofibromatosis type 2 (NF2) patients. They also develop multiple meningiomas and ependymomas, among other findings.

146. What is the difference between schwannoma and neurofibroma?
Schwannoma is a proliferation of tumor cells with Schwann cell-like cytologic features. These are eccentrically placed with respect to the parent nerve. These may also have microcysts and hemosiderin-laden macrophages. Neurofibroma is a mixture of Schwann cells, inflammatory cells (most famously, mast cells), and fibroblasts including perineurial-like cells. More frequently than schwannoma, a neurofibroma has a myxoid tumor stroma with thin strips of collagen. Unlike schwannoma, which is seen in schwannomatosis and NF2, neurofibromas are seen in neurofibromatosis type 1 (NF1).

147. Aside from multiple neurofibromas, what is another classic nervous system tumor of NF1 patients?
Optic nerve glioma, which is histologically identical to a pilocytic astrocytoma.

148. What is a hemangioblastoma?
Hemangioblastoma most typically arises as a circumscribed, partially cystic tumor in the cerebellum. These tumors are notable for a delicate capillary network and tumor cells with degenerative-type nuclear atypia that makes them appear more worrisome than they actually are. Tumor cells also contain vacuolated (or "bubbly") cytoplasm and their lipid content is highlighted by a special stain for fat called *Oil Red O*.

149. What systemic tumor does hemangioblastoma mimic? What tumor predisposition syndrome is this seen in?
Hemangioblastoma looks very similar to a low-grade clear cell renal cell carcinoma (typically a very vascular tumor that also may have bubbly cytoplasm). This differential is usually resolved by a combination of H&E features and immunostains, if these are necessary. Hemangioblastomas may arise sporadically but are associated with Von Hippel–Lindau syndrome.

150. What is a subependymal giant cell tumor (SEGA)? What syndrome is it associated with?
SEGA is characterized by sweeping fascicles of ganglion cell-like tumor cells that look similar to dysmorphic ganglion cells that would be seen in ganglioglioma of the temporal lobe or in severe cortical dysplasia in a patient with epilepsy. These tumor cells have neuronal and glial features when examined immunohistochemically and are seen in patients with tuberous sclerosis.

151. Where does SEGA occur?
SEGA occurs as an enhancing, well-demarcated intraventricular mass. Because these may look histologically very unusual, correlation with radiology is essential.

152. What other types of tumors and growths occur in the ventricular system?
Examples include intraventricular meningioma (in the atrium of the lateral ventricle), choroid plexus papilloma, xanthogranuloma, choroid plexus cyst, and ependymoma (typically in the fourth ventricle).

153. How is choroid plexus papilloma distinguished from normal choroid plexus?
Papillomas may appear very similar to normal choroid plexus architecturally (papillae with fibrovascular cores), but in addition these are more cellular with nuclear crowding. Papillomas also lack the undulating ("cobblestone") epithelial surface of normal choroid plexus as though a straight line could be drawn across the surface of the neoplastic cells.

154. What is a dysembryoplastic neuroepithelial tumor, or DNET?
A DNET most commonly presents as a nonenhancing, cortically based mesial temporal lobe nodule (or multiple nodules) in a nonsyndromic patient without seizures. These are WHO Grade I tumors that are treated by gross total surgical resection alone.

155. What is the histology of DNET?
The critical element of DNETs is the glioneuronal element, which consists of small, round tumor cells with neurocytic cytologic features (fine nuclear chromatin, discrete nucleoli, lack of fibrillary processes) aligned along axons with intervening cystic pools of mucoid material. These mucinous microcysts may contain "floating neurons," which are another nice diagnostic feature when present. Simple, complex, and nonspecific forms of DNET have all been proposed.

156. What tumor arises as an enhancing mass within the ventricle at the foramen of Monro and looks like a perfect mimic of an oligodendroglioma?
This would be the central neurocytoma, which features oligodendroglioma-like, neurocytic tumor cells that are reactive for the immunostain synaptophysin. These tumors do not demonstrate codeletion of 1p and 19q, which further distinguishes them from oligodendroglioma.

157. Primary CNS lymphoma (PCNSL) is typically what type of lymphoma?
A high-grade, diffuse large B-cell lymphoma. These may be associated with Epstein–Barr virus and/or immunosuppression.

158. Similar to glioblastoma, what unique imaging feature may PCNSLs exhibit?
Extension of enhancing tumor across the midline via the corpus callosum in the so-called "*butterfly*" pattern.

159. Describe the histology that characterizes PCNSL.
These are high-grade, diffuse large B-cell lymphomas with dyscohesive, pleomorphic tumor cells, obvious mitotic activity, apoptotic cells, and necrosis. Architecturally, the tumor cells aggregate around and within blood vessels walls (termed "*angiocentric*" *growth*). Individual tumor cells may infiltrate as single cells in brain parenchyma.

160. Besides PCNSL, what other tumors may infiltrate brain parenchyma as single tumor cells?
Infiltrating gliomas (this is their defining feature), and rarely, metastatic melanoma and metastatic high-grade neuroendocrine carcinoma.

TUMOR NEUROPATHOLOGY: PEDIATRIC TUMORS

161. What are embryonal tumors of the CNS?
These are WHO Grade IV neoplasms that typically arise in infants and young children. These include atypical teratoid/rhabdoid tumor (AT/RT), pineoblastoma, medulloblastoma, choroid plexus carcinoma, and central primitive neuroectodermal tumor (PNET). The most recent addition to this list is embryonal tumor with multilayered rosettes, which is defined by chromosome 19q13.42 amplification.

162. What is an AT/RT?
AT/RT is an embryonal tumor, typically occurring in the cerebrum or cerebellum of infants, that frequently includes poorly differentiated small blue tumor cells, as well as cells with eccentrically located nuclei and densely eosinophilic cytoplasm (so-called "*rhabdoid*" *cells*). These tumors are multiphenotypic by immunohistochemistry, staining for glial, neuronal, mesenchymal, and epithelial immunohistochemical markers (hence their designation as "teratoid").

163. What genetic alteration defines the AT/RT?
AT/RT is defined by deletions or mutations in *INI1/SMARCB1* at chromosome 22q11. On immunohistochemical examination this genetic alteration is reflected by the loss of INI-1/BAF47 protein, which is retained in nontumor cells that serve as an internal control.

164. **What is an "internal control" in immunostaining?**
As used in the previous answer, this refers to the presence of a tissue or cell type on a slide that serves as a benchmark for evaluating a stain of interest. In a patient with a poorly differentiated cerebral tumor, GFAP staining of uninvolved, gliotic brain would serve as an internal control relative to the poorly differentiated tumor cells of interest.

165. **Where does medulloblastoma occur?**
Within the cerebellum. A small blue cell tumor that looks like medulloblastoma, outside of the cerebellum, cannot be called medulloblastoma unless it represents leptomeningeal spread or a metastasis from a known cerebellar primary.

166. **Do adult medulloblastomas occur?**
Yes, but these are rare. Unlike childhood medulloblastomas, which are typically in the midline vermal cerebellum, those of adulthood involve the lateral cerebellar hemispheres.

167. **What are the prognostically favorable forms of medulloblastoma?**
The most favorable histologic form of medulloblastoma is the desmoplastic/nodular form, which features pale islands of tumor cells with neuronal differentiation and eosinophilic neuropil (appearing "pale" relative to densely cellular foci of small blue tumor cells). These pale islands represent foci of maturation and they lack a reticulin network when a reticulin special stain is performed.

168. **Desmoplastic/nodular medulloblastoma may be associated with what favorable genetic alteration?**
These may be associated with activations of the *Wnt* signaling pathway. Neuropathologists frequently perform beta-catenin immunostaining on medulloblastomas because those with *Wnt* pathway alterations will have nuclear localization of this marker (an important example of microscopic pathology predicting molecular pathology and prognosis). These tumors also have monosomy of chromosome 6.

169. **Which histologic subtype of medulloblastoma is prognostically unfavorable?**
The most unfavorable histology is that of large cell/anaplastic medulloblastoma. These rarely have *Wnt* signaling pathway alterations and are more frequently associated with *MYC* amplification (Group 3 and Group 4 tumors).

170. **What are other genetic alterations are seen in medulloblastomas?**
Activation of the sonic hedgehog pathway and isochromosome 17q.

171. **What would you call a small blue cell tumor with high mitotic activity, necrosis, and Homer Wright rosettes if it arose in the cerebral hemisphere of a child?**
A central primitive neuroectodermal tumor (central PNET). Again, *medulloblastoma* is a term reserved for cerebellar tumors.

172. **What are the characteristic features of a germ cell tumor in the CNS?**
The prototypical germ cell tumor is a germinoma of the pineal region that arises in a teenage male patient. These tumors have large polygonal cells with prominent nucleoli, similar to those seen in a high-grade lymphoma but with more cytoplasm. Characteristically, these tumors have intervening fibrous septa and admixed, mature lymphocytes. They are important to recognize because they are very sensitive to radiotherapy. Other germ cell tumors may be seen less commonly and include yolk sac tumor, teratoma, and rarely choriocarcinoma and embryonal carcinoma (actually a germ cell tumor rather than a malignancy of epithelial cells as implied in the term *carcinoma*).

TUMOR NEUROPATHOLOGY: METASTASES

173. **What distinct anatomic compartments or structures may be involved by metastases?**
Bone (cranium or vertebrae), dura, subarachnoid space, the subpial and perivascular (Virchow–Robin) spaces, CNS parenchyma, choroid plexus, pineal gland, and pituitary gland. The involvement of some anatomic compartments is stereotypic for some tumors (e.g., breast carcinomas frequently metastasizes to dura).

174. **What is the approximate ratio of supratentorial to infratentorial metastases? Which primary site tumors more commonly metastasize to infratentorial locations?**
The ratio is approximately 3-4 to 1. Pelvic organs (colorectal, ovarian, and uterine carcinomas) and breast are overrepresented in metastases of the infratentorial compartment/posterior fossa.

175. Metastases to the choroid plexus are very uncommon. Which tumor most typically does this?
Renal cell carcinoma.

176. What are the hemorrhagic metastases?
The classic list of hemorrhagic metastases includes renal cell carcinoma, melanoma, lung cancer, and choriocarcinoma. Hemorrhagic primary tumors include glioblastoma and, most famously, oligodendroglioma.

177. In the cortex, what is the typical site of metastasis that may be seen macroscopically?
The most common site of metastasis is to the frontal lobe in arterial border (watershed) zones at the junction of gray and white matter.

178. What features are unique to epidural metastases of the spine?
Epidural metastasis presents with symptoms of cord and nerve root compression with extremity weakness and sensory loss. Epidural metastases rarely penetrate through dura to involve cord parenchyma (unlike leptomeningeal metastatic disease in which invasion into parenchyma is common). Epidural metastases may also result in a compressive myelopathy that is progressive and irreversible with cavitation and necrosis of cord parenchyma, as well as spongiosis and vacuolation in ascending/descending white matter tracts of the cord.

KEY POINTS: TUMOR NEUROPATHOLOGY

1. The two major classes of glioma are infiltrating (diffuse) and circumscribed.
2. The molecular signature of oligodendroglioma is whole-arm 1p/19q codeletion
3. Glioblastoma, WHO Grade IV, is characterized by nuclear pleomorphism, mitotic activity, and either microvascular proliferation or necrosis (or both).
4. Tumors with eosinophilic granular bodies include pilocytic astrocytoma, pleomorphic xanthoastrocytoma, and ganglioglioma.
5. Tumors commonly seen with a history of chronic seizures include dysembryoplastic neuroepithelial tumor, ganglioglioma, pleomorphic xanthoastrocytoma, hypothalamic hamaratoma (with characteristic gelastic fits), and angiocentric glioma (not discussed here).

INFECTIOUS DISEASE AND RELATED NEUROPATHOLOGY

179. Describe the macroscopic ("gross") appearance of bacterial meningitis.
Bacterial meningitis typically causes marked cerebral edema (see preceding descriptions of cerebral edema), and a purulent yellow exudate accumulates along the convexities of the hemisphere. Sulci may not be well visualized due to the combination of edema and purulent exudate. Secondary infarction may occur so that large hemispheric infarcts may be superimposed on this picture.

180. What characteristic neuroimaging features are indicative of a purulent brain abscess?
These are intra-axial, circumscribed masses with significant mass effect and a smooth enhancing rim that is unlike the irregular rim of a glioblastoma. On diffusion weighted imaging these lesions demonstrate diffusion restriction due to the dense, encapsulated accumulation of necrotic tissue and cellular debris and neutrophils (this environment is not conducive to Brownian motion!).

181. If an abscess is resected, what is the expected histology?
Abscesses are multilayered, with a central purulent core surrounded by concentric layers of granulation tissue, a fibrous capsule, and gliotic brain tissue.

182. What two infectious/inflammatory processes have a predilection for the basilar meninges?
Neurosarcoidosis and tuberculosis.

183. What is the anatomic distribution of lesions in neurosarcoidosis?
The pathologic lesions of neurosarcoidosis classically occur in the leptomeninges (convexities, basilar, ventral to the pons) and in the Virchow–Robin perivascular spaces around vessels that penetrate the

brain. These lesions also are common in the subependymal region adjacent to the ventricular system, within the tissues of the sella and even within the choroid plexus. A key finding in neurosarcoidosis is that bona fide intraparenchymal lesions are rare in general and are exceedingly rare as isolated lesions in the absence of the aforementioned leptomeningeal, perivascular, and subependymal lesions.

184. What is the typical microscopic appearance of neurosarcoidosis?
Neurosarcoidosis characteristically features "tightly" formed granulomas with a cuff of lymphocytes (CD4+ T cells). Multinucleated giant cells are commonly seen. The caseating necrosis of a mycobacterial infection is not expected but can happen and does not exclude a diagnosis of neurosarcoidosis.

185. How can neurosarcoidosis and tuberculosis meningitis be distinguished reliably?
Special stains for mycobacterial organisms (acid-fast bacilli [AFB] and Fite stains), AFB cultures, and even polymerase chain reaction for mycobacterial organisms may be necessary to absolutely exclude tuberculosis.

186. What opportunistic fungal pathogens do neuropathologists commonly encounter?
Yeast forms include *Cryptococcus neoformans*, *Coccidioides immitis*, *Histoplasma capsulatum*, and *Blastomyces dermatitidis*. Hyphal forms include *Aspergillus* species and *Mucor*. *Candida* species are the most common fungal pathogen and may have both yeast and pseudohyphal forms within small microabscesses in immunosuppressed patients.

187. What fungal pathogens are angioinvasive and may lead to significant intraparenchymal hemorrhage?
Aspergillus species and *Mucor* are particularly prone to angioinvasion, leading to fibrin thrombi with either infarction or intraparenchymal hemorrhage. *Candida* species may also be angioinvasive and lead to microabscesses with foci of hemorrhage.

188. What general morphologic features do viral infections of the nervous system share?
A characteristic structure is the microglial nodule, which consists of clusters of activated microglia (rod-shaped or elongated, twisted forms) and other chronic inflammatory cells. Perivascular lymphoplasmacytic inflammation is common. Infected neurons may be surrounded by inflammatory cells and microglia in a process termed *neuronophagia*.

189. What is the characteristic microscopic appearance of West Nile virus encephalitis?
This is a viral infection with preferential involvement of neurons in the cerebral cortex, brainstem, and spinal cord. Microglial nodules, neuronophagia, and perivascular lymphocytic cuffing are all seen in this infection.

190. Which viral infections are characteristically associated with cellular inclusions?
Herpes, cytomegalovirus, and measles virus (all have intranuclear Cowdry type A inclusions), plum-colored nuclear inclusions in oligodendroglia (in progressive multifocal leukoencephalopathy, or PML), and cytoplasmic inclusions in rabies (Negri bodies) and cytomegalovirus infection.

191. What is the characteristic microscopic appearance of human immunodeficiency virus (HIV) encephalitis?
The classic histologic finding is the presence of aforementioned features of viral encephalitis but with the addition of perivascular multinucleated giant cells. These patients may also have significant white matter injury with a vacuolar myelopathy.

192. What is PML?
PML is a destructive white matter lesion that typically spares the cortex. It results from JC virus infection of oligodendroglia, resulting in the death of these cells and demyelination of the involved foci. On microscopic examination, these lesions show an alternating arrangement of reactive glial cells and histiocytes, as well as various unique glial cell types (see question below).

193. What patient population was PML originally described in?
PML was first described in patients with chronic lymphocytic leukemia. In the 1980s it became most associated with HIV/AIDS (autoimmune deficiency syndrome) and is recognized as an AIDS-defining condition. It is now recognized that patients on immunomodulatory therapy may be at risk for this condition as well.

194. What are the two unique glial cell types of PML?
The first is an oligodendroglial cell infected by the JC virus. These oligodendroglia have significant nuclear enlargement and a characteristic plum-colored nuclear inclusion (the virus is replicating within the nucleus with margination of normal nuclear chromatin to the periphery). The second is a bizarre, reactive astrocyte with very large and hyperchromatic nuclei. Unfortunately, these bizarre astrocytes are frequently positive on p53 immunostaining if one mistakenly recognizes these cells as glial tumor cells (hence, PML is an entity that should never be forgotten in an immunosuppressed patient!).

195. If bizarre astrocytes are seen in PML, then what are type II Alzheimer astrocytes?
These are astrocytes with enlarged, clear nuclei (appearing empty). These are present in the gray matter (inferior olive, globus pallidus, deep cortical laminae) of patients with hyperammonemia and hepatic encephalopathy.

196. Describe the characteristic setting and appearance of cerebral toxoplasmosis.
Cerebral toxoplasmosis occurs in patients with a compromised immune system, typically as one or more enhancing cerebral lesions with edema. Histologically, a characteristic finding is necrosis and histiocytic inflammation (even granulomatous). The bradyzoite form of the organism is most typically seen, which represents an encysted form. The "free-living" tachyzoites in brain tissue are notoriously difficult to identify without the use of special techniques.

197. What organisms should be considered in the (histologic) differential diagnosis of any neuroinfection that looks like cerebral toxoplasmosis?
The morphology of small, round organisms raises a differential that includes *Trypanosoma cruzi* (Chagasic encephalitis, the most critical differential and possibly underrecognized), *H. capsulatum*, and *Leishmaniasis* (only very rare reports exist for brain involvement).

NEUROMUSCULAR PATHOLOGY

198. What are the characteristic H&E features of "myopathic" muscle?
Muscle "degen–regen," or degeneration with fiber necrosis and regeneration (seen as basophilic fibers with prominent nucleoli). Myopathic muscle may have more internalized nuclei in fibers than usual (these should usually be subsarcolemmal), fiber size variation with both large and small fibers, and fibrosis. Macrophages are also common in various types of myopathy as these cells deal with the debris from degenerating fibers.

199. What is "dystrophic" muscle? What are its characteristic features on H&E?
Dystrophic muscle, as in Duchenne muscular dystrophy, is a subtype of myopathic muscle. This term encompasses a more limited set of diseases with onset in either childhood or early adulthood and a possible family history of muscle disease or a genetic basis for the disease. These muscles may also have all of the features of a myopathic muscle as well as significant fiber hypertrophy and fiber splitting (where a cleft develops in a hypertrophic fiber). Infiltration of the muscle by adipose tissue and lymphocytic inflammation are other features seen in dystrophic muscle.

200. What is an "inflammatory myopathy"? What are its H&E features?
Inflammatory myopathies, including dermatomyositis and inclusion body myositis, are characterized by lymphocytic inflammation, often around blood vessels (e.g., in dermatomyositis) or between muscle fibers. In addition to the inflammatory component, these muscle biopsies may have all of the features of a myopathic muscle described above (necrosis, regeneration, etc.).

201. What are the characteristic pathologic features of dermatomyositis?
Perivascular lymphocytic infiltrates, perifascicular atrophy (this is very suggestive), and variable myopathic findings. On electron microscopy these patients have unique structures termed *tubuloreticular inclusions* (*TRIs*) within their endothelial cells. Polymyositis, another inflammatory myopathy, typically lacks perifascicular atrophy and these biopsies show T lymphocytes and macrophages around and within individual muscle fibers.

202. What is the pathognomonic histologic feature of inclusion body myositis?
The "rimmed vacuole," which is demonstrated on Gomori trichrome special stain. These are seen in a background that may be similar to an inflammatory myopathy. The contents of the vacuole may also be highlighted with a variety of stains, including Congo red (for amyloid).

203. **What are the characteristic pathologic features of collagen vascular disease (lupus)?**
This may look very similar to dermatomyositis on muscle biopsy, and clinical history and serologic studies are essential. Both lupus and dermatomyositis may have interferon "footprints," or TRIs, within endothelial cells on electron microscopy. Since lupus is a vasculitis by nature it may show changes of that process with intramural inflammatory cells and fibrinoid necrosis of the vessel wall—these findings would not be typical for dermatomyositis.

204. **What are the pathologies to consider in the muscle biopsy of an infant with marked hypotonia?**
The list would include: (1) structural congenital myopathies, which are named for their salient morphologic feature (e.g., central core myopathy, centronuclear myopathy, nemaline myopathy), (2) mitochondrial myopathy, (3) spinal muscular atrophy, and (4) metabolic disease.

205. **What are the "ragged red" fibers that characterize mitochondrial myopathies?**
On Gomori trichrome stain, these are bright red subsarcolemmal crescents. On electron microscopy, these crescents are accumulations of subsarcolemmal mitochondria, which may have structural abnormalities. These appear as "blue" crescents on the nicotinamide adenine dinucleotide hydride (NADH) special stain and are also highlighted on the special stains with succinate dehydrogenase and cytochrome oxidase.

206. **What are the hallmark pathologic features of neurogenic atrophy?**
Small, atrophic, and angulated fibers that appear dark on special stain with nonspecific esterase. Grouped atrophy may also appear if innervation to an entire group of fibers is lost. Though not necessary for the diagnosis, neurogenic atrophy muscle may demonstrate "target" fibers on special stains like NADH (losing their staining in the central portion of the fiber).

207. **What conditions is selective type II fiber atrophy seen in?**
Selective type II atrophy may be seen with chronic administration of steroids and with muscle disuse. Neurogenic atrophy, in contrast, may be nonselective with atrophy of both type I and type II fibers.

208. **Myophosphorylase stain is routinely performed on muscle biopsy to identify what metabolic disease?**
McArdle's disease (myophosphorylase deficiency).

209. **Oil Red O stain is routinely performed on muscle biopsy to identify what process?**
Accumulation of lipid within muscle fascicles and muscle fibers. Increased Oil Red O staining is not specific but may be seen particularly in lipid storage diseases and with mitochondrial myopathies.

DEMYELINATING DISEASE AND WHITE MATTER NEUROPATHOLOGY

210. **What is a demyelinating disease?**
These are diseases associated with myelin loss in the central or peripheral nervous system, typically without loss of axons or neurons. The prototypical disease is multiple sclerosis (MS) (central demyelination). Charcot–Marie–Tooth disease is an example of a peripheral disturbance in myelination. Other diseases may affect both central and peripheral myelination (e.g., leukodystrophies).

211. **How does MS appear macroscopically?**
The demyelinating lesions of MS are appreciated as discolored, tan lesions in a periventricular distribution. The loss of phospholipid content in normal myelin is what gives these lesions their tan appearance. These plaques are sharply demarcated from adjacent white matter. An important finding in MS plaques is that they neither follow a vascular distribution (as would be seen in hypoxic/ischemic injury) nor occur in an anatomically restricted pathway (as would be seen in Wallerian degeneration).

212. **How do MS plaques appear histologically?**
The appearances are highly variable and depend on the age of the lesion. In general, the loss of myelin (highlighted on Luxol fast blue [LFB] special stain and also apparent on H&E) and rarefied parenchyma is sharply demarcated with respect to uninvolved white matter. At the periphery of the plaque, a proliferation of normal oligodendroglial cells may be identified. Within the area of demyelination, a mature-appearing lymphocytic infiltrate is present (usually these are T cells) in a

perivascular distribution, and plasma cells may also be present. Activated microglia and macrophages will be present with the latter engulfing myelin debris (occasionally highlighted by LFB stain as LFB-positive debris within the macrophage cytoplasm). Stains that highlight the course of axons (e.g., neurofilament) typically show that axons are intact without the axonal retraction balls seen in lesions resulting in axonal transection (exceptions do exist).

213. What is the name of the characteristic, multinucleated cell type of a demyelinating lesion? How specific is this finding?
Multinucleated, bizarre astrocytes in demyelinating lesions are named Creutzfeldt cells. Each of these cells has multiple small micronuclei and due to their abundant cytoplasm these cells can be quite large and appear alarming. These cells are not specific to MS and may be seen in glioblastoma in particular; however, for any board examination, demyelination is always the first choice if Creutzfeldt cells are present.

214. What is a demyelinating pseudotumor? Who described this entity?
This is a fulminant form of MS, also called *"tumefactive"* MS, wherein the demyelinating focus creates a tumor-like mass lesion that may be mistaken for high-grade glioma. This entity was first described by John Kepes, a Hungarian-born neuropathologist who spent the majority of his career at the University of Kansas.

215. How is demyelinating pseudotumor recognized?
The imaging is characteristic in that horseshoe- or C-shaped enhancement is identified in the cerebral white matter with the nonenhancing end directed toward the ventricular surface. Most critically, on intraoperative consultation (see preceding description of frozen sections), the critical cell of a demyelinating lesion—the macrophage—is present. This is one of the reasons why neuropathologists tread very carefully at the time of intraoperative consultation whenever a macrophage-rich lesion is identified on cytologic or frozen section preparations.

216. What serologic finding is common to neuromyelitis optica spectrum disorder?
The presence of aquaporin-4 antibodies.

217. What is the neuropathologic basis of central pontine myelinolysis (CPM)?
Classically, CPM is characterized by myelin loss with macrophage accumulation in the central basis pontis. At low-power magnification it may appear similar to a brainstem infarct. However, neuronal loss and axonal destruction, which would be expected in infarct, are *not* present in CPM.

218. What is the differential diagnosis of diffuse petechial hemorrhage involving the white matter?
The differential is extensive but includes rickettsial infection (Rocky mounted spotted fever), acute disseminated encephalomyelitis, coagulopathy, malaria, and fat emboli (as might follow a motor vehicle accident with long bone fracture).

219. What is radiation necrosis of white matter, and how does it look macroscopically and microscopically?
Radiation necrosis is necrosis of *normal* brain tissue (*not* tumor!), typically in the white matter adjacent to the angle of the lateral ventricles. It occurs in patients who have undergone radiotherapy for a high-grade glioma, metastasis, or lymphoma. Macroscopically, the tissue is necrotic appearing, friable, and yellow, similar to the appearance of cornbread dressing (minus the flavorful ingredients). Microscopically, it is characterized by bland, eosinophilic necrosis with thick-walled vessels demonstrating fibrinoid necrosis of the vessel wall and perivascular hemorrhage.

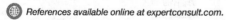 *References available online at expertconsult.com.*

BIBLIOGRAPHY

1. Dickson D, Weller RO: Neurodegeneration: The Molecular Pathology of Dementia and Movement Disorders, 2nd ed. Chichester, West Sussex, Wiley-Blackwell: International Society of Neuropathology, 2011.
2. Dubowitz V, Sewry CA, Oldfors A, Lane RJM: Muscle Biopsy: A Practical Approach, 4th ed. Oxford, Elsevier, 2013.
3. Fuller GN, Goodman JC: Practical Review of Neuropathology, Philadelphia, Lippincott Williams & Wilkins, 2001.
4. Greenfield JG, Love S, Louis DN, Ellison D: Greenfield's Neuropathology, 8th ed. London, Hodder Arnold, 2008.
5. Kovacs GG: Neuropathology of Neurodegenerative Diseases: A Practical Guide, Cambridge, Cambridge University Press, 2015.
6. Mills SE: Histology for Pathologists, 3rd ed. Philadelphia, Lippincott Williams & Wilkins, 2007.
7. Nelson JS: Principles and Practice of Neuropathology, 2nd ed. New York, Oxford University Press, 2003.

INDEX